ADVANCES IN TELEMEDICINE: TECHNOLOGIES, ENABLING FACTORS AND SCENARIOS

Edited by **Georgi Graschew**
and **Theo A. Roelofs**

Advances in Telemedicine: Technologies, Enabling Factors and Scenarios
Edited by Georgi Graschew and Theo A. Roelofs

Published by InTech
Janeza Trdine 9, 51000 Rijeka, Croatia

Publishing Process Manager Katarina Lovrecic

Technical Editor Teodora Smiljanic

Cover Designer InTech Design Team

Additional hard copies can be obtained from orders@intechopen.com

Advances in Telemedicine: Technologies, Enabling Factors and Scenarios,
Edited by Georgi Graschew and Theo A. Roelofs
p. cm.
ISBN 978-953-307-159-6

For EU product safety concerns:
IN TECH d.o.o., Prolaz Marije Krucifikse Kozulić 3, 51000 Rijeka, Croatia,
info@intechopen.com or visit our website at intechopen.com.

Meet the editors

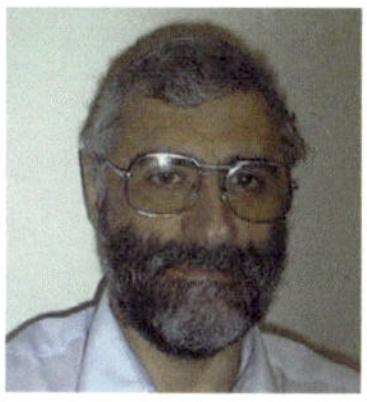

Dr. Georgi Graschew has been Scientific Coordinator of the Surgical Research Unit OP 2000 at the Max-Delbrück-Center for Molecular Medicine and the Experimental and Clinical Research Center of Charité – University Medicine Berlin (Germany) since 1993. Following his research studies at the Department for Mathematics and Natural Sciences of the Technical University Dresden (Germany) he gained his Ph.D. there in 1974. After research appointments at various international sites he became in 1987 co-founder of the Research Unit OP 2000 at the German Cancer Research Center DKFZ in Heidelberg (Germany), where he acted as its Scientific Coordinator until its transfer to Berlin. He made major contribution to numerous leading national and international telemedicine projects: SICONET, PANORAMA, GALENOS, DELTASS, MEDASHIP, EMISPHER. He has co-authored more than 360 scientific publications and presentations and holds 18 patents in Germany, the European Union, Japan and USA.

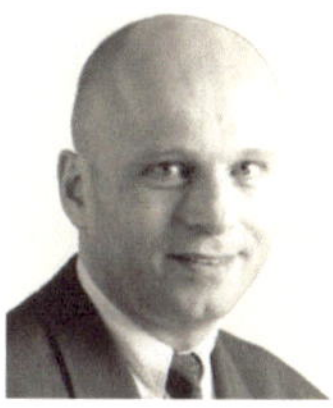

Dr. Theo A. Roelofs has been working since 1999 as Research Associate & Project Manager at the Surgical Research Unit OP 2000 of the Max-Delbrück-Center for Molecular Medicine and the Experimental and Clinical Research Center of Charité – University Medicine Berlin (Germany). He also contributed to various international Telemedicine projects (GALENOS, DELTASS, MEDASHIP) and acted as manager of the EMISPHER project. Following his studies in Molecular Sciences at the Wageningen University (Netherlands) and his Ph.D. in Biophysics (Max-Planck-Institute for Radiation Chemistry, Germany, and Free University at Amsterdam, Netherlands) he was a visiting research associate at the Chemical Biodynamics Department of the Lawrence Berkeley National Laboratory (USA, 1992-1994) and a research & education associate at the Physics Department of the Free University at Berlin (DE, 1994-1999). He has co-authored more than 140 scientific publications.

Contents

Preface

Innovative developments in information and communication technologies (ICT) irrevocably change our lives and enable new possibilities for society. One of the fields that strongly profits from this trend is Telemedicine, which can be defined as novel ICT-enabled medical services that help to overcome classical barriers in space and time. Through Telemedicine patients can access medical expertise that may not be available at the patient's site. The use of specifically designed communication networks with sophisticated quality-of-service for Telemedicine (distributed medical intelligence) contributes not only to the continuous improvement of patient care, but also to reducing the regional disparity in access to high-level healthcare. Telemedicine services can range from simply sending a fax message to a colleague to the use of broadband networks with multimodal video- and data streaming for obtaining second opinions as well as medical telepresence. Depending on the specific medical service requirements, a range of classes-of-services is used, each requiring its own technological quality-of-service.

Originally started as *interdisciplinary* efforts of engineers and medical experts, Telemedicine is more and more evolving into a *multidisciplinary* approach. Consequently, compiling a book on recent "Advances in Telemedicine" will have to cover a correspondingly wide range of topics. In addition, if each topic shall be treated in sufficient depth to allow the reader to get a comprehensive understanding of both the developmental state-of-the-art as well as the broad spectrum of issues relevant to Telemedicine, one might easily end up with a huge tome, too big to be practical in handling. Therefore, this book "Advances in Telemedicine" has been split into two volumes, each covering specific themes: Volume 1: Technologies, Enabling Factors and Scenarios; Volume 2: Applications in Various Medical Disciplines and Geographical Regions. The Chapters of each volume are clustered into four thematic sections.

The current Volume 1 "Advances in Telemedicine: Technologies, Enabling Factors and Scenarios" contains 19 Chapters clustered into the following thematic sections:

- Fundamental Technologies (Chapters 1-3),
- Applied Technologies (Chapters 4-11),
- Enabling Factors (Chapters 12-13),
- Scenarios (Chapters 14-19).

The section on ***Fundamental Technologies*** starts off with a thorough study on a novel **cross-layer design of wireless-LAN (1)** that combines the SVC extension of the H.264

video coding standard with the recent IEEE 802.11e WLAN standard. This new approach allows for the transmission of video streams over WLAN with an assigned guaranteed bandwidth (QoS) as required for telemedicine video applications in sufficiently high quality. The next study reports on the development of a **wireless cross-standard communication protocol (2)** that supports the creation of network-of-networks for e-Health applications from existing commercial (WiFi, WiMAX) and military (HIDL, Link 11) communication systems. This new protocol has been implemented in a demonstrator network that allows for the operation and investigation of various real-life healthcare scenarios. The section is closed up by extensive considerations on **safety and electromagnetic compatibility (3)** in wireless WiFi-, DECT- or GSM-based telemedicine applications. The electromagnetic environment of typical urban homes is characterised and an assessment for the potential safe use of home telemonitoring systems is presented. The need for adequate and harmonised legislation and regulation is also addressed.

The next section on ***Applied Technologies*** begins with an exploration of combining **digital video transport systems** with **global research and education networks (4)** for high quality video streaming in telemedicine. This new combination can help to overcome many of the bottlenecks in telemedicine implementation in daily routine, such as: insufficient image quality, too-high cost for set-up and operation, too difficult to use by medical experts. Next, a new algorithm for **lossless compression of medical images (5)** of various kinds using Huffman-based contourlet transform coding is presented. It is demonstrated that this new algorithm achieves higher compression ratios and yet superior image quality for different classes of medical images as compared to existing methods in the literature. The next chapter addresses the critical question as to the reliability of colour representation in transmission and display of medical videos and still images by presenting a novel sophisticated **multispectral colour reproduction system (6)**. Experimental evaluation of this new system used in video-based telemedicine applications for dermatology, surgery and general teleconsultation demonstrates that the reproduced colour is perceived as almost identical to the original, enabling improved remote diagnosis. The following chapter describes the application of Hilbert Huang transformation-based time-frequency **analysis approach for studying normal and sharp waves in electroencephalograms contaminated by transmission errors (7)**. Especially when applied as a tool to diagnose, differentiate and classify various stages of epilepsy this novel analysis approach yields more accurate results. The section continues with a presentation of three-level indexing hierarchy (TIH)-based **smart playback and recovery functions to enrich teleconsultation systems with retrieval capabilities (8)**. Thanks to the smart combination of cross-linked referencing and prioritised recovery the system allows a range of smart playback functions (e.g. replaying all the segments of a session controlled by a particular physician, or replaying all the session segments for which a particular medical image is discussed). The next chapter extensively treats a wide range of different aspects of the application of **statistics in telemedicine (9)**. It treats diverse aspects of qualitative and quantitative statistical methods in telemedicine such as for research and evaluation, for testing web-based platforms with different numbers of users, for new biomarker detection, or for electronic medical records and bio-banks. This work uncovers corresponding opportunities and challenges and provides the reader with useful guidelines. The subsequent chapter provides a survey on the technological and perceptive aspects of **video communication (10)** as used in various classes of services in telemedicine. It describes video applications ranging from simple videoconferencing up to medical telepresence and stereoscopic (3D) video communication. Technological solutions for applications in surgery, dermatology, ophthalmology and emergency medicine are presented. The section ends with a comprehensive overview of benefits and technological solutions for **broadband applications in telemedicine (11)**. Besides descriptions of suitable technologies this survey also addresses the potential benefits from the different perspectives of the various stakeholders. This chapter closes with an address of important challenges that are currently still unresolved, like privacy policies, security standards, interoperability guidelines, patients' acceptance and proof of cost effectiveness.

The section on ***Enabling Factors*** starts with a chapter on **Quality Control in Telemedicine (12)**. Describing the transposition of a corresponding Directive by the European Union into Spanish national legislation, the paper explains in detail how quality control in distant medical *service provision* has recently been legally regulated (by a CE-label instrument similar to the one for *equipment*) and points out the consequences for medical doctors and healthcare providers. It calls for and contributes to appropriate measures for corresponding training and licensing of health workers. The next chapter focuses on those complex heterogeneous factors ("work system") other than technology that are crucial for sustainable implementation of **Effective Telemedicine-based Services (13)**. Using an established approach from research on Socio Technical Systems as lens of analysis, three main levers emerge: formalisation of a clear and agreed business model between hospital unit and local health agency, involvement of a call center for service provision, empowerment of nurses. The resulting managerial implications are discussed.

The last section on telemedicine ***Scenarios*** begins with a contribution on **Real-time Interactive Telemedicine for Ubiquitous Healthcare (14)**. It describes specifically designed modules that allow for various real-time interactive scenarios: telesonography, telesurgery, telemicrobiology, distributed collaborative work, telementoring, etc. Both networks and services have been optimised and deployed for different real-life situations and shall ultimately be integrated into a Virtual Hospital. The next chapter addresses the question as to a **Possible Role for Home Telemedicine in the U.S. Medicare Program (15)**. An independent evaluation of the congressionally mandated IDEATel demonstration is presented, which includes intervention effects both on intermediate clinical outcomes and on use and costs of Medicare services, besides the cost of the demonstration itself. The evaluation results suggest that although the applied technology did not lead to a reduced use of Medicare services (and corresponding costs) and was very expensive in itself, home telemedicine might become important in the future, if legislative and market trends align to yield positive synergies. The next contribution describes a **Portable Vital Sensing System for Home Telemedicine (16)**. Integration of physiological sensing circuits, digital signal processors and wireless communication devices into a small smart unit allows for noninvasive monitoring of blood pressure, electrocardiograph and pulse wave and body temperature. Collection and processing of these data on a home medical server applying a virtual physiological model allows for health monitoring in support of the prevention of lifestyle diseases. The following chapter treats the role of **Telemedicine for Implementation of Self Management Models for Chronic Diseases in Vulnerable Patient Populations (17)**. It is described how telemedicine services, if tailored to the individual patients' needs, can lead to the empowerment of elderly, rural or underprivileged minority patient populations.

It can promote patient-centered healthcare systems by linking acute, transitional and chronic care needs, thus creating a care continuum. Also, continuous medical education of both patients and service providers becomes imperative. In the next chapter the **Telemedicine System of the Spanish Ministry of Defense (18)** is described, with emphasis on its role in tactical and strategical medical evacuation scenarios in the context of international (NATO-coordinated) interventions abroad. The standard system components have been selected to support both store-and-forward and real-time telemedical scenarios. Emphasis has been put on system standardisation according to ISO/IEEE 11073. Work in progress includes a Tele-Assistant system (for diagnostic and surgical procedures), a mobile ICU ambulance with integrated telemedicine capabilities for on-the-move scenarios, as well as a robotic tele-ultrasound examination unit. The last chapter of this book gives a presentation on a novel **Telemedicine system for hostile environments (19)** that is ontology-based and accounts for the lack of sensors or pre-defined data exchange protocols, conditions typical for these kind of settings. It implements a knowledge framework based on interrelated ontologies, a rule base and an inference engine. The implemented knowledge base is generic, scalable and open to support different telemedicine applications and services in patient-oriented scenarios.

This book has been conceived to provide valuable reference and learning material to other researchers, scientists and postgraduate students in the field. The references at the end of each chapter serve as valuable entry points to further reading on the various topics discussed and should provide guidance to those interested in moving forward in the field of Telemedicine.

We sincerely acknowledge all contributing authors for their time and effort in preparing the various chapters; without their dedication this book would not have been possible. Also we would like to thank Katarina Lovrecic from InTech Open Access Publisher for her excellent technical support during the realisation process of this book.

Georgi Graschew and Theo A. Roelofs
Surgical Research Unit OP 2000
Max-Delbrück-Center for Molecular Medicine
and Experimental and Clinical Research Center
Charité – University Medicine Berlin
Campus Berlin-Buch
Lindenberger Weg 80, D-13125 Berlin,
Germany

Email: graschew@mdc-berlin.de and roelofs@math.tu-berlin.de

Part 1

Fundamental Technologies

1

Cross Layer Design of Wireless LAN for Telemedicine Application Considering QoS Provision

Eko Supriyanto[1], Emansa Hasri Putra[2], Jafri bin Din[3], Haikal Satria[4] and Hamid Azwar[5]
[1]*Faculty of Biomedical Engineering and Health Science, Universiti Teknologi Malaysia,*
[2,5]*Telecommunication Department, Politeknik Caltex Riau,*
[3,4]*Faculty of Electrical Engineering, Universiti Teknologi Malaysia,*
[1,3,4]*Malaysia,*
[2,5]*Indonesia*

1. Introduction

Wireless Local Area Network (WLAN) have been widely utilized at this moment to support video-related applications such as video streaming, multimedia messaging, teleconference, voice over IP, and video telemedicine. This is due to WLAN constitutes a ubiquitous wireless standard solution and its implementation is not complex in terms of WLAN devices configuration and deployment. In addition, WLAN has superior characteristics compared with other wireless standard, including mobility fashions, high data rate, and low cost infrastructure.

The video-related application transmission such as telemedicine video will experience challenges including low throughput, delays, jitter and packet lost during its transmission over wireless network. This is due to wireless network or WLAN has specific characteristics which can influence the transmission consisting of time-varying channel, transmission error, and fluctuating bit rate characterized by factors such as noise, interference, and multiple fading. Thus, a video coding system for the transmission is necessary to adapt to the WLAN characteristics.

Recently, The Scalable Video Coding (SVC) standard as an extension of H.264/AVC have enabled a video bit stream to adapt to time-varying channel, transmission error, and fluctuating bit rate (Schierl et al. 2007). SVC also provides a scalability of receiver side receptions since receivers have possibly heterogeneous capabilities in terms of display resolution and processing power. In addition, SVC can support lower throughput and improve better coding efficiency compared with prior video coding techniques such as H.262/MPEG-2, H.263, MPEG-4, and H.264/AVC.

Currently, a new IEEE standard called The IEEE 802.11e is available to support Quality of Service (QoS) in WLAN. Specifically, this standard introduces a new MAC layer coordination function called Hybrid Coordination Function (HCF). Although IEEE 802.11e is more reliable than the previous standard, it still refers to OSI protocol stack in which every layer does not cooperate with each other. While wireless environments have specific

characteristics which may influence and degrade the quality level of the telemedicine application, namely time-varying bandwidth, delay, jitter and loss (Kim et al. 2006).
There are previous works which concern with cross layer techniques in wireless network. In (Choi et al., 2006), the focus was on cross layer optimization between application, data link, and physical layers to obtain the end to end quality of wireless streaming video application. A cross layer scheduling algorithm was utilized in (Kim, 2006) for throughput improvement in WLAN considering scheduling method and physical layer information. The authors utilized a H.264/AVC video coding in application layer over IEEE 802.11e EDCA wireless networks (Ksentini et al., 2006). MPEG-4 FGS video coding and FEC were utilized in application layer to deliver video application over IEEE 802.11a WLAN in (Schaar et al., 2003). In (Schaar et al., 2006), the authors utilized a MCTF video coding in application layer over IEEE 802.11 a/e HCCA wireless networks.
In this paper, a new approach in transmitting telemedicine video application over wireless LAN is performed to assign guaranteed bandwidth (QoS) for connection request of telemedicine video application. This approach utilizes a cross layer design technique based on H.264/SVC and IEEE 802.11e wireless network to optimize the existing wireless LAN protocol stack. From our results, an appropriate bandwidth could be achieved based on Quality of Service (QoS) provision for telemedicine video application during its transmission over wireless LAN.
The rest of this paper is organized as follows. The overview of telemedicine system including Telemedicine, H.264/SVC, and IEEE 802.11e Wireless Network is explained in Section II. Section III explains our proposed cross layer design of wireless LAN for video telemedicine transmission. The prototype and simulation model is described in Section IV. Results and Analysis is explained in Section V. Then, we conclude this paper in Section VI.

2. Telemedicine system

2.1 Telemedicine

Telemedicine constitutes healthcare services implemented through network infrastructures such as LAN, WLAN, ATM, MPLS, 3G, and others, to provide health care service quality especially in rural, urban, isolated areas, or mobile areas (Ng et al., 2006). Furthermore, telemedicine involves interactions between medical specialists at one station and patients at other stations and utilizes healthcare application which can be divided into video images, images, clinical equipments, and radiographic images.
The authors in (Pavlopoulos et al., 1998) have presented an example of telemedicine advantage through implementation on ambulatory patient care at remote area. Another application has been done in (Sudhamony et al., 2008) for cancer care in rural area. High technology telemedicine application in surgery has already been developed in (Xiaohui et al., 2007).
Currently, the telemedicine utilizes available wired and wireless infrastructures. Telemedicine infrastructures with wired network have been proposed using Integrated Service Digital Network (ISDN) (Al-Taei, 2005), Asynchronous Transfer Modes (ATM) (Cabral and Kim, 1996), Very Small Aperture Terminal (VSAT) (Pandian et al., 2007) and Asymmetric Digital Subscriber Line (ADSL) (Ling et al., 2005). Telemedicine has also been implemented in wireless network using Wireless LAN (WLAN) (Kugean et al., 2002), Worldwide Interoperability for Microwave Access (WIMAX) (Chorbev et al., 2008), Code Division Multiple Access (CDMA) 1X-EVDO (Yoo et al., 2005), and General Packet Radio Switch (GPRS) (Gibson et al., 2003).

Every infrastructure has its own obstacle, in particularly when implemented in a remote area. For example, Asynchronous Transfer Mode (ATM) and Multi Protocol Label Switching (MPLS) have mobility and scalability limitations, although both networks provide high Quality of Service (QoS) and have stability on delivering data (Nanda and Fernandes, 2007). The fragility of 3G UMTS network for telemedicine has been explored in (Tan et al., 2006), where the implementation costs are high and does not provide QoS.

There is a necessity of specific rule to define Quality of Services (QoS) provision of telemedicine application. In addition, parameterized QoS is a clear QoS bound expressed in terms of quantitative values such as data rate, delay bounds, jitter, and packet loss (Ni and Turletti, 2004). Thus, we refer to (Supriyanto et al., 2009) to obtain the parameterized QoS or QoS provision for telemedicine application. The desired output data rate for telemedicine system in seven medical devices can be seen in Table 1.

Devices	Data Rates	
	Good	Excellent
ECG	2 kbps	12 kbps
Doppler Instrument	40 kbps	160 kbps
Blood Pressure Monitor	1 kbps	1 kbps
Ultrasound Machine	100 kbps	400 kbps
Camera	100 kbps	2,000 kbps
Stethoscope	40 kbps	160 kbps
Microphone	40 kbps	160 kbps
Total	323 kbps	2,893 kbps

Table 1. Desired output data rate (Supriyanto et al., 2009)

Table 2 shows QoS bounds required for telemedicine application, namely throughput, delay, jitter and packet loss.

Parameter	Definition	Requirement
throughput	packet arrival rate	min 323 kbps
delay	the time taken by a packet to reach its destination	max 100 ms
jitter	time of arrival deviation between packets	max 50 ms
packet loss	percentage of non-received data packets	max 5 %

Table 2. QoS bounds for telemedicine application (Supriyanto et al., 2009)

2.2 H.264/SVC Standard

Recently, a video coding technique in wireless network has transformed into a way to optimize the video quality over a fluctuating bit rate instead of at a fixed bit rate. This due to wireless network or WLAN has specific characteristics which can influence video transmission consisting of time-varying channel, transmission error, and fluctuating bit rate characterized by factors such as noise, interference, and multiple fading. Thus, the video coding technique should adapt to fluctuating bit rate in wireless network and then reconstructing a video signal with the optimized quality at that bit rate.

Figure 1 shows a characteristic of video coding techniques consisting of non-scalable and scalable video coding. The horizontal axis means the channel bit rate, while the vertical axis means the received video quality. The distortion-rate curve constitutes an indicator of acceptable video quality for any coding techniques at fluctuating bit rate. If a video coding curve follows the movement of the distortion-rate curve, an optimal video quality will be acquired. The three staircase curves mean the performance of the non-scalable coding technique. On fluctuating bit rate conditions such as low, medium, or high bit rate, the non-scalable coding techniques try to follow the movement of the distortion-rate curve indicated by the upper corner of the staircase curve very close to the distortion-rate curve. The three staircase curves have different optimal video quality at each since every staircase curve can only achieve the distortion-rate curve either in low, medium or high bit rate. While a scalable video coding can follow the movement of the distortion-rate curve in which the scalable video coding has two layers, namely base layer and enhancement layer. Thus, the scalable video coding has the optimal video quality at each condition, either in low, medium, or high bit rate.

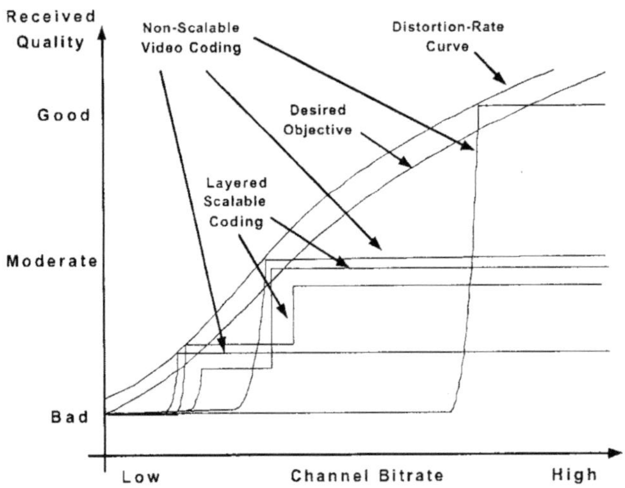

Fig. 1. A characteristic of video coding techniques consisting of non-scalable and scalable video coding (Li, 2001)

In the scalable coding technique, a video sequence is encoded into a base layer and an enhancement layer. The enhancement layer bit stream is similar to the base layer bit stream in which it is either completely received or it does not enhance the video quality at all. The base-layer bit rate constitutes the first stair while the enhancement layer bit rate constitutes the second stair as shown in Figure 1 (Li, 2001).

A Scalable Video Coding (SVC) standard constitutes an extension of H.264/AVC widely utilized for video transmission such as multimedia messaging, video telephony, video conference, Mobile TV, and other mobile networks at this time. The SVC provides scalability capability to improve features of prior video coding systems such as H.262/MPEG-2, H.263, MPEG-4, and H.264/AVC. In addition, The SVC has an adaptation capability to time-varying bandwidth conditions in wireless network, and heterogeneous receiver requirements. The time-varying bandwidth will lead to throughput variations, varying delays or transmission errors. Then, the heterogeneous receiver conditions will influence acceptable video bit stream in receiver sides limited by display resolution and processing power.

The common forms of scalability consist of temporal, spatial, and quality scalability. The spatial scalability constitutes a video coding technique in which picture size (spatial resolution) of video source is reduced. The temporal scalability means some parts of video bit stream reduced in term of frame rate (temporal resolution). Then, quality scalability constitutes a video coding technique in which the spatio-temporal resolution of video source is still the same as the complete bit stream, but fidelity is lower. The quality scalability is also commonly known as SNR scalability. Figure 2 shows a basic concept of SVC in which it combines temporal, spatial, and quality scalability.

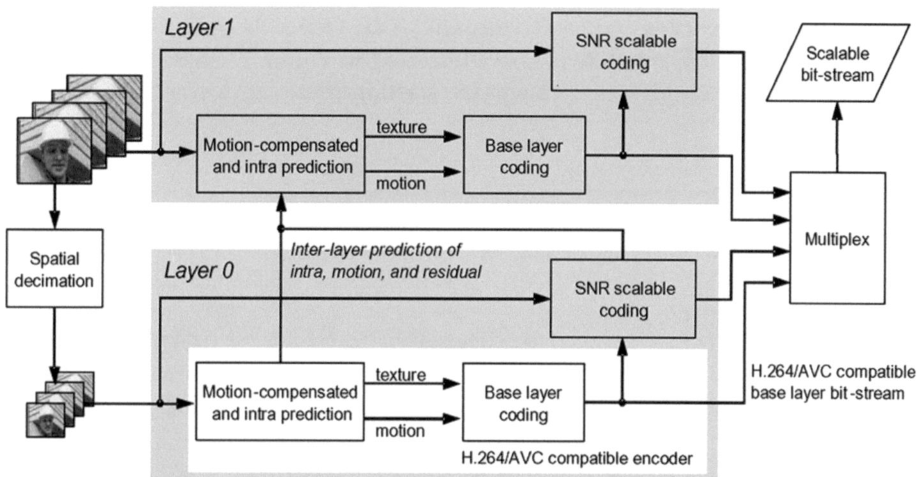

Fig. 2. SVC encoder structure (Schwarz et al., 2007)

The SVC encoder structure is arranged in dependency layers in which every dependency layers has a definite spatial resolution. The dependency layers utilize motion-compensated and intra prediction as in H.264/AVC single-layer coding and include one or more quality layers. Then, each dependency layer corresponds to a video source for a time instant with a definite spatial resolution and a definite fidelity. For more complete overview of SVC concept is referred to (Schwarz et al., 2007).

2.3 IEEE 802.11e Wireless Network

There are two different kinds of wireless network configuration. The first one is an infrastructure network, in which every communication between wireless stations is through an access point (AP). The second one is an ad hoc network, where communications between wireless stations are directly to each other, without a connection to an access point (AP). A group of stations arranged by an access point (AP) is called a basic service set (BSS), while for an ad hoc network is called independent BSS (IBSS). An area included by the BSS is referred as the basic service area (BSA), such as a cell in a cellular mobile network.

The IEEE 802.11 WLAN standard includes both datalink and physical layers of the open system interconnection (OSI) network reference model. The datalink layer intends to arrange access control functions to the wireless medium such as access coordination, addressing or frame check sequence generation. Basically, there are two medium access coordination functions, namely the basic Distributed Coordination Function (DCF) and the optional Point Coordination Function (PCF).

Recently, IEEE 802.11e standard proposed a new MAC layer coordination function in the datalink layer to provide QoS support, namely HCF (Hybrid Coordination Function). HCF consists of two channel access method, namely The Enhanced Distributed Channel Access (EDCA) and The HCF Controlled Channel Access (HCCA). Access Points (APs) and wireless stations which have supported The IEEE 802.11e standard are called QoS-enhanced AP (QAP) and QoS-enhanced station (QSTA) respectively (Ni and Turletti, 2004).

2.3.1 The Enhanced Distributed Channel Access (EDCA)

The EDCA consists of four access categories and starts from the highest priority until the lowest priority for supporting traffics of voice (AC_VO), video (AC_VI), best effort (AC_BE), and background (AC_BK) respectively, as illustrated in Figure 3. Table 3 shows relations between user priorities and access categories starting from the lowest until the highest priority.

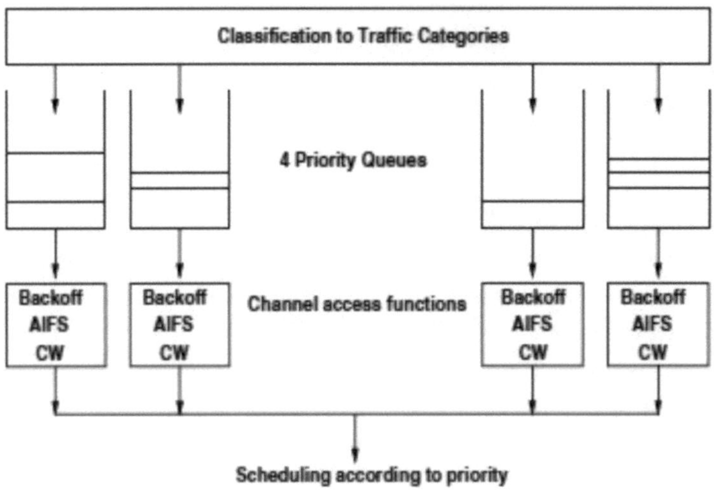

Fig. 3. The IEEE 802.11e EDCA model (Kim et al., 2006)

Priority	User Priority	802.1D Designation	Access Category	Designation
Lowest	1	BK	AC_BK	Background
	2	-	AC_BK	Background
	0	BE	AC_BE	Best Effort
	3	EE	AC_BE	Video
	4	CL	AC_VI	Video
	5	VI	AC_VI	Video
	6	VO	AC_VO	Voice
Highest	7	NC	AC_VO	Voice

Table 3. Relations between user priorities and access categories (Kim et al., 2006)

The IEEE 802.11 standard specifies four types of Interframe Spaces (IFS) utilized to define different priorities, namely Short Interframe Spaces (SIFS), Point Coordination IFS (PIFS),

Distributed IFS (DIFS), and Arbitrary IFS (AIFS). SIFS is the smallest IFS utilized to transmit frames such as ACK, RTS, and CTS. PIFS is the second smallest IFS utilized by Hybrid Coordinator (HC) to acquire the medium before any other stations. DIFS is the IFS for stations to wait after sensing an idle medium. The last, AIFS is the IFS utilized by different Access Categories (ACs) in The Enhanced Distributed Channel Access (EDCA) to wait after sensing an idle medium.

Every access categories in the EDCA contains their own Arbitrary Interframe Space (AIFS), Minimum Contention Windows (CW_{min}), Maximum Contention Windows (CW_{max}), and Transmission Opportunity (TXOP) in which the highest priority is assigned by the smallest values of AIFS, CW_{min}, CW_{max}, and the largest value of TXOP to acquire the first probability in term of channel access functions, and the lowest priority is vice versa, as illustrated in Figure 4 (Kim et al., 2006).

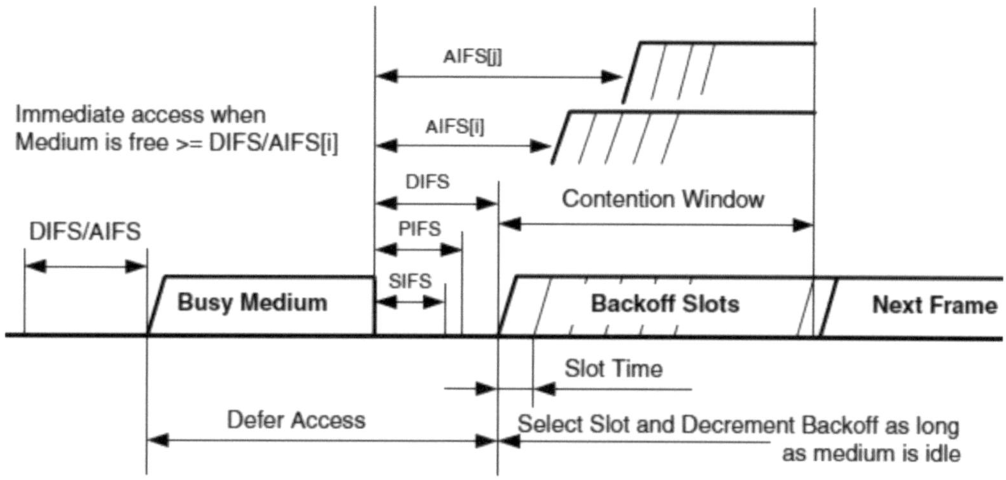

Fig. 4. Different IFS values in IEEE 802.11e EDCA (Kim et al., 2006)

2.3.2 The HCF Controlled Channel Access (HCCA)

The Hybrid Coordination Function (HCF) includes an optional contention-free period (CFP) and a mandatory contention period (CP) and contains a centralized coordinator called Hybrid Coordinator (HC). HC can perform a poll-and-response mechanism and start HCCA during CFP and CP. After optional CFP with a PCF mechanism, EDCA and HCCA mechanisms will alternate during mandatory CP. Although HCCA is better to support QoS than EDCA, the latter is still mandatory in IEEE 802.11e standard. Figure 5 shows Target Beacon Transmission Time (TBTT) interval of IEEE 802.11e HCF frame (Ni and Turletti, 2004).

When a QSTA desires to deliver data, the QSTA has to determine a Traffic Stream (TS) distinguished by a Traffic Specification (TSPEC). The TSPEC which is arranged between the QSTA and the QAP constitutes the QoS parameter requirement of a traffic stream consisting of Mean Data Rate, Delay Bound, Nominal Service Data Unit (SDU) Size, Maximum SDU Size, and Maximum Service Interval (MSI). The QSTA can deliver up to eight traffic streams and its transmission time is bounded by Transmission Opportunity (TXOP) (Cicconetti, 2005).

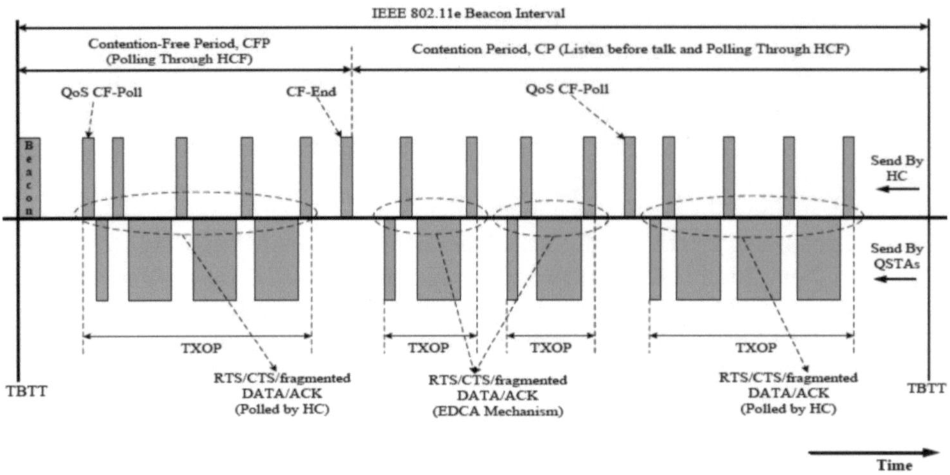

Fig. 5. The Target Beacon Transmission Time (TBTT) interval of IEEE 802.11e HCF frame (Cicconetti, 2005)

3. The proposed cross layer design

Cross layer design (CLD) is a new paradigm to optimize the existing OSI architecture. Every layer of OSI protocol stacks has tasks and services independently to each other as well as there are no direct communications between adjacent layers. It enables to provide dependencies and communications between layers to select the optimal solution. This optimization is provided to adapt to wireless environments and support QoS for telemedicine video application (Chen et al., 2008).

The Cross layer design can be split into three main ideas consisting of:

1. *Parameter abstraction:* Required information is collected from application, datalink, and physical layer through a process of parameter abstraction. The process of parameter abstraction selects specific parameters of the existing protocol layers into parameters which are possible for the cross-layer optimizer, so-called cross-layer parameters.
2. *Cross-layer optimization:* Parameters obtained through the parameter abstraction then are optimized to find a particular objective.
3. *Decision distribution:* The results of cross-layer optimization are distributed back into the related layers.

As illustrated in Figure 6, our proposed cross layer design consists of one expert station connected to an access point of WLAN IEEE 802.11g, and some patient stations will access the expert station in other side. A medical specialist in expert station side may conduct telemedicine application which involves data, video, and voice to examine patients in patient station through WLAN infrastructure.

To assign guaranteed bandwidth for connection requests of telemedicine application from a patient station to an expert station and vice versa, we perform cross layer design of the existing WLAN protocol stacks. We consider three OSI layers, namely application, datalink, and physical. We gather important information of them through a process of parameter abstraction. Then, the information is optimized to fulfil QoS provisions of telemedicine application. The results of optimizer are implemented back into application, datalink, and physical layers.

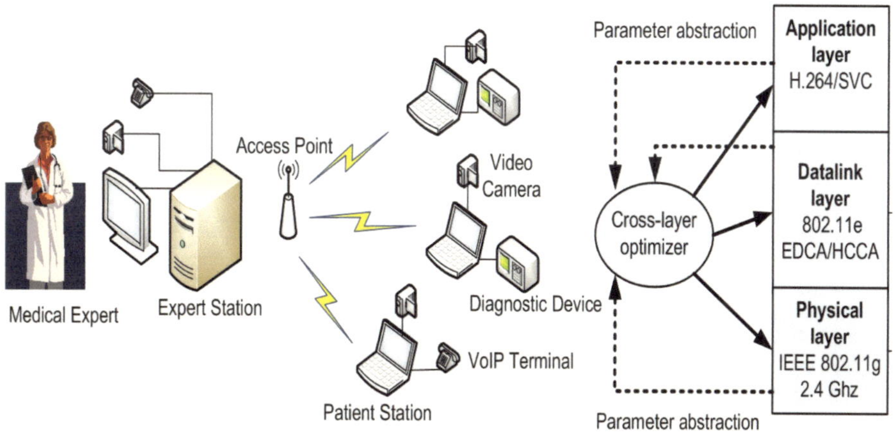

Fig. 6. Proposed Cross Layer Design of Wireless LAN for Telemedicine Video Transmission

We utilize H.264/SVC as a video coding technique in application layer due to this standard has an ability to support current technologies such as digital television, animated graphics, and multimedia application. In addition, its implementation utilizes relatively low bit rate in wireless network so it could be accessed easily by heterogeneous mobile users.

In datalink layer, we utilize a new MAC layer coordination function in datalink layer of OSI layers to provide QoS support, namely HCF (Hybrid Coordination Function). The HCF consists of two channel access method, namely The Enhanced Distributed Channel Access (EDCA) and HCF Controlled Channel Access (HCCA).

In physical layer, we utilize IEEE 802.11g standard which is currently available in many wireless LAN devices. This standard operates in 2.4 GHz radio band and supports a variety of modulations and data rates so that it can operate with its predecessor such as 802.11a and 802.11b (Labiod et al., 2007).

4. Prototype and simulation model

We have performed two NS2 simulation models to examine our proposed cross layer design of wireless LAN, namely called EDCA and HCCA simulation respectively. As explained in Section III, we utilize HCF consisting of EDCA and HCCA in datalink layer. Thus, we divide our NS2 simulation models into EDCA and HCCA simulation respectively based on the channel access method, namely EDCA and HCCA in the datalink layer. After NS2 simulations, we perform experiments of IEEE 802.11e EDCA prototype to identify and to investigate the proposed cross layer design in real wireless LAN environment. In this prototype, only EDCA scheme is utilized in the datalink layer to arrange access control functions to the wireless medium.

4.1 EDCA Simulation Model

This simulation was conducted in NS2 simulation (Ke, 2006) consisting of three steps. First step, we utilize a "Sony Demo" SVC video (Auwera and Reisslein, 2009) delivered over the proposed cross layer design. Furthermore, the "Sony Demo" video encoded with single layer H.264/AVC, temporal scalability, and spatial scalability (Auwera et al., 2008) respectively is delivered over the proposed cross layer design. In addition, we also utilize a "Jurassic Park 1" MPEG4 video (Trace, 1993) delivered over the proposed cross layer design.

Parameter	Value
Application Layer	
Video coding	H.264/SVC
Datalink Layer	
Slot time	20 μs
SIFS	10 μs
Data rate	54 Mbps
Basic rate	6 Mbps
Parameter for queue 0	
AIFS	2
CWMin	7
CWMax	15
TXOP	3.008 ms
Parameter for queue 1	
AIFS	2
CWMin	15
CWMax	31
TXOP	6.016 ms
Parameter for queue 2	
AIFS	3
CWMin	31
CWMax	1023
TXOP	0
Parameter for queue 3	
AIFS	7
CWMin	31
CWMax	1023
TXOP	0
Physical Layer	
Frequency	2.472 GHz
Preamble length	96 bits
PLCP header length	24 bits
PLCP data rate	6 Mbps

Table 4. Simulation parameters for the proposed cross layer design (the second step)

Then, the SVC video is compared with others. In this step we only utilize one QSTA and one QAP.

In the second step, there are four kinds of traffic flows between QSTA and QAP delivered over the proposed cross layer design. First flow is VoIP traffic at 64 Kbps data rate over UDP protocol and constitutes the highest priority. Second flow is video traffic in which we utilize a "Sony Demo" SVC video over UDP protocol and constitutes the second highest priority. Third flow is CBR traffic at 125 Kbps data rate over UDP protocol and constitutes the third highest priority. Forth flow is FTP traffic at 512 Kbps data rate over TCP protocol and constitutes the

lowest priority. The simulation parameters utilized in this step are shown in Table 4. In this step, we utilize five QSTAs and one QAP to increase traffic in the wireless LAN.
Third step, four traffic flows are delivered over the original IEEE 802.11b wireless LAN. First flow is VoIP traffic at 64 Kbps data rate over UDP protocol. Second flow is video traffic in which we utilize a "Sony Demo" SVC video over UDP protocol. Third flow is CBR traffic at 125 Kbps data rate over UDP protocol. Forth flow is FTP traffic at 512 Kbps data rate over TCP protocol. In this step, we also utilize five QSTAs and one QAP to increase traffic in the wireless LAN.

4.2 HCCA simulation model

In this HCCA simulation, we utilized one QAP and one QSTA in our proposed cross layer design. There is a bi-directional video flow between QAP and QSTA in which we utilize a "Sony Demo" SVC video over UDP protocol. Furthermore, we also generate other bi-directional flows consisting of VoIP, CBR, and FTP as the same way as in the EDCA simulation model to increase traffic in the network. The simulation is conducted in NS2 simulation (Cicconetti et al., 2005).

The SVC video traffic flow constitutes the highest priority for HCCA scheduler in the datalink layer. When the QSTA desires to deliver the SVC video, the QSTA has to determine a Traffic Stream (TS) characterized by a Traffic Specification (TSPEC). The TSPEC arranged between the QSTA and the QAP constitutes the QoS parameter requirement of a traffic stream consisting of Mean Data Rate, Delay Bound, Nominal Service Data Unit (SDU) Size, Maximum SDU Size, and Maximum Service Interval (MSI). Table 5 shows Traffic Specification (TSPEC) for the SVC video traffic flow.

Parameter	Value
Application Layer	
Video coding	H.264/SVC
Datalink Layer	
Service Interval (SI)	20 ms
Mean Data rate	10 Mbps
Nominal SDU size	1500 byte
Maximum SDU size	2132 byte
SIFS	10 μs
PIFS	30 μs
CWMin	31
CWMax	1023
TXOP	8.16 ms
Physical Layer	
Frequency	2.472 GHz
Preamble length	96 bits
PLCP header length	24 bits
PLCP data rate	1 Mbps

Table 5. Simulation parameters for the proposed cross layer design (HCCA simulation model)

4.3 IEEE 802.11e EDCA prototype

IEEE 802.11e EDCA prototype consists of a wireless Access Point (AP) and a wireless station (STA). A wireless Access Point (AP) constitutes a personal computer (PC) equipped with a wireless TP-LINK TL-WN551G card, and Debian 4 Linux OS, and configured as wireless Access Point (AP) through Madwifi software (Madwifi, 2009) in the PC. A wireless station is also a PC equipped with a wireless TP-LINK TL-WN551G card, and Debian 4 Linux OS, and configured as wireless station (STA) through Madwifi software in the PC. As shown in Figure 7, then the wireless Access Point (AP) is connected to the wireless station utilizing 2.4 GHz frequency with 54 Mbps data rate. The wireless station also functions as a wireless monitor to capture and analyze packets delivered over wireless LAN utilizing Wireshark software (Wireshark, 2009). Table 6 shows specifications of the IEEE 802.11e EDCA prototype.

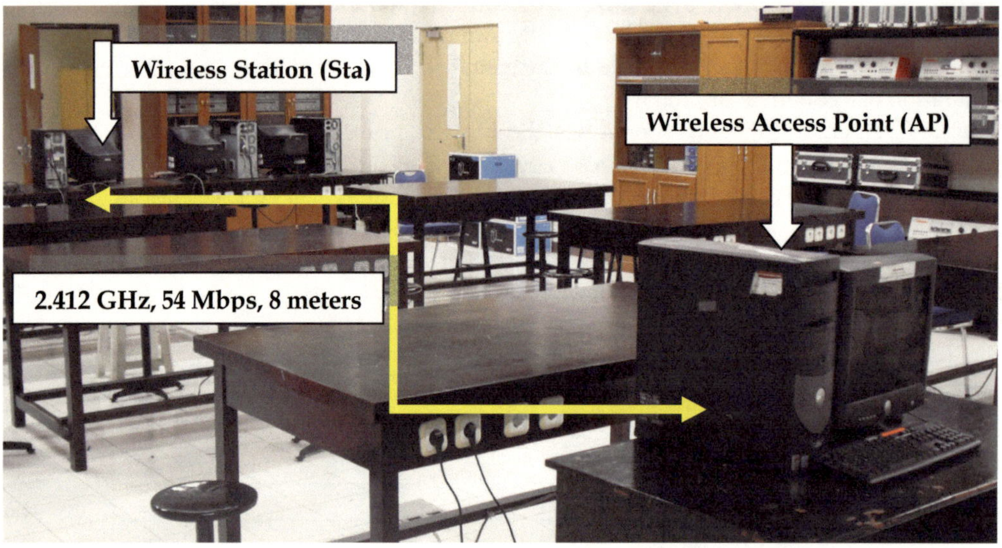

Fig. 7. The IEEE 802.11e EDCA Prototype consists of Wireless AP and wireless station

Table 7 shows Madwifi WMM/WME parameter [36] utilized in wireless AP and wireless station in which we can observe that video and voice traffic flows have smaller CWmin, CWmax, and AIFS values and higher TXOP values. Thus, the video and voice traffics will have greater probability of gaining access to the wireless medium.

To perform live video streaming application during experiments, we assign the wireless AP as a streaming server utilizing VLC software (VLC, 2009). The VLC software is also installed in the wireless station to display the live video streaming application. Then, the Foreman QCIF video is delivered over wireless LAN and the wireless station will display the Foreman QCIF video streaming utilizing the VLC media player.

All experiments performed consist of two steps. First step, we activate the WMM/WME (WiFi multimedia / WiFi multimedia extension) feature of Madwifi driver on the IEEE 802.11e EDCA prototype. Furthermore, this experiment is begun with FTP and Ping application running firstly, namely from t = 0 s to t = 4.3 s. Beginning at t = 4.3 s, the Foreman QCIF video streaming flow is begun and begins competing for channel access with the previous applications. Finally, at t = 16.46 s, the live video streaming finishes and the other applications also follow to finish after that.

Specification	Description
Wireless Access Point	
Personal Computer (PC)	Dell PC with Intel Pentium IV 2.4 GHz
Operating System (OS)	Debian 4 Linux OS
Wireless Ethernet	TP-LINK TL-WN551G
Wireless device driver	Madwifi
Applications	VLC server, Proftp server, ping
Frequency	2.412 GHz
Data rate	54 Mbps
Wireless Station	
Personal Computer (PC)	Dell PC with Intel Pentium IV 2.4 GHz
Operating System (OS)	Debian 4 Linux OS
Wireless Ethernet	TP-LINK TL-WN551G
Wireless device driver	Madwifi
Applications	VLC client, Firefox browser, Wireshark
Frequency	2.412 GHz
Data rate	54 Mbps

Table 6. Specifications of the IEEE 802.11e EDCA Prototype

Madwifi WMM/WME Parameter	Access Class			
	AC_BE	AC_BK	AC_VI	AC_VO
CWMin	4	4	3	2
CWMax	10	10	4	3
AIFS	2	7	2	2
TXOP	2048	0	3008	1504

Table 7. Madwifi WMM/WME parameter utilized in wireless AP and wireless station (Yoon, 2006)

In the first step, we perform FTP application utilizing Proftp software in which a DVD video is downloaded by the wireless station through the FTP application. We also generate background traffic utilizing ping application with 512 MB size to increase traffic load over the wireless LAN. In addition, packet analyzer software called Wireshark is operated to capture packets delivered over wireless LAN during this experiment.

Second step, we do not activate the WMM/WME (WiFi multimedia / WiFi multimedia extension) feature of Madwifi driver. We repeat procedures as the same way as the first step. Furthermore, this second step is begun with FTP and Ping application running firstly, namely from t = 0 s to t = 4.3 s. Beginning at t = 8.91 s to 20.6 s, the QCIF video streaming flow is begun and begins competing for channel access with the previous applications. Finally, at t = 20.6 s, the live video streaming finishes and the other applications also follow to finish after that.

In the second step, we also perform FTP application and generate background traffic utilizing ping application to increase traffic load over the wireless LAN. In addition, packet analyzer software called Wireshark is also operated to capture packets delivered over wireless LAN during this experiment.

5. Results and analysis

We analyze results of two NS2 simulation models, namely EDCA and HCCA Simulation, and experiments of IEEE 802.11e EDCA prototype respectively. Then, we investigate whether results of the NS2 simulation and the IEEE 802.11e EDCA prototype fulfill the QoS provision to support telemedicine application.

5.1 EDCA simulation analysis

Figure 8 shows the throughput values of five different video flows over The IEEE 802.11e EDCA wireless network. We can observe that "Sony Demo" SVC video has the lowest throughput compared with the others. This indicates that the H.264/SVC has a capability to reduce the required bit rate for the same perceptual video quality since the others require higher throughput. This also means that the H.264/SVC can improve better coding efficiency.

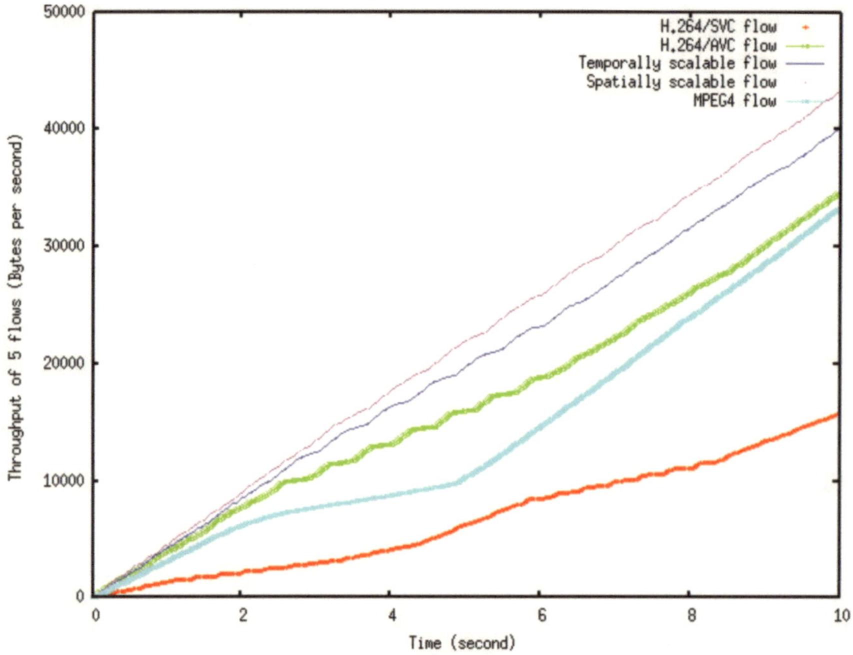

Fig. 8. The throughput values of five different video flows over The IEEE 802.11e EDCA wireless network

Figure 9 shows the throughput values of four flows with different priorities over the proposed cross layer design. We can observe that the voice and video flows acquire the assigned throughput, namely 64.13 Kbps and 309.59 Kbps respectively. In the Figure 9, the high priority streams look stable during their transmission over wireless LAN. This can happen due to EDCA scheme associates voice and video packets with access category 1 (AC1) and access category 2 (AC2) respectively so it give more channel access opportunities. In the EDCA scheme, the AC1 and AC2 have higher priority and the AC1 and AC2 are assigned with smaller CWmin, CWmax, and AIFS and longer TXOP to influence the successful transmission probability.

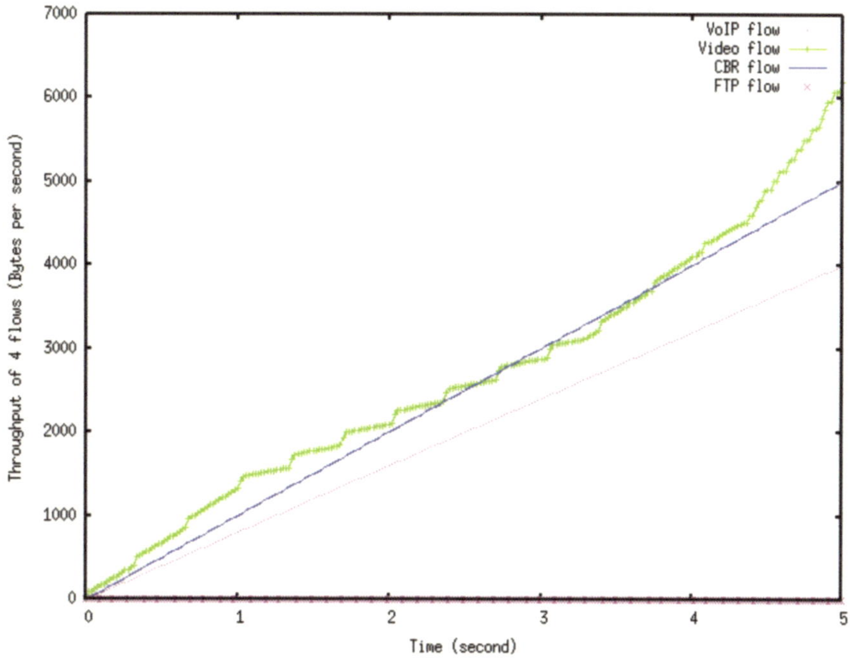

Fig. 9. The throughput values of four flows with different priorities over the proposed cross layer design.

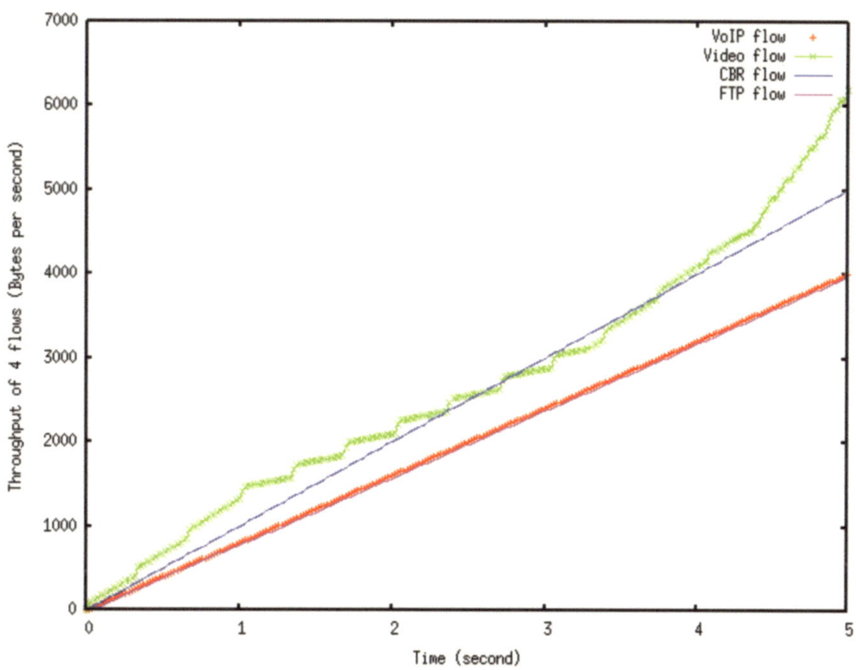

Fig. 10. The throughput values of four flows over the conventional IEEE 802.11b wireless network

Figure 10 shows the throughput values of four flows in which there are not priorities over the conventional IEEE 802.11b wireless network. We can observe that the VoIP flow has the same throughput as the FTP flow. It indicates that the delay-constrained VoIP flow competes with the non-delay-constrained FTP flow to acquire the available bandwidth. This is can happen due to there are not priorities in the wireless medium, so every traffic flow will contends each other to access to the wireless medium.

Table 8 shows the average throughput values of four flows for every video coding technique over the proposed cross layer design. We can observe that VoIP, CBR, and FTP flows are similar in term of average throughput for five video coding techniques. Furthermore, the H.264/SVC video has the lowest throughput compared with the other video coding techniques.

Table 9 shows the average throughput, delay and packet loss values of video flow for every video coding technique over the proposed cross layer design. We observe that the proposed cross layer design delivers 99.68 percent of video packets within average delay of 10.66 ms. Furthermore, the proposed cross layer design has the lowest packet loss value than the previous solutions such as Static Mapping and Adaptive Cross Layer Mapping (Lin et al., 2009). Thus, this proves that the proposed cross layer design fits to be utilized very acceptably in telemedicine application.

	Average Throughput (Bytes per second)			
	VoIP	Video	CBR	FTP
H.264/SVC	8,016.03	38,698.35	15,645.05	13.33
H.264/AVC	8,016.03	164,313.91	15,625.02	13.33
Temporal Scalability	8,016.03	185,328.26	15,625.02	13.33
Spatial Scalability	8,016.10	200,065.69	15,625.16	13.33
MPEG4	8,016.03	91,404.70	15,645.05	13.33

Table 8. The average throughput values of four flows for every video coding technique

	Average Throughput (Kbps)	Delay (ms)	Packet Loss (%)
H.264/SVC	309.59	10.66	0.32
H.264/AVC	1,314.51	11.30	52.17
Temporal Scalability	1,482.63	11.32	54.34
Spatial Scalability	1,600.53	11.42	52.46
MPEG4	731.24	10.27	0.38

Table 9. The average throughput, delay and packet loss values of video flow for every video coding technique

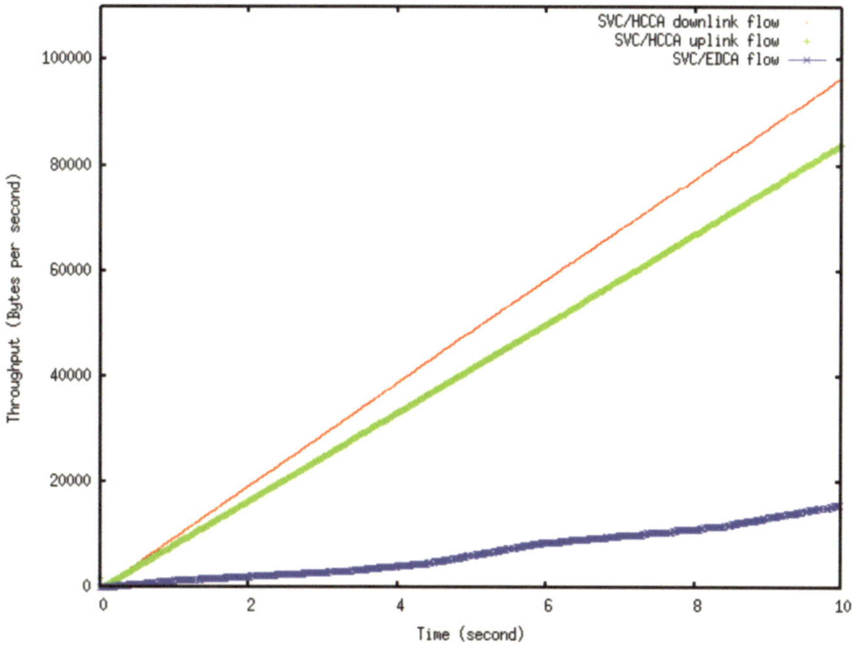

Fig. 11. The throughput values of SVC video flow over HCCA downlink, HCCA uplink, and EDCA

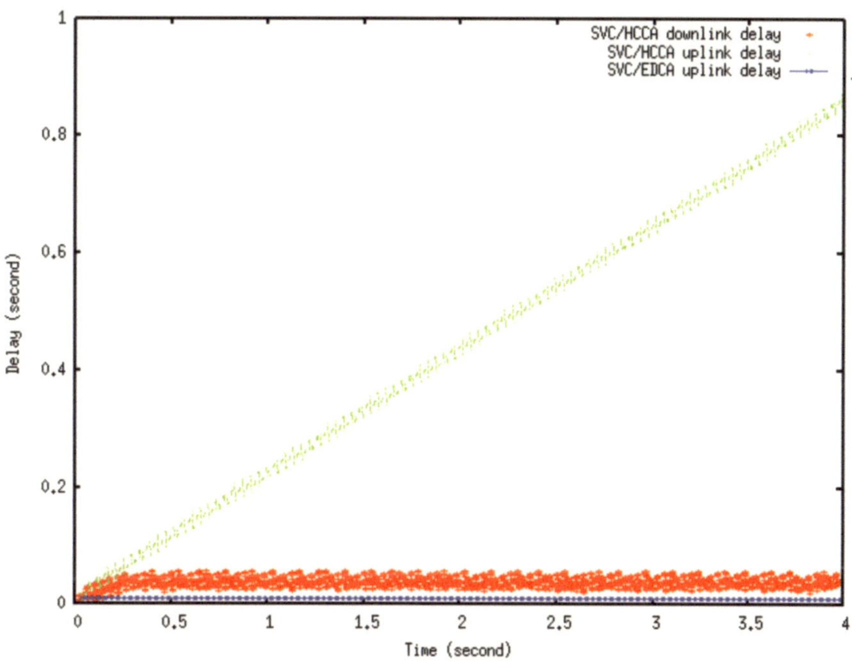

Fig. 12. The delay values of SVC video flow over HCCA downlink, HCCA uplink, and EDCA

5.2 HCCA simulation analysis

Throughput curve on Figure 11 shows that both downlink HCCA and uplink HCCA schemes succeed to acquire the required throughput for SVC video flow. In addition, SVC video flows over both HCCA downlink and HCCA uplink are more stable than SVC video flow over EDCA. This is mainly due to HCCA scheduler assigns a fixed TXOP for every SVC video traffic flow based on the required mean data rate during service interval (SI). It indicates that the reference scheduler of HCCA has a capability to support the SVC video flow with the QoS guarantee through a negotiation process of parameterized guarantee, namely Traffic Specification (TSPEC).

Figure 12 shows the delay values of SVC video flow over HCCA downlink, HCCA uplink, and EDCA. We observe that HCCA delivers 96.25 percent of the SVC video packets within average delay of 18.58 ms from the QAP to the QSTA (downlink). In addition, HCCA delivers 99.99 percent of the SVC video packets within average delay of 907.94 ms from the QSTA to the QAP (uplink). The both average delays are still in QoS provision as shown in Table 2.

Table 10 shows the throughput, delay and packet loss values of SVC video flow over HCCA downlink, HCCA uplink, and EDCA link. We can observe that throughputs of SVC/HCCA downlink, SVC/HCCA uplink, and SVC/EDCA fits to the QoS provision in Table 2. This also applies to delay and packet loss values which are suitable with the QoS provision. Furthermore, the delay values of SVC video flow over HCCA downlink, and EDCA link are lower than the delay values of the FHCF scheme (Ansel et al., 2006) and the SFS scheme (Bourawy, 2008). Moreover, the packet loss values of SVC video flow over HCCA downlink, HCCA uplink, and EDCA link are lower than the packet loss value of the SFS scheme. Thus, our proposed cross layer design fits to deliver very acceptably telemedicine application which contains delay sensitive data such as video and voice data.

	Throughput (Kbps)	Delay (ms)	Packet Loss (%)
SVC/HCCA Downlink	1,539.76	18.58	3.75
SVC/HCCA Uplink	1,669.8	907.94	0.01
SVC/EDCA	309.59	10.66	0.32

Table 10. The throughput, delay and packet loss values of video flow over HCCA downlink, HCCA uplink, and EDCA link

5.3 IEEE 802.11e EDCA prototype analysis

Figure 13 shows throughput values of video streaming flow when the IEEE 802.11e EDCA prototype utilizes EDCA scheme in the datalink layer. From t = 4.3 s to t = 5.37 s, the throughput increase quickly, and after that decrease towards the average point at 292.27 Kbps. We can observe that the bit rate requirement does not vary widely over time for the video flow. Although the video flow constitutes Variable Bit Rate (VBR) flow, the video flow is more similar to Constant Bit Rate (CBR) flow. This is mainly due to the fact that the IEEE 802.11e EDCA prototype gives more channel access opportunities (transmission) to video

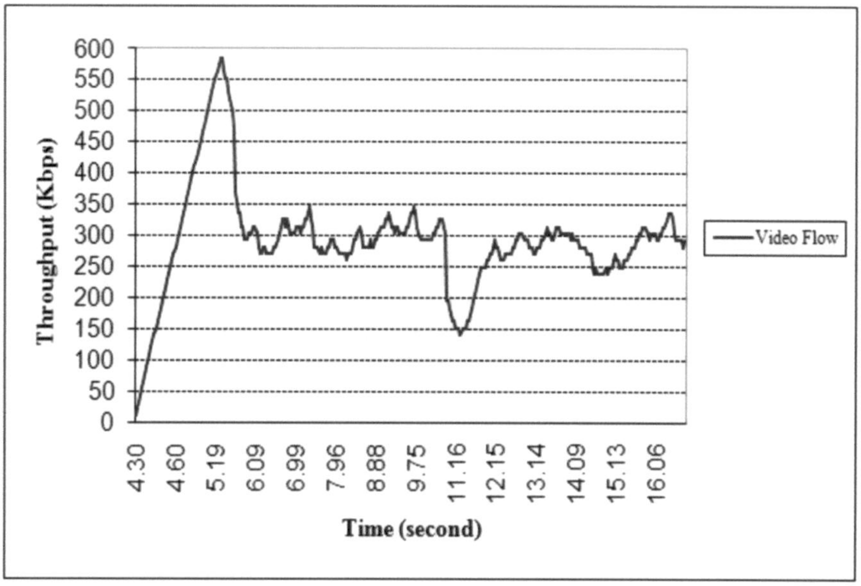

Fig. 13. EDCA throughput plot

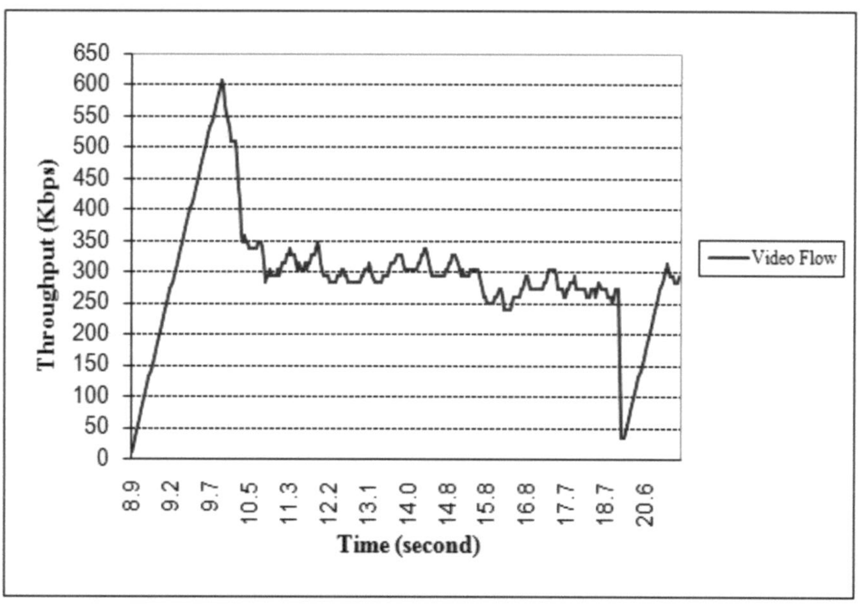

Fig. 14. Non-EDCA throughput plot

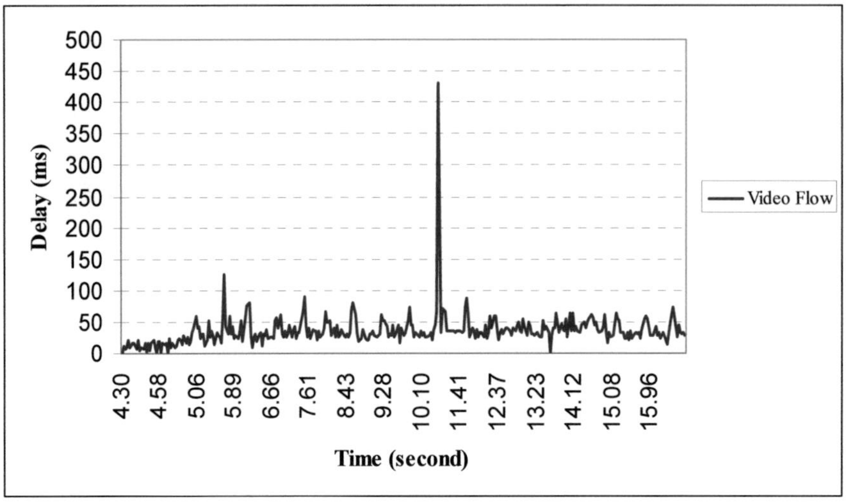

Fig. 15. EDCA delay plot

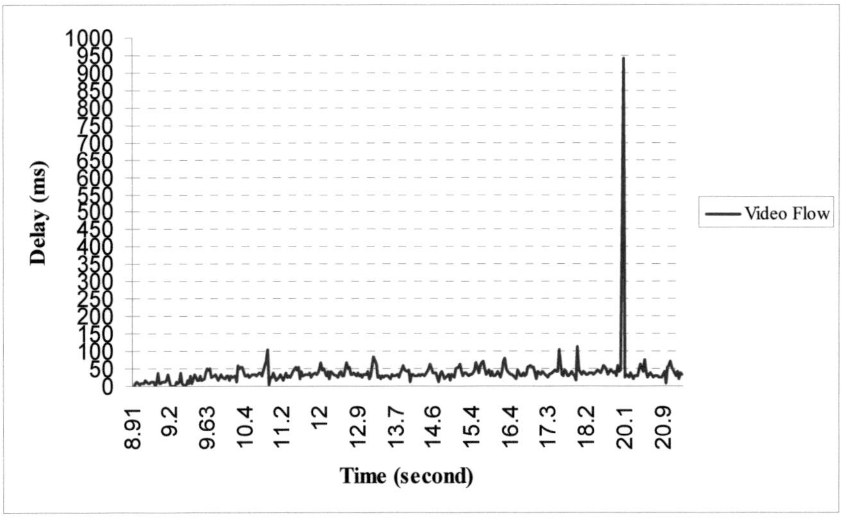

Fig. 16. Non-EDCA delay plot

flow in which video packets are assigned with smaller CWmin, CWmax, and AIFS values and higher TXOP values.

Figure 14 shows throughput value of video streaming flow over the original IEEE 802.11g wireless LAN in which we do not activate the EDCA scheme in the datalink layer. From t = 20.02 s to t = 20.25 s, the throughput decrease deeply below 100 Kbps, while the average throughput value is 292.02 Kbps. We can observe that the bit rate requirement vary widely over time for the video flow. At this duration, we can see that the video streaming experiences delay for the moment. This is can happen due to there are not priorities in the wireless medium, thus video traffic flow will contends with other flows to access the wireless medium.

Figures 15 shows delay experienced by video flow over our IEEE 802.11e EDCA prototype in which the average delay value is 36.09 ms. The IEEE 802.11e EDCA prototype reduces the delay to the minimum level, indicating that video packets are transmitted almost immediately. At t = 10.85 s, the delay increase greatly towards 431.99 ms, while the maximum delay value allowed is 100 ms. Then, the packet loss value experienced by video flow is 4.71 % and this is still in QoS provision.

Figures 16 shows delay values for video flow over the original IEEE 802.11g wireless LAN in which the average delay value is 37.17 ms. Due to video traffic has the same priority as other applications, it results in greatly increased video packet delays. This is mainly due to all packets competing with each other without restraint to acquire the shared channel medium. At t = 20.02 s, the delay increase greatly towards 942.7 ms and this is greater than the delay in our IEEE 802.11e EDCA prototype. Then, the packet loss value experienced by video flow is 7.48 % and this is out of QoS provision.

6. Conclusion

In this paper, we have implemented a proposed cross layer design of wireless LAN to deliver four traffic flows of telemedicine application with different priorities and to assign telemedicine video with QoS guarantee simulated in NS2 environment and implemented in IEEE 802.11e EDCA prototype. The NS2 simulation models are divided into EDCA and HCCA simulation respectively based on the channel access method, namely EDCA and HCCA in the datalink layer. Results of NS2 simulations and experiments of the IEEE 802.11e EDCA prototype prove that the cross layer design of wireless LAN is able to support telemedicine application acceptably during its transmission over wireless LAN based on Quality of Service (QoS) provision. Thus, the new design has a potential to be utilized in telemedicine system.

7. Acknowledgement

This work is fully support by Ministry of Science, Technology and Innovation (MOSTI) Malaysia under grant of Science Fund Vot No. 79196. The authors would like to thank to Research Management Centre (RMC) Universiti Teknologi Malaysia (UTM) for their support.

8. References

Al-Taei, M. (2005). "Telemedicine needs for multimedia and integrated services digital network (ISDN)", Proc. ICSC Congress on Computational Intelligence Methods and Applications, IEEE, Amman, Jordan.

Ansel, P.; Ni, Q.; and Turletti, T. (2006). " FHCF: A Simple and Efficient Scheduling Scheme for IEEE 802.11e Wireless LAN", Mobile Networks and Applications, 11, 391-403, Springer Netherlands.

Auwera, G.; and Reisslein, M. (2009). "Implications of Smoothing on Statistical Multiplexing of H.264/AVC and SVC Video Streams" IEEE Transactions on Broadcasting, 55(3):541-558.

Auwera, G.; David, P. T.; and Reisslein, M. (2008). "Traffic and Quality Characterization of Single-Layer Video Streams Encoded with H.264/MPEG-4 Advanced Video Coding Standard and Scalable Video Coding Extension". IEEE Transactions on Broadcasting, 54(3):698-718.

Bourawy, A. A. (2008). "Scheduling in IEEE 802.11e Networks with Quality of Service Assurance", Master of Science, Queen's University, Canada.

Cabral, J.J. and Kim, Y. (1996). "Multimedia systems for telemedicine and their communications requirements", IEEE Communications Magazine.

Cicconetti, C.; Lenzini, L.; Mingozzi, E. Stea, G. (2005) "A Software Architecture for Simulating IEEE 802.11e HCCA", Proc. 3rd Internet Performance, Simulation, Monitoring and Measurement IPS-MoMe 2005 March 14-15, Warsaw (Poland).

Chen, Y.; Feng, J.; Lo, K. T.; Zhang, X. (2008). "Wireless Multimedia Systems: Cross Layer Considerations", Taylor & Francis Group, LLC.

Choi, L.U.; Kellerer, W.; Steinbach, E. (2006). "On Cross-Layer Design for Streaming Video Delivery in Multiuser Wireless Environments", EURASIP Journal on Wireless Communications and Networking.

Chorbev, I.; Mihajlov, M.; Jolevski, I. (2008). "WiMAX supported telemedicine as part of an integrated system for e-medicine". Proc. 30th International Conference on Information Technology Interfaces, IEEE, Dubrovnik.

Gibson, O.J.; Cobern, W.R. Hayton, P.M. and Tarassenko, L. (2003). "'A GPRS mobile phone telemedicine system for self-management of type 1 diabetes", Proc. 2nd IEEE EMBSS Conference on Biomedical Engineering and Medical Physics, Birmingham.

Ke, C. H. (2006). http://140.116.72.80/~smallko.

Kim, H.; Hou, J. C.; Hu, C.; and Ge, Y. (2006) "QoS Provisionings in IEEE 802.11-complaint Networks", Elsevier.

Kim, S. W. (2006). "Cross-Layer Scheduling Algorithm for WLAN Throughput Improvement", Springer-Verlag Berlin Heidelberg.

Kim, H.; Hou, J. C.; Hu, C.; and Ge, Y. (2006) "QoS Provisionings in IEEE 802.11-complaint Networks", Elsevier.

Ksentini, A.; Naimi, M.; and Gueroui, A. (2006). "Toward an Improvement of H.264 Video Transmission over IEEE 802.11e through A Cross-Layer Architecture", IEEE Comm. Magazine.

Kugean, C.; Krishnan, S. M.; Chutatape, O.; Swaminathan, S.; Srinivasan, N.; and Wang, P. (2002). "Design of a mobile telemedicine system with WLAN, Proc. Asia-Pacific Conference on Circuits and Systems', IEEE, Singapore.

Labiod, H.; Afifi, H.; and Santis, C. (2007). "Wi-Fi Bluetooth Zigbee WiMAX", Springer.

Li, W. (2001). "Overview of Fine Granularity Scalability in MPEG-4 Video Standard", IEEE Transaction on Circuits and Systems for Video Technology.

Lin, C.-H.; Shieh, C.-K.; Ke, C.-H.; Chilamkurti, N. K.; and Zeadally, S. (2009). "An adaptive cross-layer mapping algorithm for MPEG-4 video transmission over IEEE 802.11e WLAN", Telecommunication Systems, 42, 223-234. Springer Netherlands.

Ling, L.; Dezhong, Y.; Jianqig, L.; Bin, L.; Ling, W. (2005). "A multimedia telemedicine system", Proc. 27th Annual International Conference of the Engineering in Medicine and Biology Society, IEEE.

Madwifi Project, (2009). http://madwifi-project.org/

Nanda, P.; and Fernandes, R. (2007). "Quality of Service in Telemedicine", Proc. First International Conference on the Digital Society, IEEE.

Ng, H S; Sim, M L; Tan, C M; and Wong, C C. (2006). "Wireless Technologies for Telemedicine", BT Technology Journal, Vol 24 No 2.

Ni, Q.; Turletti, T. (2004). "QoS Support for IEEE 802.11 Wireless LAN". http://www-sop.inria.fr/planete/qni/ 802.11 QoS_qni.pdf

Pandian, P. S.; Safeer, K. P.; Shakunthala, D. T.; Padaki, V. C. (2007). "Internet Protocol Based Store and Forward Wireless Telemedicine System for VSAT and Wireless Local Area Network", Proc. International Conference on Signal Processing, Communications and Networking, IEEE, Chennai.

Pavlopoulos, S.; Kyriacou, E.; Berler, A.; Dembeyiotis, S.; Koutsouris, D. (1998). "A novel emergency telemedicine system based on wireless communication technology-Ambulance", IEEE Transactions on Technology in Biomedicine, vol.2, no.4, p.261 - 267.

Schaar, M. van der; Krishnamachari, S.; Choi, S.; and Xu, X. (2003). "Adaptive Cross-Layer Protection Strategies for Robust Scalable Video Transmission Over 802.11 WLANs", IEEE Journal on Selected Areas in Communication.

Schaar, M. van der; Andreopoulus, Y.; and Hu, Z. (2006). "Optimized Scalable Video Streaming over IEEE 802.11a/e HCCA Wireless Networks under Delay Constraints", IEEE Transaction on Mobile Computing.

Schierl, T.; Stockhammer, T.; and Wiegand, T. (2007). "Mobile Video Transmission Using Scalable Video Coding", IEEE Transactions on Circuits and Systems for Video Technology, Vol 17 No 9.

Schwarz, H.; Marpe, D.; and Wiegand, T. (2007). "Overview of Scalable Video Coding Extension of The H.264/AVC Standard", IEEE Transactions on Circuits and Systems for Video Technology, Vol 17 No 9.

Sudhamony, S.; Nandakumar, K.; Binu, P.; and Niwas, S. (2008). "Telemedicine and tele-health services for cancer-care delivery in India", IET Communications, vol.2, no.2, p. 231 - 236.

Supriyanto, E.; Satria, H.; Mulyadi, I. H.; Putra, E. H. (2009). "A Novel Low Cost Telemedicine System Using Wireless Mesh Network", 3rd SEATUC Symposium.

Tan, Y. E.; Istepanian, N.P. and R.S.H. (2006). "Fragility Issues of Medical Video Streaming over 802.11e-WLAN m-health Environments", Proc. the 28th IEEE EMBS Annual International Conference.

Trace Files, (1993). http://trace.eas.asu.edu/TRACE/ltvt.html.

VLC Media Player, (2009). http://www.videolan.org/vlc/

Xiaohui, X.; Ruxu, D.; Lining, S.; and Zhijiang, D. (2007). "Internet based telesurgery with a bone-setting system", Proc. IEEE International Conference on Integration Technology, Shenzhen.

Yoo, S.K.; Jung, S. M.; Kim, B. S.; Yun, H. Y; Kim, S. R.; Kim, D. K. (2005). "Prototype Design of Mobile Emergency Telemedicine System", Proc. Computational Science and Its Applications, Springer, Berlin.

Yoon, H. (2006). "Test of Madwifi-ng WMM/WME in WLANs, NML-technical report-UM group.

Wireshark, (2009) http://www.wireshark.org/download.html.

2

Novel Wireless Communication Protocol for e-Health Applications

A. Zvikhachevskaya and L. Mihaylova
School of Computing and Communications, InfoLab21
Lancaster University
UK

1. Introduction

Evolution from wired to wireless communication systems has brought great advantages to healthcare services. Mobility support function for e-Health applications gives practitioners, medical centres, and hospitals new tools for managing patients' care, electronic records, and medical billing to ultimately enable patients to have a higher control of their own well being. E-Health and health care services are information based, hence better utilisation of information has the potential to make services more integrated, can enhance patient safety and accountability. These will have a positive impact and will increase patient's acceptance of the services. In order to make e-Health applications more integrated and acceptable for the users it is needed to improve their efficiency. All the above motivated us to research within area of wireless standards and their interconnectivity in order to provide efficient, reliable, and robust service and eliminate connectivity boundaries for e-Health applications.
In this chapter, focus is on the development and investigation of novel technologies which would allow efficient and reliable healthcare by utilising the latest wireless technologies. More specifically, research methodology and ideas, which consider the use of wireless broadband systems, commercial (such as WiFi, WiMAX) and military (such as HIDL, Link 11), in real-life healthcare scenarios are proposed and studied.

2. E-Health and Emergency Services applications interconnection

The healthcare industry includes many services, emergency services are among them. During emergency situations communication channels may suffer congestion, errors, call dropping and data loss. In contrary to commercial mobile networks the mobile network technologies for the emergency e-Health services have to be able to provide better connectivity due to sensitivity of the medical applications to data loss, corruption or delay and are expected to provide vital aid for patients.
The most common characteristic of emergency situation is mobility of involved elements (people, devices, etc) and requirements for real-time applications running over the e-Health network have to have stringent requirements in terms of delay, bandwidth, packet loss, jitter and other QoS parameters (Istepanian, et.al., 2009).
ESs must use the most reliable personal safety applications and communication channels. If military services are involved in the emergency case then they will use the military data-links

(www.synthesis.co.uk, 2006) (such as Link11, Link16 and HIDL). Link 11 (www.lm-isgs.co.uk, 2010) is a broadcast digital communications system that was designed for use over UHF or HF frequencies to exchange tactical information between units such as ships, helicopters and submarines. Link 16 (www.lm-isgs.co.uk, 2010) is a tactical data-link that provides a bigger data-rate capability than Link 11 and a more sophisticated network management system. It was designed to meet the different communications needs and a role of units within the emergency places e.g. aircraft, ships, control centres, command posts, and reconnaissance vehicles. While technically Link 16 is the messaging standard that flows over the network, for the purposes of this research it is referred to Link 16 as the data-link system as a whole (Tarter, et.al., 2008). HIDL (www.ultra-cis.com, 2010) is a command and control data-link designed for communicating with unmanned aerial vehicles and distributing situational awareness information to active and passive participants on the ground.
Interoperability between these forces is very difficult, resulting in less than optimal efficiency and effectiveness. As was shown in some well known cases (such as the 9/11 events), this lack of interoperability was the direct cause of significant loss of lives of first responders and of civilians on site.

3. System boundaries and equipment

As we are defining A New Protocol as being a method of transferring digital data from one network to another it is very hard to draw simple system boundaries. There are two main pieces: 'cross-over' nodes and terminal equipment.
The 'cross-over' nodes can be easily represented as 'black boxes' into which the terminal interfaces from multiple data-links are connected. They read the information coming out of one terminal and repackage it into a format that another terminal understands and passes it onto that other terminal. It is possible to think of this device as an operator who reads a message coming in on one radio and typing it into the terminal for transmission on another radio.
The terminal equipment can take many forms, but in essence this is the equipment that users/applications interact with that generate or receive Protocol traffic on. For units operating on a WiMAX network this will be a computer connected via an Ethernet cable to a WiMAX modem. For Link 16 it could take the format of a box/application placed between a computer and the Link 16 terminal that converts the user data generated into Link 16 compatible messages that are sent into the terminal.
Essentially they are theoretical 'bolt on' pieces of equipment that interface with the existing equipment and create this 'network-of-networks'. It should be noted that this research does not address how these 'black boxes' might be designed, manufactured or installed.

4. Data link introduction

4.1 Introduction and types of data

In order for information to be effectively communicated between two users, they must 'speak the same language'. In computing these formats are for the most part already pre-defined; video as MPEG-2/H.264/MPEG-4 (Marpe, et.al., 2006; Chiariglione, 2000), audio as MP3/WMV/AAC (Chandraiah&Domer, 2005; www.microsoft.com, 2010; www.arm.com, 2003), text as ASCII/RTF/WORD (www.asciitable.com, 2010; www.microsoft.com, 1999), etc. Computer networking has also defined protocols for transferring these formats, the ones typically used are the Internet Protocol suite e.g. Internet Protocol version 4 and 6 (IPv4, IPv6), TCP, UDP, RTP.

IPv4 is the most common network layer protocol and uses a 20 byte header for all its packets. While this works for networks such as Ethernet which can communicate packets up to 1500 bytes long, it will not work for networks such as Link 11 which is only capable of sending 6 byte packets. The computers/people generating the information do not know or think about the transmission method or protocol that is used to exchange the information only that they are able to reproduce the source data at the destination. There may be some requirements on the data such as priority, latency or data-rate, but as long as the communications medium is able to support this it does not matter how the information is transported. For the purposes of e-Health service all user data could be arranged into the three categories: Real time traffic, Priority and Best Effort.

While there may be more subcategories that these types of traffic can be divided into for the purposes of this research only these should be addressed. Real time traffic (such as audio or video) has low latency and minimum data rate requirements. If the latency increases or the data rate decreases too much then the information becomes unusable. Priority traffic (such as situational awareness updates) is typically of fixed size and has low latency, high guarantee requirements. Finally best effort traffic (such as email or file transfer) does not have any specific quality of service requirements. Therefore for each data link not only description of how to transfer digital user data is important but also how to try and provide quality of service requirements.

This subsection briefly outlines the characteristics of each data-link and its operation, including the message formats. In the next subsections an explanation is given on why and how to transport digital user data over the various data links. After explaining how each data link works and how to implement a network management system capable of supporting e-Health 'network-of-networks' the translation of information between each network will be provided and ensure compatibility on such matters as addressing and quality of service by creating an overarching network management system (NMS) separate from the individual NMSs on each network .

4.1.1 Internet protocol version 4

IPv4 is presented here before the data links as it is the worldwide standard for packetising digital user data and the message format for exchanging information not only on the Internet but also on WiFi, WiMAX, and HIDL. This means that it is the defacto message format that most PCs, routers and common terminal equipment, that will be connecting to 'network-of-networks', will be applied. Therefore this research is using it as the message format against which all of the others employ will have to be compatible with, i.e. a packet being generated in another network will have to be able to be readdressed as an IPv4 packet and vice-versa (Almguist, 1992).

IPv4 is a network layer protocol, which means it provides a mechanism for source to destination packet delivery. This includes addressing, routing, quality of service and error control. An IPv4 packet consists of a common 20 byte header and a data portion. The header includes information such as a source and destination address, a checksum and details of the underlying packet, packet length, if it has been fragmented, what type of traffic it is etc. IPv4 is being slowly phased out over the Internet in favour of IPv6. IPv6 amongst many other features has a larger address space, more features for prioritization and gives a simplified interface for processing by routers. These features are aimed primarily at large networks, which handle large amounts of traffic at high data rates, these difficulties will not be encountered in this research and thus only IPv4 will be used. This is deemed sufficient as it is possible to translate between IPv6 and IPv4 using well known techniques.

Note that an IP network does not guarantee that packets received at a destination will be received in the same sequence they were sent. It is the responsibility of the transport layer (for those transport layers that do guarantee data order such as TCP) or the application layer (if it is using a datagram protocol such as UDP) to handle mis-ordered packets.

Addressing

The pivotal role of IPv4 is that it provides a standard method of addressing which is used throughout the Internet. In fact, without it, the Internet would probably not exist as we know it today. IPv4 addressing is very similar to postal addressing; everyone has a house number, a street, a city and a country. The only difference in IP is that the information is ordered differently, an IPv4 address consists of 4 bytes which are typically written as AAA.BBB.CCC.DDD with the A's in essence denotes the country, B the city, C the street and D the house number. This subdivision of the address into 4 'octets' allows the Internet to be broken down into lots of networks of networks to facilitate with routing. Simplistically: two computers with the same A, B and C numbers will be on the same small local network, two computers with the same A and B but different C numbers will be in the same larger wide area network but different local networks, and finally two computers with just the same A numbers will probably be in the same country but on physically separated networks. Routers within this 'network-of-networks' can use subnet masks therefore to decide if they need to route a packet internal or external to the network. These subnet masks determine this via checking the source and destination addresses against the mask and if they are different then the packet is for a destination external to the network and if they are the same then it is for somewhere internal to the network. For example a typical IPv4 source address might be 192.168.20.5 and a destination address 192.15.34.140, if the router operates a subnet mask of 255.255.0.0 then the router will compare the first and second octets and if they are the same then route the packet within the network, but if they are different (as in this case) the packet is routed to the external gateway and to the correct network. The octets matching the subnet mask are referred to as the Network ID and the rest of the octets are the Host ID, in the example above the source address has a network ID of 192.168 and a host ID of 20.5. We will return to this notion of IP addresses and subnet masks later, as a mechanism for subdividing the 'network-of-networks' and thus addressing packets between different data link networks.

Header

The IPv4 header is outlined below in the table 4.1 below.

+	Bits 0–3	4–7	8–15	16–18	19–31
0	Version	Header length	Type of Service	Total Length	
32	Identification			Flags	Fragment Offset
64	Time to Live		Protocol	Header Checksum	
96	Source Address				
128	Destination Address				
160	Options				
160 or 192+	User Data				

Table 1. IPv4 Header

A quick explanation of each field is given below:
Version: This is a fixed value denoting IPv4;
Header Length: This will always be 20 for headers with no optional additions;
Type of Service: This is used to denote any quality of service requirements;
Total Length: This gives the total length of the packet - header + user data;
Identification: This gives a unique identification field and is used in fragmentation;
Flags: These denote settings for fragmentation;
Fragment Offset: Used to reconstruct a fragmented packet;
Time to Live: Gives the number of hops the packet can take from source to destination before it is dropped by the network;
Protocol: Tells the receiver the format of the user data portion is e.g. TCP/UDP/SCTP/OSPF;
Header Checksum: A checksum making sure the header is correct - note it does not protect the user data portion in any way;
Source Address: The IPv4 address of the sending computer;
Destination Address: The IPv4 address of the destination computer;
Options: This field is very rarely used, but some protocols use it to provide more information.

If a piece of information regarding the packet can be inferred without the need of the header then that information is redundant. Thus as we will see later, if we make some assumptions regarding the traffic going over the network then we limit the amount of header information we need to translate between networks.

4.1.2 Description of the military data-links

High Integrity Data Link (HIDL) Description

In Figure 1 the typical topology of the HIDL Supported Network is presented, which includes two HIDL Communities. Each of them has a timing master, Unmanned Aerial Vehicle (UAV) and a Relay terminal. Overview of the HIDL standard and characteristics of the named objects is given below in subsections below.

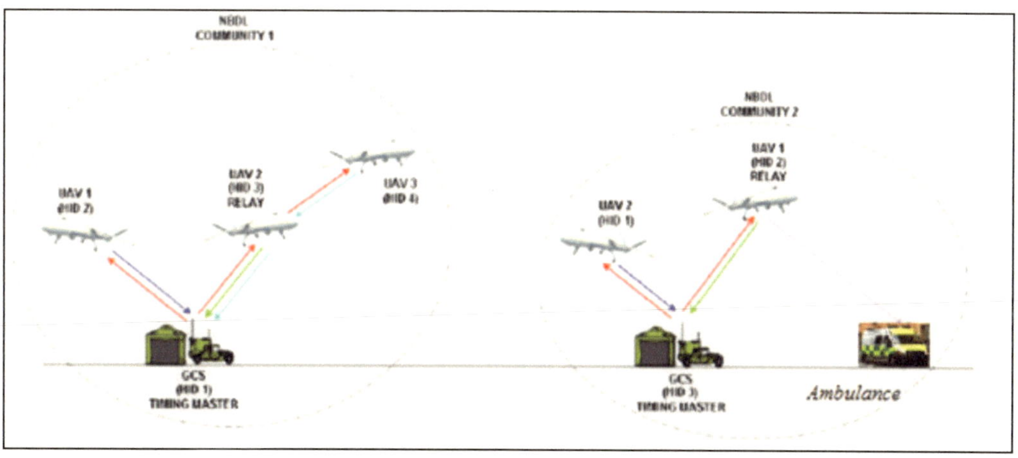

Fig. 1. Architecture of the HILD Supported Network (Tarter, et.al., 2008)

HIDL Overview

HIDL was designed to provide a near real time, high integrity data communications link between multiple nodes within an Unmanned Aerial Vehicle community. It sends command and control information from a ground station to multiple UAVs in the air. It also allows the UAVs to send information from the air to other UAVs or ground receivers.

This network can have a maximum of 5 active transmitters in the network at any one time. This effectively means 1 timing master (base station) and 4 network entrants (client units). However as explained later there can be multiple receive only passive terminals that are capable of one way communication.

Time Architecture

HIDL uses a time division mechanism to packetize the data to be transmitted, i.e. a packet of information is transmitted at a known rate (the period of the time division). The HIDL time structure divides the time domain into contiguous periods of 10ms - termed Timeslots. A group of 100 contiguous timeslots is termed an *epoch,* which is equivalent to a period of one second. These *epochs* are repeated every second, and therefore the timeslot allocation is repeated every second. It is essentially a broadcast architecture and therefore each receiver is capable of receiving every packet transmitted in an epoch as long as it is in range, and therefore while there is only ever one transmitter per timeslot there maybe multiple receivers.

As a result of this scheme multiple QoS schemes cannot be assigned to a timeslot as there is no data packet processing performed within the system, instead only bandwidth (timeslot allocation) is the only variable. Therefore voice, text and video packets are treated identically within the HIDL network; it is up to the operator to provide the required levels of network resources to meet the demands of the application. This is in contrast to Link 16 which can provide contention access as well as the dedicated access scheme which is used in HIDL. Ultimately this will mean that while real-time, priority and best effort traffic will be transported with the same level of QoS the anticipated amount of each type of traffic will be used to calculate the timeslot allocation.

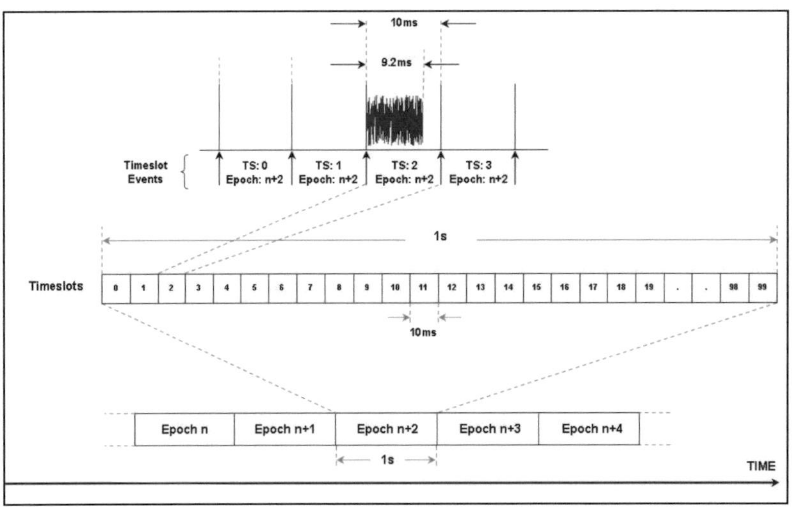

Fig. 2. The HIDL Time Architecture (Tarter, et.al., 2008)

Each timeslot in a HIDL network is assigned a 'circuit'. HIDL supports up to 15 of these 'circuits'. A 'circuit' describes the source terminal, the destination terminal(s), whether the message is to be relayed, and what the destination multicast address of the data packet in the circuit should be. As this is a broadcast radio system the list of destination terminals is really only used to filter the results (if a node is not listed as a receiver then it will not try to capture the transmission) there is no reason why they all couldn't receive the broadcast, however each circuit then need to be defined as broadcast and leave the filtering of the received packet to a higher level protocol outside of the terminal.

There are five timeslots per epoch in which no User data is allowed to be transmitted, leaving 95 timeslots per second for user data. These five timeslots are used by the control station for network management. In each user timeslot a maximum of 422 bytes of user data is allowed to be transmitted, which when Ethernet, IPv4 and UDP headers are added any Ethernet packet of up to 468 bytes can be transmitted. Of course any sized packet below this size maybe transmitted in a time slot, but only at a rate of one packet per timeslot. This gives a theoretical throughput of 355.7Kbps.

To communicate or receive data, each node must synchronise itself in time with a timing master (typically the ground station). This enables each transmitting node to operate within a synchronised global time structure and thus allow each receiving node within range to receive each packet transmitted collision free from the next packet.

Packet Format

Every packet must conform to UDP-IPv4 over Ethernet and be less than 468 bytes in total. HIDL is a very simple radio network that operates by distributing UDP/IP packets over the air. Each packet being sent must conform to UDP-IPv4 over Ethernet and be less than 468 bytes in total (the maximum transmission unit of the radio). If the packet to be transmitted is in a different format or too large (e.g. a TCP packet of 1000 bytes), then it must be fragmented and wrapped in a UDP frame and unwrapped and recreated at the other end.

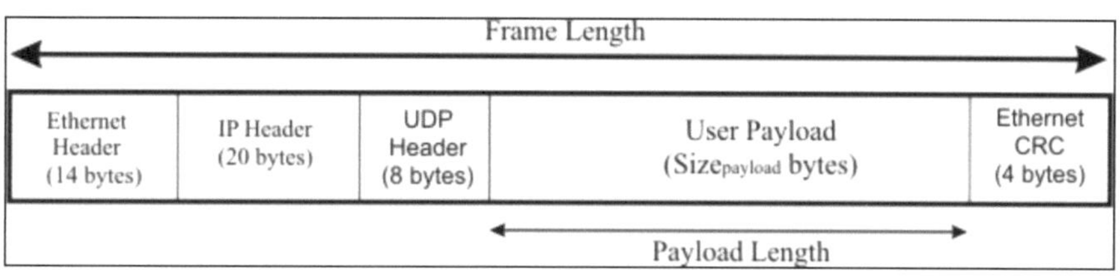

Fig. 3. The HIDL Packet Format

A HIDL terminal accepts user data packets over its Ethernet interface. The terminal recognises the associated circuit for the data via the destination IP address and puts it in the correct buffer. When a timeslot comes around that is allocated to that circuit the user data packet is read from the buffer and sent over the air. The receivers capture the packet and each one outputs it over its Ethernet interface. All circuits use multicast IP addresses for their destination address, this is to overcome the limitation that the transmitter does not know the MAC address of the receiver(s) and to reduce the overhead from the network headers, maximising user data throughput As a result any packet destined for a unicast address must be wrapped in a HIDL UDP/IP multicast packet for transmission over the HIDL network. In order to send packets to different addresses the user could send the correct packet wrapped in a multicast frame and have a receiving unit do the packet decomposition. Otherwise it could use a Network Address Translation (NAT) router that will convert the traffic to a unicast address via a Port number. While performing NAT over HIDL and 'network-of-networks' is possible, explanation of its functionality is outside the scope of this research.

Relay

HIDL provides the ability for one terminal within the network to act as a relay for other terminals too far away from the source terminal to hear its communication. As all terminals are part of the same network it is up to the network manager to ensure that there are sufficient resources (timeslots) for the relay terminal to pass on any messages destined for terminals out of range of the transmitter. However if there are not enough timeslots available to the relay to pass on the packets within an epoch some packets will get dropped. The relay unit also provides time synchronization for the nodes out of range of the ground control station, thereby ensuring that all nodes throughout the extended network are operating on the same global time structure.

Receive only units

HIDL allows for portable units to be used in receive only mode, which means that they are capable of receiving all of the messages communicated throughout the network but unable to respond. In an operational environment it is envisaged that there will be multiple ground units with these receive only terminals. This therefore means that when these ground terminals are networked to other networks as part of a larger system there will be more ways of communicating in one direction than the other.

HIDL Network Management System

Each network entrant must first communicate with the timing master in order to fully synchronise itself prior to any node-to-node communication. This process provides a registration mechanism that the network manager can use to ascertain which terminals are actively participating. The five network management timeslots already provide each client with a list of those active client nodes within the network and what their addresses are. This enables all active and passive nodes in the network to continuously have an up to date list of all active participants in the network (obviously the passive nodes are not able to declare their existence).

Resource allocation (time slots) are managed and allocated by the timing master (control station) and are fixed for the duration, unless the timing master issues a new timeslot assignment. This means that any node requiring more bandwidth will have to send a request to the network manager at the base station who will modify the timeslot allocation scheme and issue a new one.

There is no defined protocol inherent within HIDL to accomplish a change in timeslot structure, this must be done by sending over the air data messages to the controlling computer at the timing master who will then provide the timing master HIDL unit with a new timeslot allocation and instruct it to distribute it to all the nodes who will then adopt it. As these messages go over the data interface they must be compatible with the formats of messages being used for 'network-of-networks' traffic over HIDL and be identifiable to the timing master control computer that it is a resource request message. It is the recommendation of this research project to not use a separate or unique message structure for identifying these packets, but instead use a pre-existing mechanism such as UDP port numbers for identification. As long as the length of the packet is less than the maximum value that can be transmitted in one timeslot it does not matter how big the packet is, as only one packet can be transmitted in any one timeslot regardless of size.

It is also proposed that all circuits denoted for use by 'network-of-networks' compatible terminals be set to the broadcast mode, meaning that all packets transmitted by a 'network-of-networks' HIDL terminal will be received by all of the other 'network-of-networks' HIDL terminals, it will be up to each destination computer/router to decide whether or not to forward or drop the packet. There are two possible methods of implementing 'network-of-networks' over HIDL with regards to resource allocation. The first involves allocating only one circuit to each HIDL terminal for 'network-of-networks' traffic. The second involves allocating 'cross-over' nodes two circuits; the first is used to carry traffic internal to the network and the second for traffic destined for outside the network (effectively 'cross-over' to 'cross-over' communication). The second method will provide the network manager computer with more information that it can use to allocate the timeslots and balance the amount of network-to-network traffic against internal traffic. Discovery of the most effective method and resource allocation algorithm will be investigated in simulation.

HIDL Node Attrition Strategy

The HIDL network is very similar in format to a WiFi network: it requires a central base station to provide timing and network management but individual client units can talk to each other. All HIDL radio equipment is identical whether the node is to be a timing master, an active node, a relay or a passive node; therefore any node can be chosen to perform the timing master's role. It is advisable to choose a node within range of all other terminals, so as to allow synchronisation. If a node is too far away but covered by a relay node then the relay node must be in the range of the timing master. As any node can take on this role of timing master it is proposed to use the same recovery process as was outlined above in this section. Although the given scheme, will provide the ability for timing master to take over it should be noted that HIDL was designed to be a UAV Command and Control data link. As such nodes could lose contact with the timing master as a result of their location rather than the loss of the timing master. If a node falls out of link there are mechanisms such as a 're-acquisition strategy' that are performed to account for this.

Therefore it is not advised that another UAV automatically assume that the timing master has been lost and adopt its functionality, instead like WiMAX (where the role of the base station is restricted to a few units) the adoption of the timing master role should only be performed by a ground unit who should be more capable of making this assessment.

Link 16 Description

Link 16 Overview

Link 16 is one of the military's Tactical Data Links, which is to say it is primarily used to communicate tactical information between units or platforms in the battle space. This research is not aiming to investigate the benefits to be obtained from changing the equipment, but rather the benefits that could be obtained by modifying the operational use of the Link 16 standard.

Packet Format

Link 16 messages can be transmitted using either Double Pulse (DP) or Single Pulse (SP) encoding. Double pulse operation sends the same symbol packet using two pulses rather than the one used for single pulse operation. This means single pulse packets can send more data per timeslot than double pulse packets but the probability of reception is reduced. There are 4 different formats a Link 16 message can take Standard, Packed-2 SP, Packed-2 DP and Packed- 4 SP. A standard message can send 225bits/timeslot, both Packed-2 formats can send 450bits/timeslot and the Packed-4 can send 900 bits/timeslot. As there are 128 timeslots per second this gives us a data rate of 28.8, 57.6 and 115.2Kbps respectively. These numbers also depend on whether or not Error Detection Coding (EDC) is used, however this research will not be investigating their use, instead we will only use formats that do use EDC.

Each transmission in a timeslot is preceded by a Link 16 header which tells the receiver how to decode the data portion by identifying the packet format (Packed-2, Packed-4 etc), the message format (free text or fixed format), encoding (i.e. Reed Solomon) the transmitting terminal and if the message has been relayed.

There are two message formats used in Link 16: Free Text and Fixed Format. Free text messages within Link 16 do not need to follow any defined message structure; this is how voice, ASCII text and video are passed over JTIDS. Fixed format messages though need to follow the Link 16 message structure (J-Series Messages).

Access Methodologies

Link 16 operates a Time Division Multiple Access scheme (TDMA), which means that all units operating within a Link 16 network are synchronised in time and transmit and receive at predefined times.

It uses 12.8 minute epoch which is divided into 98,304 timeslots. However, this is a little unwieldy so it is broken down into 64 frames, each 12 seconds long. Each frame contains 1536 timeslots and these are used when allocating timeslots to terminals. All the timeslots in the scheme are allocated by the network manager to individual units for transmission. As all nodes know the timeslot allocation the receivers know when they should listen to receive data from any given transmitter. By increasing or decreasing a unit's timeslot allocation you are effectively changing the maximum transmission bandwidth/data-rate of the unit. Currently timeslots are first labelled according to their Network Participation Group (a mechanism for receivers to use to determine in which timeslots they need to listen) then allocated to units. This mechanism allows us to easily define a new Network Participation Group (NPG) for 'network-of-networks' network data, which will allow 'network-of-networks' to use existing hardware and maintain operational compatibility with existing systems. Those terminals not equipped to take part in the data network will not listen and will not take part in the networked data NPG and therefore will not receive any 'network-of-networks' packets and be unable to decode them. Again at the receiver, messages are output with a header defining in which NPG the packet was received in thereby allowing terminals to clearly identify 'network-of-networks' traffic from other traffic being received from the network. Users interact with Link 16 terminals by sending messages to the terminal with a header defining in which NPG the message is to be transmitted. The terminal is then left to broadcast the message in the appropriate timeslot. An interesting result of using NPGs is that the sender does not necessarily have to know who the receivers are or the route to the destination, and as it is a broadcast system, the sender can take for granted that the same timeslot allocation table has been distributed and therefore that all receivers it wants to talk to are listening in for its transmissions.

Currently Link 16 systems distribute Precise Participant Location and Identification (PPLI) messages to organise sender, receiver and route information (at least once every 12 seconds).

For data networking this concept should be utilized, although the Route Indicator Parameters do not provide enough information for this exact implementation mechanism to be used solely for 'network-of-networks' route planning. Timeslot allocation is performed via the J0.3 and J0.4 messages (TS Assignment and Radio Relay Control), these messages are used to delete assignments, add specific time slot allocations, change a terminal's operation as a relay, add or remove relay time slot allocations. When terminals receive these messages they check if the required change is valid and if so automatically inform the Network Manager that the action has been accepted, thus providing verification. Timeslots are allocated in blocks rather than as individual timeslots and a single terminal can handle up to 64 time slot blocks. These blocks define when a terminal should transmit, receive or relay some data. This places a complexity limitation on the Network Manager who must ensure that in calculating the timeslot allocation there are no more than 64 distinct blocks of timeslots (a block is a collection of timeslots that have the same parameters - e.g. type, NPG, access mode, Tx/Rx). The network manager has some flexibility over this limitation as it can describe a block's access mode as being either dedicated, contention or timeslot reallocation.
In dedicated access a timeslot is given to a single unit for transmission, this is fine when the unit always has data to send but if not then nothing is transmitted and the resource is wasted.
In contention access a block of timeslots are allocated to a number of terminals, these terminals are each given a transmission rate (a given fraction of the total number of timeslots).
The terminals are not required to transmit at this rate, but could do so if required. The terminals then use a pseudo-random function to choose the timeslots in the block that they will transmit in (up to the maximum rate granted to them). This mechanism does not guarantee the sole use of a timeslot and the likelihood of a transmission collision is a factor of the block size, number of terminals and transmission rates. Hopefully the network planning process will have reduced this probability to an acceptable maximum level.
Finally under time slot reallocation the timeslots are put together in a common pool and allocated on expected demand. At the beginning of each period terminals announce their demand using J0.7 Time Slot Reallocation messages. All other units hear these announcements and using a common algorithm in each terminal create the timeslot allocation table for the rest of the period. This allocation will not be exactly replicated across all terminals as some terminals may not have heard all of the demand announcements, even so this could still be acceptable.

Link 16 Network Management System

'Network-of-networks' proposes to use a centralised network management system for control of timeslot allocation within the network, but use a distributed scheme for allocation between 'cross-over' nodes. This means that a centralised network management system will allocate timeslots (either all of them if the system is fully automated, or the 'network-of-networks' subset if the initial allocation is done by an outside source e.g. the data links planning office) using the dedicated and contention access schemes to terminals within the network, thereby allowing current operations to continue with the minimum of impact. 'Cross-over' nodes will share a pool of timeslots which they will distribute according to the timeslot reallocation scheme. If the 'cross-over' nodes require more bandwidth than the pool is capable of supplying then they will have to negotiate with the network management system for dedicated allocation from the rest of the pool. This division of management functions means that the local network management system has ultimate control over the balance of data over its network but leaves the routing aspects between networks up to the 'cross-over' nodes. The local network management system can increase or decrease the size of the time slot reallocation pool and therefore increase or decrease the amount of utilisation of the network for 'network to network' communications.

A network is formed initially by a terminal acting as a Network Timing Reference and broadcasting a J0.0 'Initial Entry Message', network entrants then uses these J0.0 messages to synchronise in time (typically responding with a PPLI message). Other terminals can use any other active terminal to synchronise with and thus gain access to the network. There is no requirement for registering with a network manager first. This means that an up to date list of network participants is not available intrinsically from the terminals. Instead the network manager is going to have to perform this task by requiring all 'network-of-networks' Link 16 terminals to periodically inform it of their existence. Then, the network manager will then distribute this list of the participants. In order to accommodate new terminals who have yet to be granted dedicated or reallocated slots, it is recommended that the network manager always leave some timeslots in contention mode (allocated to all terminals) for network management functionality such as registration.

For standard IP traffic within the network this project would recommend using a contention access scheme. This is because IP traffic is typically bursts and a dedicated access scheme will end up with an underutilised network. Dedicated access can be used to ensure applications such as video or audio have the required bandwidth to support their use, and should only be granted on demand.

Initially the network management system will grant: a portion of its timeslots to the 'cross-over' nodes for them to use (under the time-slot reallocation scheme), a portion of its timeslots to all of the terminals within the local network under a contention access scheme, and possibly keep a portion of timeslots in reserve for requests for dedicated access. The size of these portions and the amount of timeslots held in reserve will have to be investigated and modelled using a software simulation later in this project. Obviously as the network continues to operate, terminals will request greater contention access rates, dedicated allocations and an increased pool for network-to-network communications. The network manager will have to balance the demands for resources against the utilisation of the network, the priorities of the demands and the types of traffic being sent. The network manager will allocate the timeslots and distribute that information via the current Link 16 method of using J-series messages. This will allow compatibility with non-'network-of-networks' terminals and limit the impact on continued operations.

Finally the reason for using a centralised network manager as opposed to an entirely distributed timeslot reallocation scheme is one of security and robustness. While any terminal can become the network manager and can perform its duties, completely distributing the functionality increases the risk that a mis-used terminal or spoof messaging can disrupt the consistent timeslot allocation table algorithm and thus can heavily impact the network operations

Link 16 Node Attrition Strategy

As in WiFi and HIDL any terminal can act as the Network Timing Reference (NTR) and thus take on the role of the network manager. Therefore a scheme of recovery due to node attrition similar to that outlined in 3.4 for WiFi could be utilised if another scheme has not already been outlined. Such a scheme with attrition nodes has been successfully deployed for military purposes, including a backup strategy in place that is initiated in the case of loss of a node (especially the NTR). This involves choosing the node with the closest time synchronisation to the original timing master. This thesis proposes a strategy that requires compatibility with any node that could possibly perform as the NTR be 'network-of-networks' compatible. If such an operational strategy is not required or an automatic one is required instead then as each terminal should send a PPLI message at least once every 12 seconds (frequency depends on timeslot allocation) we could use the 12 seconds frequency as a reference value. If the network manager/network timing reference does not transmit a PPLI or Initial Entry message after 48 seconds then it will be deemed to have been lost. The next terminal in the sequence should then take over. In doing so the epoch will have to begin again and units will have to renegotiate with the network manager for timeslot allocations. The reason for the renegotiation is that each node will not have the complete list of timeslot allocations, instead as explained above each node is only notified of its assignment in up to 64 blocks.

Link-11 Description

Link-11 Overview

Link 11 was the precursor to Link 16, and while its operational use is similar to that of Link 16 its technical characteristics and network operation are very different. In essence it operates very similarly to a token ring network. Nodes within the network wait until they are called upon by the Network Control Station to broadcast at which point they begin broadcasting until they have finished, at which point the Network Control Station then calls upon another node. This Roll Call mechanism is controlled by the Network Control Station and it is this NCS that controls the sequence of node transmissions. There are three methods of controlling the roll call:

- Full Roll Call - all nodes are active and are called on one by one;
- Partial Roll Call - some nodes are in Radio Silence and thus do not respond to the NCS;
- Roll Call Broadcast - the NCS broadcasts all data, and any node with new information informs the NCS of this, which the NCS then broadcasts to the rest of the network.

As we will be passing network data rather than tactical information, such as enemy/friendly positions this research does not recommend Roll Call Broadcast, instead it is proposed to use the Full Roll Call method.

This method, however, is not conducive to real-time traffic as there is no way to determine exactly when is the next time a node may be allowed to transmit (even if there is a maximum transmit window). As the information passed via Link 11 has traditionally been of use to everybody (battlefield situational awareness information) having each node transmit all of its information before releasing transmit token was acceptable. However, as we are transmitting information that might not be of use to everyone within the network this method does not seem prudent. Especially as one node that transmits a lot of data will end up monopolising the network resource. Instead one proposed method is for all 'network-of-networks' terminals within the Link 11 network to operate on a two cycle roll call. During the first roll call each terminal transmits its requirements (amount and type of data) and the network manager coordinates this information and at the end of the 1st cycle broadcasts the amount of data each terminal is allowed to transmit, each terminal then when called upon, during the second cycle, only transmits the amount of data that the network manager has decided upon.

This mechanism relies of all 'network-of-networks' terminals abiding by the allocation granted it by the network manager.

Another method may be to fix the number of Link 11 packets that each 'network-of-networks' terminal is allowed to transmit at once. This means that if a message is longer than the number of Link 11 packets a terminal can transmit at once, then it will have to wait until its turn comes round again before it may continue. In order for this method to work then each receiving terminal will have to know who has transmitted each terminal.

Link 11 Packet Format

Link 11 messages conform to the M-series messages, there is no mechanism for free text as there is with Link 16 and as such 'network-of-networks' terminals will have to conform to the M-series format in order to maintain compatibility with ongoing operations.

M-series packets are divided into two 30-bit messages, with 6 bits each used for error correction, thereby leaving 48 bits in total for the information portion. All M-series messages use the first 4 bits of the first message to denote which message type is being sent. These 4 bits are called the message number and provide for 16 different types of message. Message type 12 can be used by nations for individual systems such as 'network-of-networks'. Messages are subdivided again using a label suffix, which again is 4 bits long; in this case we propose to use M12.14.

Once the message designation has been given the rest of the 40 bits can be used for the actual information. The original use of the data-link is to pass information of use to everyone and as such there is no header field for destination - all transmissions are broadcast in essence. As can be inferred the size and nature of this data-link are orders of magnitude different to WiMAX, and thus careful consideration will have to be made in how to pass information over Link 16 networks.

Link 11 Network Management Strategy

It is proposed to use the link's Network Control Station (NCS) as the Network Manager, the NCS will either determine the maximum number of packets the terminals can send at once or collect in all of the transmission requests from each 'network-of-networks' compatible Link 11 terminal and decide on the maximum number for each terminal in the next cycle.

The NCS can operate either in Net Synchronisation or Roll Call mode. In Net Sync mode the NCS calls upon each terminal in turn to transmit and receive and thus achieve synchronisation in time with it. After network sync has been achieved the NCS moves into the normal Roll Call mode. In this mode, when the NCS polls a 'network-of-networks' terminal, which has nothing to transmit, it should answer with a zero requirement response; this will allow the NCS to determine if the node is still active and allow the NCS to skip it in the 2nd cycle. The NCS should only have to perform Net Sync at network initialisation or on command from a user; there is no automatic mechanism for a new node to register with the terminal without a user first informing the NCS that such a terminal exists and to include it in the polling loop. It is not proposed to circumvent this operation but instead to utilise it, therefore within 'network-of-networks' if a terminal wishes to join the network it must first be added manually at the NCS by an operator.

Link 11 Node Attrition Strategy

As with Link 16 a current operational Link 11 network will have a backup strategy in place that will be used in the event of the loss of a node (especially the NCS). Again it is proposed not to usurp such a strategy if one is in place. However, if an automatic solution is required the following mechanism could be used.

As this is a roll call network, where each terminal may transmit until it is finished there is not a deterministic frequency to the NCS's transmissions and thus any fixed time between control station transmissions.

5. Architecture and communication protocol of the 'Network-of-Networks'

The 'network-of-networks' is a utility that allows users of any data link network to communicate with users of any other data link network that is within the 'network-of-networks' umbrella. The information generated in one network is able to traverse the inter-networks and be consumed at any destination. This can be especially problematic if two data-link networks are fundamentally different such as HIDL and WiMAX. Each network has a different maximum packet size, data rate and network management scheme.

For instance how will Link 11 address and transport IPv4 traffic, generated in a WiMAX network or HIDL provide the QoS required for an audio stream originating in a Link 16 network? As explained in the introduction, one problem is how to label the packets so that the information is correctly routed to the destination wherever it might be, and in such a way as to enable the recipient computer to accurately reconstruct the data and communicate back in reply. To resolve this problem we propose to create a header for each data-link network so that a packet can be translated into a format compatible with any other data-link network. The conventional method is based on creating a single 'network-of-networks' header that would first wrap any packet before the data-link header (allowing compatibility with the data-link). However, as a result some information (such as a destination address) would ultimately appear twice, which for a data link (e.g. with short packages, like Link 11) might be an unreasonable amount of overhead. A new method is proposed in this dissertation which provides a translation service such that the information in a header for one network could be used to create the header for the other network. This approach would minimise the amount of duplicated network overhead information within each packet and allow packets to be re-formatted into something appropriate for that given data-link. For instance fragment a packet into smaller sizes for transmission over Link 11, but combined into a larger single packet for transmission over WiMAX.

While the header information will be useful to the 'cross-over' nodes (who will be performing the translation service) it is also required to send packetised digital data between two nodes of the same network.

Addressing

One of the main issues within 'network-of-networks' is how to address a packet of information such that it will identify a destination that may be on a different network entirely. On traditional computer networks this is done by an IP address and explained in the section 4.1.1.

It is proposed to utilise the same first two octets for each computer within the 'network-of-networks' thereby reducing the number of bits required to identify a single destination. This means that the address of each computer will only differ in the last two octets of an IPv4 address. We will use the first of these octets to identify the implementation of the data-link network that the computer resides on and the last octet to identify the computer. This ultimately means that by using this mechanism we are limited to 256 networks and 256 computers within each network or 65,536 computers in total. Of course Network Address Translation mechanisms can be employed to increase these numbers but such a technique is outside the scope of this investigation.

Figure 4 presents an example of the 'network-of-networks' where four individual data-link networks are joined together using five 'cross-over' nodes. In order to guarantee efficient communication between the users we apply the proposed translation algorithm, which is demonstrated by the following example. An Example: each computer can be addressed by the addition of two numbers, the data-link address (number in red) with the node address (number in black). Note that a 'cross-over' node has at least two addresses - one for each data link network (in this example each 'cross-over' node has the same lower octet address, though this needs not be the case. In this example if "4.3" wants to talk to "2.2" then it might send the message via "4.2" - "3.6" - "2.2". Note also that where there are two 'cross-over' nodes sharing the same data links there are two ways of communicating, one via each data link.

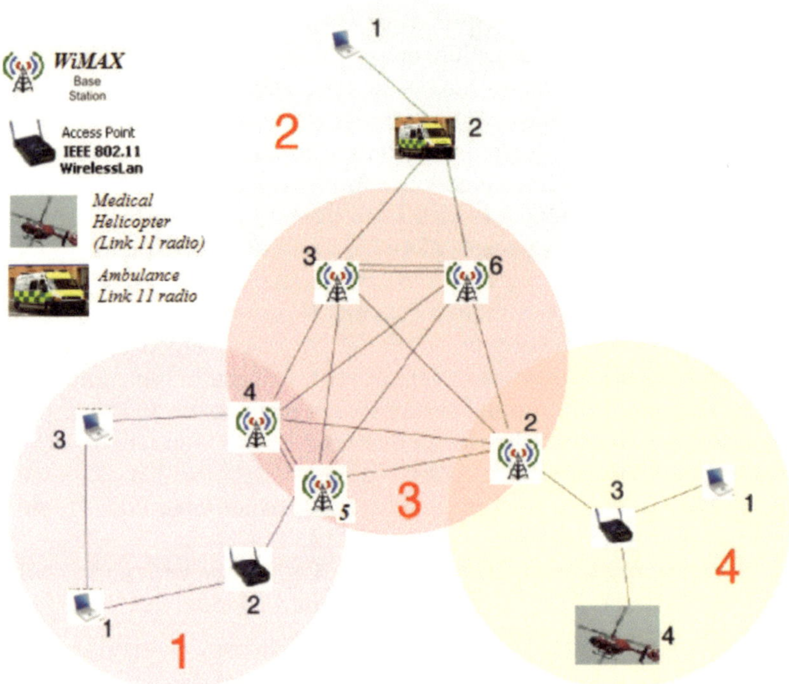

Fig. 4. Four Individual Networks Joined Together into the 'Network-of-Networks'

One of the most useful features of the IP protocol suite is the use of 'multicasting' and 'broadcasting' addressing. Using these techniques a transmitter can send a single packet that will reach multiple destinations thereby reducing the total number of packets sent.

The diversity of the developed algorithm can be another example. 'Broadcast' packets are those addresses using the '255' (or all 1's in binary) as the destination address, e.g. 172.20.255.255. With this designation any node with the same prefix before the 255s will receive the packet (e.g. all nodes with 172.20 as the leading octets of its IP address will receive a packet addressed to 172.20.255.255). A packet sent to 255.255.255.255 is a special case destined only for the local subnet (termed a limited broadcast) and will not be forwarded. This

forwarding of broadcast addresses conforms to that in outlined (Baker, 1995) and an option to prevent broadcast forwarding would be available in 'cross-over' nodes.
Multicast packets are similar to broadcast packets although they use a destination address with the first octet in the range 224 to 239. Nodes wishing to receive these packets send out requests to their routers to forward those packets onto them, who in turn pass the requests back to the sender's router, a router will then only pass on one packet for every common path to the destinations. For instance using the network above if node 1.1 is producing a multicast stream that 2.2, 4.1 and 4.4 want to receive then the following packet streams might be produced:

- 1.1 -> 1.2 -> 1.5
- Two packets are produced: 1.5 -> 3.6, 1.5 -> 3.2
- 3.6 -> 2.2
- 3.2 -> to 4.3
- Two packets are produced: 4.3 -> 4.1, 4.3 -> 4.4

The following conventions are proposed to be followed in the simulation. Firstly broadcast packets will be routed as normal using a node address of 255 to denote a broadcast packet for a given data-link network, and a data-link address of 255 with node address 255 to denote a broadcast packet to all nodes within the 'network-of-networks'. Secondly multicast routing will be done using a data-link address of 224 to 239. Due to 'network-of-networks' header compression constraints (only two byte of IP address supported), the first two bytes of a multi cast address will be repeated in the second two bytes in a 'network-of-networks' (e.g. 224.12.224.12), ensuring the address propagation across the network. The use of reserved subnets apart from theses (e.g. private, APIPA) is not recommended but it is allowed.
This will mean that the total number of data-link networks in the 'network-of-networks' at any one time will be 256 - 15 (number of multicast addresses) - 2 (0 and 255 reserved) = 239.
In order to receive the multicast packet a node will have to register its request with a 'cross-over' node.

Header Design for the 'Network-of-Networks'

In section 4.1.1 the IPv4 header is introduced, which is the predominate way of addressing packetised digital data within a computer network, and as such we need to ensure that any header that we create is cross compatible with it and that we are always able to regenerate such a header.
If we take as an assumption that we are only ever going to transport IPv4 and not IPv6 traffic then most of the IPv4 header becomes redundant. A further reduction can be made if we assume that only a few types of protocols will be transported over 'network-of-networks' e.g. TCP, UDP and routing. This means that we can use a reduced protocol field and save space. Below is the list of IPv4 header fields and a description regarding their applicability to 'network-of-networks':

- **Version:** This is a fixed value for IPv4 and therefore can be inferred;
- **Header Length:** This will always be 20 (assuming the use of no protocols with optional headers) and therefore can be inferred;
- **Type of Service**: This gives QoS requirements which will be required;
- **Total Length:** This is the total length of the datagram and can be calculated;
- **Identification**: This provides a unique ID for fragmented datagrams and will be required for IP fragments;

- **Flags:** These are used for fragmentation and in some instances can be inferred;
- **Fragment Offset**: Used to reconstruct a fragmented packet and will be required;
- **Time to Live**: Gives the number of hops the packet can take from source to destination before it is dropped by the network this can be determined by the 'cross-over' nodes;
- **Protocol**: Tells the receiver the underlying protocol which will be required;
- **Header Checksum:** A checksum for the header which can be calculated. Any transmission errors will be detected by the link layer checksum;
- **Source Address**: The IPv4 address of the sending computer which will be required;
- **Destination Address**: The IPv4 address of the destination computer which will be required;
- **Options:** This field is very rarely used and it is assumed that it is not required.

The bold fields are either required in some way or cannot be inferred about the packet, therefore any 'network-of-networks' header for any data-link must include these fields in some way to allow the (re)construction of an IPv4 header for the packet.

Quality of Service

All traffic is divided within the 'network-of-networks' network into three types:

- Real Time,
- Priority,
- Best Effort.

The Type of Service (ToS) field within IPv4 is divided into two sections: the precedence (priority) and the service type. The first three bits denote the importance of the packet and the last three bits denote low delay, high throughput and high reliability respectively. As many of the data-links provide no mechanism to affect the reliability of a packet's transmission, low delay is implicit for real time traffic and the level of throughput will be dictated by the network managers it is proposed to use 3 bits to denote QoS.

Bit 0 and 1: Denote the priority of the packet: 0 being lowest priority, 3 highest (which map to bits 1 and 2 of the ToS field)

Bit 2: 0 Indicates best effort traffic, 1 indicates real-time traffic (which maps to bit 3 of the ToS field).

Identification

Providing a unique identification number for each IP datagram will allow IP fragments to be re-assembled (as it provides a common label for all fragments). When forwarding fragmented IP packets, this *identification* field will need to be included in the compressed IP header.

Fragmentation

IPv4 datagrams are allowed to be up to 65,535 bytes long according to the standard. This is a theoretical limit; however, in the case of many computer networks as the Ethernet, WiFi and WiMAX limits are around 1500 bytes (including Ethernet headers etc). Therefore it is assumed for this simulation that there won't be any single IPv4 packets larger than 1500 bytes to begin with.

'Cross-over' nodes act like IP routers and hence would normally be required to fragment incoming IP datagrams if their length exceeds that of the network they about to traverse (Baker, 1995). However the minimum recommended MTU for IPv4 is set at 68 bytes (www.ietf.org, 1981).

Both Link 11 and Link 16 use much smaller packet sizes that this, so it is intended to fragment and re-assemble IP packets traversing these networks at the data link layer (layer 2) rather than using layer 3 (IP) fragmentation, which relies on the IP destination host to reassemble the IP fragments. A separate layer 2 fragmentation header will be defined where required for each of these 'network-of-networks' data link types. Both Link 11 and Link 16 will maintain packet order, so layer 2 fragment numbering will not be required. Fragmenting packets at layer 2 means that only the 'cross-over' nodes directly connected by the data link are involved in the fragmentation and re-assembly; the transmitting node fragments the IP packet and the receiving node re-assembles the IP packet back to the original packet received by the original node.

Packets fragmented using IP fragmentation (e.g., by an IP router) remain fragmented whilst routed across the IP network until they reach their eventual destination (e.g., an IP host computer) where the fragments will be re-assembled by the IP stack to generate the original IP datagram.

All the 'network-of-networks' must still be able to forward fragmented IP packets across their networks, so if an IP fragment is received on a 'cross-over' node, all the IP fragmentation fields must be included in the 'network-of-networks' compressed IP header. However, if the IP packet is not fragmented, no IP fragmentation information need be sent. For Link 11 and Link 16 'cross-over' nodes a 'network-of-networks' flag bit will be used to indicate if the IP packet is fragmented and the IP fragmentation data included at the end of the 'network-of-networks' IP header if so (giving a variable length header). Note that this is independent of the layer 2 fragmentation described for Link11 and Link 16.

HIDL networks have a much larger MTU (422 bytes), so IP packets over this size will use IP fragmentation before being forwarded across the HIDL network.

Time to Live

This field is used to ensure that a packet does not indefinitely flow around the network never reaching its destination. With every hop, the count is decremented by 1 and when the count reaches 0 the packet is removed. Within IPv4 8 bits are used, allowing a packet to traverse 256 networks before being dropped. It is not anticipated that the 'network-of-networks' will ever be that large, therefore it is assumed that there will never be more than 16 hops between source and destination and thus we only need 4 bits to represent the *Time to Live*. It is then proposed to ignore the most significant part of the IPv4 - *Time to Live* byte. This seems a reasonable assumption as the latency involved with traversing more than 16 hops could make the communications problematic. (Please note that this does not limit the number of networks within the 'network-of-networks' to 16, only that there will never be more than 16 degrees of separation between two networks).

Protocol

IANA defines around 140 different protocols in (Arko&Brandes, 2008) for use over IPv4, the most common for user data transfer being TCP and UDP. As 'network-of-networks' uses its own network management system and routing algorithms other protocols such as IGP, EGP, RSVP will not be needed. Therefore it is assumed that only TCP and UDP transport protocols will be used for node to node communication within 'network-of-networks'. It is also assumed that the network management functions for 'network-of-networks' (routing, resource reservation, topology discovery) will need to be identified, both for the individual and the overarching network management functions. It is therefore proposed to use 4 bits to represent the protocol field:

- 0: UDP,
- 1: TCP,
- 2: 'Network-of-Networks' internal network management traffic (individual NMS),
- 3: 'Network-of-Networks' external network management traffic (overarching NMS),
- 5: ICMP,
- 6: IGMP,
- 15: protocol defined in 8 bit (optional) header field.

'Network-of-Networks' Header

If other protocols wish to be used over the 'network-of-networks' (such as BGP or RSVP) then the protocol field will contain a special value (15) which indicates that an extra (optional) 8bit IP protocol field will be present after the main 'network-of-networks' header containing the IP protocol, adding an extra byte to the 'network-of-networks' header.

'Network-of-Networks' Headers for Particular Standards

In this Section we describe 'network-of-networks' headers for different communication standards. These headers were designed and optimised, ensuring compliance with the major 'network-of-networks' e-Health requirements.

WiFi and WiMAX 'Network-of-Networks' Header

It is proposed to continue to use the standardised IPv4 headers.

HIDL 'Network-of-Networks' Header

HIDL requires the use of UDP over IPv4 packets with a maximum user data packet size of 422 bytes. The destination addresses are limited to the multicast IP addresses described by the circuit which means that even though the packets technically use an IPv4 header, it is insufficient in its entirety for our purposes. The identification, fragmentation, time to live and source address fields within the IPv4 header can be utilised as normal, but the protocol and destination addresses are going to have to be additionally provided. Therefore all packets going over HIDL will require the following 'H.Network-of-Networks' header to be used:

Bits: 0-7	8-15	16-23
Destination Network	Destination Node	Protocol

Fig. 5. HIDL 'Network-of-Networks' Header

A full 'network-of-networks' over HIDL packet would therefore look like the following:

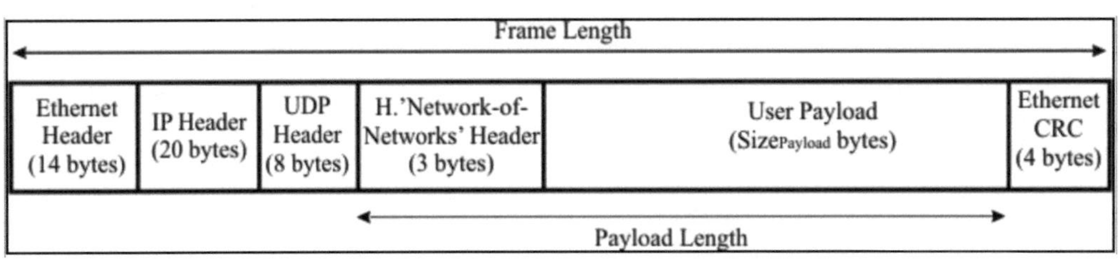

Fig. 6. Packet Format for the HIDL network within 'Network-of-Networks'

Link 16 'Network-of-Networks' Header

We proposed to use the 'Free Text' version of Link 16 which means that there are no J-series message headers for the packets we will be sending, in fact there will be no headers of any kind except to say that this packet is for transmission on the 'network-of-networks' Network Participation Group. Error correction mechanisms such as checksums and cyclic redundancy checks are not needed as they are already provided by the data-link.

Therefore, all the fields identified has to be present in a Link 16 layer 3 'network-of-networks' header. However a full IPv4 at 20 bytes would represent at least 71% of a standard message. The Link 16 'network-of-networks' layer 2 and layer 3 headers combined provide packet overhead which varies between 21 bytes = 75% (fragmented IP datagram requiring Link 16 layer 2 fragmentation) and 2 bytes = 7% (subsequent Link16 layer 2 fragments).

The Link 16 'network-of-networks' headers are formed from a layer 2 (data link) header followed by a layer 3 (compressed IP) header, both of which may contain optional fields (so they are variable length).

Layer 2 header

Optional fields are indicated by a dashed boarder and described below.

Mandatory layer 2 header fields:

- Layer 2 pkt Fragment - flag indicating this packet is a layer 2 fragment;
- Layer 2 first Fragment - flag indicating this packet is first layer 2 fragment in a sequence of fragments (only checked if Layer 2 pkt fragment flag set);
- MS bits Layer 2 fragment sequence number - Most significant 6 bits of layer 2 fragment sequence number (set to 0 if Layer 2 pkt fragment flag clear);

Optional layer 2 header fields included as follows:

- LS bits Layer 2 fragment sequence number - Least significant 8 bits of layer 2 fragment sequence number (only present if Layer 2 pkt fragment flag set);
- Layer 2 number of fragments (2 bytes) - included if Layer 2 pkt fragment flag set AND the layer 2 first fragment flag is set;
- Layer 2 IP datagram checksum (2 bytes) - included if Layer 2 pkt fragment flag set AND the layer 2 first fragment flag is set. Checksum covers the whole IP datagram including compressed IP header.

Layer 3 header

The illustration below shows the proposed Link 16 layer3 header and how it maps to the IPv4 header.

Optional fields are indicated by a dashed boarder.

Optional header fields:

Note if more than one option is present, they must be in the order shown below (shown with all optional fields present).

Optional header fields included as follows:

- IP Identification, Fragmentation Flags and Fragmentation offset (4 bytes) - included if IP pkt fragmentation flag set. Values are the same as in the original IP header.
- IP Full Protocol - included if value of protocol field is 7. Value the same as in the original IP header.

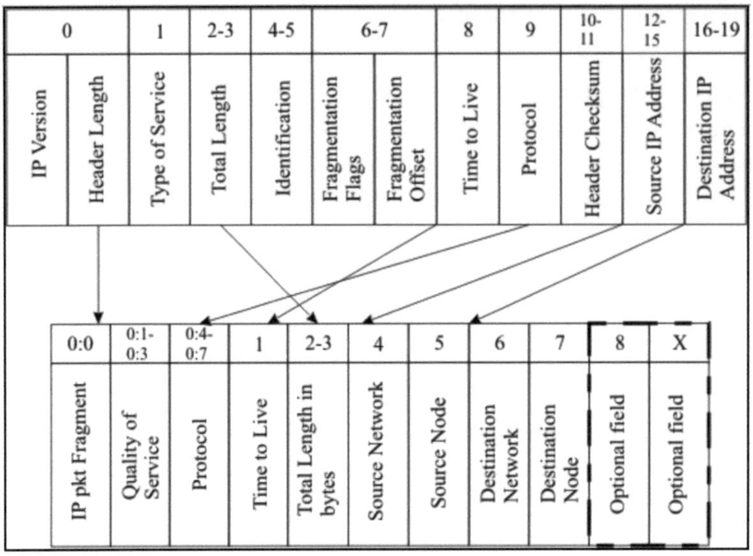

Fig. 7. Mapping Link 16 Layer3 Header to the IPv4 Header

8-9	10-13		14
IP Identification	IP Fragmentation Flags	IP Fragmentation Offset	Full IP Protocol

Fig. 8. Optional Header Fields

Link 11 'Network-of-Networks' Header

Because Link 11 uses a roll call mechanism, in which the transmitter carries on transmitting until all data is delivered and connection is completed, it means that it is not needed to provide a header to every packet we transmit, but rather send the header first and stream the data portion afterwards so the entire packet arrives all in one sequential stream. This stream may not be continuous (if other nodes transmit between portions of it), but by stitching together the transmissions from each node separately a terminal will be able to recover all packets. If the transmit window allows for multiple transmissions then it may subsequently send more header then data packet sequences. As a Link 11 packet is only 5 bytes long, the header needs to be split into 2 (or 3) packets as shown below (the destination address information arrives first thereby allowing a node to immediately determine if they should capture for the rest of the transmission or ignore it):

The layer 2 addressing for Link 11 'network-of-networks' information is mapped directly from layer 3 (the IP destination address) due to the broadcast nature of Link 11, so layer 2 and layer 3 header information are mixed together. Two bytes of layer 2 fragmentation information are always included, to assist in the identification of the first 5 byte message (which could be lost due to reception errors).

0	1:0	1:1	1:2-1:7+2	3	4
Number of data packets following	Layer 2 pkt Fragment	Layer 2 first Fragment	MS bits Layer 2 fragment sequence number	Destination Network	Destination Node

5	6	7:0	7:1-7:3	7:4-7:7	6	7-8	9	X
Source Network	Source Node	IP pkt Fragment	Quality of Service	Protocol	Time to Live	Total Length in bytes	Optional field	Optional field

Fig. 9. Link 11 Destination Identification Message

Mandatory layer 2 header fields:

- Layer 2 pkt Fragment - flag indicating this packet is a layer 2 fragment;
- Layer 2 first Fragment - flag indicating this packet is first layer 2 fragment in a sequence of fragments (only checked if Layer 2 pkt fragment flag set);
- Layer 2 fragment sequence number - 14 bits of layer 2 fragment sequence number (set to 0 if Layer 2 pkt fragment flag clear).

The optional fields consist of layer 2 optional fields followed by layer 3 optional fields.

0-1	2-3
Layer 2 number of fragments	Layer 2 IP datagram checksum

Fig. 10. Layer 2 Optional Fields

- Layer 2 number of fragments (2 bytes) - included if Layer 2 pkt fragment flag set AND the layer 2 first fragment flag is set;
- Layer 2 IP datagram checksum (2 bytes) - included if Layer 2 pkt fragment flag set; AND the layer 2 first fragment flag is set. Checksum covers the whole IP datagram including compressed IP header.

Link 11 layer 2 fragmentation works in a similar way to that described for Link 16, the major difference being that a single layer 2 fragment consists of a "stream" of Link 11 messages (as each message is only 5 bytes long). The first layer 2 fragment will have both the layer 2 header and layer 3 (compressed IP) header. Subsequent layer fragments will just have the layer 2 header bits.

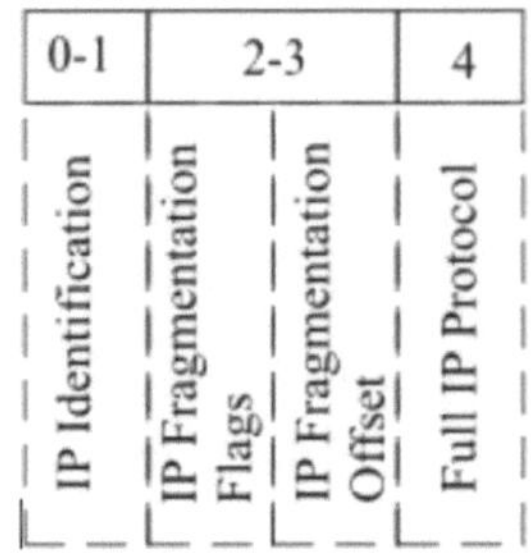

Fig. 11. Layer 3 Optional Fields are as Described for the Link 16

The layer 2 MTU size for link 11 is determined such that a 'network-of-networks' fragment will not take an excessive time to transmit, allowing other Link 11 traffic to be sent, but not too small such that the compressed 'network-of-networks' IP header is a too large fraction of the datagram. A MTU size of around 50 would take about 150ms to transmit

6. 'Cross-Over' nodes

We propose a new 'cross-over' node solution, which will ensure communication across the systems described above. However this is only half of what it is meant to do, the 'cross-over' nodes also perform an overarching network management system (O-NMS).

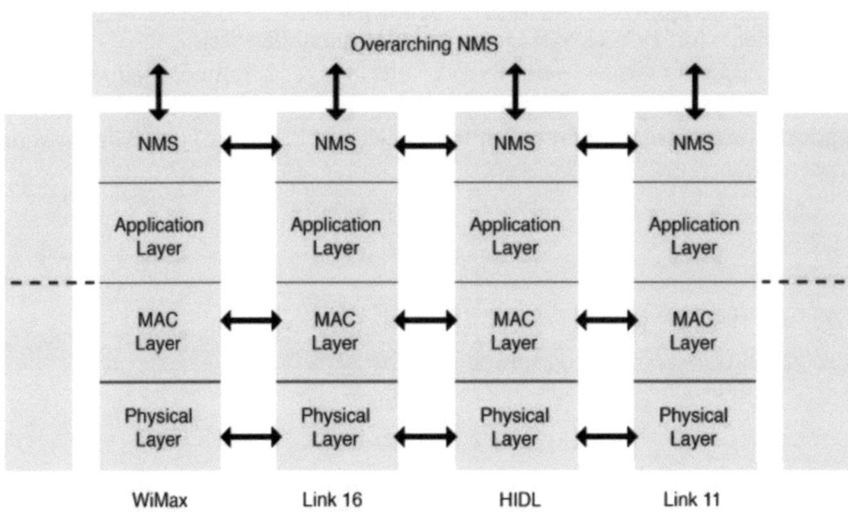

Fig. 12. Overarching Network Management System

It is shown previously how each data-link network in turn manages its own network and allocates resources, but these are narrow views of the 'network-of-networks' as a whole.
While each individual NMS maintains the allocation of resources within its own domain it is up to the Overarching NMS to try and balance the utilization and capacity of the network-of networks as a whole.
The Overarching NMS should try and make sure that not only there is no single point of failure within the large 'network-of-networks' (such as might be the case if all external network traffic is routed through the WiMAX network) but that routing information is kept

up to date and in the event of a change in the network topology (either someone joining or leaving) the routing of packets within the network reflects it.

The reason for separating the functions of the individual network management systems from the overarching network management system is that first and foremost the individual data link networks need to be able to continue functioning as they have been and provide the services they were designed for. Thus apart from a capacity utilisation impact the current data-link networks should not be further impacted. By separating the functions we are ensuring that the overarching NMS should be lost or a data-link network becomes cut off from the rest of the 'network-of-networks' it can continue operating as it has done with no noticeable effect from the point of view of non-'network-of-networks' terminals.

Centralised Overarching NMS

One method of accomplishing the task of the O-NMS is to centralise the process so that only one 'cross-over' node (per group of networks) centrally collects all the external network traffic together and re-distributes it according to the current network conditions and demands. Such a set up is shown below:

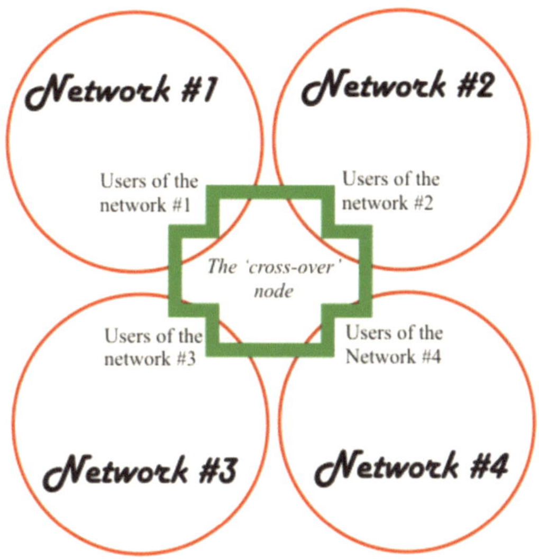

Fig. 13. Centralised Overarching Network Management System

This implementation would allow a centralised management system to request and effectively organise individual network resources so that real time and priority traffic were routed efficiently. There would also be no additional network overhead in this implementation as the O-NMS can hear all of the individual NMS's broadcasts and thus infer all the information it requires.

This central 'cross-over' node would also have a broadband link (such as WiMAX) linked to another 'cross-over' node elsewhere that controlled another separate group of networks, thereby enabling multiple groups of mini 'network-of-networks' to communicate with each other.

While there are advantages to centralised authority for communicating between networks the disadvantages are that the 'cross-over' node must be in a position to communicate with everyone within the local 'network-of-networks', and that there is a single point of failure within the system that leaves the 'network-of-networks' implementation vulnerable to node attrition.

Distributed Overarching NMS

The other option is to distribute the functionality of the O-NMS to many disparate systems and have them cooperatively perform duties such as load balancing and traffic routing. This would require multiple 'cross-over' nodes between networks at different points; there could even be the possibility of multiple 'cross-over' points between two networks. Such a set-up is shown in figure 14.
This implementation would provide a robust architecture that has no single points of failure. If one 'cross-over' node is lost there are still many other routes a packet could take from source to destination. However, in order to produce a balanced load across the 'network-of-networks' and to effectively route packets through this large network the 'cross-over' nodes will have to communicate with each other, which will mean an increased network management overhead.

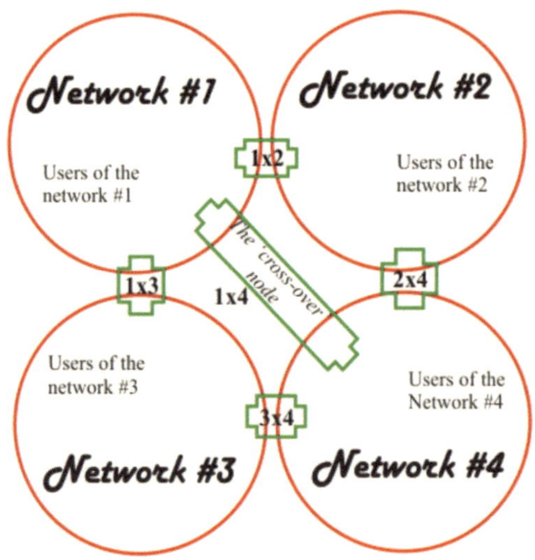

Fig. 14. Distributed Overarching Network Management System

As there are multiple routes that a packet could take and the best route for a given type of packet will depend on the current loading of the network there won't be a fixed route from source to destination. This dynamic nature may provide robustness to changing network topologies, but from the time the topology changes until the whole network is informed of this fact the network will remain in a state of flux. How changes in the topology are distributed around the network and how they will affect the routing choices of the 'cross-over' nodes will depend on the routing algorithms implemented, which will be investigated further within this research.

Routing choices

One of the most important features of IPv4 packets is that they look identical if they are addressed to a computer within the same network or to an external computer on the other side of the world. This unification of communication should be emulated within 'network-of-networks', such that a node within one network should be able to communicate in the same manner with another node regardless of its location. The only difference should be in the QoS experienced (the greater the number of hops, the greater the latency), the format should be the same.

'Cross-over' nodes as the gateways between different networks have the responsibility to forward packets between different networks, which imply that they are also capable of deciding which packets need forwarding, and onto which other network. If a 'cross-over' node only sits on two networks then it only needs to know if it needs to forward it onto the other network, however if it sits on three or more networks then it needs to also make the decision as to which interface should be used for the next hop. The goal of the 'cross-over' nodes routing therefore is twofold; first to satisfy the QoS requirements for every admitted packet/stream, and second to achieve global efficiency in resource utilisation.

A simple methodology would be to make 'cross-over' nodes forward all externally addressed packets. This approach would ensure that a packet reaches its destination, but in the process it would be replicated numerous times and would make an inefficient use of the network resources (not to mention that multiple copies of each packet would end up reaching the destination), thereby failing to meet the second goal. While this might seem reasonable for a small all-informed network the magnitude data rate differences between WiMAX and Link 11 could mean that Link 11 is swamped by external WiMAX traffic.

Another methodology would be to coordinate the actions of the 'cross-over' nodes so that they have some knowledge of the topology of the network and its current utilisation and therefore forward it on to the most appropriate next hop. Having a simple knowledge of the network topology will allow each 'cross-over' node to easily calculate the route with the least number of hops and to forward the packet onto the next hop in the sequence. However, this does not take into consideration the appropriateness of each hop in the sequence. If the traffic is real time and of a high data rate, then it does not make much sense to route it over a Link 11 network even if it may be the most direct method, instead a route with a greater number of hops may be able to provide a traffic stream with the QoS it requires. Not only does a 'cross-over' node need to make an intelligent decision regarding the routing of a packet, but it also needs to coordinate its actions with other 'cross-over' nodes within the network.

QoS Routing and 'Cost' of transmission

The routing choice a 'cross-over' node will have to make will depend on the QoS requirements of the packet and the current utilisation of the 'network-of-networks'. The 'cross-over' nodes, in their role as the O-NMS need to ensure that the network as a whole is properly load balanced, so when making their decision regarding routing they may consider the following sort of parameters:

- Type of packet (Real-time, Priority, Best Effort);
- Impact of latency on packet;
- Impact of blocking on packet;
- Individual packet or part of a stream;
- Size of packet;
- Each network's current capacity utilisation;
- Each network's data rate throughput;
- Each network's jitter;
- Each network's ability to provide QoS;
- Each network's possible Bit Error Rate;

- Each 'cross-over' node's utilisation (spare buffer capacity);
- Current traffic route patterns.

These parameters, together with a weighting value as to the importance of each parameter, can be put into a function to determine the most appropriate route for each packet type at that instant. As a result a priority labelled packet will be routed differently to a Best Effort labelled packet, which could be different again to the route for a real-time packet. The calculated weighted sum is called the 'cost' of transmission:

$$C = \alpha \bullet C1 \bullet W1 + \beta \bullet C2 \bullet W2 + ... + \gamma \bullet Cn \bullet Wn, \tag{1}$$

where C - indicates the 'cost' of transmission; Wi, i=1,...n - are the importance Weight and α, β, ..., γ are various possible QoS parameters (latency, end-to-end delay, throughput, etc.) This 'cost' function (1) is only meaningful for the current state of the network and the type of packet to be transmitted.

=For example, it is needed to transmit the delay sensitive information and there is two or more way of transmission. The cost of transmission through the first path includes

$$C_{path1} = \alpha \bullet C_1 \bullet W_1 + \beta \bullet C_2 \bullet W_2 + \xi \bullet C_n \bullet W_3 = C_1 \bullet delay \bullet 0{,}5 + C_2 \bullet blocking\_probabolity \bullet 0.1 + ... \tag{2}$$

$$C_{path2} = \alpha \bullet C_1 \bullet W_1 + \beta \bullet C_2 \bullet W_2 + \xi \bullet C_n \bullet W_3 = C_1 \bullet delay \bullet 0{,}4 + C_2 \bullet blocking\_probabolity \bullet 0.1 + ... \tag{3}$$

The parameter of weight should be chosen in respect to the type of transmitting information. When the scheme of the cost of transmission is known by the decision making mechanism, then it makes the decision about which way to transmit and initiates the transfer.

If such a cost function can be calculated for each hop through the network then a 'cross-over' node will be able to: work out the most effective route (the one with the minimum cost), ensure that it meets the load balancing requirements of the network as a whole, and route the packet accordingly.

In order for to calculate a meaningful figure the information used needs to be correct, and that means current. Using out of date information could negatively impact the network, such as route more information into an already over-congested network. 'Cross-over' nodes will therefore need to share information with each other at regular intervals. This information sharing will cause increased network overhead, which will need to be carefully balanced against the benefits the information sharing will produce. Therefore, an investigation will need to be carried out to determine which parameters and weightings will be required to effectively calculate the 'cost' of transmission for each packet type, and what update interval is most appropriate.

'Cross-Over' Node Communication Protocols

The actual message exchange will not strictly conform to a pre-existing IP protocol scheme (e.g. BGP, OSPF), this is due to the unique nature of 'network-of-networks'. 'Network-of-networks' is not trying to implement the internet, as they are orders of magnitude different and the network resources these protocols were designed around (i.e. maximum data rates, packet sizes, latencies) are very different. Instead, while the functionality may be similar the exact message structures will be different.

As described in the previous sections it is proposed to use two separate 'network-of-networks' messaging protocols: internal and external. Internal messages are used by nodes to communicate with their individual network managers, external messages are used by the 'cross-over' nodes to communicate with each other.

Internal Messages

Networks such as WiMAX and Link 16 have their own network management system communications protocols, and it is anticipated that 'network-of-networks' will continue to use them where possible. But for other messages that the current NMS protocol does not support, such as the current list of active nodes, new 'network-of-networks' NMS messages will need to be sent.

The formats of the messages should conform to the data-link network formats defined previously in this Chapter, with the protocol defined as either '2' (for 'network-of-networks' headers) or '222' for IPv4.

The following messages will be used:

Hello: Used to inform the NMS that they are present

- Node Address,
- Is it a 'cross-over' node (or not),
- The network addresses of the other networks they are attached to.

0:0-3	0:4-7	1	2:0-2	3-X
Message ID=0	Unique ID	Node Address	'Cross-over' (yes=1, no=0)	Attached Network Addressed (1/byte)

Fig. 15. 'Network-of-Networks' NMS Internal Messages (hello message)

Hello Reply: Used by the NMS in reply to a Hello message

- 'Hello' Node Address,
- NSM Node Address,
- Network Address.

0:0-3	0:4-7	1	2	3
Message ID=1	Unique ID	'Hello' Node Address	'NMS' Node Address	Network Address

Fig. 16. 'Network-of-Networks' NMS Internal Messages (hello reply message)

Active Node List: Used to distribute the list of current active nodes

- Network Address,
- Total number of Active Nodes,
- List of Active Node Addresses,
- Total number of 'cross-over' nodes,
- List of 'cross-over' node addresses,

0:0-3	0:4-7	1	2	3	4-X	(X+1)-Y
Message ID=3	Unique ID	Network Address	Number of Active Nodes	Number of 'cross-over' nodes	List of Active Nodes (1/byte)	List of 'cross-over' nodes (1/byte)

Fig. 17. Active Node List: Used to Distribute the List of Current Active Nodes

External Messages

In order to perform the required O-NMS functions the 'cross-over' nodes require two elements: some knowledge of the network topology and some knowledge of the 'cost' of traversing the network. The 'cost' can be determined by an algorithm and information exchange, but in order to know which nodes to contact and what networks are available the 'cross-over' nodes need to know the topology of the network.

There are two main methods of undertaking this, the first is for all 'cross-over' nodes to know the entire topology of the network and the other is for them to know a local portion of the network and how to route traffic to for more remote portions of the network. These two methods are born out in two styles of routing protocols; interior and exterior routing protocols. Each version requires a differing amount of network overhead, and ends up with different strengths and weaknesses.

Therefore, the two major external message types anticipated are distribution of 'cost' information, and distribution of network topology.

The exact structure of these messages and their sizes will depend on factors such as the routing algorithm, simulation implementation and network complexity. The protocol used however, should be defined as either '3' (for 'network-of-networks' headers) or '223' for IPv4.

External and Internal Messages: Resource Reservation

In order to route real-time and possibly some priority traffic some QoS requirements will need to be met for each hop from source to destination. If the route is contained within one network then this should just involve a request for resources from the Individual NMS (I-NMS). If the route involves multiple networks then each individual NMS along the route will have to be contacted and resources reserved. If resources are not available across one hop in the route, then a new route will have to be calculated and any unused reserved resources released back to their network managers. In order to fulfil our requirement that a node should be able to communicate with an external destination in the same manner as an internal one the mechanisms for the resource reservation should also be identical. This will mean that the local I-NMS will be contacted by the source requesting resources to send a traffic stream to a remote destination. The I-NMS should identify that the destination is not local to this network and allocate the necessary resources for the first hop (if possible) before sending the request to a 'cross-over' node. The 'cross-over' node will then have to decide on the appropriate route and request resources for each hop along the way. Once a route has been reserved the source will need to be informed and the stream can begin. Once the communication has been completed the source will need to inform its local I-NMS that it no longer needs the resource. Once the resources are released, the local I-NMS should inform the 'cross-over' node which will release the reserved resources along each hop. Therefore this process utilizes both internal and external messaging.

The resource reservation for each hop can either be controlled from the first 'cross-over' node or handed off to the next 'cross-over' node in turn. Which method will be more appropriate will depend on the topology and routing algorithms chosen. If the topology algorithm does not allow for complete knowledge of the network topology then the reservation process cannot be centrally managed, although if it does then the complexity of the reservation process is greatly reduced.
All individual network managers will need to monitor the utilization of all allocated resources, so that should a crucial 'cross-over' node or source node drop off the network the resources are not then reserved indefinitely.

Internal Messages

Resource Request: used to request resources from the NMS:

- Requesting Node Address,
- Destination Address (Network and Node),
- Data size in KiloBytes (or Bytes depending on the network) per frame,
- Frequency of frames per timebase (the timebase is link dependent, or for Link 11 refer to a transmission cycle),
- QoS of traffic,
- Utilisation time (units are link dependent, not required for Link 11).

0:0-3	0:4-7	1	2	3	4	5	6:0-2	6:3-7
Message ID=4	Unique ID	Node Address	Destination Network Address	Destination Node Address	Data Size	Frequency	QoS Traffic	Utilisation Time

Fig. 18. Resource Request Message: Used to Request Resources from the NMS

Resource Granted: Used to inform the node that the resource has been granted

- Requesting Node Address,
- Unique ID (used in the initial resource request),
- Destination Address (Network and Node),
- Data size granted (same as requested or less if full amount not available),
- Frequency granted (same as requested or less if full amount not available),
- Utilization time (same as requested or less if full amount not available).

0:0-3	0:4-7	1	2	2	3	4
Message ID=5	Unique ID	Destination Network Address	Destination Node Address	Data Size	Frequency	Utilisation Time

Fig. 19. Resource Granted message: Used to Inform the Node that the Resource has been Granted

Resource Denied: used when a route that can support the requested level of QoS cannot be found

- Requesting Node Address,
- Unique ID (used in the initial resource request),
- Destination Address (Network and Node),
- Reason request was denied:

1 - insufficient BW,
2 - QoS type not supported,
3 - resource temporarily unavailable.

0:0-3	0:4-7	1	2	3	4
Message ID=6	Unique ID	Node Address	Destination Network Address	Destination Node Address	Reason

Fig. 20. Resource Denied: Used when a Route that can Support the Requested Level of QoS cannot be Found

Resource Release: used by a node when it has finished with the resource

- Requesting Node Address,
- Unique ID (used in the initial resource request),
- Destination Address (Network and Node).

0:0-3	0:4-7	1	2	3
Message ID=7	Unique ID	Node Address	Destination Network Address	Destination Node Address

Fig. 21. Resource Release Message: Used by a Node when it has finished with the Resource

External Messages

Resource Request: used by the NMS to a 'cross-over' node to begin reserving resources along a route

- Unique ID (used in the initial resource request),
- Requesting Address (Network and Node),
- Destination Address (Network and Node),
- Data size in KiloBytes per frame,
- Frequency of frames per timebase (the timebase is seconds),
- QoS of traffic,
- Utilisation time (the timebase is 10 seconds),

0:0-3	0:4-7	1	2	3	4	5	6	7:0-2	7:3-7
Message ID=1	Unique ID	Request Network Address	Request Node Address	Destination Network Address	Destination Node Address	Data Size	Frequency	QoS of Traffic	Utilisation Time

Fig. 22. Resource Request External Message: Used by the NSM to a 'Cross-Over' Node to begin Reserving Resources along a Route

Resource Request: used between 'cross-over' nodes to reserve resources along a route

- Unique ID (used in the initial resource request),
- Requesting Address (Network and Node),
- Destination Address (Network and Node),
- Data size in KiloBytes per frame,
- Frequency of frames per timebase (the timebase is seconds),
- QoS of traffic,
- Utilisation time (the timebase is 10 seconds),
- Previous reserved networks (List of Network Addresses).

0:0-3	0:4-7	1	2	3	4	5	6	7:0-2	7:3-7	8-X
Message ID=2	Unique ID	Request Network Address	Request Node Address	Destination Network Address	Destination Node Address	Data Size	Frequency	QoS Traffic	Utilisation Time	Reserved Networks (1/byte)

Fig. 23. Resource Request External Message: Used between 'Cross-Over' Nodes to Reserve Resources along a Route

Resource Granted: used between 'cross-over' nodes to indicate a resources has been reserved

- Unique ID (used in the initial resource request),
- Requesting Address (Network and Node),
- Destination Address (Network and Node),
- Data size granted (same as requested or less if full amount not available),
- Frequency granted (same as requested or less if full amount not available),
- QoS of traffic,
- Utilisation time (same as requested or less if full amount not available),
- Reserved Network Address.

0:0-3	0:4-7	1	2	3	4	5	6	7:0-2	7:3-7	8
Message ID=3	Unique ID	Request Network Address	Request Node Address	Destination Network Address	Destination Node Address	Data Size	Frequency	QoS of Traffic	Utilisation Time	Reserved Network

Fig. 24. Resource Granted External Message: Used between 'Cross-Over' Nodes to Indicate a Resource has been Reserved

Resource Denied: used by a 'cross-over' node to indicate that such a request cannot be granted

- Unique ID (used in the initial resource request),
- Requesting Address (Network and Node),
- Destination Address (Network and Node),
- Denied Network Address,
- Reason (see internal message for values).

0:0-3	0:4-7	1	2	3	4	5	6
Message ID=4	Unique ID	Request Network Address	Request Node Address	Destination Network Address	Destination Node Address	Network Address	Reason

Fig. 25. Resource Denied External Message: Used by a 'Cross-Over' Node to Indicate that such a Request cannot be Granted

Resource Release: used by a 'cross-over' node release a resource:

- Unique ID (used in the initial resource request),
- Requesting Address (Network and Node),
- Destination Address (Network and Node),
- Released Network Address.

0:0-3	0:4-7	1	2	3	4	5
Message ID=5	Unique ID	Request Network Address	Request Node Address	Destination Network Address	Destination Node Address	Network Address

Fig. 26. Resource Release External Message: Used by a 'Cross-Over' Node Release a Resource

Multicast Request: used by both a node and a 'cross-over' node to register its request to receive a multicast stream:

- Unique ID,
- Requesting Address (Network and Node),
- Destination Multicast Address (Network and Node),
- Current Network Address.

0:0-3	0:4-7	1	2	3	4	5
Message ID=6	Unique ID	Request Network Address	Request Node Address	Destination Network Address	Destination Node Address	Network Address

Fig. 27. Multicast Request External Message: Used by both a Node and a 'Cross-Over' Node to Register its Request to Receive a Multicast Stream

Multicast Release: used by node to register its request to receive a multicast stream:

- Unique ID (used in the initial resource request),
- Requesting Address (Network and Node),
- Destination Multicast Address (Network and Node),
- Current Network Address.

0:0-3	0:4-7	1	2	3	4	5
Message ID=7	Unique ID	Request Network Address	Request Node Address	Destination Network Address	Destination Node Address	Network Address

Fig. 28. Multicast Release External Message: Used by a Node to Register its Request to Receive a Multicast Stream

7. Summary

This Chapter develops a wireless cross-standard communication protocol and describes the concept of 'network-of-networks' in conjunction with e-Health applications. Analysis of the legacy communication systems and their integration into a single 'network-of-networks' communication protocol is presented. Based on this analysis, the developed concept was implemented in the CLAHNS project for MOD which was supported by Lancaster University.

8. References

Arkko J., Brander S. (2008). *IANA Allocation Guidelines for the Protocol Field.* Network Working Group. February 2008. [Online]. Available: http://tools.ietf.org/html/rfc5237 [Accessed: January 2009].

Internet Protocol. Darpa Internet Program. Protocol Specification. September 1981. [Online]. Available: http://www.ietf.org/rfc/rfc0791.txt [Accessed: May 2009].

Lockheed Martin UK- Integrated Systems and Solutions. *Tactical Data Links – MIDS/JTIDS Link 16, and Variable Message Format - VMF*. [Online]. Available: http://www.lm-isgs.co.uk/defence/datalinks/link_16.htm [Accessed: March 2010].

Almquist P. (consultant) (1992). Type of Service in the Internet Protocol Suite. Network Working Group. [Online] Available: http://tools.ietf.org/html/rfc1349 [Accessed: March 2010].

ARM Technical Specification. *ARM, MPEG-4, AAC, LC Decoder Technical Specification.* Document Number: PRD10-GENC-0012884.0. Date of Issue, 19 June 2003. ARM Limited 2002-2003. [Online]. Available: http://www.arm.com/files/pdf/PRD10-GENC-001288-4-0.pdf [Accessed: March 2010].

ASCII Table and Description. www.AskiiTable.com. [Online]. Available: http://www.asciitable.com/ [Accessed: March 2010]. Available: http://iphome.hhi.de/wiegand/assets/pdfs/h264-AVC-Standard.pdf [Accessed: March 2010].

Baker F. (editor) (1995). *RFC 1812 – Requirements for IP Version 4 Routers*. Cisco Systems. Network Working Group. [Online]. Available: http://www.faqs.org/rfcs/rfc1812.html [Accessed: March 2010].

Chandraiah P., Domer R. (2005). Technical Report CECS-05-04. *Specification and Design of a MP3 Audio Decoder*. [Online]. Available at: http://www.cecs.uci.edu/technicalreport/TR05-04.pdf [Accessed: September 2009].

Chiariglione L.(2000). *MPEG-2. Generic coding of moving pictures and associated audio information. Start MPEG-2 description.* International Organisation for Standardisation. ISO/IEC JTC1/SC29/WG11 coding of moving pictures and audio. [Online] Available at: http://mpeg.chiarglione.org/standards/mpeg-2.htm [Accessed: January 2010].

Istepanian R. S. H., Philip N., Martini M. (2009). Medical QoS Provision Based on Reinforcement Learning in Ultrasound Streaming over 3.5G Wireless Systems. *IEEE Journal on Selected areas in Communications*. Vol.27, 4, pp.566-574.

Lockheed Martin UK- Integrated Systems and Solutions. *Tactical Data Links – Link 11 and 11B*. [Online]. Available: http://www.lm-isgs.co.uk/defence/datalinks/link_11.htm [Accessed: March 2010].

Marpe D., et al (2006). The H.264/MPEG4 Advanced Video Coding Standard and its Applications. Standards report. *IEEE Communications Magazine.* [Online]. Available: http://iphome.hhi.de/wiegand/assets/pdfs/h264-AVC-Standard.pdf [Accessed: March 2010].

Microsoft Corporation (1999). *Rich Text Format (RTF) Specification, version 1.6.* [Online] Available: http://msdu.microsoft.com/en-us/library/aa140277(office.10).aspx [Accessed: February 2010].

Microsoft Media. *Windows Media Video 9 Series Codecs*. [Online] Available at: http://www.microsoft.com/windows/windowsmedia/forpros/codecs/video.asp x [Accessed: February 2010].

SyntheSys. Military Systems. *UK Tactical Data Systems Reference Guide*. 2006 [Online]. Available: http://www.synthesys.co.uk/UK_Tactical_Data_Systems_Reference_Guide.htm [Accessed: September 2009].

Tarter A., et al (2008). *CLAHNS Protocol Description Document*. PD-650-50004. Issue 2. Ultra Electronics.

ULTRA Electronics Limited. Communication and Integrated Systems. *Report: High Integrity Data Links (HIDL). Mission Critical Secure Networks*. 2010. [Online]. Available: http://www.ultra-cis.com/resourses/HIDL%200909v1.pdf [Accessed: March 2010].

3

Safety and Electromagnetic Compatibility in Wireless Telemedicine Applications

Victoria Ramos and José Luís Monteagudo
Instituto de Salud Carlos III
Spain

1. Introduction

The vision of our future environment is based on Ambient Intelligence (AmI), being surrounded by various kinds of interfaces, and supported by computing and networking technology providing an intelligent, seamless and non-obtrusive assistance to people. The amount and complexity of health-related information and knowledge has increased to such a degree that a major component of any health organisation is information processing.

The health sector is clearly an information intensive sector, which increasingly depends on information and communication technologies. These technologies are supporting progress in medical research, better management and diffusion of medical knowledge, as well as a shift towards evidence-based medicine. They include tools for health authorities and professionals as well as personalised health systems for patients and citizens. Examples include health information networks, telemedicine services, personal, wearable and portable communication systems and many other information and communication technology-based tools that assist in prevention, diagnosis, treatment, health monitoring, and lifestyle management. When combined with organisational changes and the development of new skills, they can help to deliver better with even a lower cost within citizen-centred health delivery systems.

Mobile technology and wireless solutions promise to transform the healthcare industry. E-pharmacy, asset tracking, mobile voice and media-rich systems are just a few of the solutions that are enabled by those technologies. Wireless communications systems support the aggregation, analysis and storage of clinical data in all its forms; information tools provide access to the latest findings while communication tools enable collaboration among many different organisations and health professionals. Patients and health professionals are becoming increasingly mobile. Both as patients and as healthy citizens, people can benefit from better personal health education and disease prevention. They need support in managing their own diseases, risks - including work-related diseases - and lifestyles. A growing number of people are looking proactively for information on their medical conditions. Personalised systems for monitoring and supporting patients are also currently available - examples include wearable or implanted communication systems to continuously monitor patients' heart conditions. These systems can help shorten or completely avoid a patient's stay at hospital, while still ensuring monitoring of their health status. Health professionals and all the staff employed in the health sector including nursing, care, and administrative staff can also benefit.

Wireless connectivity is becoming increasingly used in Telecare application with intensive use of ubiquitous radio communications such as ZigBee, RFID, UWB (European Commission, 2001). These systems involve sensors, computing and communication devices working in increasingly dense electromagnetic environments. One emerging approach to improving the wearability of continuous ambulatory monitoring systems is to improve body-attached sensors with built-in wireless telemetry, thus freeing the user from having to carry a data recorder. For these telemetry systems, it is likely that a large number of wireless links coexist in the same area sharing the electromagnetic environment.

Nomadic technologies that work in unlicensed frequency bands are turning us into human beings with more and more devices in new electromagnetic conditions not included either in legislation concerning human exposure and the effects of long term, low intensity exposure or with regard to medical devices. Electromagnetic Interference (EMI) can be a serious problem for any electronic device, but working with medical devices can have life-threatening consequences.

Electromagnetic Fields (EMF) are present everywhere in our environment and will continue increasing. In this way, our environment will be surrounded by multiple mobile and stationary devices communicating wirelessly and working together. The level and frequency pattern of that exposure is continuously changing as technological innovation advances. Exposure of the general public and workers cannot be avoided, since various devices emitting low-level EMF are almost omnipresent in the environment, including wearable devices attached to clothes or directly to the body.

2. Antecedents / background

Patient-centred care is not new; it has been discussed for over 20 years, but only recently is it beginning to take hold. Increasingly, patients expect physicians to be responsive to their needs and preferences, to provide them with access to their medical information, and to treat them as partners in care decisions. This means that effective healthcare is now happening at the bedside, and not in the Doctor's office, which makes mobility via wireless technology an essential piece of the puzzle. Mobility used to mean doctors, nurses and medical technicians using handwritten notes on individual sheets of paper for transcription into a medical record. In addition to the high cost and delay associated with the manual transcription of patient records, there are non-productive activities such as recording redundant data, searching for misfiled and misplaced charts, and loss of important patient data.

The barriers to effective communications within a healthcare facility are numerous. Large, shift-working populations of clinical, operational and administrative personnel are mobile for much of their day; yet reliable, real-time communications is a vital requirement for them to perform their duties safely and efficiently. In a health care centre every second counts and response time is critical to how well caregivers can meet patients' needs. Multi-media communication systems that integrate wire line and wireless communications, and provide intelligent alerts, telemetry information and even location information can help clinicians evaluate patient needs and deliver appropriate care faster and more efficiently. Complete solutions enable wireless patient monitoring across the entire patient care continuum; from Emergency Care and Anesthesia to Critical Care, Perinatal Care and Home Care.

It is impossible to ignore that the everyday environments for European citizens have been in evolution since wireless technologies (DECT, landline telephones, mobile phones, UMTS,

WiFi, WiMAX, Bluetooth, baby-phones, etc.) have come into widespread use. Recognising the contribution that these new technologies can make, and their omnipresence at work or at home, also implies acceptance of the need for the devices concerned to be assessed before they are put on the market and, more generally, for thresholds to limit the degree of household exposure to RF sources.

Developments in wireless technologies have also had a huge influence in the field of medical applications, enabling wireless bio-monitoring for medical patient care or workers at risk, which can include Electrocardiogram (ECG) temperature, blood pressure, oxygen saturation, internal pressures and respiratory rate. Although the feasibility of using wireless technology to send vital signs was demonstrated more than thirty years ago, it has only been fairly recently that practical and portable devices and communications networks have become generally available. Current development combines some wireless communication technologies (e.g. GSM, Wi-Fi, WPAN, DECT and Bluetooth) to acquire physiological data, monitor patients and manage diseases in a cost-effective manner. Nevertheless, several medical applications use electromagnetic fields in the RF range whose usual frequencies are those allowed for industrial, scientific, and medical applications. There is also potential for new medical applications based on Ultra Wide Band (UWB) communications, for example in cardiology, detection of breast tumours, detection of intracranial haemorrhaging, and the use of sensory implants.

This widespread use of personal communications systems has given rise to much public concern about the possible adverse or dangerous effects of electromagnetic radiation on human health, stemming mainly from the use of mobile telephones and their associated base-station antennas. All populations are now exposed to varying degrees of EM fields. Generally, in the public arena, concern has been often expressed about potential effects of EMF exposure on children's health and on that of older and/or sick people and pregnant women (including the unborn child). This is exemplified by recent public and media concern about potential adverse health effects that might result from the exposure of young people through the rapid expansion of the use of WiFi systems in schools, libraries and universities. Additionally, the population continues to be exposed to the "more traditional sources", like those of radio and TV broadcasting, among others. Some frequencies are now experiencing decreasing usage (e.g. public exposures at 450 MHz from analogue mobile or cordless phones), but others are increasing their useage (e.g. 2.2 GHz from UMTS systems).

Scientific evidence on exposure pattern variability related to use of new wireless technologies provides tools for the better understanding of the level of risk related to those technologies, promoting actions required from decision makers to ensure public safety and increasing public trust in the quality of EMF in everyday environments and the work place (WHO, 2005).

There are several previous works of the authors (Ramos, 2005) and also European Cooperation in the field of Scientific and Technical Research - COST – as COST Action BM0704: Emerging EMF Technologies and Health Risk Management (European Commission, 2008). The Action's role, objectives and method of working is entirely harmonious in respect to sharing information and knowledge from relevant ongoing scientific studies being funded within and outside of the EU. These include, for example, the INTERPHONE Study, the mobile phone related dosimetry programme of the Mobile Manufacturers Forum (MMF) and the GSM Association (GSMA) and national programmes of EMF health-related research in EU Member States and elsewhere. The work of the Action is also complementary to the programmes of bodies providing policy-directed advice, such as the World Health Organization (WHO, 1993), (WHO, 2002), (WHO, 2006). For 10 years, the World Health Organization's EMF Project has been reviewing research needs and identifying key gaps in knowledge requiring further research. Research needs are identified through consensus meetings of internationally recognized experts for the whole EMF frequency range, as is reflected in (WHO, 2010).

3. Current state of knowledge and main objectives

3.1 Current state of knowledge

Many devices of common daily use are mobile RF transmitters. One example is mobile phones; about 3 billion people worldwide use mobile phones. The most common mobile communication technologies in Europe are the digital technologies GSM 900, GSM 1800 and UMTS, plus TETRA systems used by public services (police, fire-fighters, etc.). Nowadays, analogue technologies are rarely used in Europe. Mobile phone use is common in Europe and the proportion of users can reach values of 90 % or more. Before mobile phones can be brought into the European market they have to show compliance with the requirements of European Directives, i.e., limits for the amount of power absorbed in the human body has to be shown. Standardised methods specified by the European Committee for Electrical Standardisation (CENELEC) are used to test mobile phones in Europe. The limit for mobile phone use is the specific absorption rate (SAR) of 2 W/kg for the human head - other limits are provided for power exposing other parts of the body.

Mobile phones are tested under standardised conditions, i.e. at the highest power level, e.g., 2 W peak power corresponding to 250 mW maximum time averaged transmitted power for GSM at 900 MHz. Maximum local SAR values averaged over 10 g of tissue range typically between 0.2 and 1.5 W/kg, depending on the type of mobile phone.

In addition to mobile phones, other wireless applications like cordless phones, e.g. DECT, or WLAN systems are very common. Due to the fact that they are usually operated with lower output power compared to mobile phones the exposure is typically below the level of mobile phones. The maximum time average power level of a DECT base station is 250 mW, for a DECT handset is 10 mW. The peak value of a WLAN terminal is 100 mW, however the average power depends on the traffic and is usually considerably lower. The exposure from such systems is therefore typically below that of mobile phones, however under certain circumstances, e.g. closeness to WLAN access points, exposure due to WLAN or DECT systems can become superior compared to the exposure from GSM or UMTS mobile phones.

Anti-theft devices have become more and more common during recent years. They are typically used at shop exits or similar areas to prevent theft of goods. Some of the existing systems are operated in the RF range. The exposure depends on the type of system it is. As long as the systems are operated according to the manufacturer's requirements and the systems comply with relevant CENELEC standards, below the exposure limits. RF exposure for workers can be caused by several industrial appliances operating in the RF range, for example for heating (e.g. RF sealers) or from maintenance of broadcasting stations or radar installations. The exposure to the worker operating such systems can reach values close or even above the limits of the Directive 2004/40/EC.

Regarding the objectives of this chapter, two main RF sources are considered: those operated for general purpose far away from the human body, and those generated by medical applications.

a. Sources operated far away from the human body

Such sources are typically fixed installed RF transmitters. An example is base stations that are an essential part of mobile communication networks necessary to establish the link between the mobile telephone and the rest of the network. In most European countries, base stations have become ubiquitous in guaranteeing connectivity in large areas of the respective countries.

Other important RF sources are broadcasting systems (AM and FM radio and TV). The range of exposure is similar to analogue TV systems. However, the digital systems require more transmitters than the older analogue systems; therefore there is public concern that this can result in somewhat higher average exposure levels.

Other examples of sources relevant for far field exposure of the general population are civil and military radar systems, private mobile radio systems, or new technologies like WiMAX.

b. Medical applications

Several medical applications use electromagnetic fields in the RF range. Therapeutic applications such as soft tissue healing appliances, hyperthermia for cancer treatment, or diathermy expose the patient well above the recommended limit values to achieve the intended biological effects. These include heating of tissue (analgesic applications) or burning cells (to kill cancer cells). Therapeutic and diagnostic applications, like Magnetic Resonance Imaging (MRI), are allowed to exceed the basic restrictions of Council Recommendation 1999/519/EC as there is a benefit for the patient. In these cases exposure of therapists or other medical personnel needs to be controlled to avoid the possibility that their exposure exceeds the exposure limit values stipulated by Directive 2004/40/EC for occupational exposure. Usual frequencies are those allowed for industrial, scientific, and medical applications similar to most industrial sources. Magnetic resonance imaging devices in medical diagnostics use RF fields in addition to static and variable fields. Most actual clinical MRI devices work at 63 MHz or 126 MHz.

Concerns have been fuelled by the introduction of these technologies, often in the absence of a reliable knowledge base, on both likely exposure to people and on potential adverse health effects. This experience has highlighted the need for foresight and pro-action in dealing with the introduction of such technologies. Now, retrospectively, the results of good quality research are being published which provide a measure of reassurance as to the general low levels of exposure and to potential effects on health of some existing EMF technologies, but not for all technologies. The cost of such uncertainties and lack of foresight has been significant in respect to introducing these technologies and to health and other public authorities in dealing effectively with public concerns. In the years ahead, many new EMF related technologies will be introduced and potential health concerns should be identified and addressed through: a rigorous examination of the technologies in respect to their use and exposure to people, identification of potential adverse health effects in the light of current scientific evidence, exchanging the results of ongoing research and, overall, the provision of a focus for information exchange and research activities.

The situation of EM environments in healthcare facilities must be differentiated - where medical devices and human exposure are under control of the healthcare organization- from home and mobile situations, as is the case for a growing number of modern telemedicine applications.

Today, with the aid of telemedicine, patients can remain at home, which provides a better quality of life, especially for the prevention and management of chronic illnesses of elderly people. Telemonitoring and telecare systems are playing a key role in bringing attention to patients with mobility impairments and that require constant attention but have no doctors nearby. In contrast to the conventional use of medical devices, the latest wireless sensors are wearable and can be used intermittently over a long period of time by a large number of people.

The problem arises when wireless telemonitoring and telecommunication systems coexist in the same environment. The current electromagnetic compatibility and immunity standards do not cater for the emerging home telemonitoring scenarios. The compatibility among the new technologies of wireless communication becomes a critical issue for telemedicine applications, especially when dealing with continuous data, whose readings should not be interrupted, for example in critical cases of ECG monitoring.

3.2 Research objectives

This chapter discusses Electromagnetic Interference (EMI) by means of recognition, which involves not only the devices themselves but also the environment in which they are used, and anything that may come into that environment. Several factors make EM compatibility difficult. These include proliferation of new devices, mobility, the trend toward digital interfaces and the reliance on weak signals. Other factors are the unprecedented changes in medicine technologies as well as new wireless-frequencies management, services and technologies.

"Nomadic technologies" that help to free up our everyday lives for example microwave ovens, mobile phones, remote controls, etc. tend to utilize unlicensed frequency bands where the Resulting Electromagnetic Interferences (EMI) can have an effect on any electronic device. The result with a medical device would not only be an inconvenience but also it could potentially be life-threatening. Particularly as these telemetry systems will have to coexist in the same home electromagnetic environment as a large number of other wireless links. In the current standards, there are no quantifiable conditions regarding human exposure and long-term and low-intensity effects and medical devices Electromagnetic Compatibility (EMC).

The necessary effort to assure Electromagnetic Compatibility (EMC) of personal mobile telemedicine is motivated by the possible degradation in electronic medical devices, which could potentially result in deaths, serious injuries, or administration of inappropriate treatment. Furthermore, the electromagnetic environment continues to intensify with cellular and portable phones, wireless modems, mobile communications, paging systems, and telemetry, which share communications frequencies with home medical telemetry devices. Device users are generally not aware of the field strengths, frequency distribution, or temporal characteristics of their electromagnetic environment. The focus will subsequently shift to identify those EMF technology applications and services currently in use and/or likely to be released in the future and, where possible, to characterise likely exposures and identify potential health concerns associated with their use. Likely candidates might include, for example: so-called 4G (and further developments in mobile telephony), ad hoc networks, W-LANS, WiMax, Zigbee, Bluetooth, Wimedia, UWB, broad-band over power transmission lines, various EASD and RFID applications and further digital broadcasting.

One emerging approach to improving the wearability of continuous ambulatory monitoring systems is to improve body-attached sensors with built-in wireless telemetry, thus freeing the user from having to carry a data recorder. For these telemetry systems, it is quite probable that a large number of wireless links coexist in the same area sharing the electromagnetic environment. There is negligible or relatively little knowledge of local sources of RF radiation on close proximity to metallic implants, external or implanted medical devices.

The focus of this chapter is the characterization of electromagnetic environments currently present in urban homes in order to make an assessment for the potential safe use of home telemonitoring systems, according to the international standards for RF immunity of medical devices set by the International Electrotechnical Commision (IEC) Standard 60601-1-2. There is no regulation yet for the emerging telemedicine home scenarios.

4. Methods

Nowadays the use of RF sources is widespread in our society. Prominent examples are mobile communication, broadcasting or medical and industrial applications. Information on emissions arising from RF sources is often available and can be used for compliance assessment or similar applications such as in-situ measurements. It should be taken into account that information on the exposure of individual persons is scarce. Such information is mainly needed for epidemiological studies. There is therefore a need to optimise methodology to assess individual exposure, e.g. by using and further developing existing dosimeters.

The existing RF sources are operated in different frequency bands and emit different output power (EMF levels). Developments in wireless technologies have also had a huge influence in the field of medical applications, enabling wireless bio-monitoring for medical patient care or workers at risk (Budinger, 2003). Nevertheless, several medical applications use electromagnetic fields in the RF range whose usual frequencies are those allowed for industrial, scientific, and medical applications similar to most industrial sources.

The problem arises when wireless telemonitoring and telecommunication systems coexist in the same environment, as the current electromagnetic compatibility and immunity standards do not cater for the emerging home telemonitoring scenarios. The compatibility among the new technologies of wireless communication becomes a critical issue for healthcare environments (Urdiales-Garcia et al., 2007).

In order to assure the compatibility among wireless systems, EMF measurements have to be performed. To make EMF measurement in the frequency range 100 kHz to 300 GHz, different sets of instruments for each of the frequency spans must be used. Usually the instrumentation only covers a certain range of frequencies, for instance from 100 kHz to 30 MHz, another set goes from 10 MHz to 300 MHz and other from 100 MHz to 10 GHz. For frequencies below 300 MHz typically, both the electric and magnetic fields must be measured. Below 100 MHz there is also a need to measure both the contact and the induced current, and this demands another set of instruments.

Regarding the assessment of Electromagnetic Compatibility (EMC) in healthcare environments, several measurement procedures could be proposed. The first one is calibrated to obtain the EMF trend averages, maxima and minima over time. These values can be achieved measuring the EMF with a wide band dosimeter. In order to analyse the contribution of each emitting source over time, a second procedure based on a selective filtering of the spectrum is proposed. A dosimeter with predefined frequency bands is needed for this purpose. Finally, an ad hoc study could be performed by means of a spectrum analyser, obtaining the fundamental frequency, harmonics and emission power.

Regarding the assessment of Electromagnetic Compatibility (EMC) in healthcare environments, two different measurements have been performed. In order to analyse the contribution of each emitting source over time, measurements have been performed in urban homes using dosimeters with predefined frequency bands. The second one has been made in the laboratory, by means of measuring the radiation emitted by several RF emitters devices.

4.1 Measurements in urban homes

This research addressed the characterization of EM environments present in urban homes, regarding the assessment for potential safe use of home telemedicine systems. EM field levels have been measured with both ESM-30 "RadMan XT" Radiation Monitor and a portable device ANTENNESSA EME SPY 120, during the years 2007 and 2008. The first one used is a battery powered, portable ESM-30 "RadMan XT" Radiation Monitor (Narda Safety Test Solutions GmbH) that automatically measures and records data on site. This device measures according to the standard ICNIRP-98 in broadband and the E-field and H-field is expressed as percentages of the standard limit values in range 1 MHz - 40 GHz (see Fig.1 and Fig.2).
The second dosimeter used is a dosimeter ANTENNESSA EME SPY 120. It is a selective, isotropic personal exposure meter that has been designed for epidemiological studies. It can measure 12 frequency bands (FM, TV3, TETRA, TV4&5, GSM Rx&Tx, DCS Rx&Tx, DECT, UMTS Rx&Tx, Wi-Fi) and can identify the contribution of each emitter. This device measures the E field according to the standard ICNIRP-98 and also gives results in V/m and μW/cm^2. It has been configured to sample every 90 or 120 seconds, and the measurement period is 7 to 9 days in 16 hour segments respectively.

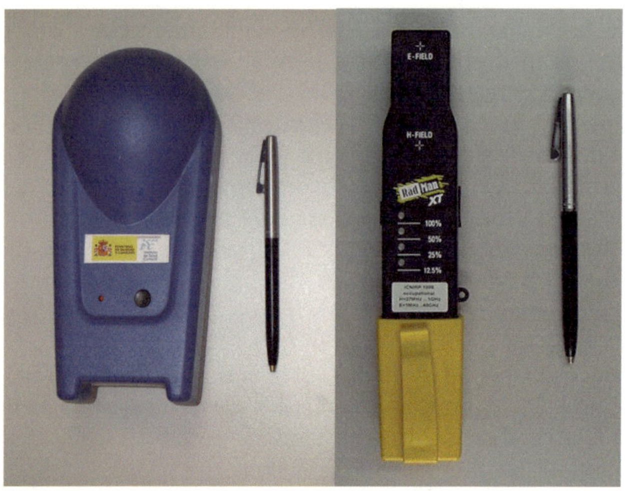

Fig. 1. Antennessa EME SPY and RadMan XT dosimeters

During the measurement time, dosimeters have been placed in different rooms of the houses. The position of the dosimeters in each room is random, although if there is any electronic device, it was recommended to place the dosimeters between 50 cm and 1 meter, in order to keep far field condition.
Data from these measurements have been saved and processed, in order to compare them with the International Electrotechnical Commission (IEC) Standard 601-1-2 (IEC, 2002) and the ICNIRP-98 standard (ICNIRP, 1998) (see Fig.2 and Fig.3). A Geographic Information System (GIS) has been used to represent obtained data (Giannopoulou, 2008).

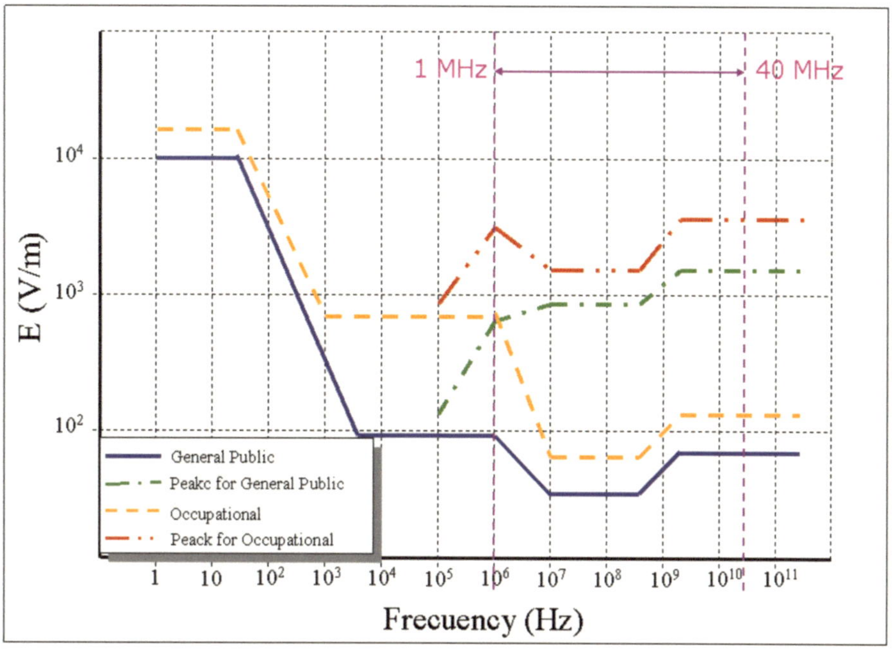

(a)

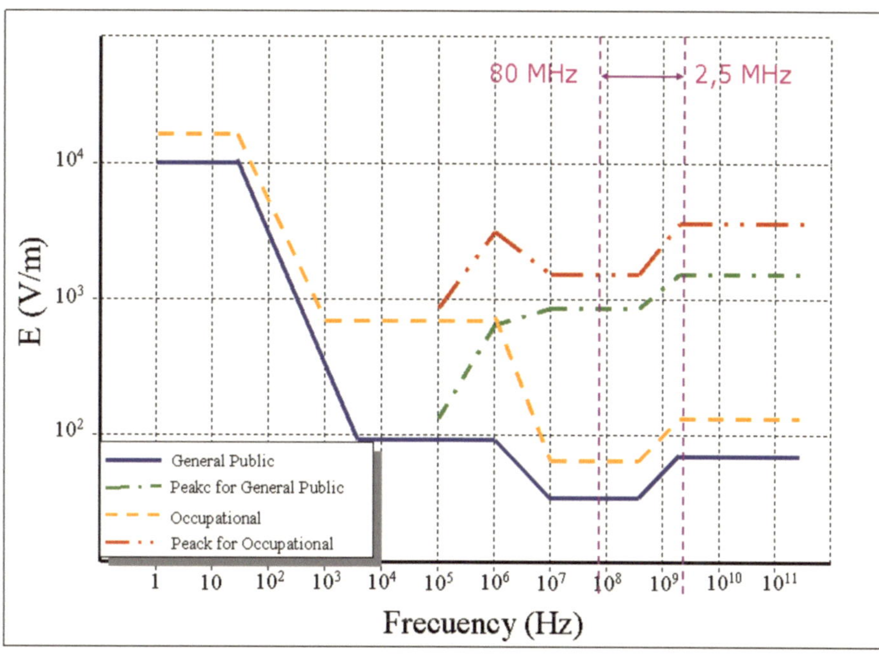

(b)

Fig. 2. E Field reference level of ICNIRP 98. Fig. 2-a-frequency band in RadMan XT and Fig. 2-b frequency band in SPY 120

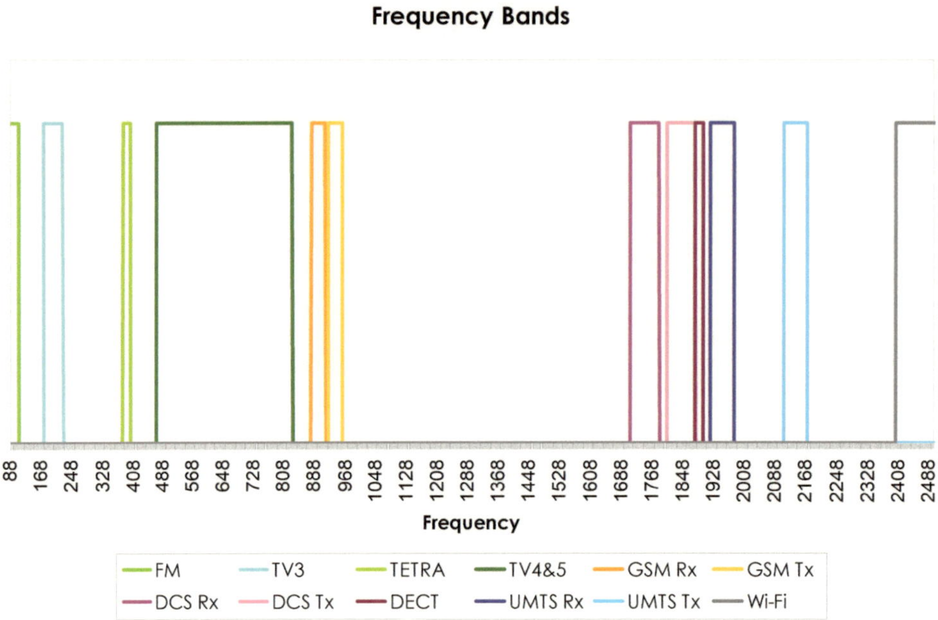

Fig. 3. Distribution of the 12 frequency measurement bands of ANTENNESSA EME SPY 120

Finally, an ad hoc study was performed by means of a spectrum analyser Rohde & Schwarz FSH6, obtaining the fundamental frequency, harmonics, emission power, signal characterization, identification of unknown signals, signal monitoring and field strength measurements. Its characteristics are: Frequency range: 100 kHz to 6 GHz, Detection limits: -80 dBm to +20 dBm, Resolution band: 100 Hz to 1 MHz.

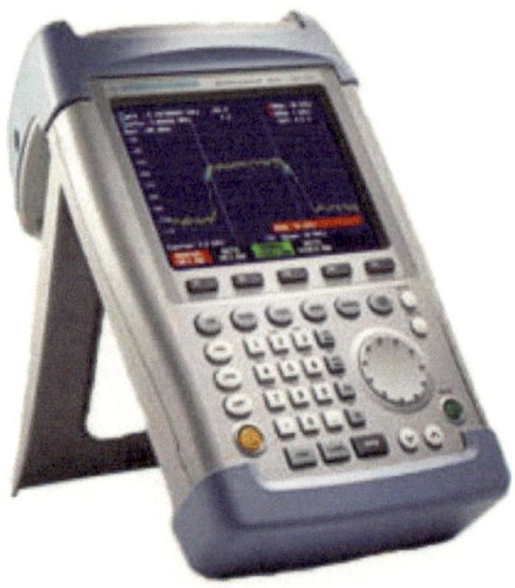

Fig. 4. Spectrum analyzer Rohde & Schwarz FSH6

4.2 Measurements in laboratory

Measurements of GSM and DECT equipments and a microwave oven have been performed. These measurements have been made in far field conditions, using the Narda Broadband Field Meter NBM-550 with the isotropic probe for electric field 1891 (NBM). The frequency range of the probe goes from 3 MHz to 18 GHz and it can measure from 600 mV/m to 1000 kV/m.

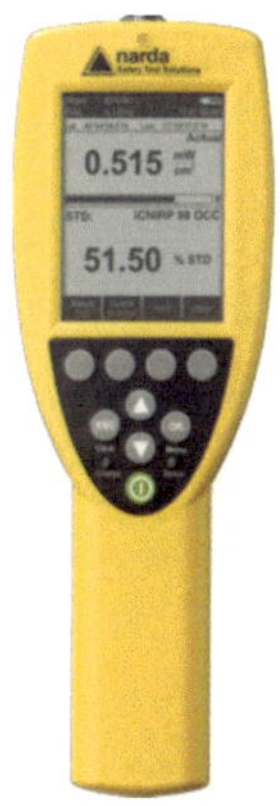

Fig. 5. Narda Broadband Field Meter NBM-550

For the GSM technology, four different measurements have been performed. The first one was made with a Nokia 6230 and Orange card, the second one with the same cellular phone but a Vodafone card, the third one with a Siemens M55 with a Movistar card and the forth one with a Samsung SGH-E250 and an Orange card. The Siemens phone is approximately 5 years old, the Nokia is 2 years old and the Samsung is about 4 months old. Measurements have been started at a distance of 3 meters, moving closer to the dosimeter at intervals of 0.5 meters until arriving at a distance of 0.5 meters (to keep the far field condition). At each distance, 4 measurements have been taken, rotating the cellular phone 90° every time. Measurements have been performed in two configurations: during the start of the call to that mobile and during a period of conversation, for 50 seconds each measurement. In the end, 48 measurements have been taken for each cellular phone.

DECT technology has been measured with two different models of phones, Siemens Giga Set A260 and Telefonica Famitel Novo. The procedure of the measurements is the same one as explained for the cellular phones, but the measurements have been repeated twice, once measuring the terminal and also measuring the base. At the end, 96 measurements have been taken for each wireless phone. A similar procedure has been adopted for measuring the microwave oven. The time of measurement has been reduced to 30 seconds, and the microwave oven has been measured in 2 angles of rotation with the same protocol explained before. Finally 12 measurements have been recorded for the microwave oven.

5. Results

Global results reported from homes studied in the metropolitan area of Madrid were analysed observing the contribution of the 12 frequency bands. Measurements made in Madrid are mapped and the maximum peak obtained in each house with the ANTENNESSA EME SPY is represented. Data from these measurements has been saved and processed, in order to compare them with the International Electrotechnical Commission (IEC) Standard 60601-1-2 and the ICNIRP-98. Then, results obtained with some of the electronic RF devices tested in laboratory will be shown.

5.1 Results of measurements in urban homes

Measurements made in Madrid during the years 2007 and 2008 are shown in the map (see Fig.6) The maximum peak obtained in each house with the ANTENNESSA EME SPY is represented in this map. Values are normalized according to the standard ICNIRP 98. The range of these values goes from 0 to 1.51, in those cases where the value limit has been gone beyond this range.

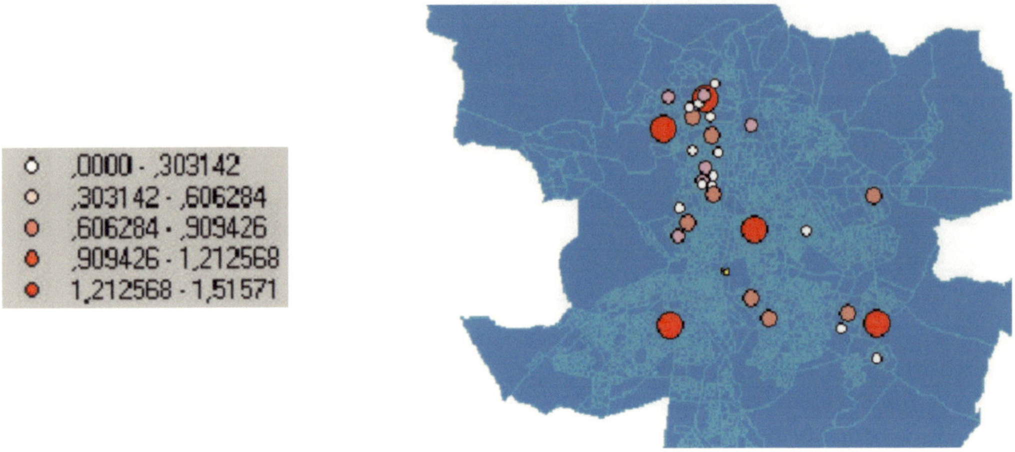

Fig. 6. Maximum peaks found (V/m)

According to the technology that causes the E Field, the distribution of number of peaks >10% ICNIRP in each home is displayed in Fig. 7. As it is shown, most of the peaks occurred because of the GSM or DCS technology. Nevertheless, in those cases where there are many peaks, the technologies causing this are FM, Wi-Fi or DECT.

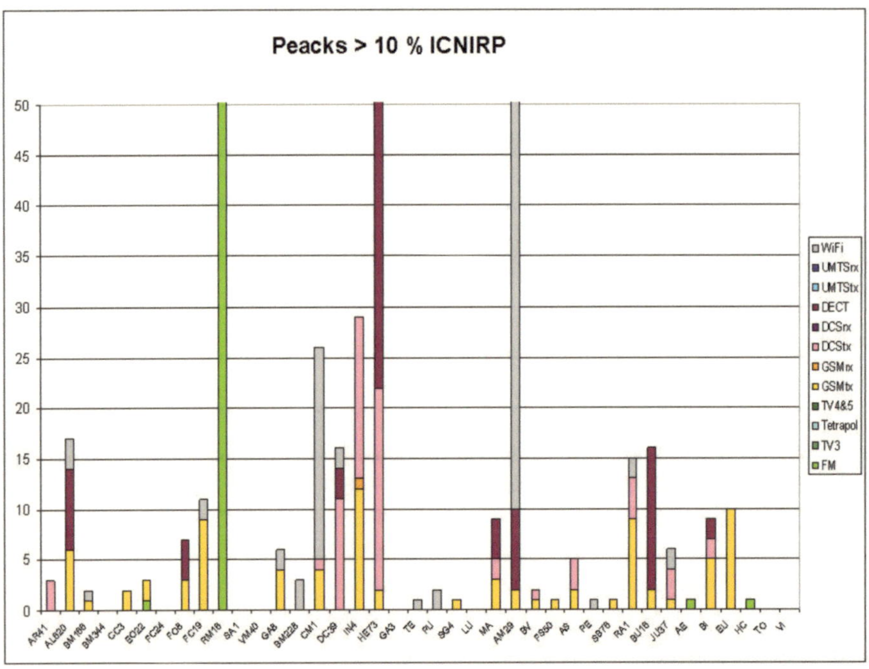

Fig. 7. Number of peaks obtained according to the technology

According to the IEC Standard 60601-1-2, a maximum E field of 3V/m is set for non-life supporting devices. Representation of the peaks higher than 3 V/m is shown in Fig. 8. As we can see, in most cases the value found corresponds to the maximum value that the dosimeter can measure (5.02 V/m). This means that these peaks are probably higher than 5.02 V/m although the dosimeter is not able to measure them.

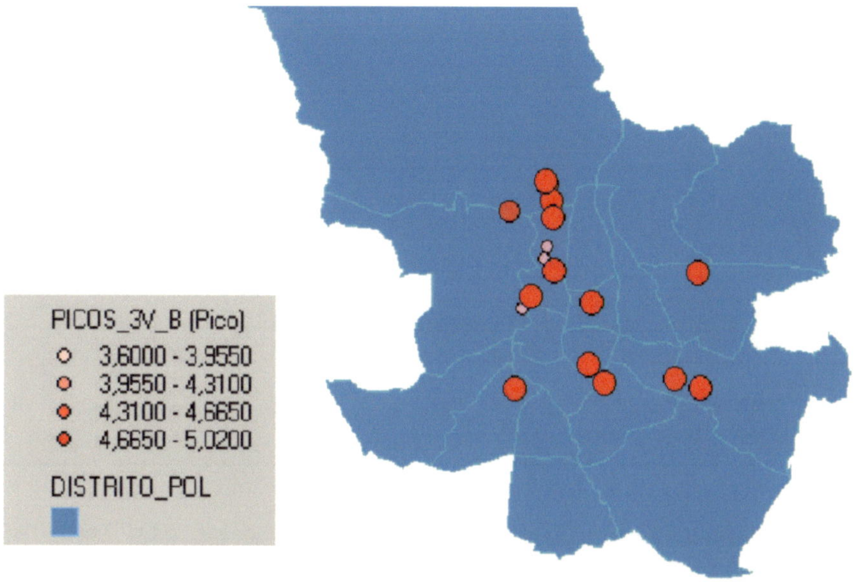

Fig. 8. Peaks higher than 3 V/m

Regarding the results obtained with the wide band dosimeter RadMan XT, no peak higher than 10% ICNIRP has been observed in any measurement. The difference between the results obtained with the dosimeter ANTENNESSA EME SPY 120 and the dosimeter RadMan XT is that in this one, measurements are made in broadband (for the E field, from 1 MHz to 40 GHz) and they are not localized in one band. Therefore, peaks obtained are much higher when the frequency bands are narrower.

Results obtained with RadMan XT did not show any important peak in the houses studied, as it is a broadband dosimeter. Baseline levels are always below the 10% of the ICNIRP standard.

Service	**Freq. band (MHz)**	**E (V/m)**	**Ref level IEC 60601-1-2 (V/m)**	**ICNIRP (%)**
Wi-Fi	2400-2500	5.02	3	68
DECT	1880-1900	5.02	3	71
GSM tx	925-960	2.36	3	34

Table 1. E Field level of some services and reference level of Medical electrical equipment standard

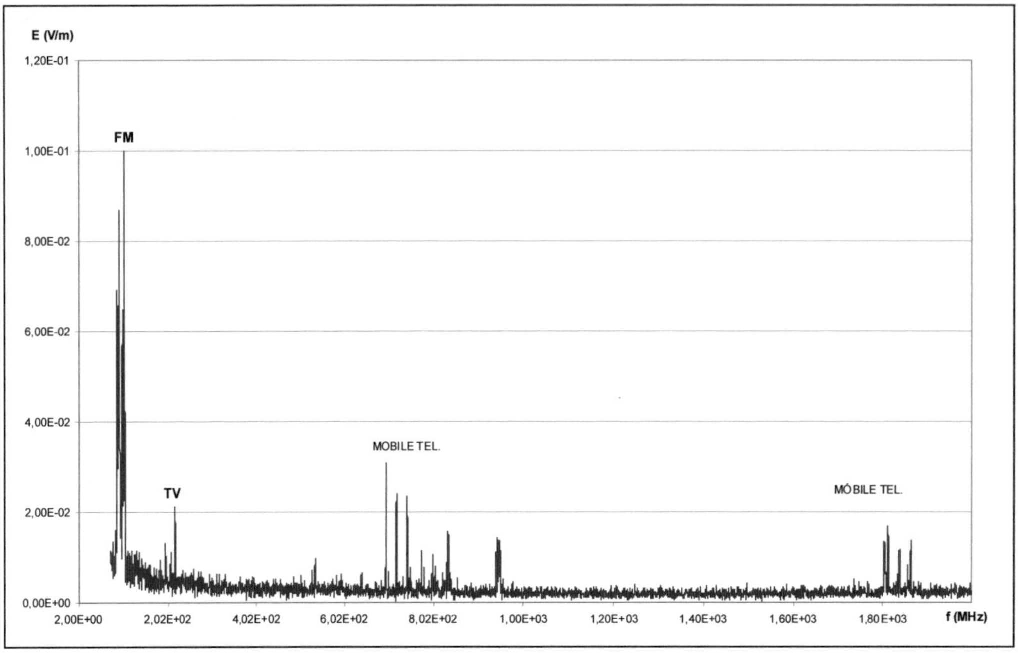

Fig. 9. Frequency composition of environmental EMF

Regarding the results obtained with the Spectrum Analyser R&S FSH6, frequency composition of environmental EMF in the area of observation is fixed by technologies used in the area. The presented frequency spectrum in Fig. 9 is typical for urban areas.

These results obtained with all the technologies measured are similar to other measurements of indoor passive RF-exposure of children (Decat et al., 2008). This study's conclusion was that within a radius of 1.60m, the exposure is substantially higher than the total field generated by all the indoor and outdoor wireless sources put together. These results are also in line with other work (Karpowicz, 2010) concluding that increased level of EMF, even EMF of level > 3 V/m might exist in the vicinity of EMF sources and special attention is needed in case of propagation difficulties for mobile phone devices. A significant difference in the median level of registered E-field should be noted - the shorter the increased E-field in the environment, the lower the hazard of unwanted exposure results in both humans and electronic devices. Potential interferences could vary from one location to the next, depending on combination, type and even the electronic equipment in use.

5.2 Results of measurements in laboratory

The most characteristic results obtained in the laboratory are shown in this section. As explained before, all these measurements have been done with the Narda Broadband Field Meter NBM-550 with an isotropic probe for the electric field.

Fig.10-a) shows the results obtained from the Nokia 6230 mobile phone terminal during the start of a call. The maximum, average and minimum electric field can be observed. The peak has a value of 3.5 V/m approximately, while the distance is 0.5 meters. Fig.10-b) shows the strength of the E-field depending on the position of the phone. Results on the electric field during a conversation are not shown because the levels of the field are lower than those of Fig.10-a).

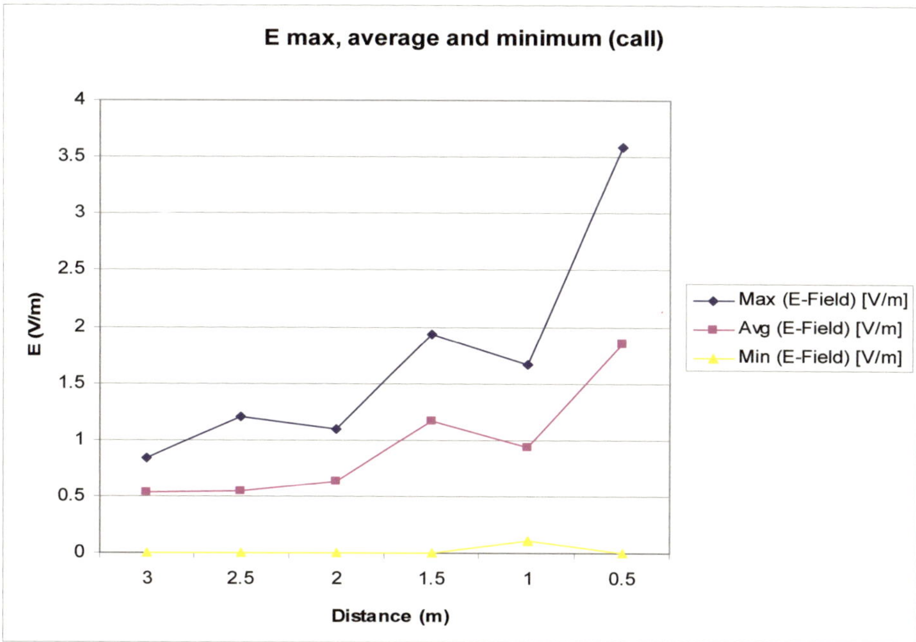

Fig. 10. a) Maximum, average and minimum E field measured, during a starting call to the Nokia 6230.

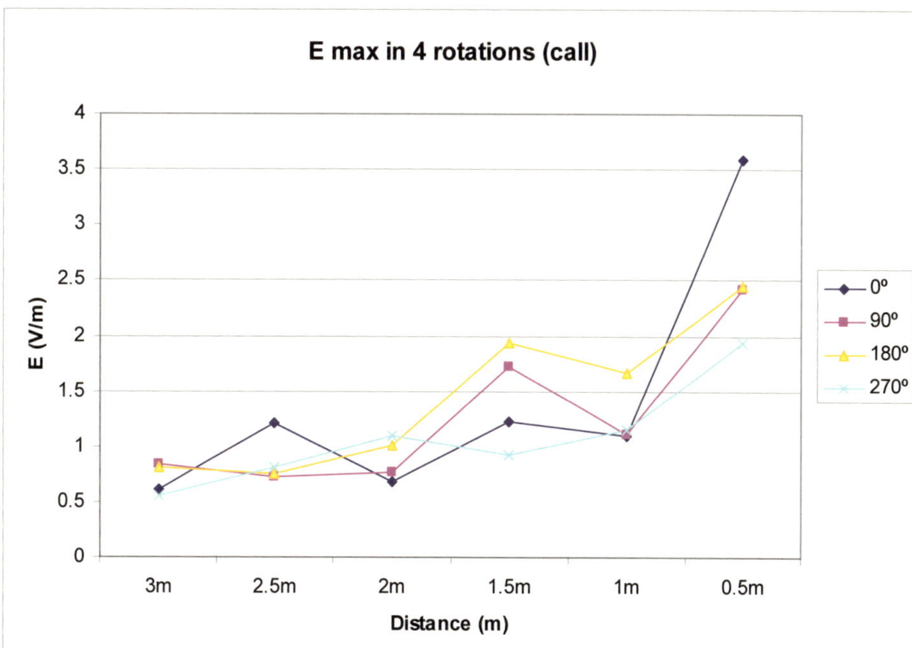

Fig. 10. b) Maximum E field according to the position of the phone, during a starting call to the Nokia 6230.

Comparing results obtained from the four performed experiments, we can observe that the oldest cellular phone (Siemens M55) is the one with the highest peaks of E field, reaching 7 V/m at a distance of 0.5 meters. The other experiments reach values of about 3.5 or 4 V/m at the same distance (see Fig. 11-a). In Fig.11-b) the SAR (specific absorption rate) for each model of phone measured is shown. In this case, the newest phone is the one that has less SAR. According to the distance from the different antennas (Orange, Vodafone and Movistar) to the laboratory, the Vodafone one was the nearest (266 meters) while the Orange and Movistar are at 468 and 462 meters respectively. Observing the data in the figure, the distance to the antenna is not relevant because the phone with the Vodafone card has the same levels as the same one using the Orange card.
The following evaluation was done with the E field radiated by a microwave oven. This microwave oven was chosen among those measured with the ANTENNESSA EME SPY, because of its high levels present (approximately 70% of the ICNIRP standard, at a distance of 0.5m). In this case, the levels are already higher than 3 V/m at a distance of 2.5 meters, reaching 7.8 V/m at 0.5 meters. As we expected, at the back of the oven, the fields emitted are a bit lower (see Fig. 12).
Fig. 13 shows the results obtained from the two different models of wireless phones with DECT technology. Measurements have been made in call and conversation mode, measuring separately the handset and the base. Levels have reached a maximum of 1.2 V/m for the handset and 1.4 V/m for the base, so they are always under the levels specified by the standard 60601-1-2 for immunity for medical devices.

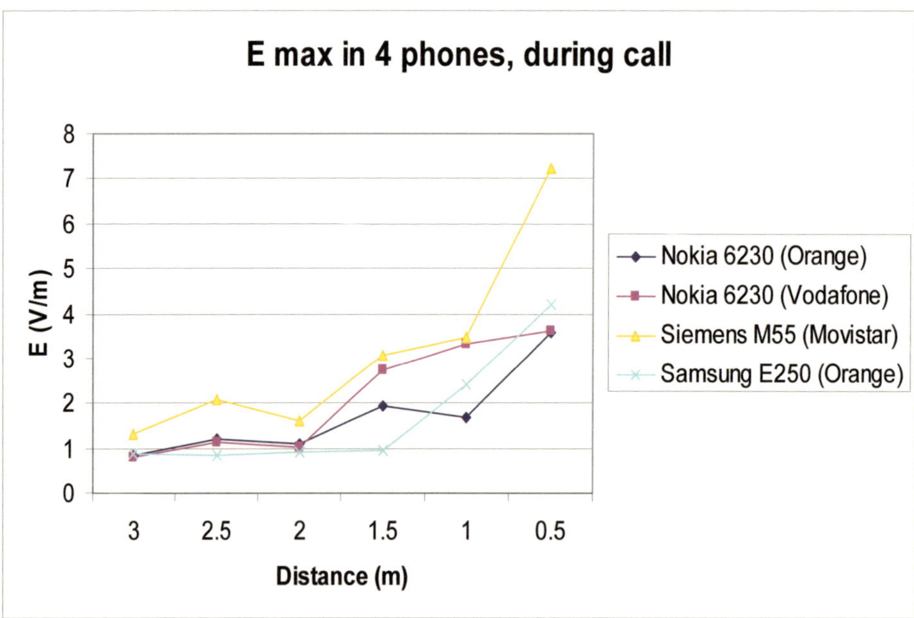

Fig. 11. a) Maximum E field for the 4 experiments with cellular phones.

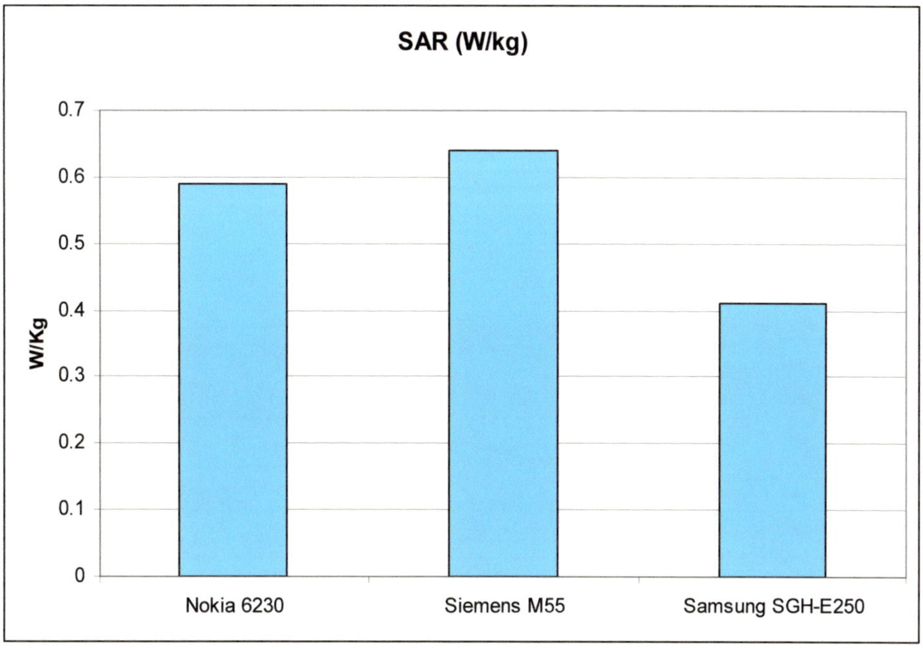

Fig. 11. b) SAR of each model.

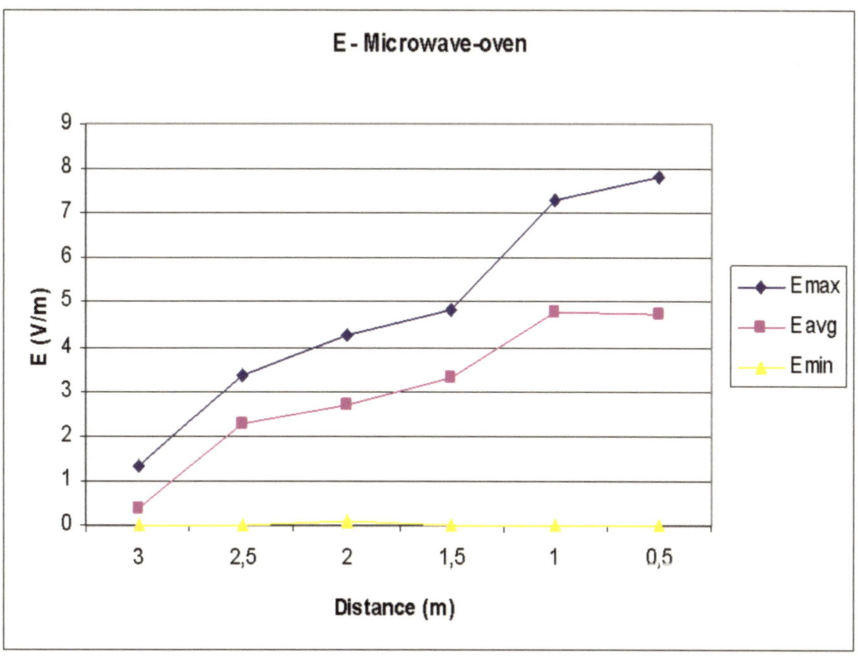

Fig. 12. a) Maximum, average and minimum E field measured in a microwave-oven.

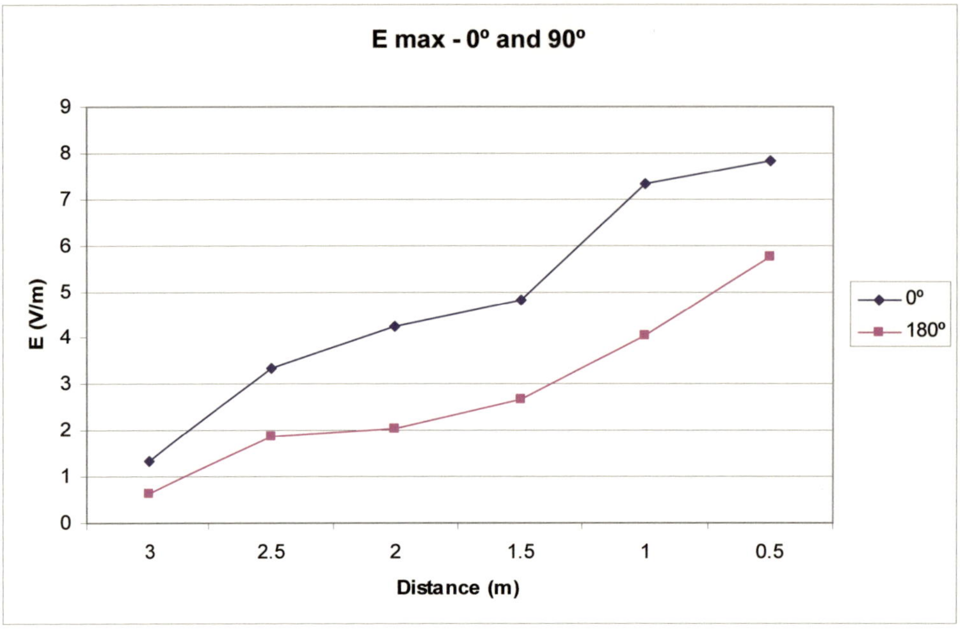

Fig. 12. b) Maximum E field measured in 2 positions (front and back side of microwave oven)

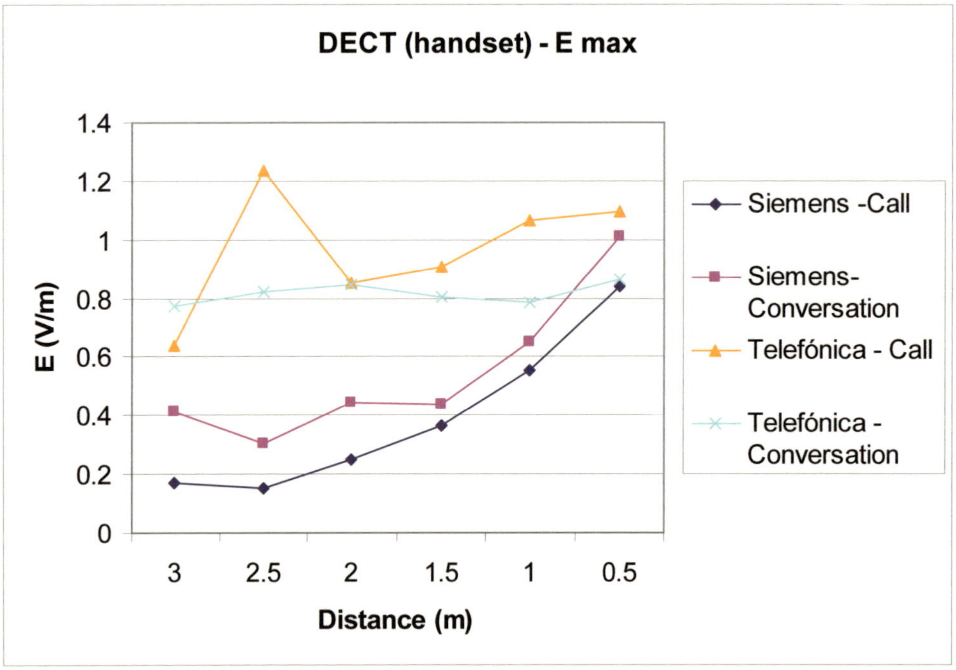

Fig. 13. Maximum E field measured in two different models of wireless phones with DECT technology. Fig.13-a) in the handset

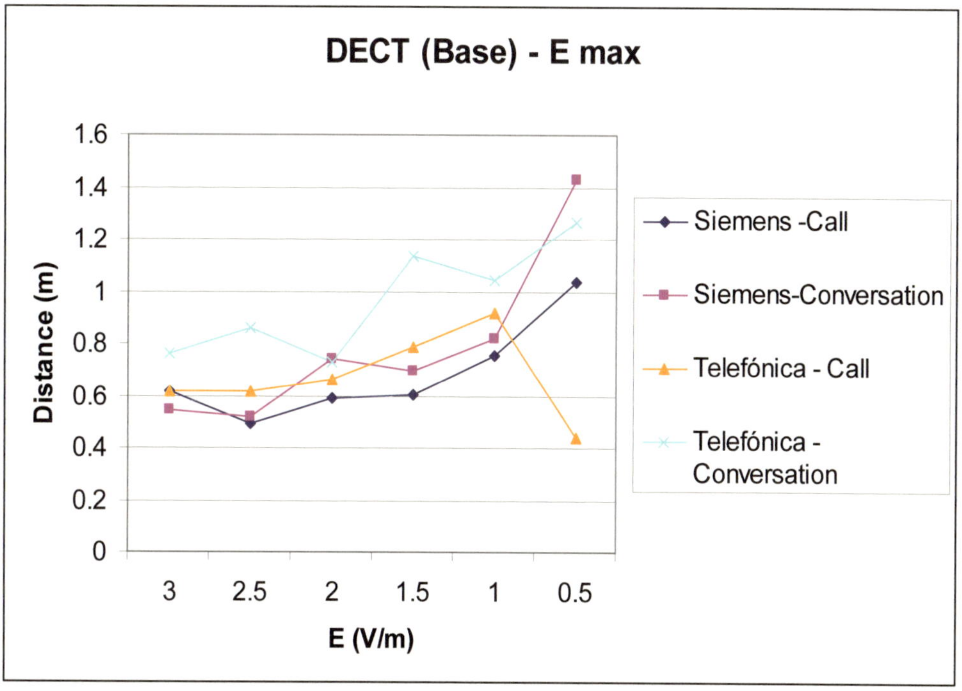

Fig. 13. b) in the base station.

6. Discussions

Real time, reliable, safe, interoperable, fully integrated wireless medical systems are expected to be widely deployed for home and personal care. The new solutions must be considered issues with respect to electromagnetic compatibility and regulatory compliance (COMAR, 2005).

With the increased use of radio networks in the proximity of home medical devices, it will be important to determine the zone/s with higher levels of exposure as well as the relative contribution of auxiliary antennas that may be installed in the proximity (even with no license or not in a permanent basis).

The European Union has recognized the importance of EMC, and all products sold in Europe must now meet the essential requirements of the EMC Directive. The IEC electro medical devices standard, IEC 60601-1-2 (IEC, 2002), permits radiated-immunity testing of non-life-supporting and life-supporting equipment from 80 MHz to 2,5 GHz, and Safety Distance Limits for patient-coupled devices.

ICNIRP-98 and the Council Recommendation 1999/519/EC (European Commission, 1999), of 12 July 1999, on the limitation of exposure of the general public to electromagnetic field (0

Hz to 300 GHz) outline a set of basic restrictions and reference levels for the Member States to follow. Compliance with these guidelines may not necessarily preclude interference with, or effects on, emerging home telemedicine systems.
According to the research results observed by the authors, the base line EM levels are below the security threshold stated by ICNIRP-98. It means E field levels in urban home environments are apparently safe in accordance with health and safety requirements, regarding the patients' exposure to the risks arising from electromagnetic fields. Nevertheless, data compared with ICNIRP standard for human exposure show high levels in Wi-Fi, DECT and GSMtx bands. That can be seen in Fig.10, Fig.11, Fig.12 and Fig.13.
The detected presence of quite high levels in some frequency bands reveals the need to pay attention to potential Electromagnetic Interference (EMI) problems in particular cases, where there is the possibility of RFI problems with medical devices. It makes it necessary to assess local EM conditions regarding home telemedicine risk analysis.
Proper design and installation of medical devices, coupled with proper characterization and management of potential sources of electromagnetic emission in the local environment, can protect against EMI.

7. Conclusion

Mobile phone technology relies upon an extensive network of fixed antennas, or base stations, relaying information with RF signals. Other wireless networks that allow high-speed internet access and services, such as Wireless Local Area Networks (WLANs), are also increasingly common in homes, offices, and many public areas (airports, schools, residential and urban areas). As the number of RF sources rises; so does, in some cases, the RF exposure of the population, depending on a variety of factors such as the proximity to the transmitter and the surrounding environment.
International and national bodies have set different limit values for permissible electromagnetic radiation levels in various standards and regulations. The European Union has recognized the importance of EMC, and all products sold in Europe must now meet the essential requirements of the EMC Directive. Compliance with these guidelines may not necessarily preclude interference with, or have effects on, emerging telemonitoring applications used at home outside of hospitals.
New wireless solutions must be considered issues with respect to electromagnetic compatibility and regulatory compliance. It would make a local assessment necessary and risk analysis prior to the installation of a home telemonitoring application. The degree and type of EMF exposure currently encountered in domestic settings needs to be characterized, in order to ensure that the equipment operates properly and exposure guidelines are not exceeded.

8. References

Budinger, T.E. (2003) "Biomonitoring with wireless communications," *Annual Review of Biomedical Engineering, vol. 5*, pp. 383-412.

COMAR Reports. (2005) Committee on Man and Radiation. COMAR Technical Information Statement the IEEE exposure limits for radiofrequency and microwave energy. *IEEE Engineering in Medicine and biology*. March/April 2005 pp. 114-121.

Decat, G., Deckx, L., and Maris, U. (2008) Personal exposimetry for measuring the indoor exposure of children to ELF, VLF and RF-field generated by internal and external electromagnetic field sources, *Environment health Unit of the Department of Environment, Nature and Energy*, Flemish Government, Belgique.

European Commission (1999) Recommendation 1999/519/EC], of 12 July 1999 on the limitation of exposure of the general public to electromagnetic field (0 Hz to 300 GHz)

European Commission (2001) Community Research. 'ISTAG Scenarios for Ambient Intelligence in 2010' User-friendly information society.

European Commission (2008) COST Action BM 0704 Emerging EMF Technologies and Health risk management.
http://www.cost-bm0704.org/

ICNIRP (1998) Guidelines for limiting exposure to protection time-varying electric, magnetic and electromagnetic fields (up to 300 GHz). International Commission on Non-Ionizing Radiation

IEC (2002) International Electrothecnical Commission (IEC) Standard IEC 60601-1-2 Electromedical devices.

Giannopoulou, E.G. (2008) Data Mining in Medical and Biological Research. Ed: *IN-TECH* ISBN 978-953-7619-30-5

Karpowicz, J. (2010) Electromagnetic fields in home and public environment and home care devices ISSN: 1559-9450 Symposium PIERS 2010. Cambridge, USA, 5-8 July Published by The Electromagnetics Academy

Monteagudo, J.L. and Reig, J. (2004) E-health and the elderly, a new range of services?, The *IPTS Report*, Sevilla.

Ramos, V. (2005) Electromagnetic Compatibility and safety in wireless personal networks for biotelemetry. PhD. Dissertation, University of Alcala, Spain.

Urdiales-Garcia, C., García-Sigler, F., Domínguez-Duran, M., de-la-Torre, J., Coslado-Aristizabal, F., Pérez-Parras, S., Trapero-Miralles, R., and Sandoval-Hernández, F. (2007) On practical issues about interference in telecare applications based on different wireless technologies, *Telemed J E Health*, vol. 13, pp. 519-33.

WHO, World Health Organization, (2005) *Report on Research Needs, Environment and Health Implications of Electromagnetic Field Exposure* - EMF-NET/WHO COMMITTEE –, Available in:
http://web.jrc.ec.europa.eu/emf-net/doc/reports/EMF-NET%20Research%20Needs%20August%202005.pdf (accessed 17 August 2010)

WHO, World Health Organization, (2006) *Framework for developing health-based EMF standards*. Geneva.

WHO, World Health Organization, (2010) *WHO research agenda for radiofrequency fields* WHO Library Cataloguing-in-Publication Data, ISBN 978 92 4 159994 8 Geneve. Available in:
http://whqlibdoc.who.int/publications/2010/9789241599948_eng.pdf (accessed 19 August 2010)

Part 2

Applied Technologies

4

High-Quality Telemedicine Using Digital Video Transport System over Global Research and Education Network

Shuji Shimizu[1], Koji Okamura[2], Naoki Nakashima[3], Yasuichi Kitamura[4], Nobuhiro Torata[5], Yasuaki Antoku[6], Takanori Yamashita[7], Toshitaka Yamanokuchi[8], Shinya Kuwahara[9] and Masao Tanaka[10]

[1,2,3,5,6,7,8,9,10]*Telemedicine Development Center of Asia, Kyushu University Hospital,*
[1]*Department of Endoscopic Diagnostics and Therapeutics, Kyushu University Hospital*
[2]*Research Institute for Information Technology, Kyushu University*
[3,6,7,8]*Department of Medical Informatics, Kyushu University Hospital*
[4]*National Institute of Information and Communications Technology*
[9]*Kyushu Electric Power Company*
[10]*Department of Surgery and Oncology, Kyushu University Graduate School of Medical Sciences*
Japan

1. Introduction

Extraordinary advances in communication and information technologies have brought about dramatic changes in our daily lives, including the overwhelming prevalence of emails, web homepages, and mobile phones, all of which are now indispensable both at home and at work. The medical community is no exception, in that the emergence of electronic recording systems, picture archiving and communication systems (PACS), and various digitalized medical equipment has had an enormous impact on clinical practice. Associated with these large waves of technological development, telemedicine has recently been gaining in popularity. It covers a variety of fields including home health care, remote patient monitoring, telementoring and telesurgery, and also encompasses a wide range of sectors from rural health to advanced treatments (Anvari et al., 2005; Hazin et al., 2010; Hu et al., 2009).

However, many doctors are still unfamiliar or unhappy with telemedicine, and the applications are limited to a very small part of daily practice and medical education. What are the reasons for this? We believe there are three key factors. First, the quality of images is critical for accurate diagnosis and appropriate treatment, yet conventional telemedicine often transmits compressed images, inevitably with degraded quality (Demartines et al., 2000; Rabenstein et al., 2002). This is especially true when sending images of surgery and various other medical procedures, because of the limitations of the transmittable bandwidth. Doctors will never be satisfied with these degraded videos, since the fine anatomy of thin membranes or tiny vessels is not clearly distinguishable. The second reason relates to cost. To participate in telemedicine, special teleconferencing equipment needs to be purchased, and this could lead to major reservations in many hospitals (Augestad et al., 2009). Third, the installation and administration of the system is difficult for many doctors and they usually do not have the time to struggle with it. In addition, the medical community is often physically separated from technological departments and they tend not to know the right technical people who would be able to assist them.

A completely new telemedicine system comprising two key technologies, namely, a digital video transport system (DVTS) and the research and education (R&E) network, has been designed to solve all these problems. Here, we introduce the system in sufficient detail to enable readers to set it up themselves and to join our worldwide activities that now cover a variety of medical application fields.

2. Digital Video Transport System (DVTS)

2.1 What is DVTS?

DVTS is software developed by the "WIDE Project" in Japan that can transfer digital video (DV) signal through Internet Protocol (IP) networks using video cameras connected to personal computers (PCs) with an IEEE 1394 cable (Ogawa et al., 1999). By sending and receiving DV streams via the Internet, which employs differentiated data transmission, such a system has the ability to send full resolution videos to remote stations.

2.2 Advantages and Disadvantages of DVTS

The advantages of DVTS are as follows.

1. High quality transmitted images:
   DVTS can preserve the image quality by skipping the compression process. This means that the transmitted video is the same quality as the original source.
2. Low cost:
   Although it is powerful and internationally authorized by the International Telecommunication Union, DVTS software is free of charge. Moreover, regular PCs and DV cameras found in a hospital or at home can be used for setting up the system without the need for purchasing any special videoconferencing equipment.
3. Minimal time delay:
   This can also be achieved because of the omission of the complicated and time-consuming compression process. The time delay under well prepared conditions is only 0.3 sec between international connections.

However, the following issues must also be considered.

1. As much as 30 Mbps network bandwidth is required for each DV stream. Furthermore, not only must the bandwidth be large enough, but there must also be a very stable network for the DVTS to work properly. Quality of service for Internet is very important.
2. There are no sound adjustment functions in the DVTS software. In contrast with conventional videoconferencing systems, which include a sound mixer or echo canceller, DVTS is a simple system merely for sending video together with sound. Microphones and other means to control sound need to be prepared and adjusted separately.

2.3 DVTS software

The DVTS can be installed on a PC running Windows, Mac, or Linux OS platforms from http://www.sfc.wide.ad.jp/DVTS/index.html. DVTS for Windows 0.0.2 (Development build) is the latest version for Windows XP as of June 2010.

The setup window depicted in Fig. 1 is displayed when the DVTS software is executed. For sender setup, input the IP address for the destination at (C) and select the DV device at (D). The default port is 8000 and the settings at (A) need to be changed.
Check the preview monitor at (G) and push "Start send" at (H) to start sending.
For receiver setup, check monitor output at (J), fix the settings at (I), and push "Start Receive" at (M) to start receiving. Use the default port 8000, unless there is a reason for another assignment.
"IEEE1394 Output" at (L) is used to export the DV stream to a DV device (Analog - digital video converter (ADVC), etc.) connected to the port. Another DV device needs to be prepared for the receiver PC, since it is impossible to share the DV device connected to the sender PC.

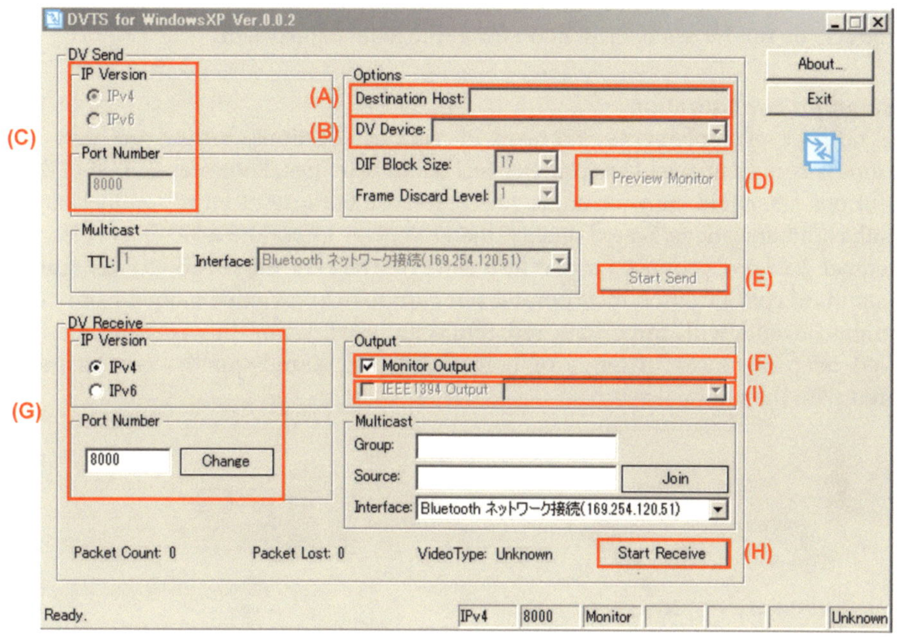

Fig. 1. DVTS window detail

2.4 Equipment and local setup for DVTS

2.4.1 Minimal configuration

Fig. 2 shows the minimal configuration for the DVTS. A DV camera with external microphone is connected to a PC through an IEEE1394 interface for DV image transmission.

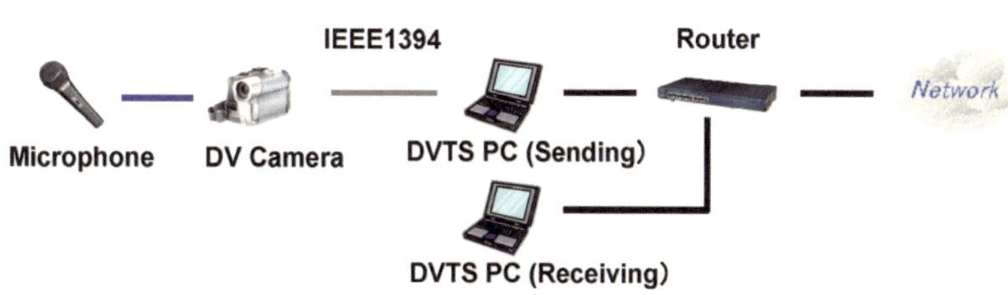

Fig. 2. Minimal configuration for DVTS setup

Although the minimal configuration should be good enough to perform the first local test to get used to the system, it does not provide adequate performance for use in teleconferencing events, because of the following problems.

1. IEEE1394 cable:
   The IEEE1394 cable benefits from the advantages of a direct connection between the DV camera and PC in terms of ease of setting up and simple configuration, but the disadvantages include the limitation of cable length, problems with unplugging because of the plug form, and unavailability of audio and visual mixing.
2. Sound level adjustment:
   Audio trouble is often caused by unsatisfactory audio devices. With the minimal configuration, it is difficult to control the sound level, since the sound comes from the microphone, which is connected via an external microphone plug, and most consumer products do not have a control knob for audio level adjustment.

2.4.2 Standard configuration

As the number of conferences increases at various locations, setting up new member institutions is becoming one of the primary foci of our activities. Poor preparation of the sound system at one site could ruin the entire teleconference because of an uncomfortable echo or unsmooth communications. Sound quality, therefore, is as important a factor as video quality.
In December 2007, we proposed a standard configuration for the DVTS as illustrated in Fig. 3. The standard configuration incorporates our complete knowledge gained from more than one hundred events with three hundred connected sites. Using this configuration, greatly improved teleconferences in terms of both video and sound quality, can be performed compared with the minimal setup.

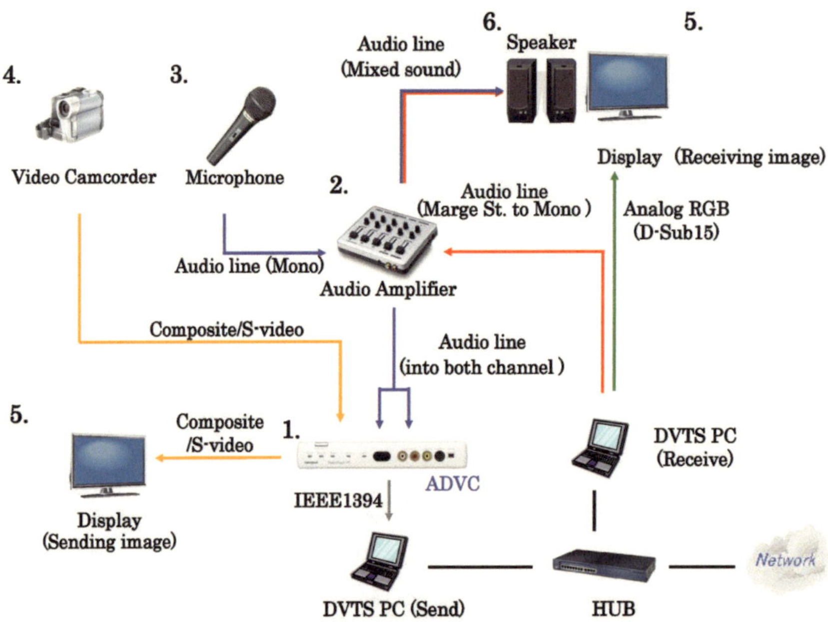

Fig. 3. Standard configuration: 1. Analog-Digital Video Converter (ADVC), 2. Audio amplifier, 3. Microphone, 4. Video camera, 5. Display, 6. Loud speaker

The areas improved are the following.

1. Audio and visual sources are separately connected to the ADVC.
2. Various image inputs from video cameras or medical devices are supported without the use of IEEE1394.
3. Sound echo is reduced by using the "minus one sound" setting.

"Minus one sound" is the fundamental sound setting method for teleconferencing. A configuration that can control transmission and reception of sound sources separately is crucial for avoiding echo noise. Fig. 4 illustrates the "minus one sound" setting. The sound source from the microphone (5) is connected to the ADVC as the sender sound (8). On the other hand, both sound sources (microphone and reception sound (4)) are connected to the loudspeakers (7).

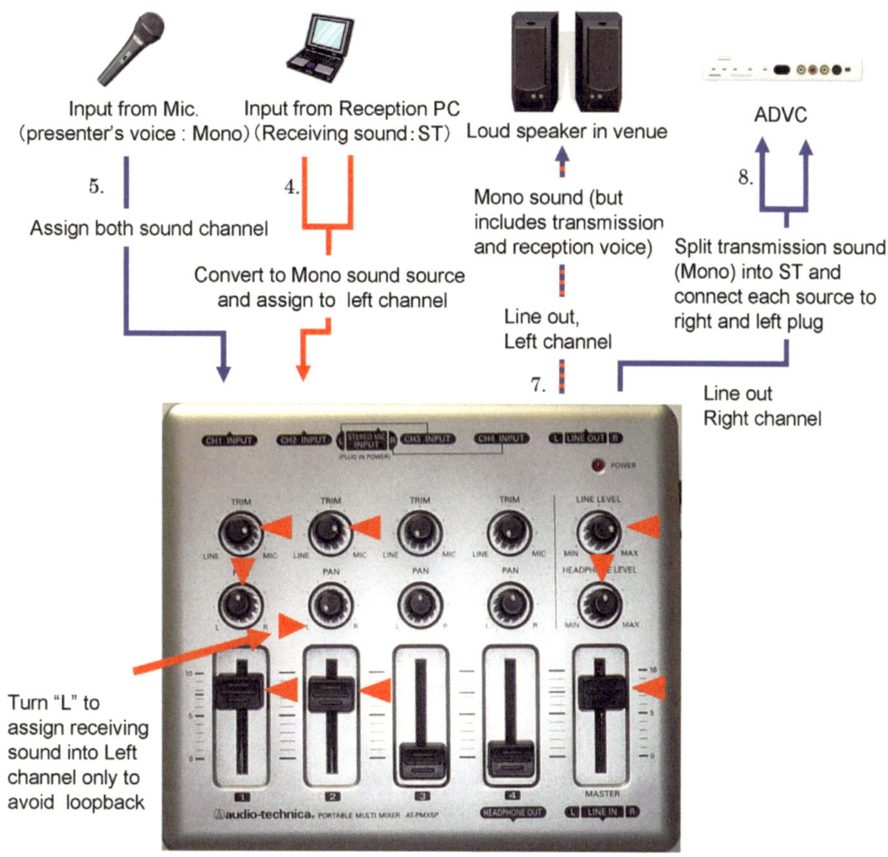

Fig. 4. Configuration diagram for setting audio

2.5 Multi-connection for DVTS

2.5.1 Multi-point control unit (MCU) for DVTS

Currently, all DVTS applications are implemented based on RFC 3189 and 3190, which are international standards for video and audio formats, respectively, for transmitting DV data over the Internet. This means that applications have the ability to transmit DV data to a specified IP address, but do not have features for session control or multi-party connections

as in H.323. Therefore, when a user starts transmitting DV data, the session begins even if the receiver is not yet ready, because of the lack of standard session control for DVTS. Of course, an implementation of the MCU (Multi-Point Control Unit) for DVTS is possible, even though this is not a standard session control and is incompatible with other MCUs.
A connection between multiple sites using DVTS had long since been awaited when the new technological breakthrough was introduced at the end of 2004. We successfully set up our first three-site connection using a commercially available MCU for DVTS, the QualImage/Quatre system (Information Services International-Dentsu, Ltd., Tokyo, Japan). The DV image transmitted from each station is digitally merged at the server, and the combined image is sent back to all stations. Once connected, participants at all sites can communicate in real-time with all other stations thereby enabling interactive discussions.

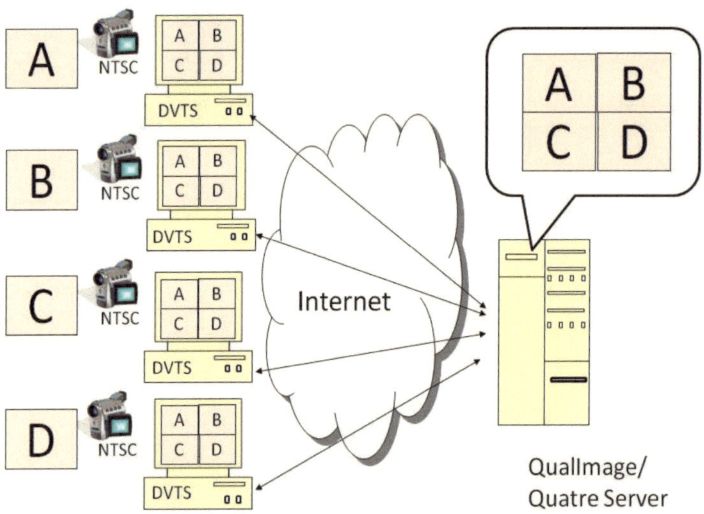

Fig. 5. Mechanism provided by QualImage/Quatre system

However, users must learn how to use the MCU carefully. Quatre runs on Linux and only uses 16 bit Audio and NTSC Video signals, as determined by its implementation. Fixing the audio and video format in this way is reasonable in order to achieve fast processing of the multiple DVTS streams under non-standard procedures. This is in contrast to a standard MCU that has the ability to resize multiple screens and is compatible with various formats resulting in the consumption of much more CPU power and poor performance. Quatre, which is the current version in use, has a web interface and a multi-party session using DVTS can be started immediately after inputting the IP addresses for the transmitting and receiving PCs.

2.5.2 Common audio-visual problems in multi-station setup

The following issues must be carefully considered in a multi-station setting. These problems do not occur in a one-to-one connection without Quatre.

1. Video format:
   TV signal can have one of three formats, NTSC (National Television System Committee), PAL (Phase Alternating Line) and SECAM (Séquentiel couleur à mémoire), but Quatre supports only NTSC. At the receiving end, this problem does not occur

because PCs support all TV signal decoding, but at the transmission end, all stations must have an NTSC camera available.

2. Audio format:
   Loss of audio transmission is encountered because of incompatibility of the audio format between DV and Quatre. Because there are two audio formats, 12 bit/32 kHz and 16 bit/48 kHz in DV signals, but Quatre supports only 16 bit, no sound is audible from a station sending 12 bit audio format.

2.6 Security of patient privacy

Protecting patient privacy is of the utmost importance during live demonstrations or tele-consultations. IPSec/VPN is a suitable means for encryption during transmission, with the performance of the processing IPSec determined by the quality of the VPN hardware for processing the encryption. In addition, all the VPN equipment should be the same model from a single vendor, because the session initiation procedure differs among IPSec/VPNs. For our own activities, we used an AR550S (AR750S is the corresponding international model) from AlliedTelesis K.K., Japan, as the IPSec VPN router. The AR550S has special hardware for IPSec and the throughput is about 150 Mbps. Thus, one AR550S can process two bi-directional DVTS streams. The setup of these routers can be done remotely once they are connected online.

3. Research and education network

3.1 What is the "research and education network"?

When the Internet service started, all the networks were for research and education activities. In 1989, the first commercial Internet service provider, UUNET, was established and the Internet Services Provider (ISP) service became popular. After the National Center for Supercomputing Applications (NCSA) released Mosaic, the first sophisticated web browser, those responsible for communication realized that a testbed for research and education was still required to provide advanced technologies of the Internet in a non-profit testbed environment. At that time, the testbed project was known as the next generation Internet (NGI), and was being championed by national governments. The first NGI testbed, established by the Group of Seven (G7), was called the Global Interoperability for Broadband Networks (GIBN). GIBN was a collaboration project between the commercial ISPs and government networks. However, owing to differences in the management policies, it became clear that a research and education environment had to be established solely by non-profit organizations or governments. The very high-performance Backbone Network Service (vBNS) (US) and TEN-34 (EU) were the first next generation Internet testbed environments or R&E networks.

In R&E networks, the backbone network is based on advanced technologies and generally provides excessive bandwidth. In about 1997, while regular Internet users were accessing the Internet at 28.8 Kbps, the R&E networks were providing 622 Mbps or more. The advanced Internet technologies, such as protocols or applications, deployed or developed on the R&E networks, are later incorporated for regular use. Border Gateway Protocol (BGP) routing, multicast Border Gateway Protocol (mBGP) routing, Internet Protocol Version 6 (IPv6), and video transmission over IP are all good examples of this.

R&E networks are typically managed on an institutional basis. Most of the customers and researchers are not concerned with payment. Nevertheless, because of the institutional based management, technical support for such R&E networks is often only provided to the edge of the individual campus networks. In other words, customers have to maintain their own circuits. Use of an R&E network requires close collaboration between the network researchers and local engineers.

3.2 Major networks world-wide

R&E networks are generally managed either by non-profit organizations or by one of the divisions in the government and can be divided into two categories. One is the national research and education network (NREN), while the other is the international research and education network. The international networks provide interconnectivity for the NRENs and other international R&E networks.

In fact, the major international R&E networks are APAN, TEIN3, Internet2 Network, GEANT2, and RedCLARA. These international R&E networks connect the NRENs or regional networks in their areas.

3.2.1 APAN (http://www.apan.net)

The Asia-Pacific Advanced Network (APAN) provides interconnectivity for the NRENs in the Asia Pacific area. Table 1 lists the NRENs of APAN members.

NREN	Country/Region	URL
AARNET	Australia	http://www.aarnet.edu.au
CERNET	China	http://www.edu.cn/english_1369/index.shtml
CSTNET	China	http://www.cstnet.net.cn/english/index.htm
SINET3	Japan	http://www.sinet.ad.jp/?set_language=en
JGN2plus	Japan	http://www.jgn.nict.go.jp/english/index.html
MAFFIN	Japan	http://nausicaa.maffin.ad.jp/Welcome.html
ThaiREN	Thailand	www.thairen.net.th/NewThaiRen/Thai/index_th.php
ThaiSARN3	Thailand	http://thaisarn.nectec.or.th/htmlweb/index.php
UniNet	Thailand	http://www.uni.net.th/UniNet/Eng/index_eng.php
KOREN	Korea	http://www.koren.kr/koren/eng/index.html
KREONET*	Korea	http://www.kreonet.re.kr/english
TANET2	Taiwan	http://www.tanet2.tw
TWAREN	Taiwan	http://www.twaren.net/english
ASGC	Taiwan	http://www.twgrid.org
PREGINET	The Philippines	http://www.pregi.net
HARNET	Hong Kong	http://www.jucc.edu.hk/jucc/harnet.html
LEARN	Sri Lanka	http://www.ac.lk
VINAREN	Vietnam	http://english.vinaren.vn
KAREN	New Zealand	http://wwwkaren.net.nz/home
SingAREN	Singapore	http://www.singaren.net.sg
NREN	Nepal	http://www.nren.net.np
MYREN	Malaysia	http://www.myren.net.my
PERN	Pakistan	http://www.pern.edu.pk
ERNET	India	http://www.ernet.in/index.html

Table 1. List of NRENs in APAN *International part is known as KREONET2.

APAN provides the transit service for other international R&E networks (Fig. 6).

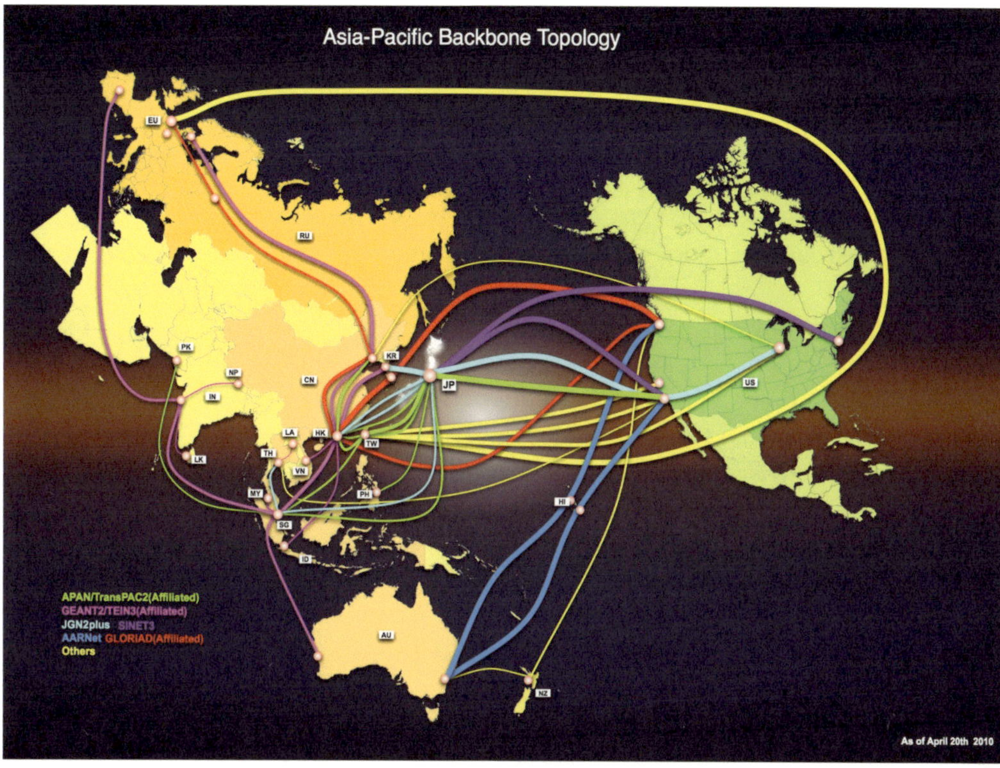

Fig. 6. R&E network map in the Asia-Pacific area (http://www.jp.apan.net/NOC/)

3.2.2 TEIN3

The Trans-Eurasia Information Network third generation (TEIN3) provides interconnectivity for the NRENs in South and Southeast Asia. TEIN3 also provides a transit service at Mumbai, Singapore, Hong Kong and Beijing with APAN and GEANT2 (Fig. 7).

3.2.3 Internet2 network

The Internet2 network (http://www.internet2.edu) provides interconnectivity for the regional networks and universities in the USA (Fig. 8). Its members represent a wide range of research and academic disciplines from over 300 member institutions, and the complete member list is available at http://www.internet2.edu/resources/listforweb.pdf. The Internet2 network has some international exchange points and a direct connection with the international R&E networks and direct circuits of NRENs. Its international partner organizations are listed at http://internet2.edu/international/partners/.

3.2.4 GÉANT2

GÉANT2 (http://www.geant2.net) is the second generation of ultra high speed international networks in Europe. It connects NRENs across 34 countries (Fig. 9). Since each NREN connects research and educational institutions within its own country, GÉANT2 provides connectivity to more than 30 million research and educational end users in over 3,500 institutions across Europe. The details of these NRENs are available at http://www.geant2.net/server/show/nav.00d009001.

3.2.5 RedCLARA

RedCLARA (http://www.redclara.net/index.php?lang=en) provides interconnectivity in Central and South America and is operated by Cooperacion Lationo Americana de Redes Avanzadas (CLARA). RedCLARA has a collaboration with the ALICE project in Europe and the WHREN project in USA (Fig. 10). Details of the member countries are listed at http://www.redclara.net/index.php?option=com_content&task=view&id=33&Itemid=217.

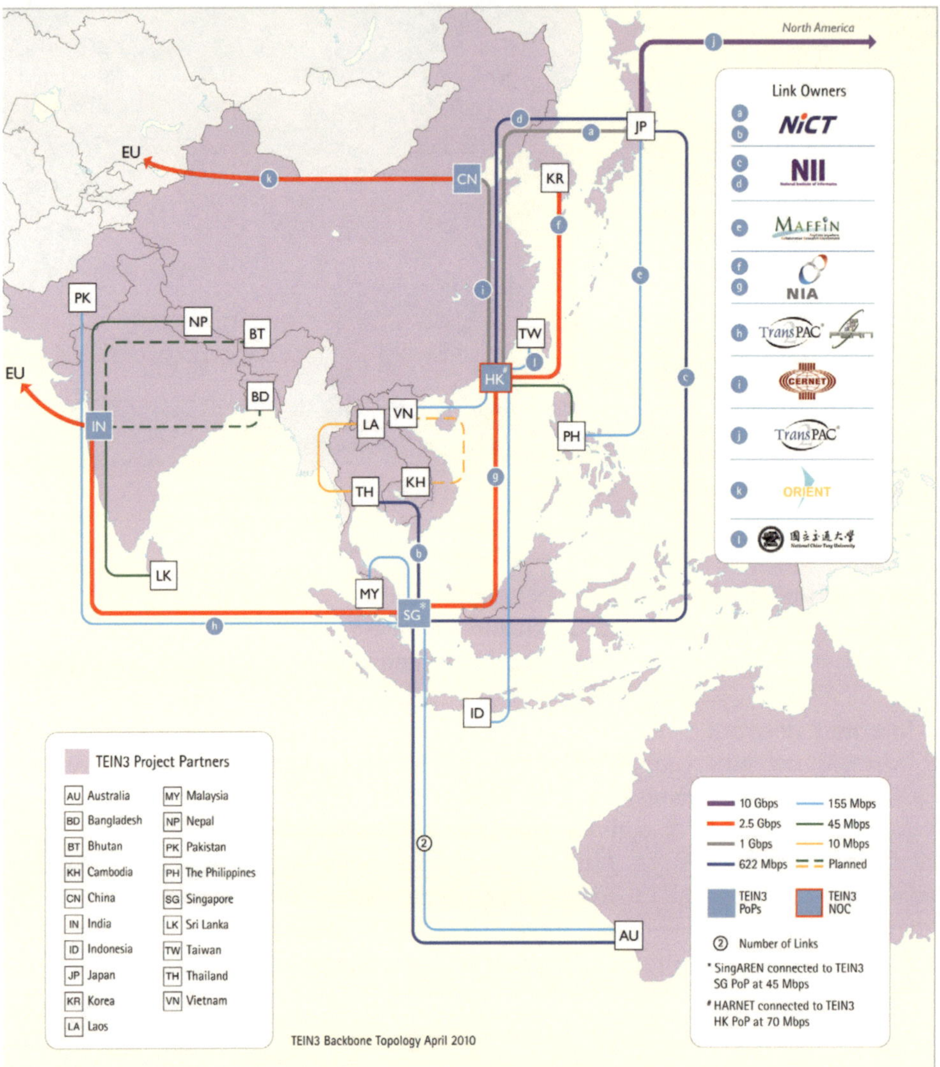

(http://www.tein3.net/upload/img/TEIN3_Topology_04.10_A4_300dpi.jpg)

Fig. 7. TEIN3 topology map

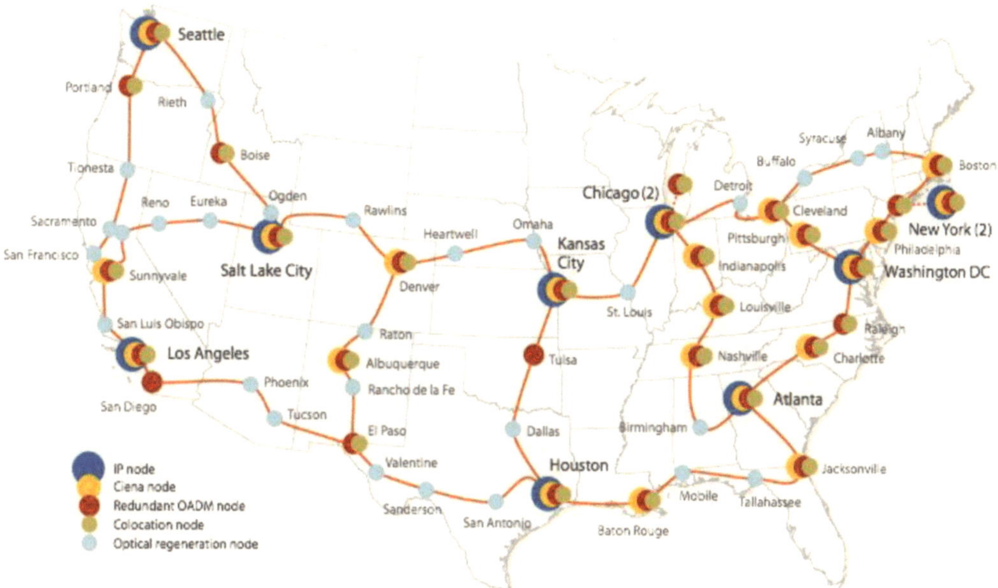

Fig. 8. Internet2 network topology (http://www.internet2.edu/network/)

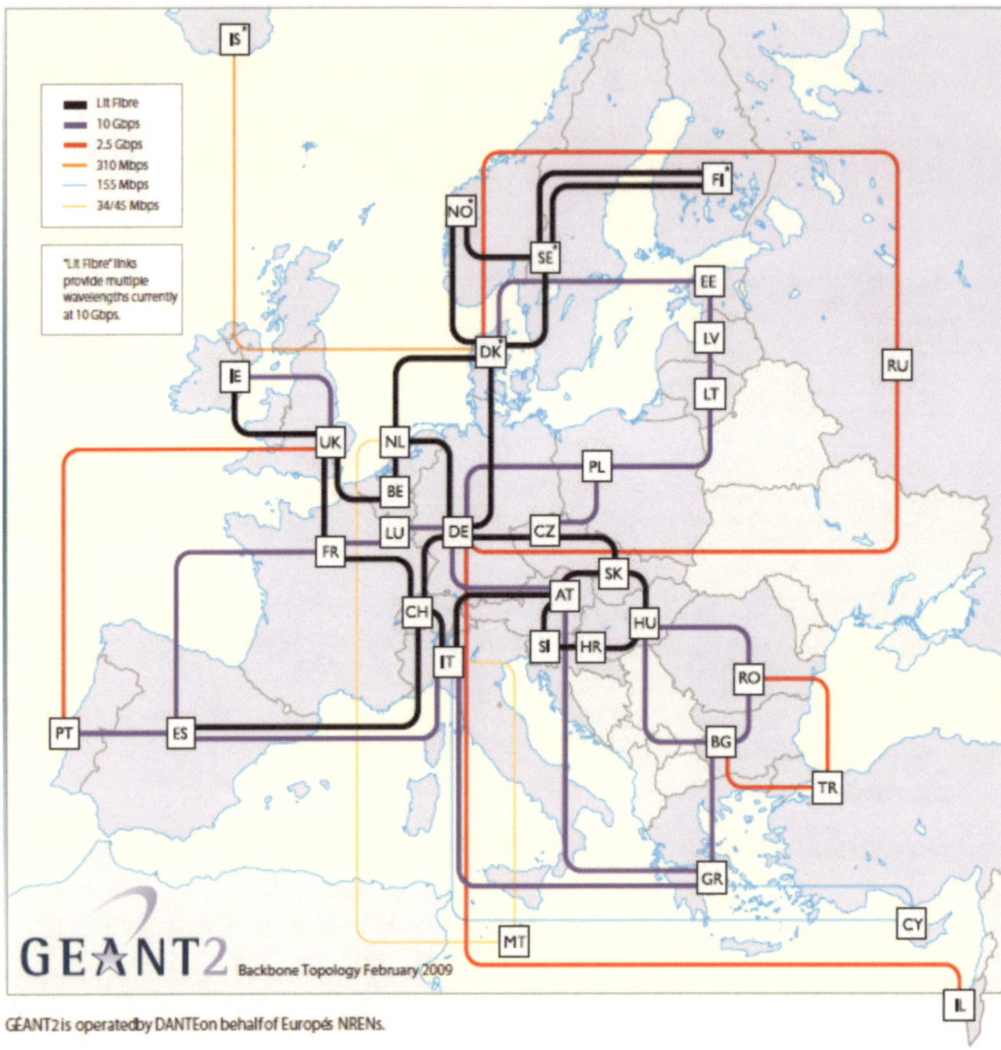

(http://www.geant2.net/upload/pdf/GN2_Topology_Feb_09.pdf)

Fig. 9. GÉANT2 topology map

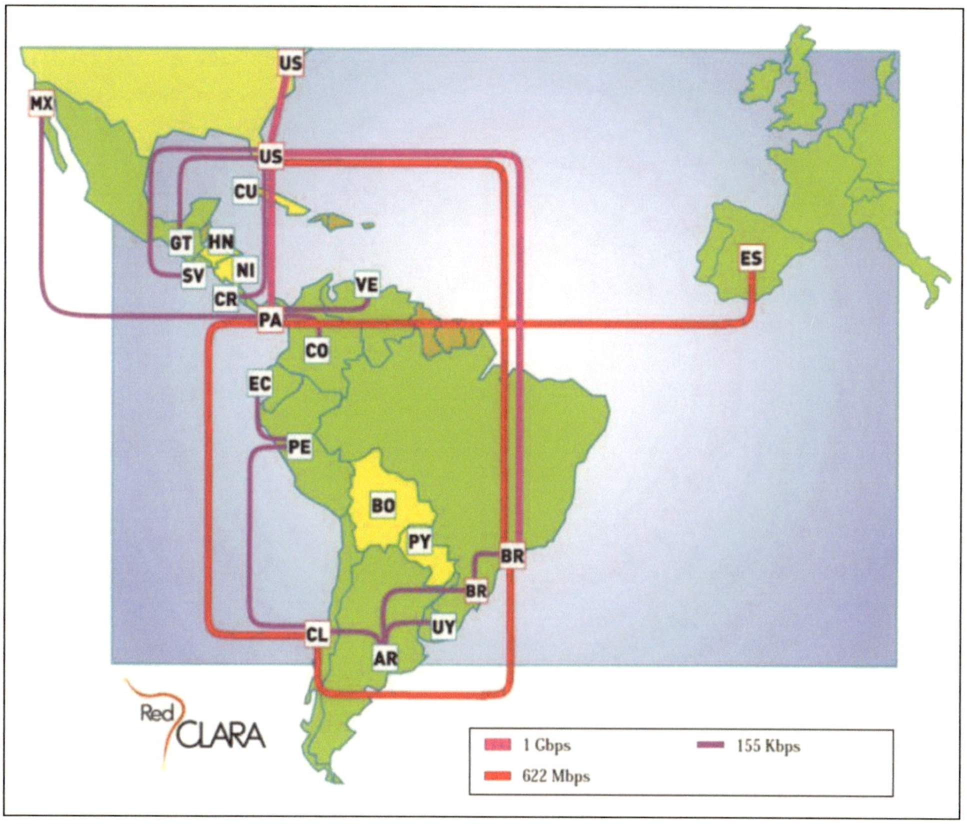

(http://www.redclara.net/doc/topology_RedCLARA_March2010.pdf)

Fig. 10. RedCLARA topology map

3.2.6 Africa

The northern part of Africa is covered by the European R&E project, EUMEDCONNECT2 (http://www.eumedconnect2.net/). Egypt also has a direct connection with Internet2. On the other hand, South Africa has a collaboration with Europe at 155 Mbps. Countries with established NRENs include Egypt, Tunisia, Algeria, Morocco, Kenya, and South Africa.

Actually, some cable systems have recently been established around Africa with huge bandwidth. Africa now has the chance to use such bandwidth (Fig. 11).

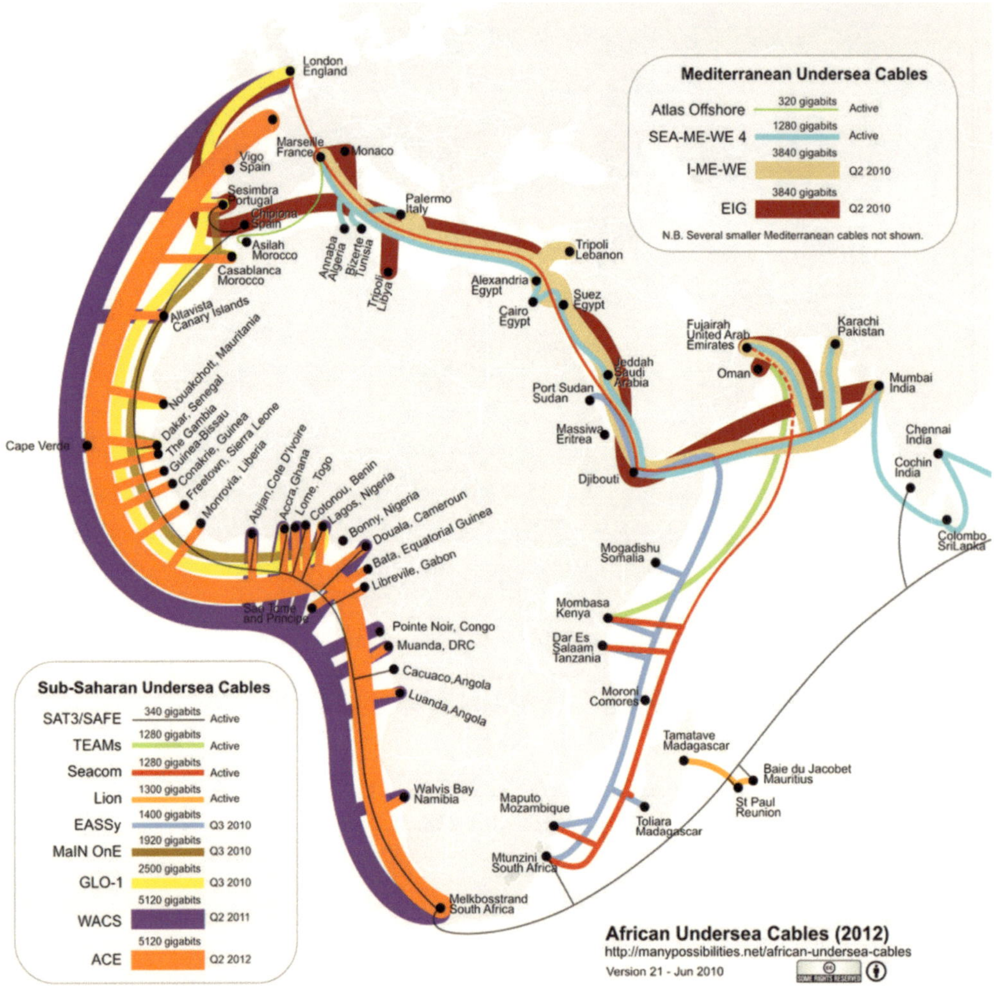

(http://manypossibilities.net/african-undersea-cables/)

Fig. 11. African undersea cable system map

3.3 How to check connectivity and create a new connection to a hospital

Each R&E network has its own management polices and these are not the same. But in general, universities and research institutions are connected with the R&E networks. Because of the campus management policies, however, all the departments in a university or research institution may not be able to use the R&E network. Thus, as a first step, please confirm whether your university or institution is listed as a member of the R&E network on the respective homepage, for example, APAN
(http://www.apan.net/home/membership/members.php) and Internet2
(http://www.internet2.edu/membership/index.cfm).
The tables should reflect the current situation, but some of the connection lists are not updated that frequently. You can, however, also check the connectivity yourself. "Traceroute" is a command in the BSD OS and its clones. Similar commands are available in other OSes as well. This command shows the route a communication takes. You should try to check the routes to some well-known universities (Fig. 12).

```
traceroute to www.internet2.edu (207.75.165.151), 30 hops max, 40 byte packets
 1  losa-tokyo-tp2.transpac2.net (192.203.116.145)  115.666 ms  115.674 ms  115.740 ms
 2  nlr-1-is-jmb-776.sttlwa.pacificwave.net (207.231.241.14)  143.236 ms  143.426 ms  142.948 ms
 3  denv-seat-58.layer3.nlr.net (216.24.186.6)  175.285 ms  171.899 ms  171.668 ms
 4  chic-denv-36.layer3.nlr.net (216.24.186.4)  197.273 ms  197.107 ms  196.841 ms
 5  tenge0-0-0-3x2087.nw-chil.mich.net (192.122.183.181)  185.242 ms  188.435 ms  185.270 ms
 6  tenge0-0-0-0x76.aa2.mich.net (198.108.23.10)  200.504 ms  200.453 ms  200.552 ms
 7  mam-77.merit.edu (192.122.200.77)  200.297 ms  200.299 ms  200.392 ms
 8  webprod0.internet2.edu (207.75.165.151)  200.260 ms !<10>  202.883 ms !<10>  201.309 ms !<10>
```

Fig. 12. Example of "traceroute" from APAN Tokyo XP to www.internet2.edu

If the names of the R&E networks are visible in the command output, these R&E networks are available at your site. If you cannot see any R&E network names, the R&E network services are probably not available at your site.
In this case, you need to establish a new connection to an access point of the R&E network. If you belong to a university or research institution, please take this issue up with the respective computer centre. The staff should know how to deal with this.
If your university or institution has a connection with the R&E network, you can discuss with the staff of the computer centre how to extend the connection to your own department or even your office. The IT staff will be able to advise you on the network configuration and network equipment required. If you cannot understand how to implement what the IT staff suggest, you should seek assistance from your colleagues who are more comfortable with IT concepts.
If your university or institution does not have a connection with an R&E network, it will be a little more complicated to set up, because most R&E networks require connections to be made at an institutional level.
Some of the R&E networks have a solution for this problem.

- Establishment of a temporary connection to the access points
- Establishment of a temporary connection to another institution as a sub-branch

Fig. 13 shows the process flow of the procedure discussed in this section.

4. Applications

We started this advanced telemedicine system as an activity in the Japan-Korea industry-government-academic joint project in 2003, with the aim of exchanging information in various fields such as education, business, culture as well as medicine over optic fiber

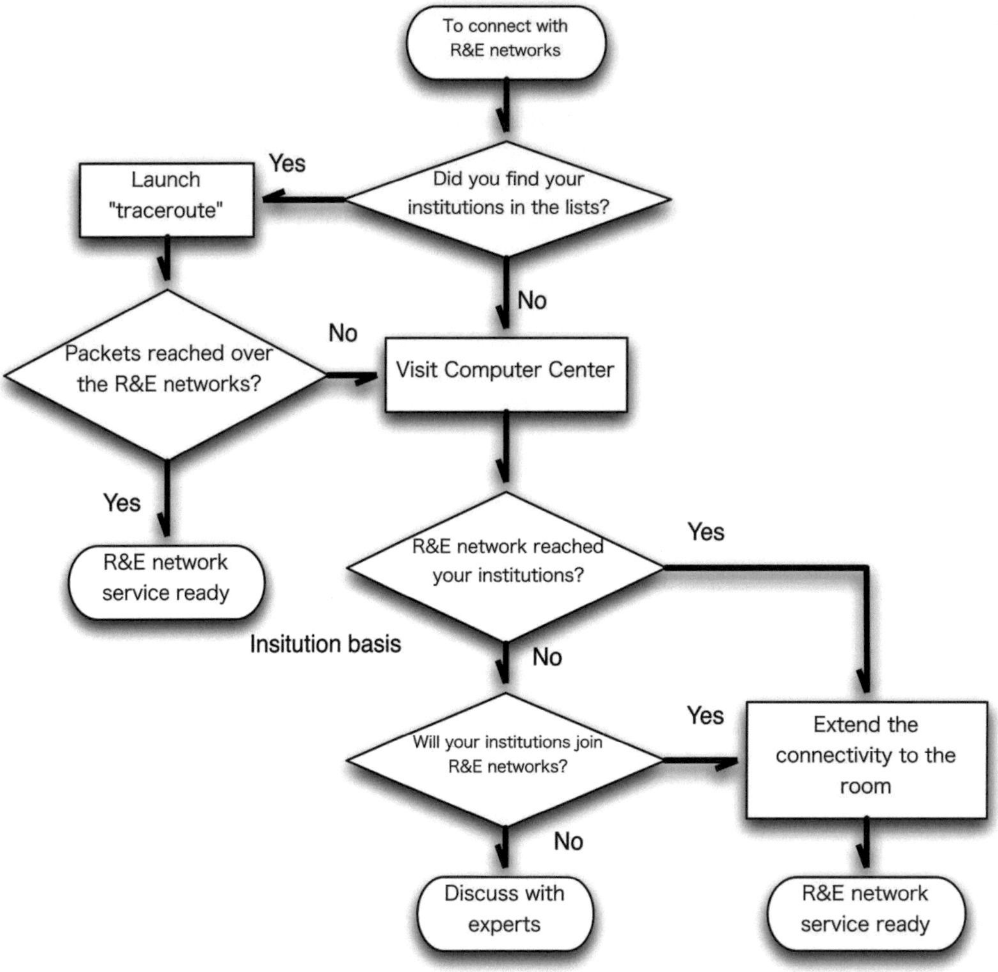

Fig. 13. Flowchart showing how to connect with an R&E network. Some R&E networks have help desks that can be contacted for assistance.

running under the strait between the two countries (Shimizu et al., 2006). This huge broadband cable, 250 times more than the conventional lines, was laid when the countries co-hosted the Soccer World Cup in 2002. We accumulated much experience and know-how from the first remote medical conference using DVTS. Moreover, because this system was found to be very useful and cost-effective, the activity was soon expanded outside the two countries, reaching China in Oct 2004, Southeast Asia in Jan 2005, Australia in Nov 2005, India and the USA in Jan 2007, and Europe in Aug 2007 (Carati et al., 2006; Huang et al., 2008; Shimizu et al., 2009). In May 2009, Egypt joined as the first country in Africa, with Brazil following suit in July 2009 as the first from South America.

Of the 223 telecommunications thus far, 78 were live demonstrations of surgery or endoscopy, for example, and 145 were teleconferences using video and slide presentations. In total, 726 universities and hospitals were connected. The details are given in Table 2 with some pictures of our recent events shown in Figures 14 and 15.

Contents	Country and region*																
	JP	KR	CN	TW	TH	SG	PH	VN	ID	IN	MY	AU	NZ	EU	NA	SA	AF	Total
Live demonstration																		
Surgery	61	39	19	4	4	7	4	1		4	1	6	2	4	2			158
Endoscopy	28	10	11	3	5	1		3			1	3		1				66
Hematology	5	3			1													9
Cardiac intervention	6	1	1															8
Others	2	1	1															4
Subtotal	102	54	32	7	10	8	4	4	0	4	2	9	2	5	2	0	0	245
Teleconference																		
Surgery	52	24	6	6	3	7	6	4			1	3		7	1		1	121
Endoscopy	76	23	14	13	11	5	1	2			3	3		6	9	2	2	170
Healthcare	17	7	2	1	3	1	1	1	2	2	1	3			7			48
Transplantation	16	6	4	3								1						30
Nursing	25		1					1	1									28
Medical informatics	6	7		1		1				2		3	1		2			23
Hepatobiliarypancreas	10	9		1														20
Others	20	5	2	3	3	2				1	1				4			41
Subtotal	222	81	29	28	20	16	8	8	3	5	6	13	1	13	23	2	3	481
Total connected stations	324	135	61	35	30	24	12	12	3	9	8	22	3	18	25	2	3	726

Table 2. List of activities and connected countries/regions (as of June 2010). *KR, Korea; CN, China; TW, Taiwan; TH, Thailand; SG, Singapore; PH, the Philippines; VN, Vietnam; ID, Indonesia; IN, India; MY, Malaysia; AU, Australia; NZ, New Zealand; EU, European Union; NA, North America; SA, South America; AF, Africa

The most active countries/regions are Japan and Korea, followed by China, Taiwan, Thailand, Singapore and Australia. These Asia-Pacific institutions often collaborate with their North American and European counterparts. The most common fields for live demonstrations are surgery and endoscopy, where clear moving images are of utmost importance for precise and adequate understanding. Quality evaluations have been reported by Eto et al. (2007) and Kaltenbach et al. (2009) in the fields of surgery and gastrointestinal endoscopy, respectively.

For the first couple of years, DVTS connections were possible only between two sites, or between several stations with multiple one-to-one connections. Since the emergence of Quatre as described in the previous section, however, real and practical multi-site connections have become possible and have rapidly increased in number. There has been a total of 92 two site and 131 multiple site connections, with the latter increasing to around 80% of the total connections in the last two years (Fig. 16). In these events, real-time discussions take place between all the connected stations, and interactive questions and answers are possible at multiple stations. The major collaborating societies include both national and international groups, such as the World Gastroenterology Organization (WGO), International Association of Surgeons, Gastroenterologists, and Oncologists (IASGO), Asia-Pacific Hepatobiliary Pancreatic Association (APHPBA), Endoscopic and Laparoscopic Surgeons of Asia (ELSA) 2006 & 2010, Korean Society of Gastroenterology, Thai Association of Gastroenterology, Japan Surgical Society 2009, and many others.

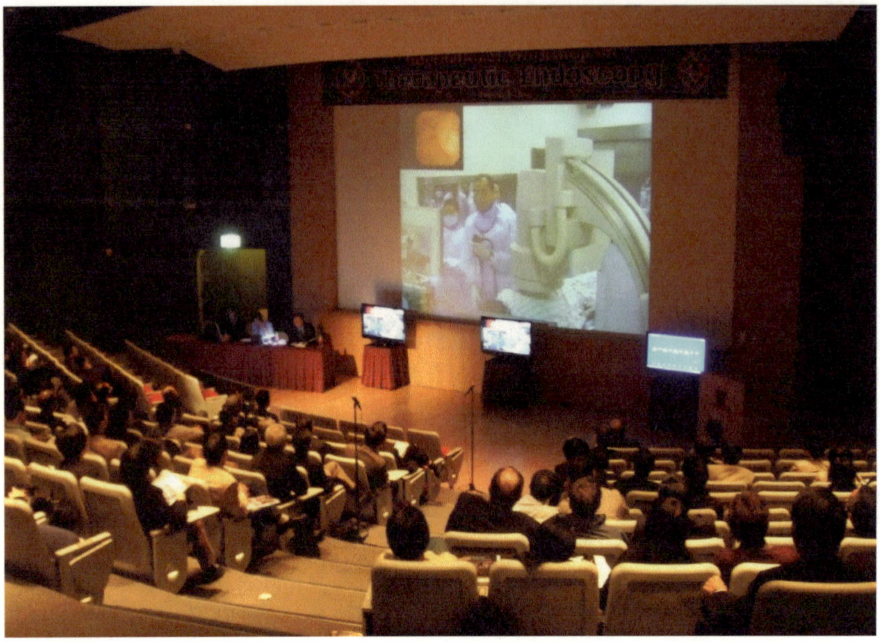

Fig. 14. Live demonstration of endoscopy at the Prince of Wales Hospital in the Chinese University of Hong Kong, connecting Xian and Shanghai in China, and Fukuoka, Japan.

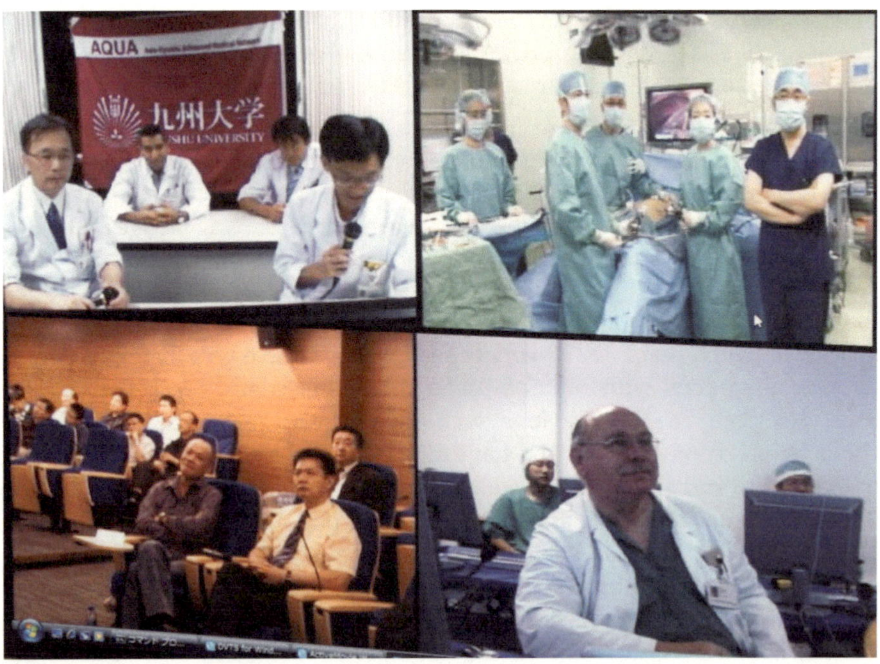

Fig. 15. Live surgery transmitted from the Cancer Institute Hospital in Tokyo, Japan (top right), to Fukuoka/Japan (top left), Shanghai/China (bottom left), and Trondheim/Norway (bottom right), with interactive discussions.

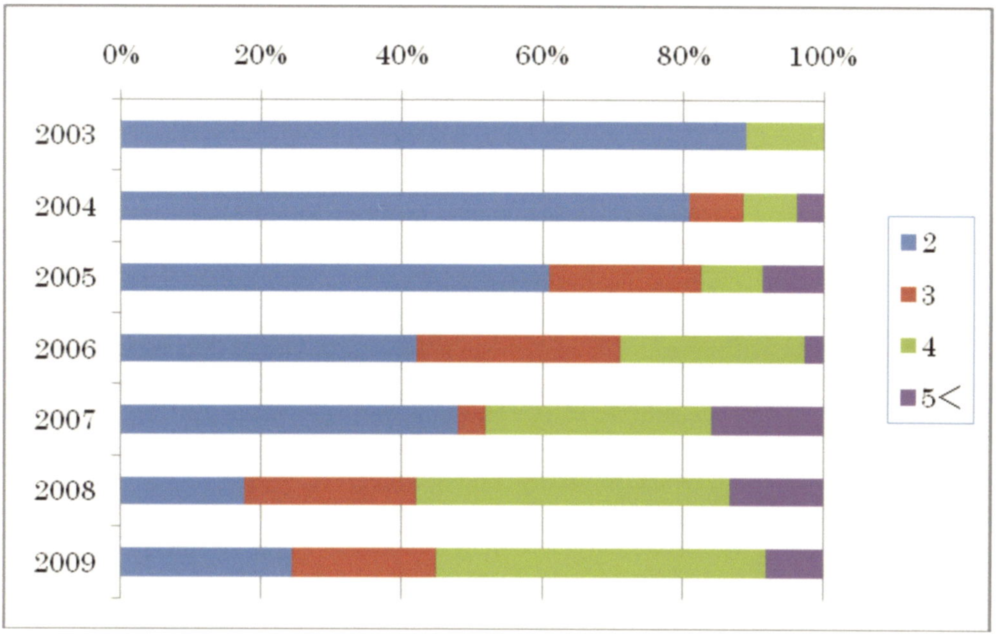

Fig. 16. Ratio of multiple connections

Currently, a main organizer of all these activities is the Medical Working Group in APAN, collaborating with other worldwide networks. The Telemedicine Development Center of Asia (TEMDEC), which was formally established at the Kyushu University Hospital, Japan, acts as the secretariat to lead the program preparations and technical arrangements. (http://www.aqua.med.kyushu-u.ac.jp/)

As of June 2010, the number of member institutions was 125 hospitals and institutions in 26 countries and regions, consisting of 31 in Japan, 19 in Korea, 10 in Australia, 9 in mainland China, and other major ones as shown in Table 3.

5. Discussion

5.1 Current problems

At the beginning of our telemedicine project, stable network conditions between remote stations were the most important concern for us. In fact, we had many experiences of teleconferences with image noise and jerky sound because of packet losses. Since then, network quality has improved very rapidly and widely, allowing stable connections to be established and many institutions to participate year after year. Nevertheless, there are still some issues that need to be solved and considered. The first is the limitation of Quatre, the only MCU currently available for DVTS. Although the participants find the multiple connections very attractive and more and more hospitals want to join the same conference, in practice, eight is the maximum number of stations that can be connected, because of the heavy load on the server. Another limitation of this MCU is that it is compatible only with NTSC video format which is mainly available in North America and East Asia and cannot be connected with PAL, which is popular in Southeast Asia and European countries. The availability of Quatre only in Japan also limits the multi-connections in other areas. The second issue is the fact that there are many hospitals that are not yet connected to the R&E

Country and region	Name of hospital or institution
Japan	Hokkaido University, Iwate Medical University, Tokyo Medical and Dental University, The Cancer Institute Hospital, Tokyo Science Foundation, Fujita Health University, Kyoto University, Kyoto Second Red Cross Hospital, Kobe University, Hiroshima University, Yamaguchi University, University of Occupational and Environmental Health, Kyushu University, Fukuoka University, Oita University, Saga University, Nagasaki University, Kyushu International College of Nursing, Fujimoto-Hayasuzu Hospital
Korea	Seoul National University, Bundang Hospital, Hanyang University, Ehwa Women's University, Yonsei University, Korea University, National Cancer Center, Asan Medical Center, Catholic University St. Mary's Hospital, Konkuk University, Chungnam University, Chungbuk University, Gyeongsang University
China	Tsinghua University, Peking University, Peking Union Medical College Hospital, Shanghai Jiaotong University Hospital, The Fourth Military University affiliated to Xijing Hospital, Chinese University of Hong Kong
Taiwan	National Taiwan University, Taipei Veteran General Hospital, Taichung Veteran General Hospital, National Central University
Thailand	Mahidol University Siriraj Hospital, Chulalongkorn University, Rajavithi Hospital, Pramongkutklao University Hospital
Singapore	National University of Singapore
Indonesia	University of Indonesia, Institute Technology of Bandung
Philippines	University of the Philippines, UP Manila General Hospital
Vietnam	National Hospital of Pediatrics, Backmai Hospital, No 108 Hospital, Choray Hospital
Malaysia	MYREN office
India	Tata Memorial Hospital
Australia	Flinders University, Australia National University, Concord Hospital, Royal Brisbane University Hospital
New Zealand	University of Auckland
USA	Stanford University, Florida International University, University of California Irvine, Seattle Science Foundation, University of Hawaii
Mexico	Universidad Nacional Autonoma de Mexico
Germany	University Hospital of Eppendorf in Hamburg
France	Bordeaux2 University
Italy	University of Rome3, Monaldi Hospital
Spain	Hospital Clinic I Provincial De Barcelona, University of Malaga
Norway	St Olavs University Hospital
Egypt	Cairo University, Theodor Bilharz Research Institute
Morocco	Mohamed V Souissi University
Brazil	University San Paolo Ribeirão Preto

Table 3. Major institutions linked by R&E networks using DVTS

network and have only a limited commercial network available, despite the fact that the R&E network is rapidly expanding in both bandwidth and location. These unconnected hospitals have to pay a network charge to the nearest point of the R&E network as previously described in Section 3. The third issue concerns the standardization and quality control of the local systems. The condition of intra-hospital networks and maintenance of audio-visual equipment should always be checked carefully by technicians in each institution.

5.2 New communication tools and demands for high-definition quality

With the rapid development of technology, there are other emerging options for remote communication other than DVTS. Skype is free software that is easily installed on a computer and widely used on a personal basis. However, Skype is mainly utilized for sound transmission instead of telephone and thus the image quality is far from perfect. Conventional H.323 videoconferencing systems like Polycom (Picturetel Corp. Danvers, MA) have also gained in popularity with their biggest advantage being the ease of handling and preparation. Furthermore, they provide all-in-one equipment, so there is no need to prepare microphones or cables to connect PCs. Nevertheless, once again the video image quality is only good enough for remote sites to recognize the person at the other end. The transmission of surgical videos would result in degraded and sluggish moving images without good recognition of fine anatomical structures, despite the initial high cost of the equipment (Shimizu et al., 2010).

Meanwhile, demands for even better quality video than that provided by DVTS are increasing rapidly, owing to high-definition (HD) quality medical equipment now being widely used in clinical settings. Although we succeeded in an international transmission of live surgery with uncompressed high-definition quality, we required extraordinarily expensive equipment with huge bandwidth such as 1.6 Gbps, which is more than 500 times larger than that necessary for DVTS (Shimizu et al., 2007). The transmission of compressed types of high-definition video may be an alternative, but the longer time delay would be detrimental to the comfortable interactive nature of the experience. In addition, the initial cost for the high-end equipment is prohibitive, which is exactly the same problem encountered with satellite connections. Although standard quality digital video (720 × 480 dpi) is gradually being replaced by HD quality (1920 × 1080 dpi) and the IEEE1394 interface by HDMI, DVTS will remain the best alternative in telemedicine until HD teleconferencing equipment becomes much more reasonably priced.

5.3 Tele-consultation

Because of the usefulness of high-quality video transmission in medicine, the system has been applied to various fields as listed in Table 2. Although current experience is not much, interventional cardiology looks promising and is expected to be one of the next major applications together with remote education for nurses and medical students. Disparity in medical services around the world is still very high, not only in terms of techniques and technology, but also in treatment strategies and ethical decisions. To standardize these issues, showing advanced operations and examinations using new medical equipment by means of live transmission, together with the possibility of interactive communication, seems to be very effective. This can provide a powerful, yet simple tool for learning advanced skills and new medical procedures across country borders. It is expected that telemedical education will be further developed in a variety of fields in the global range.

The applications mentioned above are all classified as remote education between healthcare providers. At present, tele-consultation is seriously being considered for use with this system as another target area where connections are made between doctors and patients (Kroenke et al., 2010; Mayes et al., 2010; Wei et al., 2008). Telemedical consultation, including diagnosis and second opinions, can provide expert opinions to remote general physicians, as well as support for the progressively aging society in the rural areas by the decreasing younger generation in the city. In addition, in cases of emerging infectious diseases, medical doctors in countries that have never been affected by the disease, can obtain "real" clinical experience and know-how for treating these diseases by viewing the treatment of remote patients in affected countries without the risk of getting infected. In order to make a tele-consultation as accurate as a face-to-face one and to implement tele-consultations in the social system, discussions involving government and healthcare organizations are truly necessary.

6. Conclusion

Considering all the aspects, we believe that DVTS is currently the best choice in terms of both quality and cost for telemedicine, where it is useful to explain various procedures by means of video and where image quality is a key factor. There is no doubt that DVTS has provided an efficient and practical communication means for exchanging medical knowledge and skills with medical-proof moving images on the R&E network and with minimal cost. However, medical personnel are not at all familiar with the two technologies, DVTS and the R&E network, and the initial setup of DVTS and handling of large networks is beyond their ability. Prevalence of these new technologies in the medical community and establishment of good cooperation between the two different groups of people, doctors and IT technicians, is essential to expand the telemedicine activity into daily practice, thereby finally providing better healthcare worldwide.

In the same way that our activity started when high-speed Internet was connected between Japan and Korea at the time of the Soccer World Cup in 2002, so too has South Africa, the World Cup host country in 2010, brought many new connections to Africa. The whole continent is now practically connected. We have organized a very active telemedicine society in the Asia-Pacific area under the leadership of the APAN Medical Working Group, and the establishment of two other key organizations, one in Europe/Africa and the other in North/South America, is now underway to coordinate global telemedicine.

7. Acknowledgement

The authors sincerely appreciate the commitment of the entire medical and technical staff of all the participating universities, institutions, and organizations and their kind cooperation and support, with special thanks to the APAN NOC team for their network expertise.

This project was funded in part by the Core University Program of the Japan Society for the Promotion of Science (JSPS) and the Korea Science and Engineering Foundation; the Asia Core Program of JSPS and the National Research Council of Thailand; the Japan-China Medical Exchange Program of JSPS and the China Academy of Medical Sciences; and Grant-in-Aid No. 20406027 from the JSPS.

8. References

Anvari, M.; McKinley, C. & Stein, H. (2005). Establishment of the world's first telerobotic remote surgical service: for provision of advanced laparoscopic surgery in a rural community. *Ann Surg,* 241, 3, 460-4

Augestad, K.M. & Lindsetmo, R.O. (2009). Overcoming distance: video-conferencing as a clinical and educational tool among surgeons. *World J Surg,* 33, 7, 1356-65

Carati, C.; Shimizu, S.; Okamura, K.; Lomanto, D.; Tanaka, M. & Oouli, J. (2006). High definition digital video links for surgical training. *J Telemed Telecare,* 12, S26-28

Demartines, N.; Mutter, D.; Vix, M.; Leroy, J.; Glatz, D.; Rösel, F.; Harder, F. & Marescaux, J. (2000). Assessment of telemedicine in surgical education and patient care. *Ann Surg,* 231, 2, 282-91

Eto, M.; Lee, T.Y.; Gill, I.S.; Koga, H.; Tatsugami, K.; Shimizu, S.; Ukimura, O. & Naito, S. (2007). Broadcast of live endoscopic surgery from Korea to Japan using the digital video transport system. *J Endourol,* 21, 12, 1517-20

Hazin, R. & Qaddoumi, I. (2010). Teleoncology: current and future applications for improving cancer care globally. *Lancet Oncol,* 11, 2, 204-10

Hu, S.W.; Foong, H.B. & Elpern, D.J. (2009). Virtual Grand Rounds in Dermatology: an 8-year experience in web-based teledermatology. *Int J Dermatol,* 48, 12, 1313-9

Huang, K.J.; Qiu, Z.J.; Fu, C.Y.; Shimizu, S. & Okamura, K. (2008). Uncompressed video image transmission of laparoscopic or endoscopic surgery for telemedicine. *Telemed e-Health,* 14, 5, 479-485

Kaltenbach, T.; Muto, M.; Soetikno, R.; Dev, P.; Okamura, K.; Hahm, J. & Shimizu, S. (2009). Teleteaching endoscopy: feasibility of real-time uncompressed video transmission by using advanced network technologies. *Gastrointest Endosc,* 70, 5, 1013-1017

Kroenke, K.; Theobald, D.; Wu, J.; Norton, K.; Morrison, G.; Carpenter, J. & Tu, W. (2010). Effect of telecare management on pain and depression in patients with cancer: a randomized trial. *JAMA,* 14, 304, 2, 163-71

Mayes, P.A.; Silvers, A. & Prendergast, J.J. (2010). New direction for enhancing quality in diabetes care: utilizing telecommunications and paraprofessional outreach workers backed by an expert medical team. *Telemed J E Health,* 16, 3, 358-63

Ogawa, A.; Kobayashi, K.; Sugita, K.; Nakamura, O. & Murai, J. (1999). Design and implementation of dv stream over internet. *Proceedings of Internet Workshop IWS'99,* pp. 255-260, ISBN 0-7803-5925-9, Osaka, Japan, Feb 1999, IEE Publications, New York.

Rabenstein, T.; Maiss, J.; Naegele-Jackson, S.; Liebl, K.; Hengstenberg, T.; Radespiel-Tröger, M.; Holleczek, P.; Hahn, EG. & Sackmann, M. (2002). Tele-endoscopy: influence of data compression, bandwidth and simulated impairments on the usability of real-time digital video endoscopy transmissions for medical diagnoses. *Endoscopy,* 234, 9, 703-10

Shimizu, S.; Nakashima, N.; Okamura, K.; Hahm, J.S.; Kim, Y.W.; Moon, B.I.; Han, H.S. & Tanaka, M. (2006). International transmission of uncompressed endoscopic surgery images via super-fast broadband internet connections. *Surg Endosc,* 20, 1, 167-170

Shimizu, S.; Han, H.S.; Okamura, K.; Yamaguchi, K. & Tanaka, M. (2007). Live demonstration of surgery across international borders with uncompressed high-definition quality. *HPB (Oxford),* 9, 5, 398-399

Shimizu, S.; Nakashima, N.; Okamura, K. & Tanaka, M. (2009). One hundred case studies of Asia-Pacific telemedicine using digital video transport system over research and education network. *Telemedicine J E Health,* 15, 1, 112-117

Shimizu, S.; Han, H.S.; Okamura, K.; Nakashima, N.; Kitamura, Y. & Tanaka, M. (2010). Technologic developments in telemedicine: State-of-the-art academic interactions. *Surgery,* 147, 5, 597-601

Wei, Z.; Wu, Y.; Deng, R.H.; Yu, S.; Yao, H.; Zhao, Z.; Ngoh, L.H.; Han, L.T. & Poh, E.W. (2008). A secure and synthesis tele-ophthalmology system. *Telemed J E Health,* 14, 8, 833-45

5

Lossless Compression Techniques for Medical Images in Telemedicine

Dr.J.Janet, Divya Mohandass and S.Meenalosini
Dean,Computing,Veltech Dr.RR&Dr.SR Technical Univerity,
Research Scholar,St.Peter's University&Asst.Professor,SKREC,
Asst.Professor,Veltech Dr.RR&Dr.SR Technical University,
India

1. Introduction

Telemedicine is telecommunication technology integrated with the advancements in information technology. The main purpose is to enhance health care delivery to a wider population. This telemedicine technology supports the transfer of pathological and imaging reports of patients across the telemedicine networks, so as to provide consultation by specialists located in geographically different locations. The integration of mobile communication and biomedical instrumentation technology plays an important role in Telemedicine as doctors away from the system can also get the health status of their critical patients (AlfredoI.Hernandez et al., 2001).

Advances made in the field of biomedical engineering, has lead to the development of more accurate biomedical instrumentation to measure vital physiological parameters and the development of interdisciplinary areas to fight the effects of body malfunctions and disease.

The chapter is organised as follows. Subsections under 1 describe the application of telecommunication technology to health care and the necessity of telemedicine in India. The challenges pertaining to telemedicine have also been identified and addressed accordingly. Section 2 briefs on the concepts of effective medical image compression. The effectiveness of Huffman Compression in telemedicine and related work is presented in Section 3. Section 4 describes transform based image compression. The basics of contourlet coding and global thresholding based on Otsu's method is described in Sections 4.2 and 4.3 respectively. The algorithm steps of Contourlet based Joint Medical image compression is presented in 4.5.Section 5 gives the results obtained on applying the algorithm. The conclusion is presented in Section 6.

1.1 Applying telecommunications to health care

The term telecommunications generally means electronic transmission of information over a distance. We can use modern telecommunication and information technologies for the provision of clinical care to individuals at a distance. This application is very efficient since patient records, stored electronically, can be made available through the Internet, resulting in the elimination of the need for physical storage and transfer of records. Furthermore, images and video can be included and transmitted as part of a computerized file. Hence, the patient's history can include previous examinations, lab test results, X-rays, etc. in addition to textual descriptions of the results from previous health care. Records on remote sites can also be accessed. This will greatly enhance the chances of correct diagnosis of a particular illness and possibly suggest courses of treatment. Health information of the patient, collected in digitized form, can be easily transmitted without requiring his/her physical presence for the examination. The support of video conferencing through the Internet allows a health care professional to observe and interact with the patient who is not in the same physical location. E-mail or Video Recording could be used for asynchronous discussions. Patient records, lab results and images from detailed examinations can be stored in computer file format, making them easier to search and transfer to distant locations when needed.

E-mail and Internet access for regional and rural medical centres and hospitals could be extremely useful. The benefits from connecting as many hospitals and medical centres as possible to the medical information system would be:

- Improved standard of medical practice
- Improved epidemiological and other reporting
- Educational benefits for doctors and medical staff in distant medical centers, continuous medical education.

Therefore, the telecommunication partners of these telemedicine projects will be a key factor for the future extension of telemedicine services. Successful introduction of telemedicine services require more than just the delivery of the right equipment to the users.

The Internet is already changing the way in which telemedicine is deployed and the extent to which it becomes widely available. The focus should be on low-cost, low-bandwidth Internet applications that facilitate discussion and the transmission of text, data and images (AlfredoI Hernandez et al., 2001, J.A.Mockzo et al., 2001).

Telemedicine can help to develop new ways to deliver medical and health education to professionals and to the community and improve the continuing medical education.

1.2 Technology behind telemedicine

Most of the telemedical applications use one of the two widely available technologies. The store and forward technology transfers digital images from one location to another. The other popular technology is the two-way interactive television (IATV). This is used when a 'face-to-face' consultation between the health expert and the patients become mandatory. It is usually between the patients and their provider in one location and a specialist in another location. Videoconferencing equipment at both locations allows a 'real-time' consultation to take place (K.Hung, YT Zhang 2003). The technology has decreased in price and complexity over the past five years, and many programs now use desktop videoconferencing systems. This includes transfer of basic patient information over computer communication networks, exchange of images such as radiographs or pathologies among geographically separated specialists, remote patient interviews and examination through activities. A telemedicine system enables 'virtual consultation' wherein the local doctor plays the role of a remote medical expert and implements effective decision making and treatment. Telemedicine bridges gap between specialist doctors and patients, thereby overcoming the barriers of distance and time. Health care in isolated areas are improved by enhancing continuing care.

Modern telecommunication and information technologies could be used for the provision of clinical care to individuals at a distance. Patient records, lab results and images from detailed examinations could be stored in computer file format, making them easier to search and transfer to distant locations when needed.

Thus telemedicine technology offers the following benefits:

- Reduction in time and cost incurred in travel
- Easy and quick access to specialist
- Cost effective post treatment consultation
- Efficient use of medical resources.

The major areas of telemedicine technology are

- Tele-consultation
- Tele-diagnosis
- Tele-treatment
- Tele-education
- Tele-training
- Tele-monitoring
- Tele-support

Figures 1 and 2 depict the scenario in a telemedicine setup (Anunay Nayak et al.)

1.3 Necessity of telemedicine in India

The geographical set up of India provides an ideal setup for telemedicine to be implemented in the sub-continent. India's huge population makes it difficult for health care facilities to be made available for everybody and at any place.

India is characterized by low penetration of healthcare services. 80% of secondary & tertiary healthcare facilities lie in cities and towns, distant from rural India where 70% of the population resides. Primary health care facilities for rural population are highly inadequate.

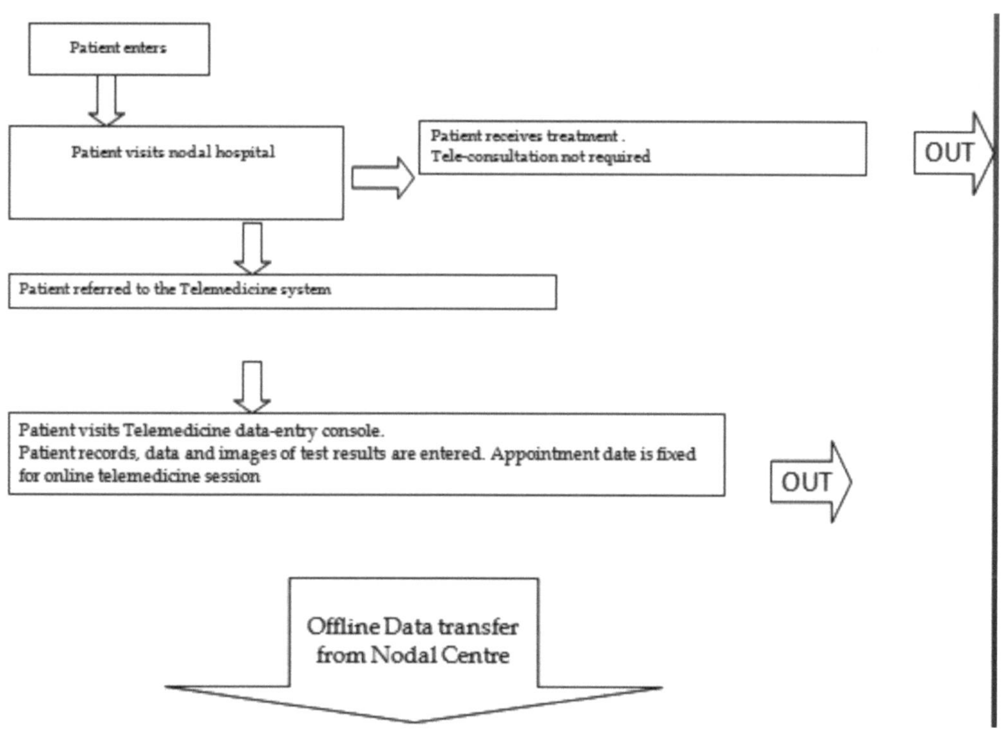

Fig. 1. Day 1 of a Telemedicine consultation (Anunay Nayak et al.)

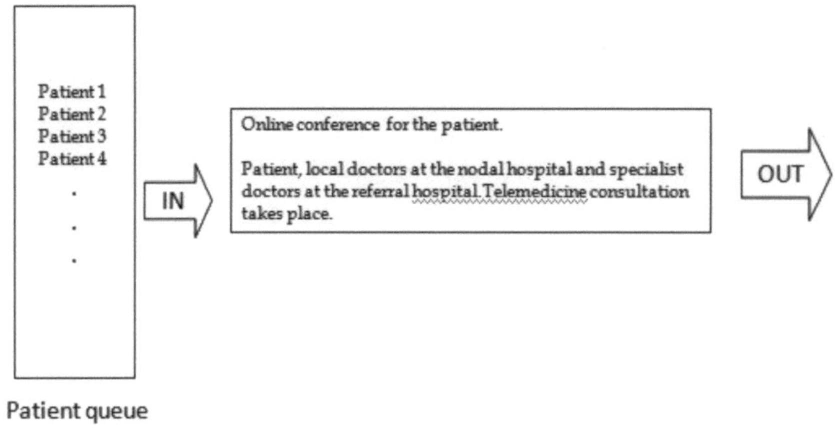

Fig. 2. Day 2 of a telemedicine consultation

Studies reveal that the rural population, though with the same disease than their urban counterparts faces twice the risk of death, due to inexperienced and poor medical facilities in the rural areas. Despite several initiatives by the Government and private sectors, the rural and remote areas continue to suffer from absence of quality healthcare. Telemedicine attempts to narrow the gap underlying urban and rural counterparts, in terms of quality health care.

India has begun to make remarkable progress in the fields of telemedicine and e-health. Indian Space Research Organization ISRO and the Department Of Information Technology provide the infrastructure to support tele applications. One of ISRO's first successful ventures to implement telemedicine in the country was in the year 2001, linking Apollo Hospital in Chennai to a rural hospital in Aragonda village in Andhra Pradesh. Later, in March 2002, Karnataka Telemedicine project linked a super speciality hospital in Bangalore to a small district hospital. The successful implementation of these pilot projects was ISRO's initial steps contributing to the growth of telemedicine in India.

Fig.3 shows the Telemedicine link provided by the Indian Space Research Organisation. These projects are implemented through the State Governments (S.K.Mishra). There is active participation from the Government and Private sectors to bridge the gap in the quality of health care facilities between the urban and rural Indians, through setting up of telemedicine networks.

ISRO has established a telemedicine network for 300 hospitals. A total 257 remote/rural district hospitals and health centres have been connected to 43- super specialty hospitals located in major states. Ten mobile tele-ophtamology units are also present. A majority of the State Governments have collaborated with the Department of IT, in setting up telemedicine networks with the state specialty hospitals and smaller district centres (Saroj Mishra et al., 2008)

The growing need of telemedicine in India can be traced back to the works of (Amrita Pal et.al 2005), where a telemedicine setup in India is absolutely essential.

There has been a number of situations in which telemedicine has been successfully implemented. The Online Telemedicine Research Institute OTRI provided telemedicine links for teleconsultation in Bhuj during the earthquake in Gujarat in the year2001.Asia Heart Foundation has been successfully practising tele-cardiology between Bangalore and cities in Eastern India.The last decade witnessed many more success stories (S.P.Sood, 2002).

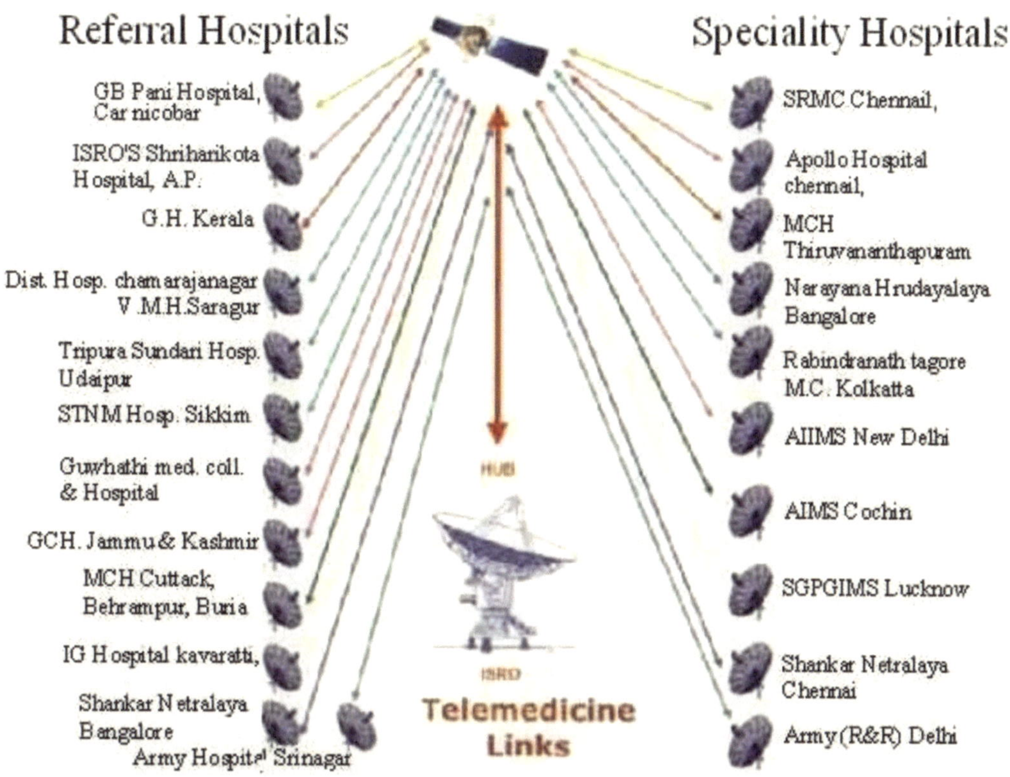

Fig. 3. Telemedicine links provided by Indian Space Research Organisation (ISRO) (S.K.Mishra)

1.4 Challenges identified in telemedicine technology in India

- A multifunctional Telemedicine facility is necessary which would enable the monitoring of the patient through a virtual instrument fed with physiological signals. This enables real time health monitoring of critically ill patients.
- To aid in decision-making, an automated decision support system can be developed which encompasses the principles of artificial intelligence and knowledge based expert system. This system could be of good use as a decision support tool to the physician.
- To improve the quality of decision making, image segmentation algorithms can be developed which take medical images as input and segment them to produce a well-defined area in that image. The same can be transmitted to the remote medical center for effective diagnosis.
- The medical images have to be transmitted across telemedicine network to remote medical centre for diagnosis. In this connection, effective loss-less compression algorithms can be developed which result in saving of storage space and better utilization of bandwidth and speed of data transmission.
- The existing image compression algorithms can be analyzed over several parameters and constraints like noise analysis. The outcome of this research will throw light on the most effective compression technique for various categories of images.
- In the present chapter, specific needs are identified and discussed hereunder. The needs are:

- An automated segmentation of two-dimensional data such as ultrasound images.
- Compression of the above data for quick and reliable transmission.

1.5 Significance of image segmentation in telemedicine

Segmentation of medical images is one of the interesting applications of image processing techniques and has attracted a significant amount of attention in the past few years(Lei Ma et al, 2005). It is a technique for partitioning the image into meaningful sub regions or objects with same attributes, and usually is image and application dependent. Several segmentation methods have been proposed in medical images and especially in ultrasound images (Wy Ma, B.S.Manjunath, 2000). A number of algorithms based upon approaches such as histogram analysis, region growing, edge detection, and pixel classification have been proposed in the past. Generally speaking, these methods make use of local information (i.e., the gray-level values of the neighbouring pixels) and/or the global information (i.e., overall gray-level distribution of the image) for image segmentation. Some algorithms using neural network approach have also been investigated in image segmentation problems (Kuo Sheng Cheng et al, 1996).

A large number of different approaches are employed recently on segmenting images. The methods for ultrasound medical image segmentation rely on five main approaches, namely, thresholding technique, boundary-based method, region based methods, and hybrid techniques that combine boundary and region criteria and active contour based approach.

Ultrasound imaging has been used extensively for detecting cysts. The Radiologist scans the body for detection of cyst and reports the features of cyst.

In general, the diagnosis of illness involves two basic tasks of collection of information about the patient and analysis of that information to arrive at a conclusion about the type of the illness. An automated model that receives information about the cyst and produces segmented output of cyst image will be of immense help in the future. These segmented images can be transmitted through the network to the medical center where the analysis is carried out and suitable medical recommendations provided by the decision support tool at the distant medical center.

Thus, there remains a tremendous need for creation of knowledge based artificially intelligent decision support system for detection and diagnosis of diseases and incorporating this model into telemedicine technology. This is achievable given the advances made in the field of information technology and medical imaging.

1.6 Significance of image compression techniques in telemedicine

1.6.1 Compression techniques

Data Compression is one of the most renowned branches of Computer Science. Over the years, extensive research has been done in this field and many standards have been developed to compress data in several ways (A.K.Jain, 1981).

Data Compression can be defined as reducing of the amount of storage space required to store a given amount of data. Data compression comes with a lot of advantages. It saves storage space, bandwidth, cost and time required for transmitting data from one place to another. Compression can be lossy or loss-less. With a loss-less compression and decompression, the original and decompressed files are identical bit per bit. On the other hand, compression efficiency can be improved by throwing away most of redundant data, without however losing much quality.

There are many loss-less compression techniques such as Arithmetic coding, Run Length Encoding, Huffman Coding and some famous Dictionary based algorithms like Lempel-Ziv-Welch (LZW) coding, though Huffman Coding forms the basis of many compression algorithms. JPEG, MPEG, which are lossy compression methods use Huffman coding. Even the new proposed algorithms like JPEG-2000, Burrows-wheeler transformations (Bwt) and BTTC use Huffman coding in the final stages.

1.6.2 Compression for medical images

Medical images give information of shape and function of organs of human body, this being one of the most important means for diagnosis. An expert physician uses images for diagnosis, together with other information. In most cases it is qualitative and subjective evaluation. The information conveyed by medical images is very difficult to exploit quantitatively and objectively. Increasingly, medical images are acquired or stored digitally. This is especially true of the images that are used in radiology applications.

1.6.3 Reasons for choosing a loss-less technique

Medical images are compressed due to their large size and repeated usage for diagnosing purposes. Certified radiologists and doctors assess the degree of image degradation resulting from various types and amounts of compression associated with several different digital image file formats. A qualitative, rather than a quantitative approach is normally chosen because radiologists typically evaluate images qualitatively in their day-to-day practice and, also, because common metrics used for comparing images pre- and post compression, e.g., mean pixel error, root mean square error, maximum error, etc., may not correlate well with visual assessment of image quality.

BMP (bitmapped picture) is Microsoft Windows device-independent bitmap standard for loss-less format. Users of this format can depend on images being displayed on any Windows device. BMP supports 24-bit images. Loss-less compression is possible, using Huffman algorithm. Images compressed in loss-less manner occupy less space than the originals. No image data are lost during loss-less compression. Decompression restores the original image without loss of fidelity.

We have dealt with the above said concepts and challenges In the present chapter, we address the research issues pertaining to effective compression of medical images.

2. Effective medical image compression

Medical images should be subjected to loss-less compression, a technique that stems from mathematical theory of communication (Shannon, 1948**)**. Loss-less compression techniques use variable length codes, proposed by Huffman (David Huffman, 1952). Compression ratio achieved is not very satisfactory in Huffman. Hence modifying Huffman's technique and optimizing it, yields a more effective compression algorithm that increases the compression ratio on medical images. Compression ratio and storage space are inversely proportional. Hence effective compression technique results in a reduction in storage space, thereby improving the bandwidth and speed of transmission of medical images with no added complexity and resources.

As far as medical images are concerned, several research processes are reported for effectiveness of loss-less compression. One such paper evaluated the effectiveness of traditional and state of the art approaches of loss-less compression of grayscale medical images. The new JPEG-LS process (ISO/IEC 14495-1), and the loss-less mode of the proposed JPEG 2000 scheme (ISO/IEC CD15444-1), which are new standard schemes that may be incorporated into DICOM, was evaluated. Three thousand, six hundred and seventy-nine (3,679) single frame grayscale images from multiple anatomical regions, modalities and vendors, were tested. For all images, combined JPEG-LS and JPEG 2000 performed equally well. Both out-performed existing JPEG.It was found that the use of standard schemes could achieve state of the art performance, regardless of modality. Further, it was found that JPEG-LS is simple, easy to implement, consumes less memory, and is faster than JPEG 2000, though JPEG 2000 will offer lossy and progressive transmission(D.A.Clunie,2004).

Another interesting paper performed loss-less medical image compression by building a modified S-tree structure to make each block contain similar pixels. The medical images have a very close pixel-to-pixel correlation. In order to preserve this characteristic, a loss-less medical image compression method was developed. It was found that this method could reduce the required number of bits to record those pixels. The experimental results also show that this method is better than other methods in almost all cases (Chi-Shiang Chan, Chin-Chen Chang, 2005).

In another paper, a design of ultrasound data compression in a tele-ultrasound system was presented. It underlines the benefits of tele-ultrasound that may not be available in locations, which lack high bandwidth transmission channels. Because of the importance of speckle structure in the ultrasound image, standard compression algorithms like conventional JPEG are not suitable for ultrasound images. This design of compression was tested on those locations, which has band limited signal channel (R.Mir et al, 2003).

Other approaches for image compression use Wavelet transform-based image compression algorithms, which are recognized as a superior method to compress, archive, and electronically disseminate medical imagery. This class of algorithm is now available to a wider medical system user base with the approval of JPEG2000 as an accepted image compression option by the DICOM Working Group 4 (compression group) (M.A Ansari, R.S. Anand, 2005).

Although, new techniques that provide better compression ratio are developed now, a careful study into the Huffman Compression technique reveals the scope for improvement in terms of compression ratio and computationally simpler code. Such an algorithm is developed which optimizes the existing Huffman's variable length codes and produces an effective compression technique for medical images. This is discussed in 3.2

3. Related work-effectiveness of Huffman compression in telemedicine

3.1 Huffman – A basic compression technique

Huffman codes are digital data compression codes resulted from the excellent piece of work by Prof. David A. Huffman. Huffman codes exploit the entropy of the message to give good compression ratios.

Huffman coding is a statistical coding technique that forms the basis for many compression techniques. Huffman compression techniques consist of techniques guaranteed to generate an exact duplicate of input data stream after an expand cycle. This type of compression is used when storing database records, spreadsheets, or word processing file and image formats. In these applications, the loss of even a single bit could be catastrophic. Huffman algorithm can be used in the case of medical image compression where there should not be any loss of information during compression that will affect proper diagnosis.

3.2 Improved Huffman compression Algorithm (An introduction to the existing work)

The Huffman Coding can be refined to generate a new effective compression algorithm, which will give improved compression ratio and at the same time maintain the quality of the original image like Huffman.

The core concept of the algorithm is based on building up a collection of n-length patterns in the image. The basic model of new compression algorithm is similar to that of the Huffman encoder except for the pattern finder (J.Janet, T.R.Natesan, 2005). The operation of the pattern finder is to find the best pattern, which is the most frequent occurring pattern. Therefore the best pattern will also be an input to the encoder. The output of the encoder will be the code along with footer information.

3.2.1 Working steps for IHC (Improved Huffman Compression) Algorithm

There are four basic considerations for implementing this new compression method. However, they do not impose an added complexity to the existing system.

These restrictions include:

- The pattern is restricted to 3-length patterns.
- The first and last characters in the pattern must not be same as the second (middle) character to be replaced by Footer information.
- The pattern once traced for its positions must not be traced again. (i.e.) Each pattern must be traced only once.
- Positions of the patterns and sub patterns traced must be accurate.

3.2.2 Pattern recognition

The idea is based on the redundant nature of character or signals in the data encountered. Consider for example a 3-length pattern commonly occurring in text files say "ABC". Here, considering the sub pattern "AC" of length 2, all 3- length patterns such as "ABC" patterns can be encoded as "AC" in the corresponding compressed version. To differentiate between "ABC"s and "AC"s in order to bring out the exact original file on decoding, the concept of a new feature called "Footer Information" is introduced. Through this footer information bits, "1"s indicate the presence of "B" in "ABC" and "0"s denote the absence of "B" in the sub patterns "AC"s. These bits are added at the last of compressed file after coding other characters in the file. These extra sets of bits are called footer bits, as they resemble the footer note of a word document that is added at the end of a page. Generally to identify the start of Footer bits from the normal compressed bits codes are added for first and third characters found in the pattern being selected (i.e.) codes of "A" and "C" are added in footer information. They also help in the identification of the sub patterns between which the reduced character namely "B" (here) have to be inserted during decompression.

3.2.3 Search of best patterns

The original medical image considered for compression can be of any type namely scans images, or x-ray or MRI etc. As the first step, all the characters are read with an initial note of forming the frequency table. The count for each character is entered in their corresponding ASCII position in the output file. Now the file is searched for 3-length patterns with the initial conditions stated above. This aim for finding the patterns forms the basic differences from original method. The positions of occurrence of each and every pattern throughout the file are stored with their count of occurrence. Each and every pattern has its corresponding sub pattern formed by their first and last character (i.e.) omitting their middle character. These sub patterns are also searched for its occurrence throughout the file. Their positions and their count are stored along with their corresponding pattern's positions and count.

After tracing the patterns, selection is made for the best pattern that can yield the maximum amount of bits that can be reduced. Hence, an array is constructed which holds the total bits that can be reduced for each and every pattern. The total bits that can be reduced are calculated by computing the product of the code length of the middle character of each and every pattern of length 3 that are being stored and their count. Hence a tree data structure is constructed. Based on the codes formed for middle character for the patterns, the maximum bits that can be reduced are noted. Then this large sum is subtracted from the number of footer bits being added to the file. This is obtained by computing the sum of counts of occurrences of the pattern and its corresponding sub pattern. The total number of bits that can be reduced for each pattern is then stored in a new array for each pattern. The patterns are then sorted in the descending order to decide for the best pattern.

Once the best pattern is decided, footer bits are identified. Any footer information starts with the codes for the first and the third character of the chosen pattern. The remaining bits are formed based on the position of occurrences of the selected pattern and its corresponding sub pattern. This is obtained by finding the index of the best pattern from the stored pattern array. Based on this index, 1 is added to the footer information if the first encountered position is from patterns list, else a zero is added if the first encountered position belongs to that of sub patterns.

The normal Huffman method is followed if the best pattern cannot be found. The compressed file is formed by replacing each character with their codes except the middle characters in the chosen pattern, which are checked by their positions already traced. The footer bits are added at the last after adding compressed codes. The set of bytes so formed make up a compressed file. The compressed file includes an extension ". hff1" to the original bmp file. As the compressed file size gets reduced further, the amount of compression done here increases in comparison to Huffman model.

3.3 Optimization

In the optimization part, the new compression algorithm is improved further by selecting out two best patterns each of length three but assisted via a single set of footer information. In simple words it is the extension to one pattern replacement. This part helps in increasing the compression percentage by 2-3% more than the single pattern and by 4-5% than the Huffman method. The research was further extended to search for 3 best patterns, which yield better compression ratios than existing methods (Divya Mohandass, Dr.J.Janet, 2010). The 3pattern Huffman compression algorithm as depicted in Fig. 4.can be applied to all types of medical images namely CT, MRI and ultrasound images. Experimental results indicate improved compression ratios without compromise on image quality.

However, at a particular point in time, as the numbers of best pattern search increases, a slight degradation in the image quality is observed. The threshold value' n' is computed, where there is some complexity in pattern search and image quality. The value of n is found to be 5.

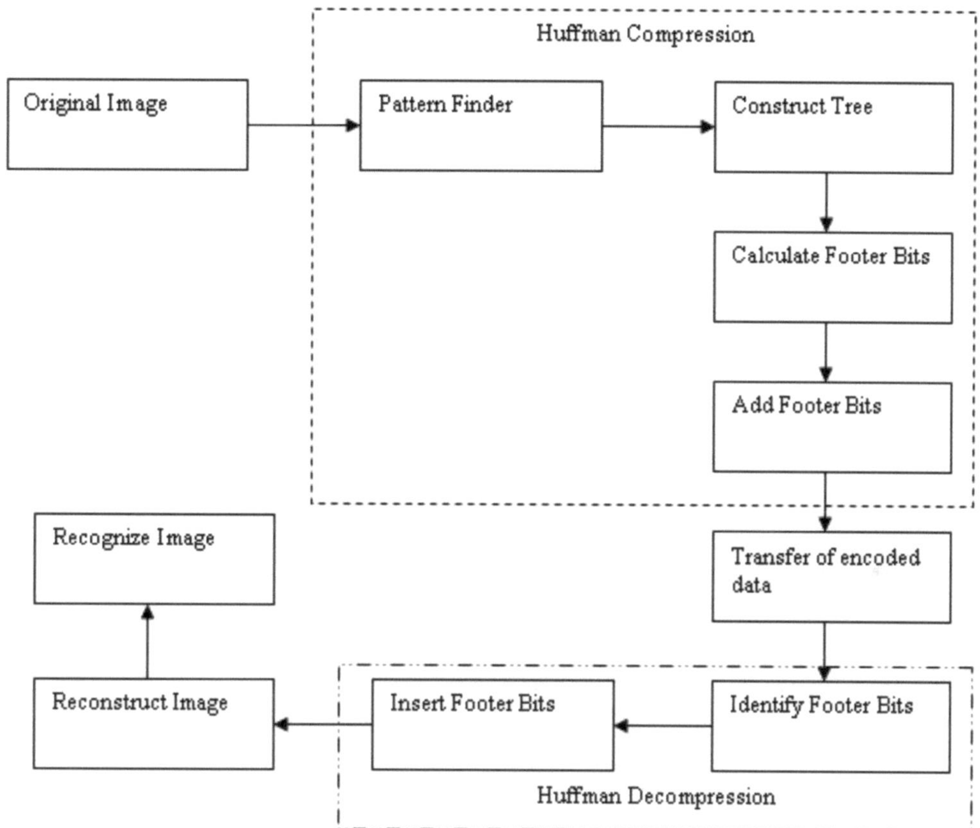

Fig. 4. 3-pattern Huffman compression algorithm

Increasing the value of n to be greater than 5 introduces complexity in computation of footer bits. Increasing size of footer bits causes a reduction in the compression ratio. Hence, it has been observed that the search for best patterns is restricted to 5.

A hybrid compression technique (Divya Mohandass, Dr.Janet,2010) was also implemented. The input to the system was an ultrasound medical image.The image was segmented into ROI and non-ROI using Canny Edge Detction Algorithm.The ROI was compressed using 4-pattern Huffman compression algorithm and the non-ROI was compressed using lossy baseline JPEG algorithm. Another challenge pertaining telemedicine namely image segmentation has been addressed with the design of a hybrid algorithm (Divya Mohandass, Dr.J.Janet,2010).The hybrid algorithm has been tested on ultrasound images with cyst. The input algorithm was introduced to enhance the amount of compression still further.

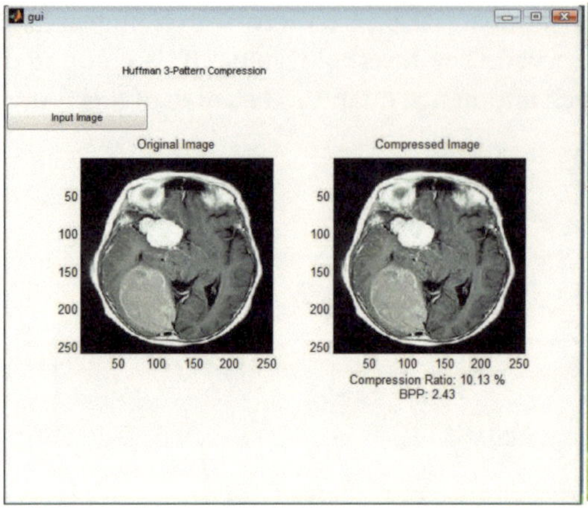

(a)

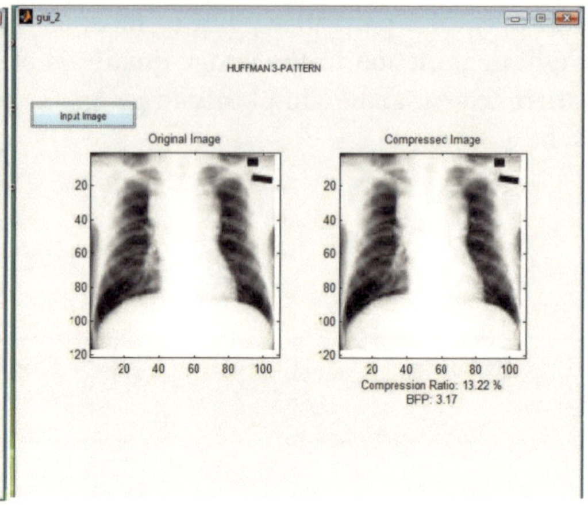

(b)

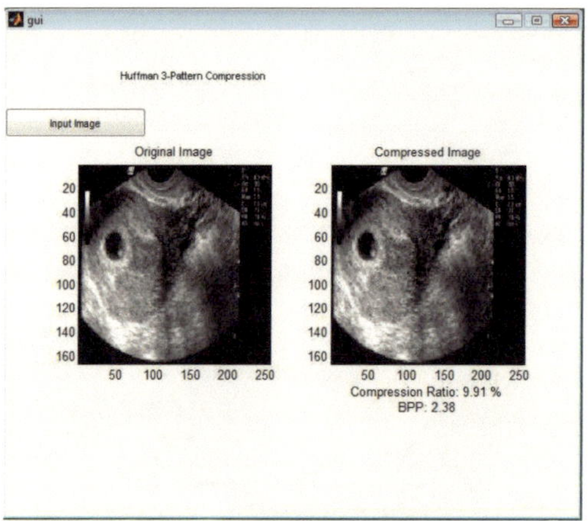

(c)

Fig. 5. 3 Pattern Huffman Compression results a) MRI Brain image b) X-ray chest image c) Ultrasound abdomen image

4. Transform based image compression

The focus on image compression algorithms lie on the fact that image should be represented with a minimum number of bits while maintaining a desirable quality. A number of methods are available in literature. Transform coding is a widely used method of compressing medical images.2-D images from the spatial domain are mapped to the frequency domain and concentrates vital information into few transform coefficients. The generalized transform-based image compression method works as follows:

a. Image Transform: This operation aims to decorrelate pixels of the image. This operation is reversible and does not cause any loss of information in the image. Examples of such a transform operation are cosine transform, wavelet transform and contourlet transform.
b. Quantization: This operation is irreversible and represents the lossy stage in the compression process. It maps a large set of input image values to a smaller set of quantized values.

c. Encoding: This process removes redundancy of the output of the quantizer. The most common entropy coding techniques are Run-Length Encoding (RLE), Huffman coding, arithmetic coding and Lempel-Ziv- Welsh methods.

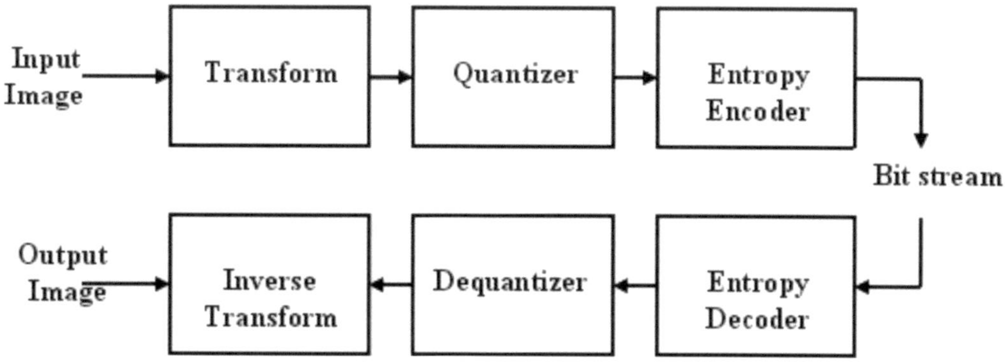

Fig. 6. Transform based image compression

4.1 Proposed strategy

In this chapter, a Joint compression method based on contourlet and built upon the well known Huffman encoding is proposed. The basic characteristics of contourlet transform and the details of the proposed strategy are presented in detail.

4.2 Contourlet coding

Contourlet transform is an extension to the existing wavelet transform. They use non-separable and directional filter banks. Recent studies reveal the lack of directionality caused by wavelets. (M.Do.and M.Veterelli,2005) have proposed the concept of contourlet in representing contours and other fine details in an image, which was a drawback in the wavelet methods.Moreover,unlike other transforms, contourlet is easily implemented by a filter bank (S.Esakkirajan et al.,2006).

Contourlet transform comprises two blocks, a Laplacian pyramid (LP), introduced by (Burt and Adelson,1983) and a directional filter bank (DFB). The LP decomposition at each level generates a signal by means of a low pass filter and down sampling. This coarse version is then sampled up and filtered to predict the original image. The prediction residual constitutes the detail signal as seen in Fig. 7. This procedure can be repeated iteratively in order to obtain a multiresolution decomposition.

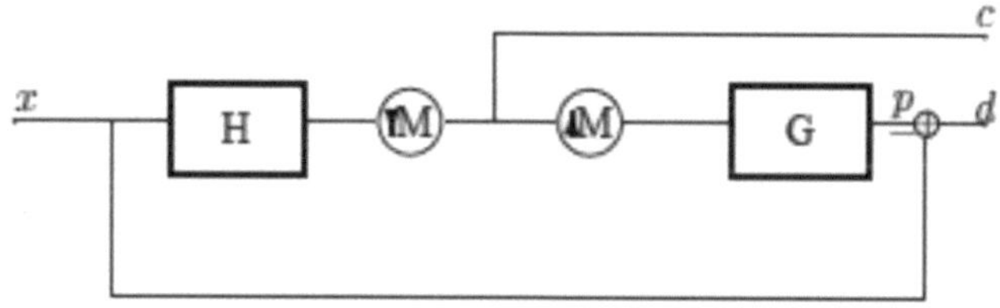

Fig. 7. Laplacian pyramid

In contourlet decomposition, a directional filtering is performed on the band pass versions of input signal. Hence, it needs a decomposition that permits further sub band decomposition of its band pass images. LP has two advantages. First, it generates only one band pass version, second, it does not suffer from the frequencies "scrambling

In contourlet scheme, a structure which implements the dual frame reconstruction has been implemented because it is an optimal choice in presence of noise.

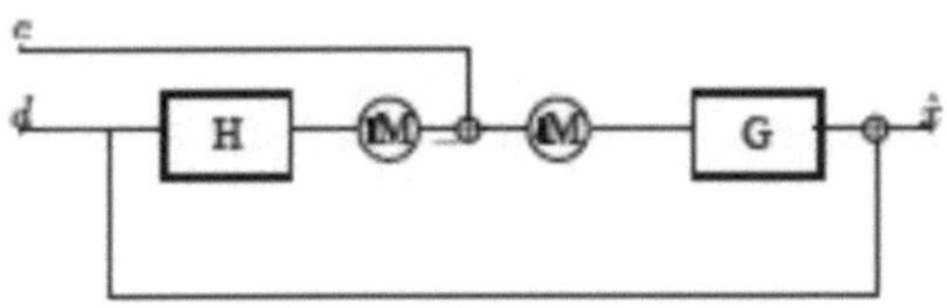

Fig. 8. Directional filter bank

The second block of contourlet decomposition is a directional filter bank that singles out directional components, with a number of directions that can vary as a power of two. Bamberger and Smith introduced a perfect reconstruction directional filter banks (DFB) that can be maximally decimated, implemented via an l-level tree-structured decomposition that leads to 2l sub bands with wedge-shaped frequency partition. Fig.9 shows an example of DFB frequency partitioning with l = 3, the sub bands 0-3 correspond to the mostly horizontal directions, while sub bands 4-7 correspond to the mostly vertical directions.

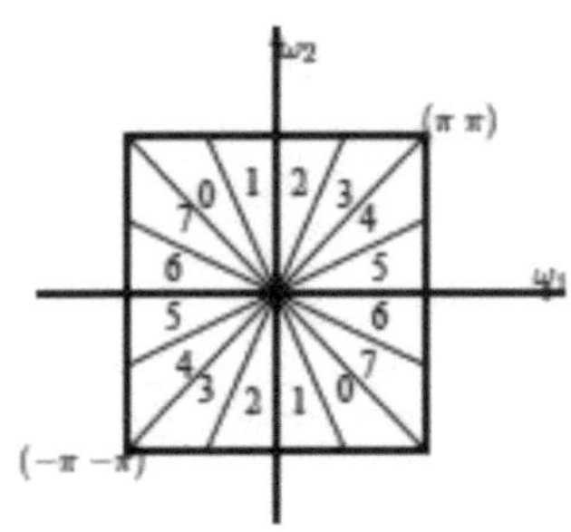

Fig. 9. DFB frequency partitioning with l=3

4.3 Global thresholding and Huffman encoding

The proposed approach involves the computation of threshold using the Otsu's method. (N.Otsu,1979) proposed the widely used binarisation method. If a binarization method computes threshold for an entire image, it is known as a global method.Local thresholding is more adaptive, by selecting different threshold for each area in the image, according to the image characteristics.

In this method, we can directly calculate the threshold without pre-treatment to histogram. This algorithm is simple and is a remarkable method for selecting the threshold. The fundamental principle is given.

The gray value of a grey-scale map is 0~255.The total number of pixels is defined as N, n_i is the number of pixels which's gray value is i. By normalizing the histogram, the following equations could be obtained.

$$\sum_{i=0}^{255} n_i = N \tag{1}$$

$$p_i = \frac{n_i}{N} \tag{2}$$

p_i is the probability of the pixels which's gray value is i. The threshold of the image segmentation is defined as m, then the probability θ and mean value μ of the background can be obtained through the following equations:

$$\theta_0 = \sum_{i=0}^{m} p_i \qquad \mu_0 = \frac{\sum_{i=0}^{m} ip_i}{\theta_0} \tag{3}$$

The probability and typical value of the target also can be obtained:

$$\theta_1 = \sum_{i=m+1}^{255} p_i \qquad \mu_1 = \frac{\sum_{i=m+1}^{255} ip_i}{\theta_1} \tag{4}$$

The variance between the background and target is defined as σ^2

$$\sigma_B^2 = \theta_0(\mu_0 - \mu_T)^2 + \theta_1(\mu_1 - \mu_T)^2 \tag{5}$$

$$\mu_T = \sum_{i=0}^{255} ip_i \tag{6}$$

By computing the equation (3), (4), (5) and (6), the following equation (7) could be obtained.

$$\sigma_B^2 = \theta_0\theta_1(\mu_0 - \mu_1)^2 \tag{7}$$

Variance is a metric of the uniformity of distribution, the greater the variance yields, the greater the difference between the target and the background. Therefore, the threshold which makes the variance yields maximal is the optimal threshold.

4.4 Contourlet based joint medical image compression

A simple block diagram of the proposed strategy is depicted in Fig. 10. The input to the system is a gray scale image. A 2-dimensional contourlet transform is applied to the acquired input medical image. The image is split into 8 subbands. Global Thresholding and Huffman encoding is applied to the lower frequency sub bands and the compression percentage is calculated.

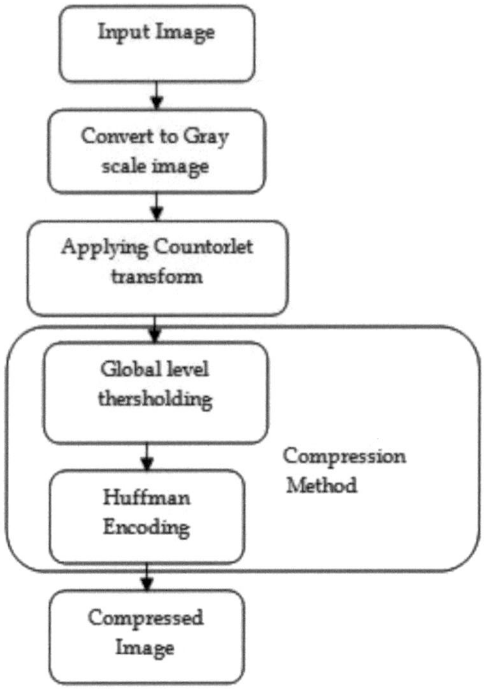

Fig. 10. Block diagram of proposed system

4.5 Algorithm Steps of Joint Contourlet based Medical Image Compression

Step 1. Input Medical image
Step 2. Convert Gray scale image
Step 3. Contourlet transform
    Level = 3
Begin contourlet (Input image, Level)
CT = nsctdec (Input image, Level)
for x = 1:2^Level
    Add the all contourlet subband images
end
End Contourlet (Input image, Level)
Step 4. Step 4: Compress technique
    Method name = 'gbl_mmc_h'
    option = 'c'
Begin Compress (Method name, option, Input image)
    1. Calculate size of output image.
    2. Calculate compression percentage.
End Compress (Method name, option, Input image)

5. Experimental results and discussion

The proposed algorithm was tested on 256x256 CT, MRI medical images. Simulation results reveal the compression ratios and PSNR values of the tested input images.

$$\text{Compression Ratio} = \frac{\text{Compressed Size}}{\text{Uncompressed Size}}$$

Thus a representation that compresses a 10MB file to 2MB would yield a space savings of 1 - 2/10 = 0.8, often notated as a percentage, 80%.
PSNR expanded as Peak Signal To Noise ratio is a metric used to determine the quality of reconstruction in any compression method. For a considerably good quality image reconstruction, the PSNR ranges from 20 to 40. Experimental results reveal that our method shows good compression ratios and PSNR values.The compression ratio and PSNR values were computed on various test images and calculated.

Test Image	Compression Ratio	PSNR value(db)
Image1	11.78	34.03
Image2	13.84	33.39
Image3	10.76	35.53
Image4	17.93	35.61
Image5	14.27	34.68
Image6	15.2	35.07
Image7	15.53	32.8

Table 1.Compression ratio and PSNR values of test images

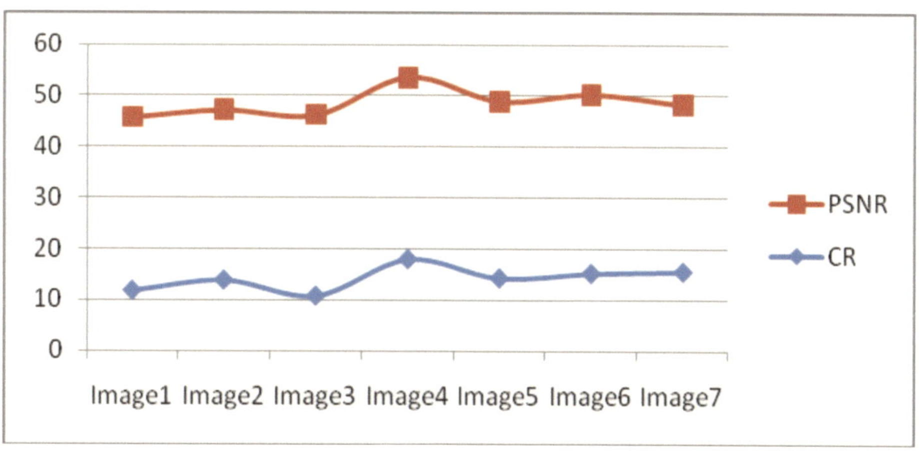

Fig. 11. Graph plot of CR and PSNR of test images

6. Conclusion

In the present chapter, a joint medical image compression scheme based on contourlet transform was proposed. The outcome obtained on applying most of the image processing algorithms is that they give different results when applied to different classes of medical images. The algorithm was applied to various medical images, collected from a database of CT, MRI modalities. Better image reconstruction is possible, on account of the application of the contourlet transform Telemedicial applications require images to be transferred without loss of information.Hence, lossless methods are applied. The proposed system is a purely lossless technique in which the experimental results reveal improved compression percentages, than the existing methods in literature, thereby making it suitable for telemedicine applications and for the medical fraternity. In future, the joint medical image compression technique could be applied on different transforms namely directionlets and curvelets , and the compression percentage could be evaluated.

7. References

Alfredrol. Hernandez, Fernando Mora, Guillermo Villegas, G. Passariello, Real Time ECG Transmission Via Internet for Non Clinical Applications. IEEE Transactions on Information Technology in Biomedicine,Vol.5,No.3, September 2001, pp.253-257.

Ansari.M.A, Anand.R.S, Performance Analysis of Medical Image Compression Techniques with respect to quality of compression, Proceedings of ICTES 2007, Chennai, India, December,2007,pp.743-750, ISSN:0537-9989.

Anunay Nayak,Jayanta Mukherjee, Arun Kumar Majumdhar, Telemedicine: A low cost Solution, www.facweb.ernet.in.

Amrita Pal, Victor W. A. Mbarika, Fay Cobb-Payton, Pratim Datta, and Scott McCoy, Telemedicine Diffusion in A Developing Country: The Case Of India(March 2004), IEEE Transactions On Information Technology In Biomedicine,Vol.9, No.1,March 2005, pp59-65,ISSN:1089-7771

Burt.P.J., Adelson.E.H., The Laplacian pyramid as a compact image code, IEEE Transactions on Communication,Vol.31,No.4,1983,pp532-540,ISSN:0090-6778.

Chi-Shiang Chan, Chin Chen Chang, A Loss less Medical Image Compression Scheme Using Modified S-Tree Structure,19th conference on Advance Information Networking and Applications(AINA'05),Vol.2,pp.75-78,ISSN:1550-445X.

Clunie, DA,Lossless compression of grayscale medical images – effectiveness of traditional and state of the art approaches, SPIE International Conference on Medical Imaging,San DIEGO , CA,Feb 2000 ,pp 74-84,ISBN:0-8194-3597-X.

David .A.Huffman, A method of construction of minimum redundancy codes, Proceedings of I.R.E.,September 1952.

Divya Mohandass, J.Janet, An Improved Three Pattern Huffman Compression Algorithm For Medical Images In Telemedicine", Proceedings of the International Conference On Business Administration And Information Processing (BAIP'20107),March 2010,pp 263-268,ISBN:978-3-642-12213-2.

Divya Mohandass, J.Janet, Design And Implementation Of A Hybrid Compression Technique For Ultrasound Images In Telemedicine, Vol.2, No.7, pp112-117,ISSN print:2076-2739.

Do.M.N.,and Vetterli.M, The contourlet transform: an efficient directional multiresolution image representation, IEEE Transactions. Of ImageProcessing, vol.14, no.12, Dec 2004, pp. 2091-2106, ISSN:1057-7149.

Esakkirajan.S, Veerakumar.T, Senthilmurugan. V and Sudhakar.R., Image Compression using contourlet transform and multistage vector Quantization. *GVIP Journal*, Volume 6, Issue 1, July 2006,pp19-28,ISSN Print:1687-3998.

Hung.K,Zhang YT, Implementation of a WAP -based telemedicine system for patient monitoring, IEEE Transactions on Information Technology in Biomedicine, Vol 7, No.2, June 2003,pp.5019-5029,ISSN Print:1089-7771.

Jain A.k, Fundamentals of Digital Image Processing, Prentice Hall, Information and System Science Series, Eaglewood Cliffs, NJ, USA,1989, ISBN:0-13-336165-9.

Janet.J, Natesan T.R., Effective image compression technique for medical images in Telemedicine, Asian Journal Of Information Technology,Vol.4,No.12, pp1180-1186,ISSN Print:1682-3915.

Kuo Sheng Cheng, Jzau-Lin, and Chi-Wu Mao, The Application of Competitive Hop Field Neural Network to Medical Image Segmentation. IEEE Transactions on Medical Imaging, Vol 15, No.4, August 199, pp, 560-567, ISSN:0278-0062.

Lei Ma, Xiao-Ping Zhang, Jennie Si, and Glen .P.Abousleman, Bi-directional Labeling and Registration Scheme for GrayScale Image Segmentation, IEEE Transactions on Image Processing, Vol.14,Vol.12,December 2005,ISSN:1057-7149.

Ma.W.Y., Manjunath.B.S, Edge Flow: A Technique FOR Boundary Detection and Image Segmentation. IEEE Transactions on Image Processing, Vol.9,No.8,August 2000,pp.1375-1388,ISSN:1057-7149.

Mir.R, S.k.Setarehdan, and P.J.Maralani (Iran), Ultrasound Data Compression in a Tele-Ultrasound system, Proceedings from IASTED conference on Biomedical Engineering, 2003, pp.386-396.

Mishra S., Ganapathy. K, Baljit Singh Bedi, The Current Status of ehealth initiativesIn India, Bellagio, Italy, August 2008.

Mishra S.K, "India Country Report On Tele health initiatives http://mohfro.nic.in/NRHM/presentations/India ehealth status.pps.

Mockzo.J.A, L.Kramer, A.Gacek, J.Jezewski, Virtual instrumentation in medical investigations and diagnosis support , Proceedings of 23rd Annual International Conference of the IEEE on Engineering in Medicine and Biology Society, October 25-28,2001,pp.1881-1891.

Otsu.N., A threshold selection method from gray-levelhistograms. IEEE Transactions on Systems Man, Cybernet pp-62-66,ISSN:0018-9472.

Shannon, C.E. A mathematical Theory of Communication, Bell System Technical Journal, Vo..27, July 1948, pp 379-423, ISBN:0-25-272548-4.

Sood, S.P., India telemedicine venture seeks to improve care, increase access. TeleMedicine Today, Oct/Nov 2002, pp.25-26.

6

Video-Telemedicine with Reliable Color Based on Multispectral Technology

Masahiro Yamaguchi[1], Yuri Murakami[1], Yasuhiro Komiya[2], Yoshifumi Kanno[3], Junko Kishimoto[3], Ryo Iwama[4], Hiroyuki Hashizume[5], Michiko Aihara[6] and Masaki Furukawa[6]

[1]Tokyo Institute of Technology,
[2]Olympus Co.,
[3]NTT DATAi Co.,
[4]NTT DATA Co.,
[5]Kasaoka Daiichi Hospital,
[6]Yokohama City University
Japan

1. Introduction

Videos and still-images play quite important role in telemedicine, such as dermatology, teleconsultation, endoscopy, and surgery video. However, one of the problems is the lack of color reproducibility, since it is difficult to reproduce the original color of the object in conventional color imaging systems based on RGB (red, green, blue). Although the color management technology enables to deal with color as device independent information, the color reproduced on the monitor still does not agree with the original object.

For the solution to such problem, the spectrum-based technology, instead of conventional RGB based methods has been developed aiming at high-fidelity color reproduction in both video and still image systems. By using multispectral image capture, illumination spectrum measurement, spectrum-based color conversion, and multiprimary color display, the colors of real object can be faithfully reproduced on a display. The technology is called "natural vision (NV)" (Yamaguchi et. al., 2008). The advantages of multispectral technology in various possible applications, such as telemedicine, digital archives of historical heritage or art works, electronic commerce, educational video contents, and high-quality color printing, have been shown in the literature.

In this chapter, we introduce the system developed for video-based telemedicine with reliable color, and demonstrate the results of experimental evaluation for the telemedicine applications including dermatology, surgery video and the video-based teleconsultation between a general hospital and a clinic.

2. Related works

The color of the medical images was not paid strong attention until now, but the color information is quite important in many cases. In dermatology, the color of skin has critical

information for diagnosis (Numahara, 2001), and attempts to calibrate the color imagnig device have been presented (Herbin et. al., 1990; Haeghen et. al., 2000; Maglogiannis, 2004). In 2008, American Telemedicine Association published practice guidelines for teledermatology, in which the technique to maintain the color quality was described Krupinski et. al., 2008).
Color video are also used in telemedicine; both store-and-forward and real-time teleconferencing, such as teledermatology (Loane et. al., 2000; Maglogiannis, 2004), telesurgery (Demartines, et. al., 2000; Rafiq, et. al., 2004; Augestad, et. al., 2009), tele-endoscopy (Wildi et. al., 2004), emergency telemedicine (Gállego, et. al., 2005; Bolle, et. al., 2009), telecare for chronic disease (Nilsson, et. al., 2009), and telepsychiatry (Yellowlees, et. al., 2010). Image quality issues in video telemedicine have been studied (Hanna and Cuschieri, 2001), such as the dependence on the image compression (Broderick, et. al., 2001; Duplaga, et. al., 2008) or the comparison of different equipments (Berci, et. al., 1995). However, no report is found on the quantitative analysis of color fidelity in video.
It has been pointed out that there is a limitation in the color reproduction capability of RGB-based imaging system, and the application of multispectral imaging have been suggested (Burns and Berns, 1996; Hill, 1998; Yamaguchi, et. al., 1997). There have been proved that the high accuracy can be achieved by applying multispectral imaging. In the display industry, the multiprimary color approach becomes one of the choices for expanding color gamut (Ueki, et. al., 2009), but it is difficult to take full advantage of multiprimary color technology with conventional RGB image capture, because a wide gamut image is not available by RGB cameras. There have been proposed the systems for color management including spectral information for hardcopy applications (Rosen, et. al., 2001; Derhak and Rosen, 2004) and image displays (Hill, 1998; Yamaguchi, et. al., 2008). Using spectrum-based color management, the color of the original object can be reproduced in high-accuracy. As for medical application, the multispctral imaging was applied to dermatology (Tomatis, et. al., 2003; Yamaguchi et. al., 2005) and pathology (Levenson, et. al., 2003; Abe, et. al., 2005), providing the benefit of color reproducibility as well as the quantification of color information in the medical color images.
The applications of multispectral video for color reproduction have been studied in our group; such as apparels, video production especially for science and art, and videoconferencing (Yamaguchi, et. al., 2008) It enables high-fidelity and wide-gamut video creation and will enhance the visual communication in both professional and consumer applications. Telemedicine is one of the most important application areas of multispectral video technology, and this research focuses on the application of multispectral video to the color reproduction in dermatology, surgery, and rural patient care. Through the experiments in these fields, this work addresses the question: does the use of multispectral technology provide any benefit from the viewpoint of color reproducibility? For this purpose, both objective and subjective evaluations of color reproducibility were performed. There was no such report on the evaluation of the color reproducibility of multispectral imaging in telemedicine.

3. Spectrum-based color reproduction system

3.1 Overcoming the limitation of RGB trichromatic scheme

The color of images we see on display is based on the "additive color mixture," and all the conventional color imaging technology stands on trichromatic color system, especially using RGB. There are however, limitations of conventional RGB trichromatic systems, and it is quite difficult to realize high-fidelity color reproduction in the video or still-image communication systems. An approach to overcome such limitations and to realize high-fidelity color reproduction is going beyond RGB, namely, adopting a spectrum-based system instead of RGB. NV provides the method for systematizing the multispectral and multiprimary color imaging technologies, including image capture, processing, storage, printing, and display. Followings are the details of how the spectrum-based approach can overcome the limitation of conventional RGB scheme.

1. The RGB values in conventional systems have different meanings, depending on the device characteristics or color processing. For example, consumer color cameras are usually designed for user preference, and the RGB values do not represent objective color information. In order to deal with the color information independent on the devices, the color management technology should be employed, such as the color conversion using ICC (International Color Consortium) profile. However, there still remains the problem; since the spectral sensitivity of a color camera is different from that of human vision, the RGB signal does not have one-to-one correspondence to the tristimulus values perceived by human vision. Using MS image capture and appropriate color processing, it becomes possible to realize the spectral sensitivity that is equivalent to human vision.
2. When the illuminant of the image capture environment is different from that of display observation, white balance adjustment is performed in conventional color imaging systems. The white balance can adjust white, but other colors often change, since the spectral reflectance of object and the illuminant spectrum are required in principle in order to derive the color under the different illuminant. In such case, it is reasonable to reproduce the color as if the object were placed at the site of the observer. The reproduction of the color under different illuminant is possible based on the spectrum-based color conversion.
3. In the color image display, the color gamut is usually inside the triangle spanned by RGB primary colors, and does not cover all the existent colors; thus some high-saturation colors cannot be reproduced. Recently wide-gamut displays are commercially available, with using purer RGB primaries or multiprimary colors. Even if the display gamut is enlarged, the color signals represented in conventional color space, such as sRGB (equivalent to the color space defined in ITU-R BT.709) do not support a wider gamut. Wide gamut color spaces have recently become available, such as AdobeRGB and xvYCC, but most of the color input devices cannot capture high-saturation colors correctly, because the error described in (1) tends to large in high-saturation colors.
4. It is known that the spectral sensitivity of human vision, or color matching function, varies depending on individuals (Alfvin and Fairchild 1997). Therefore, when the color displayed on a monitor is compared with the real object, the perceived colors may disagree with each other even if the colorimetric accuracy is high. Such phenomenon is called observer metamerism. The multispectral and multiprimary approach can solve this problem by reproducing the spectral color reproduction (Murakami, et. al., 2004).
5. In most RGB-based color imaging systems, RGB does not represent the color attribute of an object, because the RGB values depend on the illumination light and/or the device characteristics. Thus the utilization of color information is limited in the image analysis, archive, or database. In contrast, the spectral information can represent the original attribute of an object that generates color. The quantitative spectral attributes of object, useful for the analysis or the recognition of object, are captured and preserved. Moreover, the exploration of invisible features becomes possible from spectral images.

3.2 The principle of spectrum-based color reproduction system

In this subsection, let us briefly review the principle of spectrum-based color reproduction (Yamaguchi, et. al., 2008). In the spectrum-based color reproduction system, the spectral radiance, reflectance, transmittance, or colorimetric tristimulus values under arbitrary illumination are estimated from the camera signal with using the input device profile and the spectral information of illuminant, as shown in fig.1. Using multispectral cameras with larger number of bands for the image capture, higher accuracy can be realized.

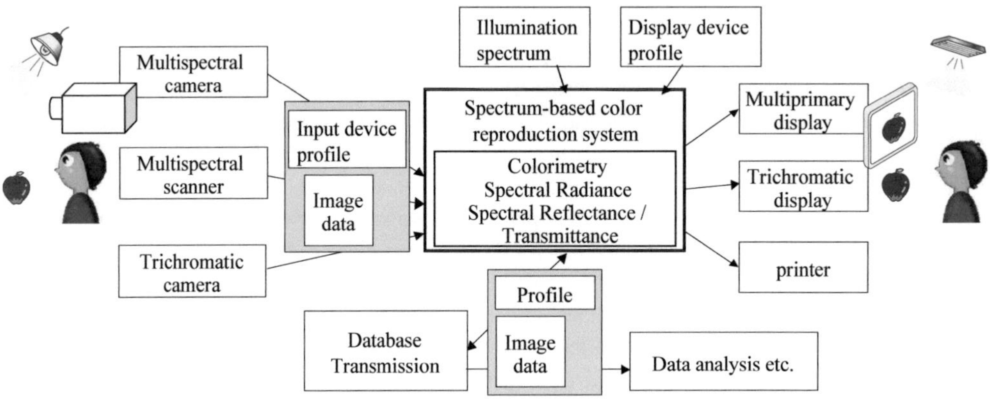

Fig. 1. The spectrum-based color reproduction scheme

Consider a certain point on the object, and its spectral reflectance sampled and denoted as **f**, which is an L-dimensional column vector. k-th element of **f** represents the reflectance of k-th wavelength λ_k, where

$$\lambda_k = \lambda_{\min} + k\Delta\lambda, \quad (1)$$

and $\lambda_{\min}$ and $\Delta\lambda$ are the minimum wavelength of visible range and the sampling interval in wavelength, respectively. Assuming linear response of the image sensor, the observed MS image **g**, represented by N-dimensional column vector, is given by

$$\mathbf{g} = \mathrm{S}\,\mathrm{E_c}\,\mathbf{f} + \mathbf{n}\,, \quad (2)$$

where S is a matrix with NxL elements and each row of S holds the discretized spectral sensitivity of the color camera, $\mathrm{E_c}$ is a diagonal matrix with LxL elements, and the diagonal elements corresponds sampled version of spectral radiance of illumination light at the image capture, **n** is a column vector which represents the noise in the observed image **g**, respectively. For the color reproduction under arbitrary illuminant, the colorimetric tristimulus values, such as CIE (Commission Internationale de l'Eclairage) 1931 XYZ, are required. Let a 3-dimensional column vector **x** be the XYZ values of the corresponding object under certain illuminant $\mathrm{E_r}$, which is called rendering illuminant hereafter, then **x** is given by

$$\mathbf{x} = \mathrm{C}\,\mathrm{E_r}\,\mathbf{f}\,, \quad (3)$$

where C is a matrix with 3xL elements, where each row represents CIE 1931 XYZ color matching function. Then the task for high-fidelity color reproduction is to derive **x** from **g**.

There have been reported various methods for this purpose, and one of the common approaches is a linear estimation, like

$$\hat{\mathbf{x}} = \mathrm{Q}\mathbf{g}, \tag{4}$$

where $\hat{\mathbf{x}}$ is the estimated tristimulus values, and Q is an estimation matrix with 3xM elements. Also a typical way to determine Q is Wiener estimation, given by

$$\mathrm{Q} = \mathrm{CE_r R_f E_c S}^t(\mathrm{SE_c R_f E_c S}^t + \mathrm{R_n})^+, \tag{5}$$

where R_f is the correlation matrix of **f** in LxL elements, R_n is the correlation matrix of noise in NxN elements, respectively. Additionally Q_s can be defined as,

$$\begin{aligned} &\mathrm{Q} = \mathrm{CE}_r\mathrm{Q_s} \\ &\mathrm{Q_s} = \mathrm{R_f E_c S}^t(\mathrm{SE_c R_f E_c S}^t + \mathrm{R_n})^+ \\ &\hat{\mathbf{f}} = \mathrm{Q_s}\mathbf{g} \end{aligned} \tag{6}$$

$\hat{\mathbf{f}}$ is the estimate of the spectral reflectance of the object, namely, Q_s is the matrix for spectral estimation.

In order to estimate the tristimulus values from the camera output using the eqs. (4) and (5), we need S, E_r, E_c, R_f, and R_n. The spectral sensitivity of the camera, S, can be obtained by using monochrometer and spectroradiometer. For example, a standard white diffuser is irradiated with the monochromatic light of every wavelength generated by the monochrometer, and is captured by the camera and the spectroradiometer. By normalizing the output signal value of each band of the camera, the spectral sensitivity is obtained. E_c and E_r are the spectral radiance of illumination light, measured by spectrometer at the image capturing and observation sites. As the correlation matrix R_f of the object spectral reflectance, there are several choices; if it is measured from the real object, the estimation accuracy is high, but is not always possible to get it. Instead, sometimes the correlation matrix derived from a color chart, such as GretagMacbeth ColorChecker, is used, and it gives fairly good performance. Another design of R_f is based on the 1st order Markov random field (MRF) model for the spectral reflectance. Since the spectral reflectance of most objects is smooth in the wavelength axis, MRF also gives good performance (Platt and Mancill, 1976). The noise correlation, or the covariance R_n, can be usually substituted with diagonal matrix, where each diagonal element is the noise variance of corresponding spectral channel. Another choice is to assume the noise variance to be constant over all channels, or just it can be omitted if the noise level is satisfactory low.

In the imaging model of eq.(2), the camera output is assumed to be linear to the light energy. In fact, when the input-output characteristics of the camera cannot be treated as linear, the tone reproduction curve of the camera is measured by capturing the gray-scale chart. The dark current of the sensor, such as CCD (Charge Coupled Device), should be also considered. It can be measured by placing a cap to the camera lens, and the average signal level is subtracted.

For the color image display, the characterization of display device is also required. It can be performed by using the commercial tool for making ICC profile, though the accuracy depends on the devices (both display device and characterization device). In the spectrum-based system, it is required to reproduce the XYZ tristimulus values regardless of the white point setting of the display device. For this purpose, the chromaticity coordinates of three primary colors and the tone reproduction characteristics of the RGB channels are measured, and we can obtain the 3x3 matrix and lookup tables for color conversion. As an alternative way, the white point of the display device can be set to the ambient illumination, such as the

standard D65 illuminant, and then the commercial color management scheme using ICC profile can be employed. The case of multiprimary color displays is discussed later.
Based on the above theory for spectrum-based color reproduction, the color under the illuminant of observing environment can be faithfully reproduced, and the observer perceives realistic color images as if the object were placed at the observer's site.

3.3 Multispectral image capture

Using multispectral image capture, i.e., using more than 3-bands, is beneficial for higher accuracy in spectral and color estimation. Some multispectral input devices suitable for color reproduction have been developed in several groups, and it has been shown to realize the color estimation in high-accuracy a. In the work explained in this paper, 6-band HDTV camera shown in fig.2 was developed for the acquisition of multispectral motion picture (Ohsawa, et. al., 2004).

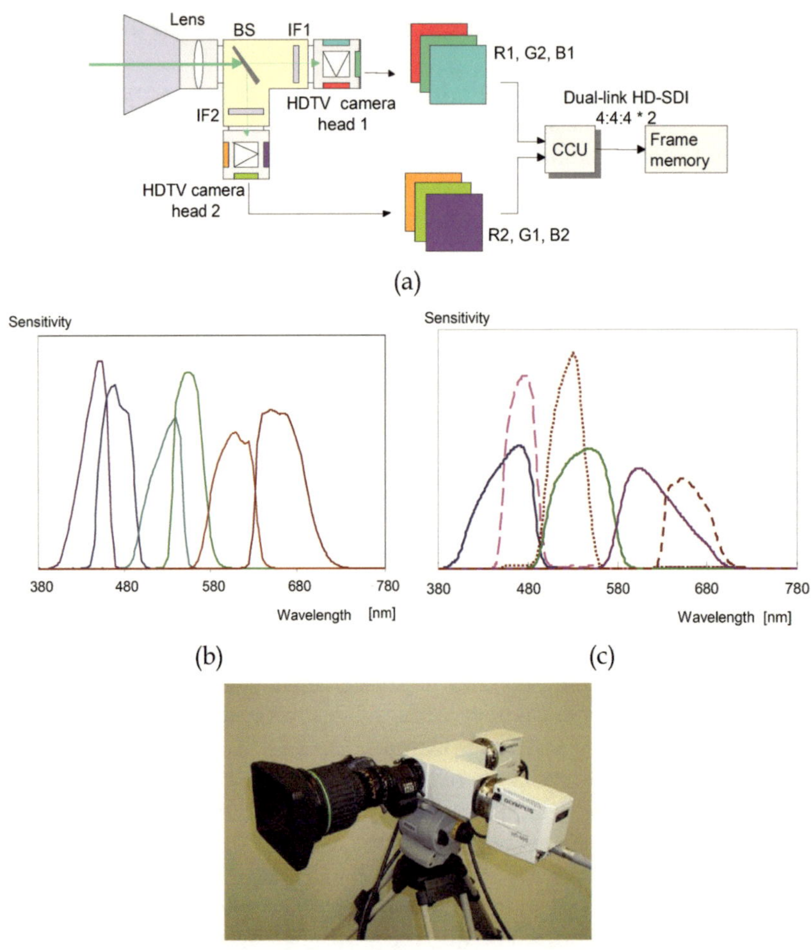

Fig. 2. Six-band video camera. (a) System configuration, (b) spectral sensitivities of 6-bands, and (c) photograph of the camera. BS: beam splitter, IF1, IF2: interference filters.

The 6-band camera consists of two 3-CCD HD cameras, a single imaging lens system, a beam splitter, and two different spectral filters (interference filters) that trim the spectral sensitivities of RGB channels. Two cameras output 3-band images of different RGB sensitivities, and combining them yields 6-band images. Two different versions are experimentally developed; one that is shown in fig.2(a) and (b), and another one IF2 in fig.2(a) is removed so that the spectral sensitivity becomes different as shown in fig.2(c). In the latter camera, a set of three channels has the spectral sensitivity identical to original RGB camera, and was used for the comparison of 6-band and 3-band capabilities.

It was reported that the average and maximum error (CIELAB ΔE) of GretagMacbeth ColorChecker estimated from the 6-band camera image (the case of fig.2(b)) were 1.43 and 4.24, while they were 4.12 and 8.22 in 3-band camera. The colorimetric accuracy is considerably improved by 6-band system, almost less than the color discrimination capability of human vision. The spectral sensitivities and the tone reproduction curves of the 6-band camera (camera profile) were measured in advance, as shown in fig.2(b), for spectrum-based color reproduction.

3.4 Multispectral video conferencing system

Fig.3 shows the system configuration for multispectral video recording and conferencing with high-fidelity color reproduction, especially employed in the experiments presented in the sections 5 and 6 (Yamaguchi, et. al., 2009). For the image input, a 6-band HD (high-definition) camera, a 3-band video camera, and a 6-band still camera were employed. In addition to the multispectral camera with more than 3-band, 3-band camera can be also employed in NV color reproduction even though the color accuracy is lower than 6-band case. The spectral sensitivities and the tone reproduction curves of these cameras (camera profile) were measured in advance, for spectrum-based color reproduction. The colorimetric signal for transmission was generated by the color converter set-top box, using the camera profile and the illumination spectrum measured by a compact spectrometer shown in fig.4.

The spectral reflectance of the object was estimated by Wiener estimation technique, which can be implemented with 6x3 or 3x3 matrix multiplication. The gray levels of video signal of camera output is encoded by 10-bit, where the color conversion process is operated with 12-bit signal. The output of color converter was a colorimetric signal in wide-gamut color space, and encoded by the H.264/AVC encoder. The maximum rate determined by the encoder is 15Mbps. Flat-panel liquid crystal displays (LCDs) are used in this experiment, while multiprimary color displays are considered to be applied in the future.

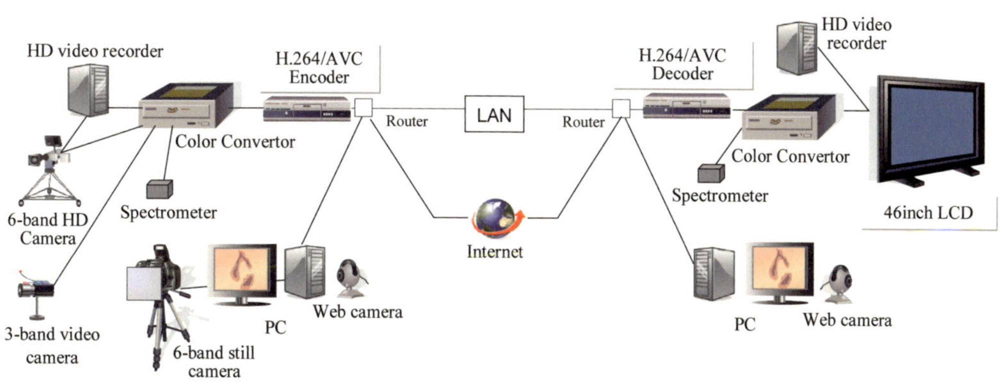

Fig. 3. System overview used in the experiments.

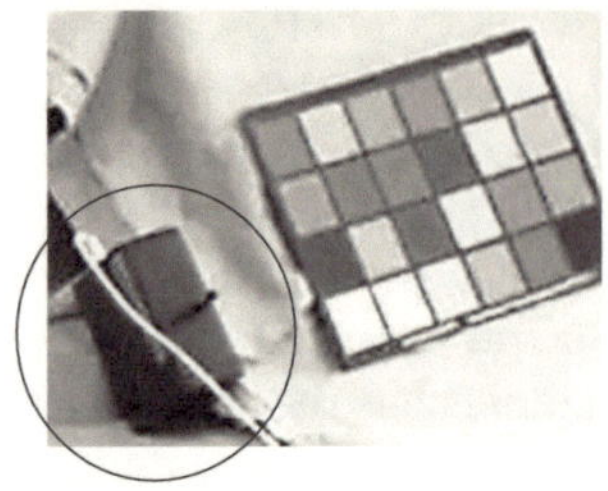

Fig. 4. Compact spectrometer for illumination spectrum measurement.

4. Experimental evaluation for the color reproducibility of skin lesions

This section briefly introduces the experiments, performed to evaluate the spectrum-based system in the dermatology department, Yokohama-city University Hospital, Yokohama, Japan (Yamaguchi, et. al., 2006). Instead of real patient, the erythema artificially produced by prick test was used, as its color can be considered as a good replication of typical flare such as urticaria. Fig.5(a) shows an example of the target arm with erythema. Prick tests of histamine, cedar pollen and mite allergens are performed onto 18 arms from 9 healthy volunteers. The experiment is composed of following 4 steps;

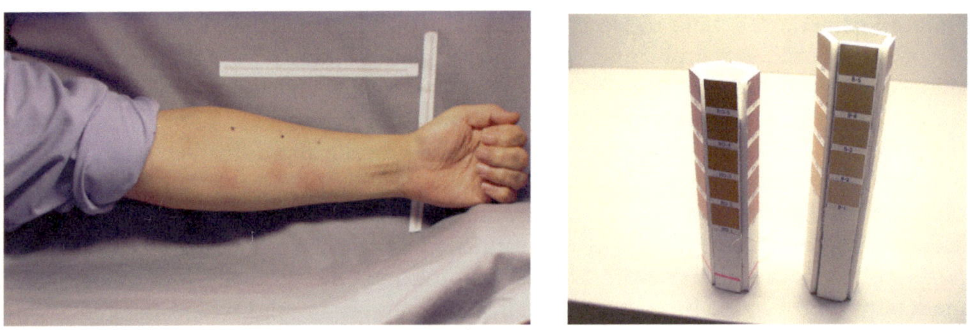

(a) (b)

Fig. 5. (a) Photograph of target arm with erythema by prick test. (b) Skin color chips on pentagonal cylinders used in the experiment.

1. Colorimetric evaluation, in which the colors of target skin and reproduced images were measured by a spectroradiometer to check the colorimetric accuracy. The CIELAB (ΔE^*ab) color differences between corresponding points were calculated, but it was confirmed that good color reproducibility is realized in 6-band system, i.e., average $\Delta E^*ab = 3.5$, where $\Delta E^*ab = 11$ in 3-band case, for both normal skin and flare regions.
2. Visual evaluation by dermatologists.
   For the color matching between the reproduced image and the real object, we prepared 25 color chips, printed by an inkjet printer and attached on a handy pentagonal cylinder as shown in fig.5(b). The colors are selected from the preliminary measurement of skin colors; they are distributed around the normal and flare skin colors. The average spacing between the neighboring color chips is $\Delta E^*ab = 3 - 5$ in CIELAB color space.
   In the first step of this experiment, the real skin was observed at first, and a best-matched color chip was determined by the mutual agreement among three

dermatologists. Next, the erythema was shot by 6-band camera and the image for 6-band and conventional RGB system are prepared. In this case the camera shown in fig.2(c) was used and a set of three channels corresponds to the conventional RGB signal.

The colors of target skin and reproduced images from 6-band and conventional RGB cameras were visually compared with a set of color chips by dermatologists to find the best-matched color chip. Then to see if the dermatologists perceive identical color from the reproduced image, the color difference between the color chips matched with the reproduced image and the real skin is illustrated in fig.6. The color chips selected from the observation of 6-band system distribute within ΔE*ab < 4 - 5 range, while in the observation of RGB system, the center of distribution is shifted and the color difference becomes about ΔE*ab = 7 - 8. As the tristimulus values of color chips matched to the target skin and reproduced images are satisfactory close each other, it can be said that the dermatologist perceives almost same color in the case of 6-band system.

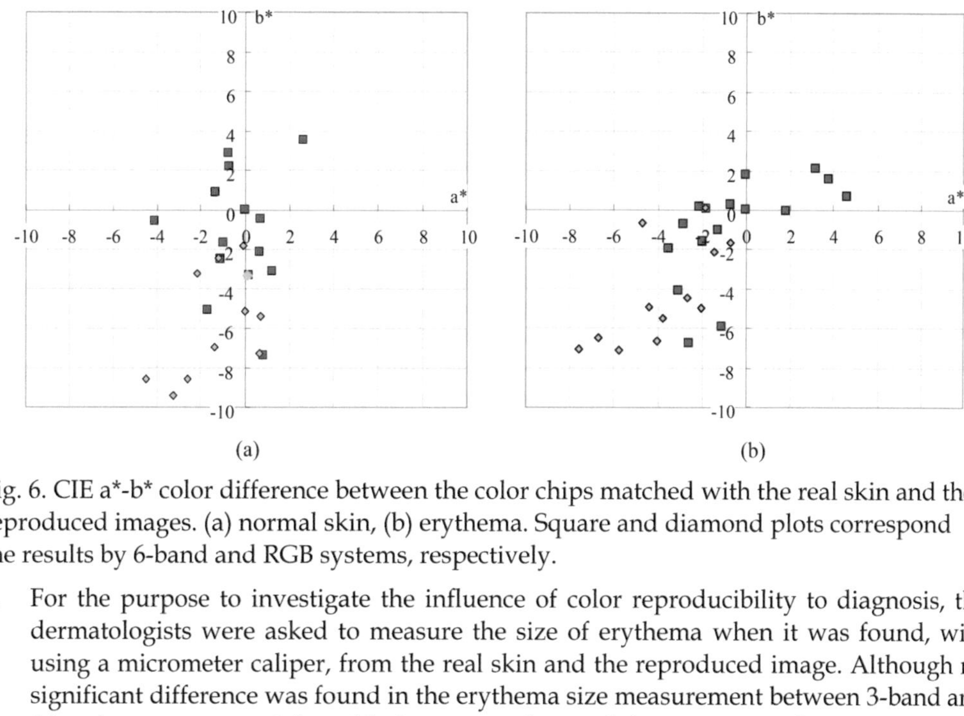

Fig. 6. CIE a*-b* color difference between the color chips matched with the real skin and the reproduced images. (a) normal skin, (b) erythema. Square and diamond plots correspond the results by 6-band and RGB systems, respectively.

3. For the purpose to investigate the influence of color reproducibility to diagnosis, the dermatologists were asked to measure the size of erythema when it was found, with using a micrometer caliper, from the real skin and the reproduced image. Although no significant difference was found in the erythema size measurement between 3-band and 6-band systems, oversights of lesions were observed; in some cases the sizes were not measured from the observation of RGB system because the erythema was not found. Three dermatologists dealt with 60 cases in total, and 8 cases were not judged as flare, though they were found in direct observation. This indicates the possibility that the natural color reproduction capability reduces the oversights of skin lesions.
4. After the overall evaluation with observing the real-time video reproduction, following comments were obtained from the participated dermatologists;
   a. The color reproduction by RGB system is not sufficient especially in reddish colors, and is not suitable for the diagnosis of subtle flare such as measles, virus infection, and drug allergy.

b. The image color in 6-band system looks natural, and the reddish and yellowish colors can be easily discriminated. Then the profile of the erythema is clearer in the image of 6-band system.
c. The dilatation of blood capillary can be clearly observed in 6-band system.

	6-band	Conventional HDTV
Oversight	0	8
Total Obsrvation (3 Dermatologists)	80	60

Table 1. Oversight in the conventional HDTV system (Erythema sizes were not measured).

5. Evaluation for the color reproducibility in surgery video

5.1 The system for surgery video recording and evaluation

The NV technology was also applied to the video capture of open surgery and medical doctors visually evaluated the reproduced image quality (Yamaguchi, et. al., 2010). The system configuration used in the experiment is shown in fig.7. For the image input, a 6-band HD camera of fig.2(b) was used. The 6-band camera was installed on a camera stand and set in the operation room as shown in fig.8(a). Seven cases of hand operations were captured and recorded in a hard disk video recorder in an uncompressed format. The spectrum-based color conversion was applied in the manner explained in the section 2. The illumination in the operation room was a mixture of fluorescent and surgical light (Stryker, Visum Surgical Light, halogen lamp mounted). Its spectral energy distribution is shown in fig.8(b), which was measured by a spectroradiometer (Topcon SR-3) and a standard white diffuser.
For the image display, a flat-panel LCD (liquid crystal display, Sharp, Information Display PN-455) was used. The resolution of the LCD panel was HD format (1920×1080 pixels). The ambient illumination of the viewing environment was fluorescent lamp, and the irradiance around the monitor was about 300 lx, which is almost equivalent to the typical office environment. In the subjective evaluation, the observation distance was 5H, where H is the height of the image displayed on the monitor. Although the standard observation distance is 3H in HD television system, the standard for SD (standard-definition) was used here since the image resolution was almost equivalent to SD image. In the second experiment subsection 5.3, the observation distance was 3H since the image was HD format. For the evaluation of compressed video, H.264/AVC software codec (MainConcept H.264 Encoder / Decoder) was applied to the signal after the color conversion from the 6-band image.
For comparison with the 6-band images, a consumer HD digital camcoder of high-end specifications was simultaneously used as shown in fig.7(a). Both the 6-band and RGB camera were mounted on the camera stand and operated by two engineers to adjust the image. After the observation of captured image, the images of conventional video showed apparently different color, it was difficult to be employed for the subjective evaluation in comparison with 6-band image. Thus the image captured by operating room camera was used as the conventional image in the evaluation experiment described in the subsection 5.3. The camera was attached to the flexible arm and its position was occasionally adjusted by a nurse to keep the best view. The video sequence was compressed about 1/70 by the encoder included in the camcoder product.

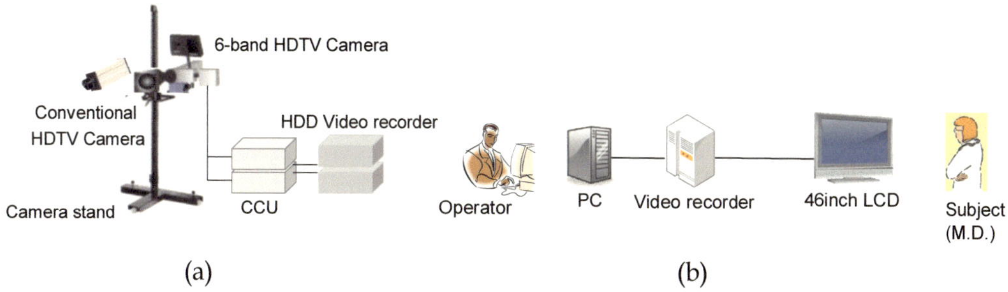

Fig. 7. The system configuration used in the experiment for (a) image capture and (b) subjective evaluation. CCU: Camera control unit.

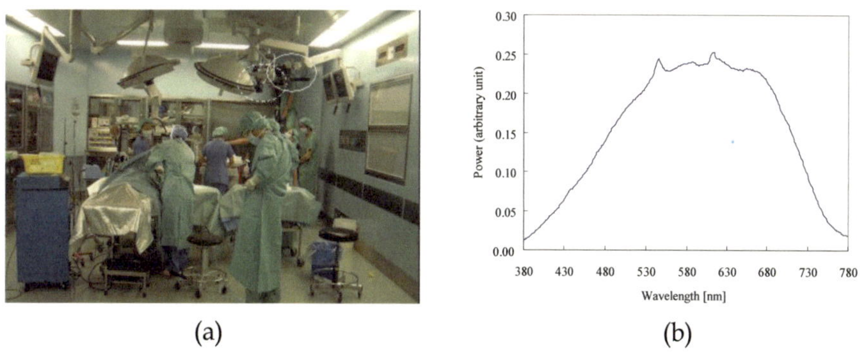

Fig. 8. (a) The operation room after the 6-band video camera installed. (b) The illumination spectrum of the operation room.

5.2 The color distribution of organs and tissues

The image data captured by 6-band camera have quantitative spectral information, which can be utilized for the tissue classification or visualization. As a preliminary investigation, the colorimetric information captured by 6-band camera with high accuracy was derived. Fig.9 shows the colors of the tissue elements on CIE xy-chromaticity coordinates. The colors of tissues distributes from red to yellowish white. Tendon, fat and fascia are yellow-white, and muscle and blood are reddish, while the slightly different red colors of muscle and blood are myoglobin and hemoglobin. The colors were also affected by the deeper organs because some of the tissues are semitransparent.

This shows the possibility of discriminating the tissue elements using the spectral information in the image data for the support of the observation. It is observed that the color of blood exceeds the color gamut of conventional RGB space. It is expected to employ a wide color-gamut display especially in the deep red region for reproducing blood color. In the following experiment, however, we used a flat-panel LCD with normal color gamut, since practical wide-gamut display suitable for this experiment was not available.

5.3 Evaluation of subjective image quality

The videos captured by 6-band (raw and 1/70 compression) and conventional RGB (1/70 compression) cameras were reproduced on a 45inch LCD and the image qualities were evaluated based on Scheffe's paired comparison test. A HD video camera furnished in the

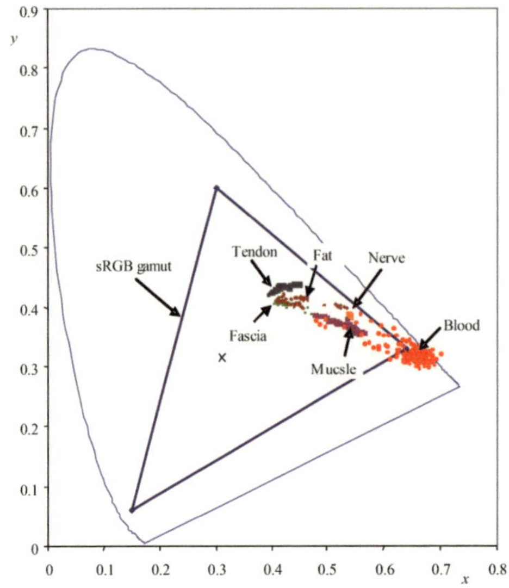

Fig. 9. The color coordinates of the tissues captured by 6-band camera (CIE xy chromaticity coordinates)

operation room was used as the conventional camera. Three doctors (a surgeon and dermatologists) participated in the experiment as the observers. The observers viewed a pair of video (A and B) sequentially and scored 8 items for evaluation into 6 levels (extremely A, much A, slightly A, slightly B, much B, extremely B). The result is summarized in fig.10. Among the evaluation items, 6-band systems were rated significantly higher in "color reproducibility," "fidelity," and "material appearance" at 95% confidence level. It shows that the appearance of the field of operation is superior for the doctors in the 6-band video reproduction than that of the conventional system.

5.4 Evaluation of perceptual color difference

In the experiment described in this section, it was tested if the color difference reproduced by video systems would be perceivable by the medical doctors. For this purpose, the image reproduced by a conventional RGB system was artificially generated from the 6-band image, where the color reproduction from the 6-band image was considered to be a gold standard. In addition, the spectrum-based color reproduction from 3-band camera was artificially generated and compared with 6-band.

In the evaluation, two images (6-band and RGB, or 6-band and 3band) were displayed side by side, without notifying the observer which was the 6-band image. Then the observer answered the color difference was perceivable or not, scoring into 5 levels (5:identical, 4:perceivable but not annoying, 3:slightly annoying, 2:annoying, 1:completely different). The resultant scores for every observer is shown in fig.11, and it can be seen that the differences in (6-band vs. RGB) and (6-band vs 3-band) are significant.

According to the comments from the participants, the most apparent difference was the color of skin. The color difference of tumor was noticeable as well. Human vision is generally sensitive to the skin color variation, and it was confirmed that the color reproduction of skin is quite difficult. Although it cannot be said whether the color difference would give rise to error in diagnosis or decision from this experiment, significantly noticeable errors were observed in the reproduced image. In order to find the cases in which the color accuracy is critical, much more cases should be acquired by multiband camera in future.

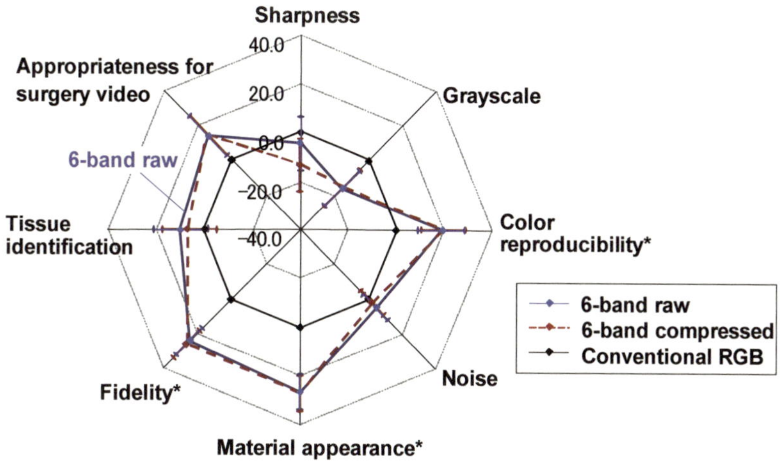

Fig. 10. Result of subjective evaluation. Each score is relative amount where the score of conventional RGB is zero.

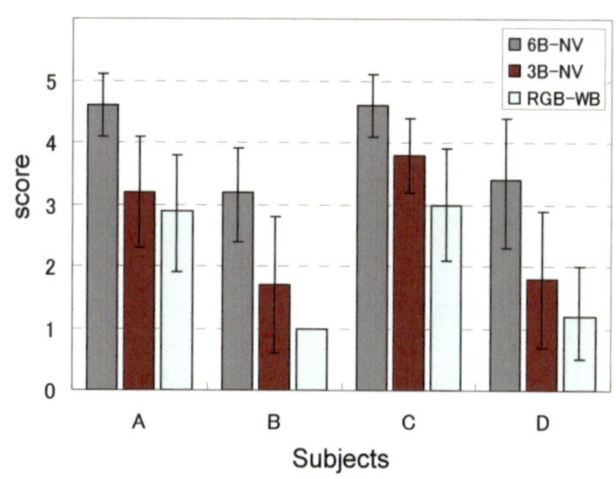

Fig. 11. Result of subjective evaluation of color difference. The error bars indicate the 95% confidence interval.

5.5 Transmission through LAN

To demonstrate the applicability of the high-fidelity color reproduction system using multiband camera to telemedicine, such as telementoring or telesurgery, the color video generated from 6-band data were transmitted through local network using the system shown in fig.3. HD size (1920×1080 pixels) 6-band video clips were stored in video recorder, and converted to the standard color signal (xvYCC color space) in real-time by the color convertor set-top box developed for 6to3 color conversion. The color signal was compressed by H.264/AVC hardware encoder and transmitted though local area network (LAN). The receiver was located in a different room in the same hospital. The received stream was decoded by a decoder, and the display RGB signal were generated by another color converter. The maximum bit-rate of transmission was limited by the encoder up to 15Mbps, and the compression rate could be varied. The image was reproduced on the same LCD of 1920×1080 pixels. Then the doctors observed the images for the informal evaluation, and followings are the discussions based on the comments from participated doctors;

The distortion due to the compression was not so problematic for the physicians when the transmission rate was 15 Mbps. In the case of 4 Mbps, the distortion considerably affected the image quality but it would be usable as the HD video, and the image strongly degraded in 2 Mbps case. Relatively lower bit-rates were accepted, as the motion in the image was small in the surgery video. As a result, it can be said that telementoring or telesurgery system with HD video would work with the transmission rate 10~15 Mbps approximately.

The delay due to the codec was 0.5~1.0 sec, which may obstruct real-time communication. The delay was caused by the color conversion, codec process, and network, and that by codec was considered to be dominant. The reduction of delay time and the investigation of acceptable delay time are one of the important issues.

The material appearance in the field of operation was evaluated to be much better than the conventional video and quite similar to the direct vision, and therefore the multiband system will be effective in case archives, conferences and demonstration. For the practical use, it is required to address some problems, such as the widespread monitors are not usually calibrated, and the H.264 codec is not implemented in the common PCs. The introduction of color management in the medical display is required.

In monitoring surgeries from remote site, in addition to the high-fidelity video of the field of operation, it is desired to view the image of whole operating room or the operator's situation, in which the image quality may not be high. Thus it is recommended that the conventional videoconferencing system for whole operating room and the high-fidelity video transmission for the field are concurrently used, and probably displayed PinP (picture in picture) mode. Moreover, though naturally, the system should be applied to the endoscopic and laparoscopic images.

6. Remote teleconsultation experiment

The system was also tested in the video-based teleconsultation experiment, in which the system was installed at real hospital and clinic sites (Kasaoka Daiichi Hospital and Manabeshima island clinic, Kasaoka, Okayama Pref., Japan) (Yamaguchi, et. al., 2009). Manabeshima island is located about 20km distant from mainland in Setonaikai sea. A doctor usually visits once a week to the clinic, thus improved care service is demanded, and a constant support through teleconsultation would be quite valuable.

The system configuration shown in fig.3 was used in the experiment. For low-bandwidth live-view, 3-band camera was also tested with spectrum-based color processing, along with the 6-band HD camera explained before. A still camera with 6-band capability was employed in addition to the video systems. It was an experimental system with using high-end commercial digital still camera (Olympus E-3), and two pictures were shot for an object; one is normal RGB image, and another one was captured with a color filter in front of the lens. The filter characteristics were similar to the ones shown in fig.2(c). The two pictures were synthesized into a 6-band image, and the spectrum-based color reproduction was applied. The image resolution was 3900x2616 pixels and the image was obsrved with changing the window and the magnification.

Before the remote teleconsultation experiment, a dermatologist tested the video-based teleconsultation by NV technology inside the hospital. The dermatologist overviewed a volunteer patient thoroughly with using the video, and high-resolution 6-band images were captured with 6-band still-camera when suspicious feature was found. Then the magnified still-image was carefully observed to give the final decision.
In the experiment at the real site, the network was provided by cable TV line, where the connection between the mainland and the island was radio transmission. The transmission rate was about 2-10Mbps depending on the weather condition. Ahead of the consultation, the images reproduced by NV and conventional system were compared as shown in fig.12 (left). Two identical skin color charts were kept at both sites, and the image of the color chart was reproduced on the monitors reproduced by NV technology and conventional RGB. In the case of NV, the color reproduced on the monitor almost agrees with the real chart, which was confirmed by the participated doctors. The color difference in the conventional system was evident. After that, a simulated patient at clinic site was consulted by doctors in the hospital through the NV video and still image transmission system [fig.12 (right)]. When using 3-band live-view system, a doctor in the hospital instructed the assistant in the remote clinic to show the part of interest, and high-resolution image was captured by 6-band still camera.
Doctors commented that the NV system provides more natural and realistic images. It was also pointed out that the combined use of normal-resolution video and high-resolution 6-band still image seemed to be practical to observe the patient situation in detail.

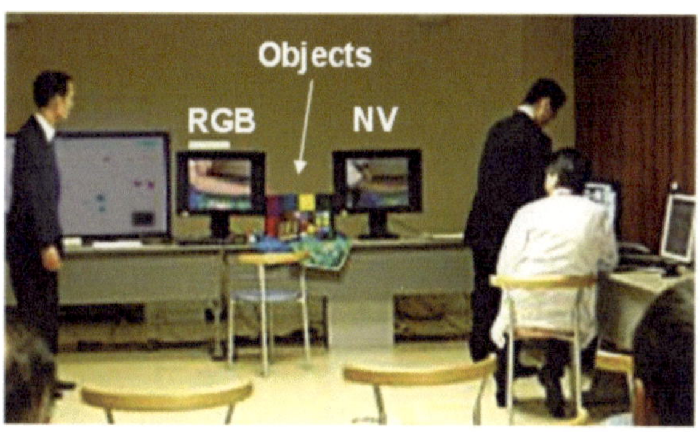

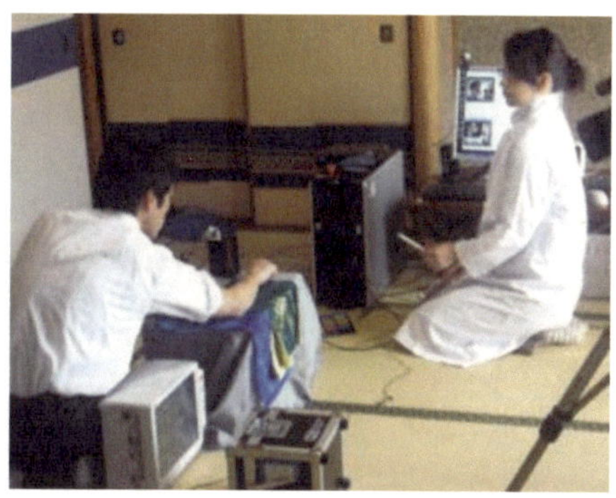

Fig. 12. Left: Hospital site. Doctors were viewing the images reproduced by NV and RGB schemes. Color charts were placed at the center for a reference. Right: Clinic site. A patient is showing his arm to the 6-band camera according to the doctor's direction in the hospital site. The person in front of the patient is a technical operator. The color chart is not seen in this photograph.

7. Conclusion

By the use of spectrum-based color reproduction technology, the color reproduced on a display is perceived almost identical to the original, and the advantage of the system was proved in dermatology, surgery video, and teleconsultation. Through the experimental evaluation, in addition to the color reproducibility, the reality, the discriminability of skin lesions and material appearance are significantly improved in the spectrum-based system. In the remote teleconsultation experiment, the video was transmitted through the internet with H264/AVC coding, and the reality of the reproduced image was highly evaluated by the participated medical doctors. For the practical use of the system, it is necessary to develop compact and high-quality multiband camera with better usability.

8. Acknowledgement

The authors greatly acknowledge the members of Natural Vision project for the great contribution to this work. This work was supported by NICT (National Institute of Information and Communications Technology) Japan, and the Natural Vision Promotion Council.

9. References

Abe, T., Murakami, Y., Yamaguchi, M., Ohyama, N., Yagi, Y., "Color correction of pathological images based on dye amount quantification," Opt. Rev. Vol. 12, (2005), 293-300

Alfvin, R. L., and Fairchild, M. D., "Observer variability in metameric color matches using color reproduction media," Color Res. Appl. Vol. 22, (1997), 174-188

Augestad, K. M., and Lindsetmo, R. O., "Overcoming distance: video-conferencing as a clinical and educational tool among surgeons," World J. Surg., Vol. 33, No. 7, (April 2009), 1356-1365

Berci, G., Wren, S. M., Stain, S. C., Peters, J., Paz-Partlow, M., "Individual assessment of visual perception by surgeons observing the same laparoscopic organs with various imaging systems," Surg. Endosc., Vol. 9, No. 9, (1995) 967-973

Bolle S. R., Larsen F., Hagen O., Gilbert M., "Video conferencing versus telephone calls for team work across hospitals: a qualitative study on simulated emergencies," BMC Emerg. Med., Vol. 9, No. 22, (November 2009)

Broderick, T. J., Harnett, B. M., Merriam, N. R., Kapoor, V., Doarn, C. R., Merrell, R. C., "Impact of varying transmission bandwidth on image quality," Telemed. J. e-Health, Vol. 7, No. 1, (2001), 47-53

Burns, P. D., Berns, R. S., (1996) "Analysis of multispectral image capture," Proceedings of IS&T/SID 4th Color Imaging Conference, pp.19-22

Demartines, N., Mutter, D., Vix, M., Leroy, J., Glatz, D., Rösel, F., Harder, F., Marescaux, J., "Assessment of telemedicine in surgical education and patient care," Ann. Surg., Vol. 231, No.2, (February 2000), 282-291.

Derhak, M., and Rosen, M., (2004) "Spectral colorimetry using LabPQR - an interim connection space," Proceedings of IS&T/SID 12th Color Imaging Conference, pp. 246–250.

Duplaga, M., Leszczuk, M. I., Papir, Z. Przelaskowski, A., "Compression evaluation of surgery video recordings retaining diagnostic credibility (compression evaluation of surgery video)," Opto-Electronics Review, Vol. 16, No. 4, (September 2008), 428-438

Gállego J. R., Hernández-Solana A., Canales M., Lafuente J., Valdovinos A., Fernández-Navajas J., "Performance analysis of multiplexed medical data transmission for mobile emergency care over the UMTS channel," IEEE Trans. Inf. Technol. Biomed., Vol. 9, No. 1, (March 2005) 13-22.

Hanna, G., and Cuschieri, A., "Image display technology and image processing," World J. Surg., Vol. 25, No. 11, (September 2001), 1419-1427

Herbin, M., Venot, A., Devaux, J. Y., Piette, C., "Color quantitation through image processing in dermatology," IEEE Trans. Med. Imaging, Vol. 9, No. 3. (September 1990), 262-269

Hill, B., (1998). "Multispectral color technology: a way towards high definition color image scanning and encoding," Proceedings of SPIE, Vol. 3409, pp.2-13

Krupinski, E., Burdick, A., Pak, H., Bocachica, J., Earles, L., Edison, K., Goldyne, M., Hirota, T., Kvedar, J., McKoy, K., Oh, D., Siegel, D., Antoniotti, N., Camacho, I., Carnahan, L., Boynton, P., Bakalar, R., Evans, R., Kinel, A., Kuzmak, P., C. Madden, B., Peters, S., Rosenthal, L., Simmons, S., Bernard, J., Linkous, J., "American Telemedicine Association's Practice Guidelines for Teledermatology," Telemedicine and e-Health, Vol. 14, No. 3, (April 2008), 289-302.

Levenson, R., Cronin, P. J., Pankratov, K. K., (2003), "Spectral imaging for brightfield microscopy," Proceedings of SPIE, Vol. 4959, 27-33

Loane, M. A., Bloomer, S. E., Corbett, R., Eedy, D. J., Hicks, N., Lotery, H. E., Mathews, C., Paisley, J., Steele, K., Wootton, R., "A comparison of real-time and store-and-forward teledermatology: a cost-benefit study," British Journal of Dermatology Vol. 143, (2000), 1241-1247.

Maglogiannis, I., "Design and Implementation of a Calibrated Store and Forward Imaging System for Teledermatology," Journal of Medical Systems, Vol. 28, No. 5, (2004), 455-467

Murakami, Y., Ishii, J., Obi, T., Yamaguchi, M., Ohyama, N., "Color conversion method for multi-primary display for spectral color reproduction," J. Electron. Imaging, Vol. 13, (2004), 701-708

Nilsson M., Rasmark U., Nordgren H., Hallberg P., Skönevik J., Westman G., Rolandsson O., "The physician at a distance: the use of videoconferencing in the treatment of patients with hypertension," J. Telemed. Telecare, Vol.15, No. 8, (2009), 397-403.

Numahara, T., "From the standpoint of Dermatology," in Digital Color Imaging in Biomedicine, H. Tanaka, Y. Miyake, M. Nishibori, and D. Mukhophadhyay, (Ed.), Digital Biocolor Society, (October 2001) 67-72, http://biocolor.umin.ac.jp/book200102/din01022812.pdf, Tokyo

Ohsawa, K., Ajito, T., Fukuda, H., Komiya, Y., Haneishi, H., Yamaguchi, M., Ohyama, N.,"Six-band HDTV camera system for spectrum-based color reproduction" .J. Imag. Sci. and Tech., Vol. 48, No. 2, (2004) 85-92

Pratt W. K., and Mancill, C. E., "Spectral estimation techniques for the spectral calibration of a color image scanner," Appl. Opt., Vol. 15, (1976), 73-75

Rafiq, A., Moore, J. A., Zhao, X., Doarn, C. R., Merrell, R. C., "Digital video capture and synchronous consultation in open surgery," Ann. Surg., Vol. 239, No. 4, (April 2004), 567-573

Rosen, M., Imai, F., Jiang, X., and Ohta, N., (2001). "Spectral reproduction from scene to hardcopy II: Image processing," Proceedings of SPIE, Vol. 4300, pp. 33-41

Tomatis, S., Bono, A., Bartoli, C., Carrara, M., Lualdi, M., Tragni, G.., Marchesini, R., "Automated melanoma detection: multispectral imaging and neural network approach for classification," Med. Phys., Vol. 30, No.2, (2003), 212-221

Ueki, S., Nakamura, K., Yoshida, Y., Mori, T., Tomizawa, K., Narutaki, Y., Itoh, Y., Okamoto, K., (2009). "Five-primary-color 60-inch LCD with Novel Wide Color Gamut and Wide Viewing Angle," SID 2009 Digest, Paper No. 62.1

Haeghen, Y. V., Naeyaert, J. M., Lemahieu, I., Philips, W., "An imaging system with calibrated color image acquisition for use in dermatology," IEEE Trans. Med. Imaging., Vol.19, No.7 (July 2000); 722-730.

Wildi, S. M., Kim, C. Y., Glenn, T. F., Mackey, H. A., Viator, G. E., Wallace, M. B., Hawes, R. H., "Tele-endoscopy: a way to provide diagnostic quality for remote populations," Gastrointestinal Endoscopy, Vol. 59, No. 1, (January 2004), 38-43

Yamaguchi, M., Haneishi, H., Ohyama, N., "Beyond red-green-blue (RGB): spectrum-based color imaging technology," J. Imag. Sci. Technol., Vol. 52, No. 1, (January 2008) 010201

Yamaguchi, M., Iwama, R., Kanazawa, H., Fujikawa, N., Fukuda, H., Haneishi, H., Ohyama, N., Wada, H., Kambara, T., Aihara, M., Yamakawa, Y., Nemoto, A., Furukawa, M., and Ikezawa, Z., (2006). "Color reproducibility of skin lesions in multispectral video: Experimental evaluation," Proceedings of IS&T/SID 14th Color Imaging Conference, pp. 8-13

Yamaguchi, M., Iwama, R., Ohya, Y., Obi, T., Ohyama, N., Komiya, Y., Wada, T., (1997). "Natural color reproduction in the television system for telemedicime," Proceedings of SPIE, Vol. 3031, pp. 482-489

Yamaguchi, M., Kishimoto, J., Komiya, Y., Kanno, Y., Murakami, Y., Hashizume, H., Haneishi, H., Yamada, R., Miyajima, K., (2009). "Video-based telemedicine with reliable color: Field experiments of natural vision technology," Proceedings of the 3rd International Universal Communication Symposium, IUCS 2009, pp. 150-153

Yamaguchi, M., Mitsui, M., Murakami, Y., Fukuda, H., Ohyama, N., and Kubota, Y., (2005). "Multispectral color imaging for dermatology: application in inflammatory and immunologic diseases," Proc. IS&T/SID 13th Color Imaging Conference, pp. 52–58.

Yamaguchi, M., Murakami, Y., Hashizume, H., Haneishi, H., Kanno, Y., Komiya, Y., (2010). "High-fidelity color video reproduction of open surgery by six-band camera," Proceedings of SPIE, Vol. 7627, 762707

Yellowlees, P. M., Odor. A., Parish, M. B., Iosif, A. M., Haught, K., Hilty, D., "A feasibility study of the use of asynchronous telepsychiatry for psychiatric consultations," Psychiatr. Serv. Vol. 61, No. 8, (August 2010), 838-840

7

Sharp Wave Based HHT Time-frequency Features with Transmission Error

Chin-Feng Lin[1], Bing-Han Yang[1], Tsung-Ii Peng[2], Shun-Hsyung Chang[3], Yu-Yi Chien[2], and Jung-Hua Wang[1]
[1]*Department of Electrical Engineering, National Taiwan Ocean University*
[2]*Department of Neurological Division, Chang Cung Memorial Hospital, Keelung Branch*
[3]*Department of Microeletronic Engineering, National Kaohsuing Marine University*
Taiwan

1. Introduction

Signal analysis is a field of study that attempts to extract information features from various physical phenomena. Fourier transform (FT), wavelet transform (WT), and Hilbert-Huang transformation (HHT) are the 3 major approaches used in signal analysis (Huang et al., 1998) (Yan & Gao, 2007). FT is a global energy-frequency distribution approach that is suitable for analyzing linear, strictly periodic, and stationary signals. In contrast, HHT is a good method for analyzing non-linear and non-stationary signals, such as those associated with wind, earthquakes, electrocardiographs (ECGs), and electroencephalograms (EEGs). This method can also used to describe the local features of dynamic signals, and illustrate the energy-frequency-time distribution of these signals. The 2 principal steps employed in HHT are empirical mode decomposition (EMD) and Hilbert spectral analysis, EMD is used to decompose local signals to finite data sets, which are referred to as intrinsic mode functions (IMFs), and Hilbert transforms (HTs) are used in conjunction with the obtained IMFs to determine the instantaneous frequencies (IFs), time-frequency-energy distributions of the local time signals. A number of studies have been performed to elucidate various aspects of signal analysis. Cohen reviewed the fundamental ideas, methods, and characteristics of the time-frequency analysis approaches employed until 1989 (Cohen, 1989). Blanco *et al.,* used the Gabor transform (GT) time-frequency analysis approach to facilitate identification of the source of epileptic seizures (Blanco et al., 1997). The GT approach is similar to the fast FT approach, but GT offers the advantage of allowing the analysis of the frequencies and their time evolution. Blanco *et al.,* adopted GT to achieve maximal concentration of the time and frequency characteristics for epilepsy and obtain accurate information on the time evolution of the frequency epileptic activity. Tzallas *et al.,* used short-time Fourier transform and 12 different time-frequency distributions for studying epilepsy classification problems and discussed the obtained sensitivity, accuracy, and selectivity results, and the characteristic data features for the detection of epilepsy (Tzallas et al., 2009). However, they did not use the HHT-based time-frequency analysis approach to define epileptic sharps. Sharabaty *et al.,* used the HHT signal-analysis approach to determine the alpha and theta localizations for estimation of the vigilance level, and proposed an alpha/theta localization algorithm for EEG signal analysis (Sharabaty et al., 2006). Wang *et al.*, extracted the data features from C3 and C4 EEG signals to design a Brain-Computer Interface (BCI) (Wang & Xu *et al.*, 2008). They discussed the accuracy of a classification system based on imagery-movement tasks and analyzed the average marginal spectra at electrode C3 and C4 during each imagery task. Wang *et al.*, also used HHT to automatically remove ocular artifacts in contaminated EEGs (Wang & Liu et al., 2008). The authors described EEGs contaminated with ocular artifacts, IMFs and the residual artifacts from FP2, and also elucidated the differences between the contaminated FP2 EEGs and the corrected EEGs. Further, they determined the differences between the power spectra for the corrected EEGs and the contaminated FP2 EEGs. In our previous studies, we have discussed the design concept for mobile telemedicine and chaos-based encryption mechanisms for biomedical signals (Lin & Chang et al., 2006)(Lin & Chang et al., 2007)(Lin & Chang, 2008)(Lin & Li, 2008)(Lin & Chung et al., 2008)(Lin & Chen et al., 2008)(Lin et al., 2009)(Lin, 2010)(Lin et al., Online First) (Lin, Online First) (Lin & Wang, Accept). In 3 previous studies, we have described the HHT-based time-frequency characteristics of the FP1 EEG signals recorded from normal and alcoholic observers watching a single picture and 2 different pictures (Lin et al., 2008) (Lin et al., 2010)(Lin et al., Online Book, 2010). In this paper, we analyzed the sharp and normal waves with a transmission bit error rate (BER) of 10^{-7} in the EEGs obtained for epilepsy patients. The IMFs, IFs, and the time-frequency-energy distributions of these EEG signals are studied. In section II, the concept of HHT is presented, and in section III we describe the simulation results and discuss the application of HHT in the analysis the sharp waves of EEG signals obtained from patients with epilepsy. In section IV and V, we present our discussions and conclusions, respectively.

2. Method

In the HHT temporal frequency-energy-time signal analysis technique, EMD is used to perform IMFs decomposition, and HT is used to obtain the IFs, and time-frequency-energy distributions of these EEG signals.

The following procedure is employed for analyzing the IMF using EMD:

Step 1. initially assume $r_o = x(t)$ and i=1;

Step 2. analyze the ith IMF;

- a. initially assume $h_{i(k-1)} = r_i$, k=1;
- b. analyze the local maximum and minimum for $h_{i(k-1)}$;
- c. construct the upper-limit and lower-limit envelope for $h_{i(k-1)}$ by performing additional sampling;
- d. calculate the-mean $m_{i(k-1)}$ of the upper-limit and lower-limit envelope for $h_{i(k-1)}$;
- e. $h_{ik} = h_{i(k-1)} - m_{i(k-1)}$;
- f. if h_{ik} is the IMF, then $IMF_i = h_{ik}$; alternatively, refer to step (b) and consider k = k+1;

Step 3. define $r_{i+1} = r_i - IMF_i$;

Step 4. if r_{i+1} has at least 2 extreme values,
refer to step 2 or consider that the analysis procedure is complete and that r_{i+1} is the residual signal;

In such cases, IMF is defined by 2 conditions:

Condition 1: The difference between the crossing with zero and the local extreme value of the entire data shall be equal or the difference with 1.

Condition 2: The mean of any point is the average of the local maximum and minimum envelope.

In addition, the HHT-based time-frequency analysis scheme is performed on the basis of 4 assumptions:

Assumption 1: At least 2 extreme value for the signals, i.e. maximum and minimum values, are present.

Assumption 2: The scale size of the characteristic time is selected according to the extreme values and the temporal interval.

Assumption 3: If that the data to be analyzed have no extreme values but contain identifiable points that can be expressed as extreme points of single or multiple analyses, and accompany with an increase in the number of analyses, the maximum/minimum points gain significance.

Assumption 4: The final result should be the sum of the above stated composition. Thus, the single channel EEG wave can be defined as function $x(t)$, and function $x(t)$ can be expressed as the following empirical mode function to analyzes the IMF.

$$x(t) = \sum_{i=1}^{n} IMF_i(t) + r(t) \tag{1}$$

where, $IMF_i(t)$: the ith IMF

r(t): attribution function(residual)

Then

$$z(t) = x(t) + jy(t) = x(t) + jHT\{x(t)\} = a(t)e^{j\theta(t)}$$

HT{}:Hilbert Transformation

$$a(t) = \sqrt{x^2(t) + y^2(t)}$$

$$\theta(t) = \arctan(\frac{y(t)}{x(t)}) \tag{2}$$

Thus, the IF of a single channel EEG signal can be analyzed using the following equation:

$$f(t) = \frac{1}{2\pi}\frac{d\theta(t)}{dt} \tag{3}$$

Using the HHT-based time-frequency analysis technique, the time-frequency characteristic vector of the EEG signal for epilepsy can be acquired, and the frequency characteristics, amplitude characteristics, time-dependent temporal-spatial frequency correlation, and correlation of the EEG signal to the clinical characteristics can be analyzed. Furthermore, this approach can allow determination of statistically common and abnormal points, generalization of a standard by comparison with a normal sample, augmentation the efficiency of observation, and analysis of the HHT time-frequency-energy characteristics corresponding to sharp wave.

3. Simulation results

We have used an HHT-based time-frequency analysis to analyze the sharp waves in the EEG obtained for epilepsy. A sharp EEG signal was obtained from the T3 channel from a clinical patient presenting with epilepsy; the transmission BER of the EEG was 10^{-7}. Figure 1 and Figure 2 show the sharp and normal waves, respectively. Two hundred and fifty samples per second were used to generate the sharp and normal waves. The sharp wave was generated in the interval of 0.324 and 0.444 *s*, its length was 120 *ms*, and its amplitude was 73.63 mV. Tables 1, and 2 show the statistical characteristics of the IMFs of the sharp and normal waves, respectively; we assume that the received EEG signals had a transmission BER of 10^{-7}. The maximum amplitude of the sharp wave (76.64 uV) was larger than that of the normal wave (20.7 uV). We analyzed the IMFs, IFs, and time-frequency-energy distributions for the sharp and normal waves. Figure 3 and Figure 4 show the IMFs and residual function for the sharp and normal waves, respectively; these IMFs were obtained using EMD. In these examples, 4 IMFs and a residual function were decomposed for the sharp and normal waves. In these IMFs, the amplitudes of the sharp signals were higher than those of the normal waves. The analysis results show that the ratios of the energy of a sharp wave to its total energy for IMF3 and IMF4 were 34.55%, and 33.73%, respectively. Further, the ratios of a normal wave to its total energy for IMF4, and the residual function were 43.25%, and 37.63%, respectively. The ratio of the energy of a sharp wave to its IMF4 energy for δ (0.5 *Hz*-4 *Hz*) band was 98.4%, the similar ratio of a normal wave was 82.2%. Figure 5 and Figure 6 show the IFs corresponding to the sharp and normal waves, respectively. Tables 3 and 4 show the statistical characteristics of the IFs of the sharp and normal waves, respectively. The mean frequencies of the IFs of the normal waves were larger than those of the IFs of the sharp waves. The frequency-energy distributions corresponding to the sharp and normal waves in the IMF3, IMF4, and the residual function are shown in Tables 5, 6, and 7, respectively. From Table 5, the maximum energy of the sharp and normal waves in IMF3 appeared in the θ and δ bands, and they are 25374.79 uV^2 and 1336.66 uV^2, respectively. From Table 6, the maximum energies of the sharp and normal waves are 40853 uV^2 and 7696 uV^2, respectively, and they appeared in IMF4 in the δ bands. From Table 7, the maximum energies of the sharp and normal waves in the residual function are 14421.09 uV^2, and 7714.66 uV^2, respectively, in the δ bands. The time-frequency-energy distributions of sharp waves in IMF3, and IMF4 are listed in Table 8 and 9, respectively, while those of normal waves in IMF4, and the residual function are listed in Table 10 and 11, respectively. This is because the maximum energy distributions of sharp and normal waves are in IMF3, and IMF4, and IMF4, and the residual function, respectively. For IMF3, the energies of the sharp wave in the δ band and the interval of 0.3-0.5 *s*, and the θ band in the interval of 0.4-0.7 *s*, are 15247.30 uV^2, and 22203.43 uV^2, respectively, as shown in Table 8. The energies of IMF4 of the sharp wave in the δ band in the intervals of 0.1-0.2 *s*, 0.3-0.4 *s*, and 0.7-0.9 *s* are 6789.34 uV^2, 6003.27 uV^2, and 11534.98 uV^2, respectively, as shown in Table 9. In contrast, the energies of IMF4 of the normal wave in the δ band in the interval of 0-0.1 s, 0.1-0.3 s, 0.8-0.9 s, and 0.9-1 s are 1940.13 uV^2, 2554.11 uV^2, 1056.87 uV^2 and 2614.52 uV^2, respectively, as shown in Table 10. The energies of the residual function of the normal wave in the δ band in the intervals of 0.1-.0.2 *s*, 0.3-0.4 *s*, 0.5-0.6 *s*, and 0.7-0.9 *s* are 1348.84 uV^2, 1045.06 uV^2, 1229.81 uV^2, and 2307.81 uV^2, respectively, as shown in Table 11. These results indicate the distinct differences between the time-frequency-energy distributions of sharp and normal waves with a transmission BER of 10^{-7} in the EEG for epilepsy.

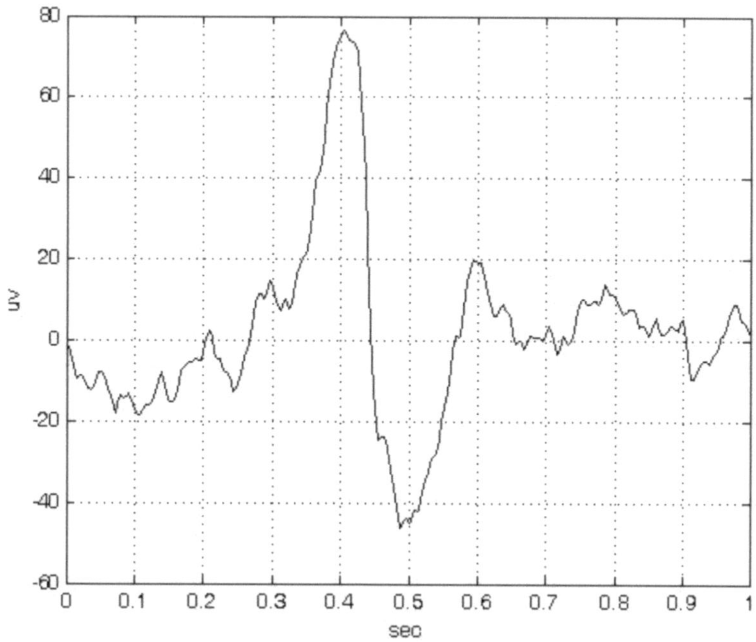

Fig. 1. Sharp wave with a transmission BER of 10^{-7} .

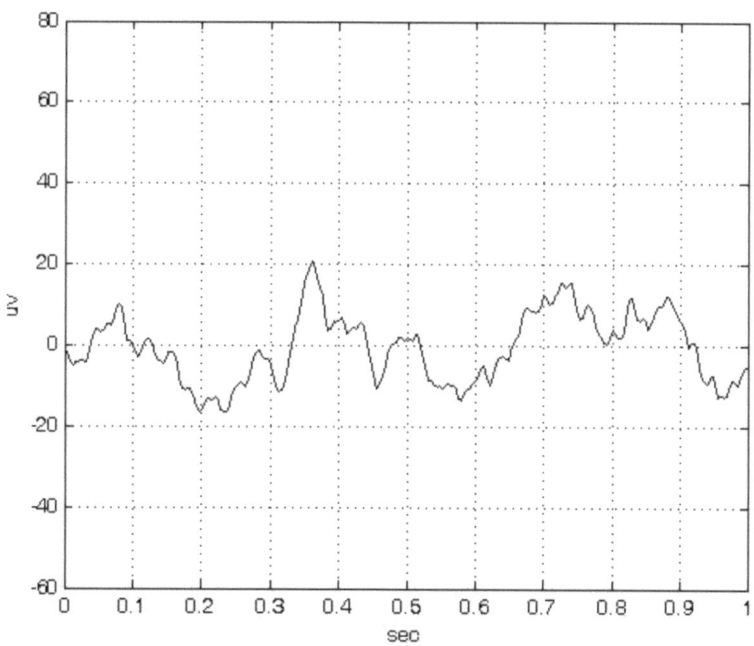

Fig. 2. Normal wave with a transmission BER of 10^{-7} .

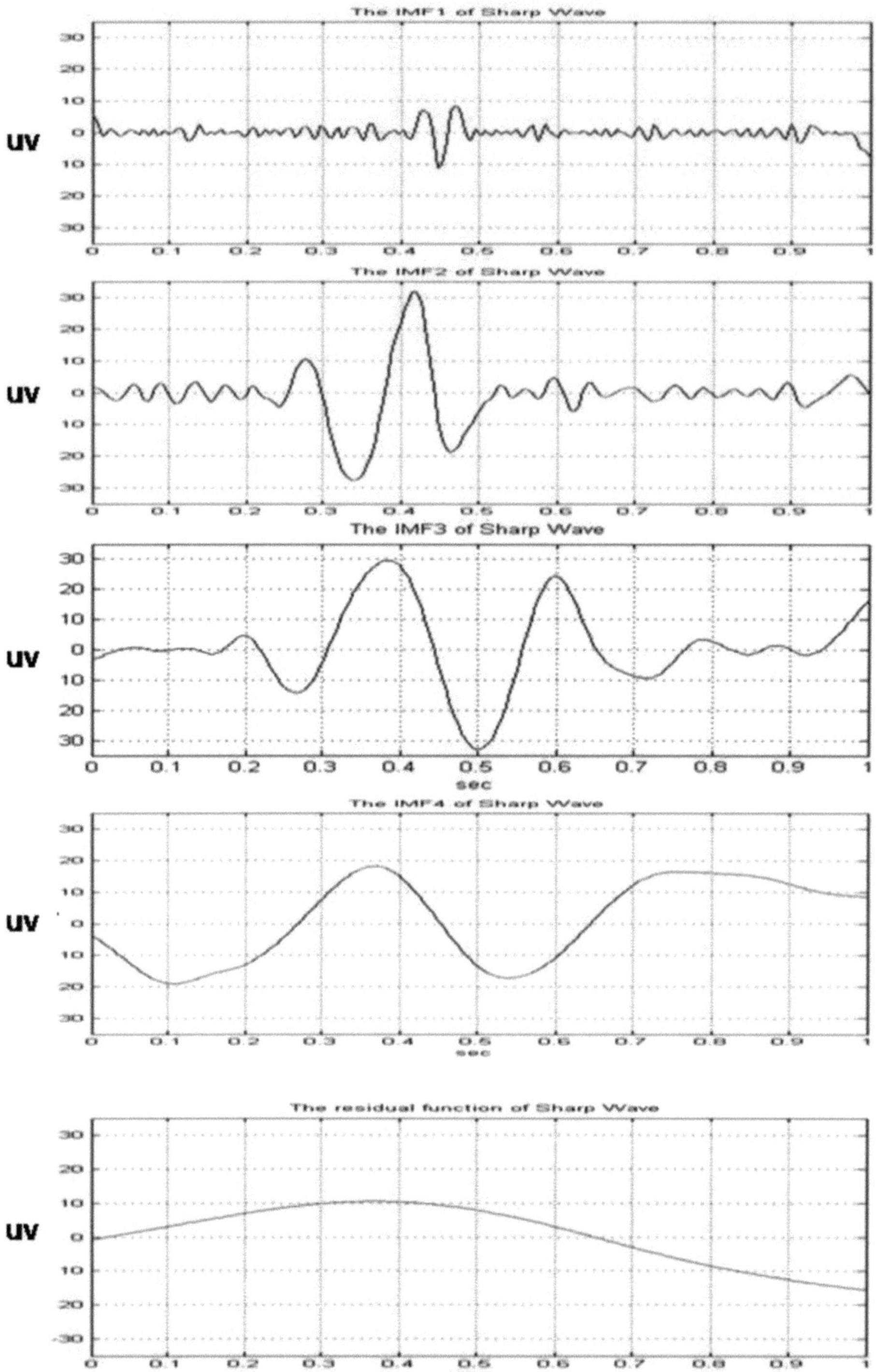

Fig. 3. IMFs and the residual function of the sharp wave with a transmission BER of 10^{-7}.

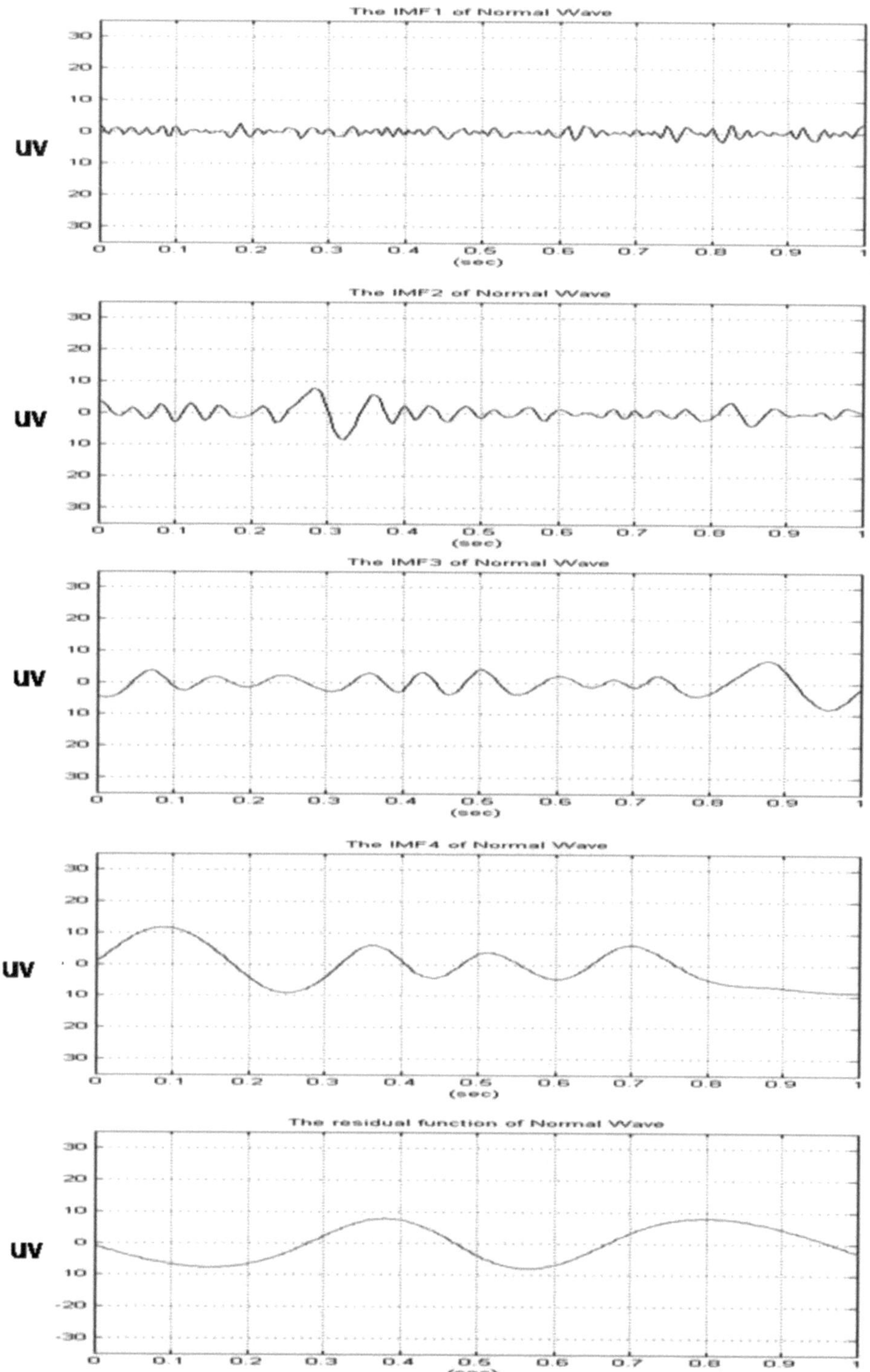

Fig. 4. IMFs and the residual function of the normal wave with a transmission BER of 10^{-7}.

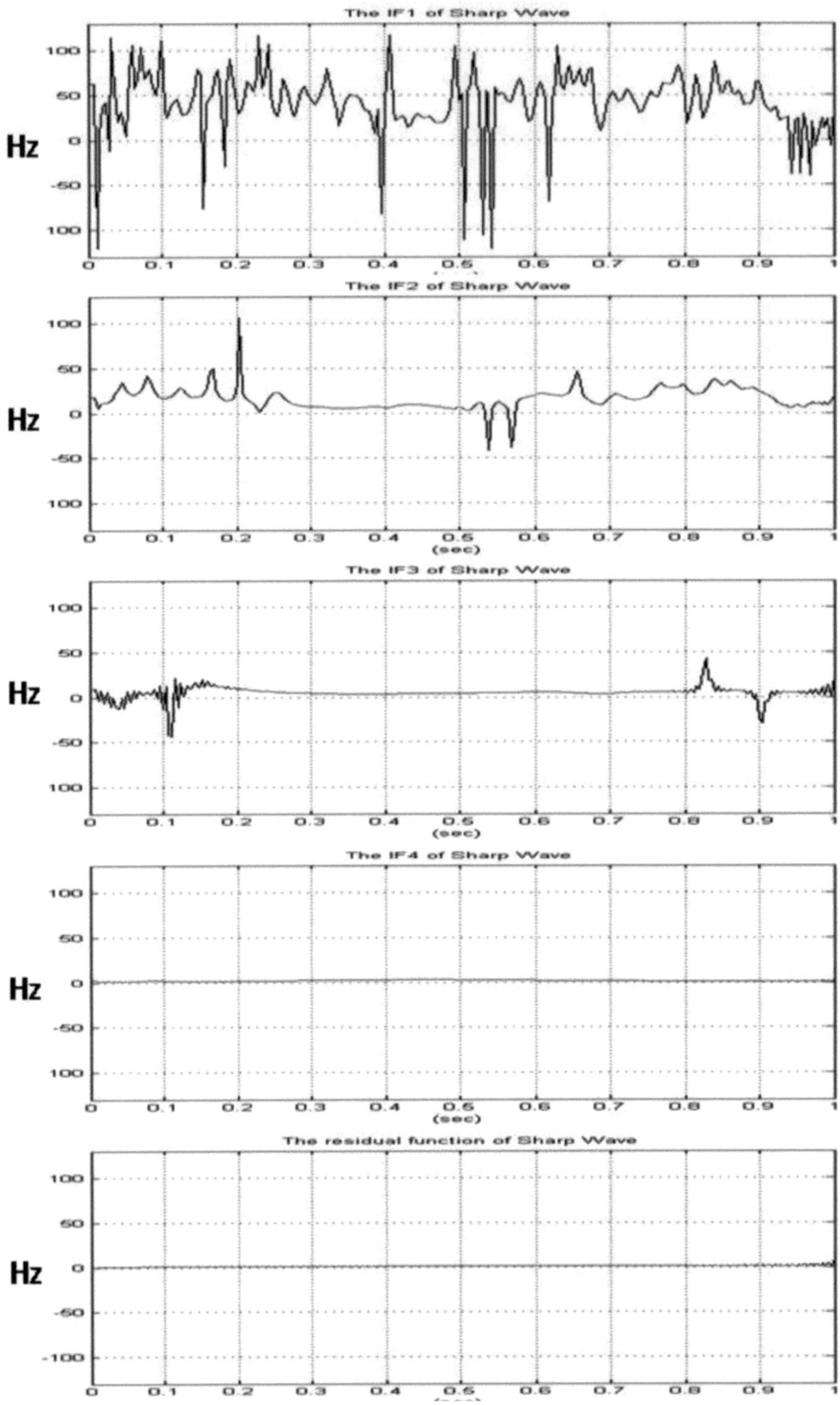

Fig. 5. IFs of the sharp wave with a transmission BER of 10^{-7}.

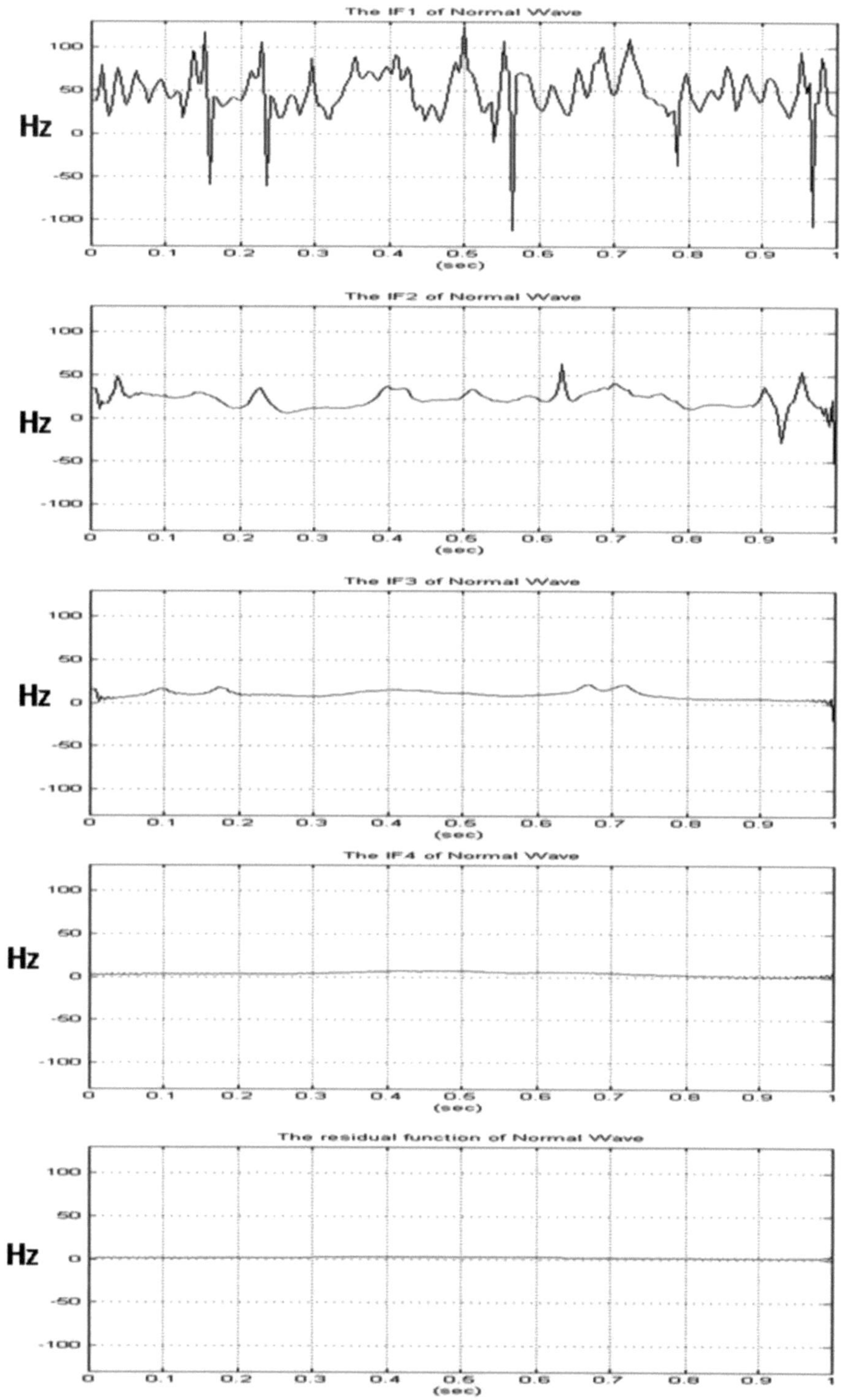

Fig. 6. IFs of the normal wave with a transmission BER of 10^{-7} .

	Mean (uv)	Std (uv)	Max (uv)	Min (uv)	Eng (uv^2)	Eng (%)
sharp wave	**1.95**	**22.72**	**76.64**	**-46.22**	**123340**	**100**
IMF1	**0.02**	**2.2**	**8.35**	**-11.07**	**1208.3**	**0.98**
IMF2	**-0.71**	**9.06**	**31.84**	**-27.68**	**20604**	**16.7**
IMF3	**0.79**	**13.08**	**29.55**	**-32.98**	**42764**	**34.67**
IMF4	**0.95**	**12.87**	**18.05**	**-19**	**41510**	**33.75**
residual function	**0.89**	**8.27**	**10.47**	**-15.57**	**17256**	**13.99**

Table 1. Statistical characteristics of the sharp wave IMFs with a transmission BER of 10^{-7}.

	Mean (uv)	Std (uv)	Max (uv)	Min (uv)	Eng (uv^2)	Eng (%)
normal wave	-0.48	8.53	20.70	-10.60	20499	100
IMF1	0.02	1.08	2.67	-2.75	293.8	1.43
IMF2	0.14	2.32	7.65	-8.49	1349.2	6.57
IMF3	-0.36	2.98	7.07	-8.13	2253.3	10.99
IMF4	-0.62	5.93	11.65	-9.16	8877.8	43.31
residual function	-0.02	5.57	8.02	-7.90	7726.9	37.69

Table 2. Statistical characteristics of the normal wave IMFs with a transmission BER of 10^{-7}.

	Mean (*Hz*)	Std (*Hz*)	Max (*Hz*)	Min (*Hz*)
IF1	42.04	34.37	116.40	-121.49
IF2	16.25	12.55	106.70	-41.33
IF3	4.89	7.52	42.84	-43.76
IF4	1.94	0.73	3.75	0.23
residual function	0.91	0.67	8.6	-0.16

Table 3. Statistical characteristics of the sharp wave IFs with a transmission BER of 10^{-7}.

	Mean (Hz)	Std (Hz)	Max (Hz)	Min (Hz)
IF1	49.04	28.28	124.40	-112.08
IF2	21.96	11.57	63.22	-75.62
IF3	10.10	4.83	22.04	-26.8
IF4	3.93	1.90	7.48	0.52
residual function	2.04	0.55	5.53	0.05

Table 4. Statistical characteristics of the normal wave IFs with a transmission BER of 10^{-7}.

IMF3	<0.5Hz	δ	θ	α	β	γ
sharp	0.31	16497.95	25374.79	381.41	509.35	0.17
Normal	773.28	1336.66	117.95	25.45	0.00	0.00
sharp (%)	0.00	38.58	59.34	0.89	1.19	0.00
normal (%)	34.32	59.32	5.23	1.13	0.00	0.00

Table 5. Frequency-energy distributions of IMF3 of the sharp and normal waves with a transmission BER of 10^{-7}.

IMF4	<0.5Hz	δ	θ
sharp	663.00	40853.00	0.00
normal	0.00	7696.00	1580.89
sharp(%)	1.60	98.40	0.00
normal(%)	0.00	82.20	17.80

Table 6. Frequency-energy distributions of IMF4 of the sharp and normal waves with a transmission BER of 10^{-7}.

residual function	<0.5Hz	δ	θ
sharp	2356.10	14421.09	236.54
normal	3.73	7714.66	8.52
sharp(%)	13.65	83.57	1.37
normal(%)	0.05	99.84	0.11

Table 7. Frequency-energy distributions of the residual function of the sharp and normal waves with a transmission BER of 10^{-7}.

sharp IMF3 (sec)	<0.5 Hz	δ	θ	α	β	γ
0-0.1	0.31	5.63	4.51	21.60	0.23	0
0.1-0.2	0	0.20	0	76.66	25.07	0.06
0.2-0.3	0	0	2217.07	41.63	0	0
0.3-0.4	0	11983.3	96.602	0	0	0
0.4-0.5	0	3264.05	8076.35	0	0	0
0.5-0.6	0	0	11104.50	0	0	0
0.6-0.7	0	427.44	3022.18	0	0	0
0.7-0.8	0	166.66	741.86	0	0	0
0.8-0.9	0	3.88	22.00	9.85	1.99	0.11
0.9-1.0	0	646.75	89.73	231.66	482.06	0

Table 8. Time-frequency-energy distributions of IMF3 of the sharp waves with a transmission BER of 10^{-7}.

sharp IMF4 (sec)	<0.5Hz	δ
0-0.1	0	4429.30
0.1-0.2	0	6789.34
0.2-0.3	0	1288.18
0.3-0.4	0	6003.27
0.4-0.5	0	1870.42
0.5-0.6	0	5935
0.6-0.7	0	1232.43
0.7-0.8	0	6105.55
0.8-0.9	0	5429.43
0.9-1.0	662.79	1764.27

Table 9. Time-frequency-energy distributions of IMF4 of the sharp waves with a transmission BER of 10^{-7}.

Normal IMF4 (sec)	δ	θ
0-0.1	1940.13	0
0.1-0.2	1125.07	0
0.2-0.3	1429.04	17.67
0.3-0.4	0	409.96
0.4-0.5	0	201.27
0.5-0.6	0	239.73
0.6-0.7	0	401.12
0.7-0.8	188.11	158.76
0.8-0.9	1056.87	0
0.9-1.0	1557.65	152.39

Table 10. Time-frequency-energy distributions of IMF4 of the normal waves with a transmission BER of 10^{-7}.

normal residual function (sec)	<0.5Hz	δ
0-0.1	3.73	523.16
0.1-0.2	0	1348.84
0.2-0.3	0	358.32
0.3-0.4	0	1045.06
0.4-0.5	0	439.20
0.5-0.6	0	1229.81
0.6-0.7	0	329.76
0.7-0.8	0	1138.58
0.8-0.9	0	1169.23
0.9-1.0	0	132.69

Table 11. Time-frequency-energy distributions of the residual function of the normal waves with a transmission BER of 10^{-7}.

4. Discussion

Hilbert-Huang transformation (HHT) is one of the major time-frequency analysis methods and is suitable for the analysis of local time signals. In this article, we use HHT-based method to analysis the signal deemed of the sharp wave. In addition, we describe the features of a sharp wave recorded and a normal wave recorded with a transmission bit error rate (BER) of 10^{-7} for patients with epilepsy by using HHT analysis method. Simulation results shows that the performance of the sharp wave based HHT time-frequency characteristics is not affected under the transmission BER of 10^{-7} assumptions. We present the intrinsic mode functions (IMF), instantaneous frequencies (IF), time-frequency-energy distributions for the sharp and normal waves. Clear energy-frequency-time variations of the sharp waves and normal waves with a transmission BER of 10^{-7} are shown. There are 4 IMFs and a residual function of the sharp and normal waves by using the HHT analysis. Analysis results show that the ratio of the energy of a sharp wave with the IMF3 and the total energy of a sharp wave, the ratio of the energy of a sharp wave with the IMF4 and the total energy of a sharp wave, the ratio of the energy of a normal wave with the IMF4 and the total energy of a normal wave, the ratio of the energy of a normal wave with the residual function and the total energy of a normal wave are 34.55%, 33.73%, 43.25%, and 37.63%, respectively. The ratio of the energy of the IMF4 of a sharp wave with δ (0.5Hz-4Hz) band and the total energy of the IMF4 of a sharp is 98.4%. The ratio of the energy of the IMF4 of a normal wave with δ (0.5Hz-4Hz) band and the total energy of IMF4 of a sharp is 82.2%. The mean IF of the IMF4 of a sharp wave is smaller than the mean IF of the IMF4 of a normal wave. From these analysis results, we observe that the HHT-based time-frequency characteristics of the sharp waves with a transmission BER of 10^{-7}.

5. Conclusion

The HHT-based time-frequency analysis approaches are suitable for studying the local and non-stationary normal waves and sharp waves in EEGs for epilepsy. We obtained the IMFs, and IFs to analyze the energy-frequency-time distributions of normal waves and sharp waves with a transmission BER of 10^{-7} in the EEG. The mean IF of IMF4 of a sharp wave is smaller than the mean IF of IMF4 of a normal wave. In addition, the substantial energies of IMF3 of the sharp wave are the δ band in the interval of 0.3-0.5 s, and the θ band in the interval of 0.4-0.7 s. The substantial energies of IMF4 of the sharp wave are the δ band in the intervals of 0.1-0.2 s, 0.3-0.4 s, and 0.7-0.9 s. In contrast, the substantial energies of IMF4 of the normal wave are the δ band in the intervals of 0-0.1 s, 0.1-0.3 s, and 0.8-1 s. The substantial energies of the residual function of the normal wave are the δ band in the intervals of 0.1-.0.2 s, 0.3-0.4 s, 0.5-0.6 s, and 0.7-0.9s. These observations show that the sharp signal characteristics and the IMFs, IFs, time-frequency-energy distributions of sharp-related and normal signals can be distinguished from each other, thereby ensuring more accurate diagnosis of patients with an epilepsy-related sharp.

6. Acknowledgements

The authors acknowledge the support of National Taiwan Ocean University, Center for Marine Bioscience and Biotechnology and the Chang Cung Memorial Hospital, Keelung Branch Research Project 98529002k8, The Ministry of Education of Cross fields learning projects of personnel training of 99A1 in NTOU, Taiwan, National Taiwan Ocean University, Center for Teaching and Learning, Telemedicine Teaching and Learning Probject, the grant from the National Science Council of Taiwan NSC 98-2221-e-022-018, NSC 93-2218-e-019-024, and the valuable comments of the reviewers.

7. References

Huang, N. E.; Shen, Z.; Long, S. R.; Wu, M. C.; Shih, H. H.; Zheng, Q.; Yen, N. C.; Tung C. C. & Liu, H. H. (1998). The empirical mode decomposition and the Hilbert spectrum for non- linear and non-stationary time series analysis. *Proceedings of the Royal Society of London Series A – Mathematical Physical and Engineering Sciences*, 903-995.

Yan, R. & Gao R. X. (2007). A tour of the Hilbert-Huang transform: an empirical tool for signal analysis. *IEEE Instrumentation & Measurement Magazine*, 11-15.

Cohen, L. (1989). Time-frequency distributions-a review. *I Proceedings of the IEEE*, 941–981.

Blanco, S.; Kochen, S.; Rooso, O. A.& Salgado, P. (1997). Applying time-frequency analysis to seizure EEG activity. *IEEE Engineering in Medicine and Biology*, 64-71.

Tzallas, A. T.; Tsipouras, M. G. & Fotiadis, D. I. (2009). Epileptic seizure detection in EEGs using time-frequency analysis. *IEEE Trans. Information Technology in Biomedicine*, 703-710.

Exarchos, T. P.; Tzallas, A. T.; Fotiadis, D. I.; Konitsiotis, S. & Giannopoulos, S. (2006). EEG transient event detection and classification using association rules. *IEEE Trans. Inf. Technol. Biomed,* 451–457.

Williams, W. J.; Zaveri, H. P. & Sackellares, J. C. (1995). Time-frequency analysis of electrophysiology signals in epilepsy. *IEEE Eng. Med. Biol,* 133–143.

Sharabaty, H.; Martin, H. J.; Jammes, B. & Esteve, D. (2006). Alpha and theta wave localisation using Hilbert-Huang transform: empirical study of the accuracy, *Proceedings of IEEE Int. Conf. Information and Communication Technologies,* 1159-1164.

Wang, L.; Xu, G.; Wang, J.; Yang, S. & Yan, W. (2008). Application of Hilbert-Huang transform for the study of motor imagery tasks, *Proceedings of IEEE Int. Conf. EMBS,* 3848-3851.

Wang, Y. L.; Liu, J. H. & Liu, Y. (2008). Automatic removal of ocular artifacts from electroencephalogram using Hilbert-Huang transform, *Proceedings of IEEE Int. Conf. ICBBE,*2138-2141.

Lin, C. F.; Chang, W. T.; Lee, H. W. & Hung, S. I. (2006). Downlink power control in multi-code CDMA mobile medicine system. *Medical & Biological Engineering & Computing,* 437-444.

Lin, C. F.; Chang, W. T. & Li, C. Y. (2007). A chaos-based visual encryption mechanism in JPEG2000 medical images. *J. of Medical and Biological Engineering,* 144-149.

Lin, C. F. & Chang, K. T. (2008). A power assignment mechanism in Ka band OFDM-based multi-satellites mobile telemedicine. *J. of Medical and Biological Engineering,* 17-22.

Lin, C. F. & Li, C. Y. (2008). A DS UWB transmission system for wireless telemedicine. *WSEAS Transactions on Systems,* 578-588.

Lin, C. F.; Chung, C. H.; Chen, Z. L.; Song, C. F. & Wang, Z. X. (2008). A chaos-based unequal encryption mechanism in wireless telemedicine with error decryption. *WSEAS Transactions on Systems,* 49-55.

Lin, C. F.; Chen, J. Y.; Shiu, R. H. & Chang, S. H. (2008). A Ka band WCDMA-based LEO transport architecture in mobile telemedicine, In: *Telemedicine in the 21st Century,* Lucia Martinez and Carla Gomez, (Ed.), 187-201, Nova Science Publishers, USA.

Lin, C. F.; Chung, C. H. & Lin, J. H. (2009). A Chaos-based visual encryption mechanism for EEG clinical signals. *Medical & Biological Engineering & Computing,* 757-762.

Lin, C. F. (2010). An Advance Wireless Multimedia Communication Application: Mobile Telemedicine. *WSEAS Transactions on Communications,* 206-215.

Lin, C. F.; Hung, S. I.; & Chiang, I. H. (Online First). 802.11n WLAN Transmission Scheme for Wireless Telemedicine Applications. *Proceedings of the Institution of Mechanical Engineers, Part H, Journal of Engineering in Medicine.*

Lin, C. F. (Online First). Mobile Telemedicine:A Survey Study. *Journal of Medical Systems.*

Lin, C. F. & Wang, B. S. H. (Accept). A 2D Chaos-based Visual Encryption Scheme for Clinical EEG Signals. *Journal of Marine Science and Technology.*

Lin, C. F.; Yeh S. W.; Peng, T. I.; Chien, Y. Y.; Wang, J. H. & Chang, S. H. (2008). A HHT-based time frequency analysis scheme in clinical alcoholic EEG signals. *WSEAS Transactions on Biology and Biomedicine,* 249-260.

Lin, C. F.; Yeh, S. W.; Chang, S. H.; Peng, T. I. & Chien, Y. Y. (2010). An HHT-based time-frequency scheme for analyzing the EEG signals of clinical alcoholics. In: *Advances in Medicine and Biology, Volume 11,* Leon V. Berhardt, (Ed.), Nova Science Publishers, USA.

Lin, C. F.; Yeh, S. W.; Chang, S. H.; Peng, T. I. & Chien, Y. Y. (2010). *An HHT-based Time-frequency Scheme for Analyzing the EEG Signals of Clinical Alcoholics,* Online Book, Nova Science Publishers, USA.

8

Teleconsultation Enhanced via Session Retrieval Capabilities: Smart Playback Functions and Recovery Mechanism

Pau-Choo Chung and Cheng-Hsiung Wang
National Cheng Kung University
Taiwan

1. Introduction

With the widespread deployment of the Internet nowadays and the increasing power and sophistication of network communication technologies, many collaborative systems have been proposed to support users in geographically dispersed areas in transmitting and sharing multimedia data (Huang et al., 2007; Li et al., 2004; Marsh et al., 2006). One area in which collaborative systems have found particular use is that of telemedicine and teleconsultation, and it is now common practice for physicians to use such systems as a means of analyzing medical images, discussing patients' symptoms, consulting with other medical experts, and so forth (Vazquez et al., 2007; Lee et al., 2004; Lo et al., 2000; Shah et al., 1997; Paul et al., 1998; Guerri et al., 2003; Kholief et al., 2003; Kim et al., 2001). By fully exploiting real-time videoconferencing and medical information sharing, conventional medical teleconsultation systems may satisfy the requirement of providing the interactive discussion environment, but lack session retrieval capabilities that are addressed in terms of session-replay and session-recovery in this chapter.

In medical teleconsultation systems, the ability to replay sessions on demand is of crucial importance since it provides the opportunity to resolve arguments relating to the corresponding case and enables the multimedia content within the session to be used for teaching purposes. However, in the majority of the telemedicine and teleconsultation systems presented in the literature, playback functions are addressed only in passing or have no more than a limited functionality. Shah et al. presented a telemedicine consultation playback system in which a discrete event system specification (DEVS) approach was used to couple the data objects within the system and to model their behavior over time (Shah et al., 1997). However, whilst this approach enabled a synchronization of the various data objects during the playback sequence, the provision of specific playback functions was not considered. In the telemedicine systems (Paul et al., 1998; Guerri et al., 2003), playback functions were provided, but were restricted to chronological order only since all the communication packets within the session were time-stamped to facilitate their synchronization during playback. The event-based and event-tree systems (Kholief et al., 2003; Kim et al., 2001) provide a greater playback flexibility than these time-stamping methods, but lack time-related descriptions and indexes of the objects in the session, and are therefore unable to support playback from randomly specified time points. The ***PlayWatch*** scheme (Tanaka et al., 2005) adopts a chart-style semantic indexing method to locate video scenes and allows users to jump directly to a particular scene simply by selecting an appropriate predefined keyword. However, the system lacks a time index, and thus the process of advancing to a particular time position within video scenes is very slow. The recent MPEG-7 standard (Chang et al., 2006) defines a set of descriptors for describing and indexing video sequences. However, the contents of most video sequences are relatively static, i.e. they do not vary over time. By contrast, medical teleconsultation sessions comprise both image contents and a sequence of commands imposed upon these contents. As a result, the contents of typical medical teleconsultation sequences vary dynamically in accordance with the particular sequence of commands applied to them. Consequently, the scene-based descriptors defined in MPEG-7 are inappropriate for describing and indexing medical teleconsultation sessions.

In developing playback functions for medical teleconsultation sessions, two fundamental issues must be resolved. Firstly, when a playback function is selected, the indexing mechanism of the teleconsultation system must locate the appropriate cut-in point within all the various types of data (e.g. image data, audio data, and so on) which constitute the corresponding scene before the replay process can commence. To reduce the ***restart-latency time*** (i.e. the delay between the moment at which the playback function is invoked and the moment at which playback actually commences), the indexing mechanism must maintain an appropriate cross-linkage amongst the various multimedia data within the session in order to determine the cut-in point in the most efficient manner possible. Secondly, as described above, typical medical teleconsultation sessions involve the use of multiple image processing commands, many of which change the contents of the images within the session. For example, a physician may use a drawing tool to circle a ROI (region-of-interest) on an image and then use a text editing tool to append relevant comments. Furthermore, the modified image contents may be further changed by the invocation of additional commands later in the session. As a result, a strict dependency exists between the image contents and the type and sequential order in which the image processing commands are applied. Consequently, once a suitable cut-in point for a playback function has been located, it is necessary to carry out an appropriate restoration process to restore the image contents from their current condition to that which existed at the cut-in point in the original session.

As mentioned in the above paragraph, the contents of teleconsultation sessions depend critically on the type and sequence of the image processing / analysis commands used during the course of the session. Thus, the reliability of the network connecting the various participants in the session is critical in ensuring that each participant receives a consistent and continuous view of medical images during the on-going session. In practice, however, the network may fail for a variety of hardware or software-related reasons, and thus one or more of the participants are obliged to drop out of the session and re-enter it later. In addition, while some participants take part in a session for its entire duration (e.g. the physician with the overall responsibility for a particular case), others may participate only at a later point in the discussions (e.g. a consultant with input to only one medical image, a physician with the results obtained from medical tests, and so on). For both these "late" users and the "re-entrant" users described above, it is necessary to reconstruct the session contents in such a way that they are able to catch up with the on-going discussions in shortest time as possible.

To support this requirement, some form of "fast forwarding" mechanism is used to advance the re-entrant / late users' view of the session from its initial state to the current state. This is commonly achieved by using a centralized content-recording scheme to record the changes in the session contents over the course of the session such that they can be re-executed at the user end as and when required. Existing content-recording schemes can be broadly classified as either checkpoint schemes or message-logging schemes. The former schemes (Gropp & Lusk, 2004; Johnson & Zwaenepoel, 1987; Elnozahy et al., 2002) take periodic snapshots of the session contents and use the latest snapshot as the synchronization point in the restoration process. This method is particularly common in videoconferencing systems in which the session contents at any particular moment in time are independent of the video and audio signals transmitted previously. However, in medical teleconsultation systems, the session contents are critically dependent on the type and sequence of the commands used by the various participants over the course of the session, and thus ensuring the consistency of the session views amongst all the session participants is far more complex. For example, when using the checkpoint scheme to restore the session contents for a re-entrant / late participant, a *rollback propagation* problem (Elnozahy et al., 2002) arises in that it is necessary to rollback the session contents of all the users to the synchronization point. In other words, the restoration process not only causes the on-going session to be suspended, but also loses any updates after the synchronization point. Moreover, the need to back up the entire session contents at each checkpoint incurs a significant overhead. As a result, a tradeoff exists between the frequency at which the checkpoints are refreshed and the performance of the restoration process. Moreover, when the session contents are backed up on a frequency basis in order to ensure the quality of the restoration results, it is possible that in the worst case scenario, the effect of suspending the session for even a very short period of time may result in missing a time-critical aspect of the medical image under discussion.

In contrast to the checkpoint content-recording schemes described above, the message-logging schemes (Elnozahy et al., 2002) sequentially record every message transmitted in a session and reconstruct the session contents from scratch by re-executing each of these messages in the same sequential order. Compared to checkpoint schemes, message-logging schemes not only avoid the worst case scenario described above, but also allow the session to continue without interruption for all the participants other than those for which the restoration process is actually being performed. However, the restoration process is inevitably time consuming since it is necessary to re-execute each and every recorded command for every re-entrant / late user in order to restore the image contents to their current condition. To address this need, a high ***recovery-latency*** delay is induced between the moment at which the re-entrant / late user joins the on-going session and the moment at which the restoration process is completed so that he or she can actively participate in the session. From the above discussions, it is clear that two fundamental issues must be resolved for developing content-recording and restoration schemes for medical teleconsultation sessions. First of all, in restoring the image contents for re-entrant / late users, it is essential that the dependency existing between the image contents and the type and sequential order in which the image processing commands are used must be preserved in order to ensure that each session user has a consistent and up-to-date view of the current session contents. Secondly, the restoration process should be completed as rapidly as possible such that a delay for the re-entrant / late users joining the on-going session can be minimized. Thus, upon implementing restoration schemes for teleconsultation sessions, it is essential to construct an efficient content-recording structure which minimizes the ***recovery-latency*** delay incurred in the restoration process.

Therefore, to design playback functions and recovery mechanism for the teleconsultation sessions, this chapter proposes an enhanced content-recording scheme designated as ***three-level indexing hierarchy*** (***TIH***) which utilizes an efficient cross-linkage design to maintain the dependency between the image contents and the sequential order as the image processing commands are used. As shown in Fig. 1, the ***TIH*** architecture comprises a single *SessionNode* in the first level, a series of *DataNodes* distributed in the time domain in the second level, and a *CommandNode, PictureNode* and *UserNode* under each *DataNode* in the third level. Furthermore, ***TIH*** utilizes the command file (Wang et al., 2005) as a ***Command-Record*** file to record all the commands invoked throughout the teleconsultation session, e.g. "mouse move", "mouse click", "draw line", "vertical/horizontal flip", "zoom in/out", "rotation", and so forth. Of these commands, only a limited subset (e.g. "vertical / horizontal flip" and "zoom in / out") actually affect the image appearance. Utilizing a novel cross-linkage design, the ***TIH*** architecture indexes these commands (referred to henceforth as "image-affect commands") such that they can be rapidly identified in the event that a playback function is invoked or a restoration process is required.

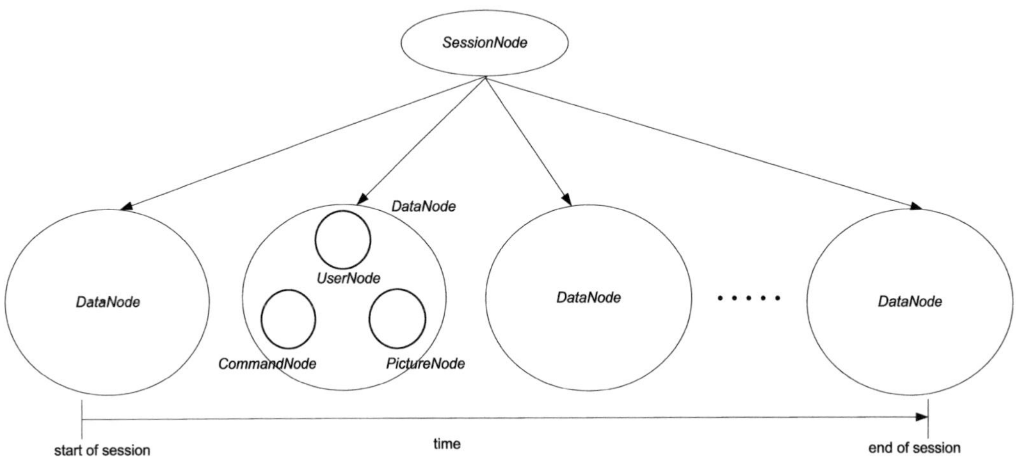

Fig. 1. Illustration of ***TIH*** architecture showing *SessionNode* and *DataNodes* comprising *UserNode, CommandNode* and *PictureNode.*

With the help of ***TIH***, four smart playback functions are supported for medical teleconsultation systems, namely (1) replaying the session from a specified point in time, (2) replaying all the segments controlled by a particular physician, (3) replaying all of the segments associated with a specific medical image, and (4) playing a montage of the entire session in order to show its major features. As for the recovery mechanism, the ability of re-entrant / late users to catch up with the on-going discussions in a timely manner can be improved by restoring the foreground image (i.e. the image under current discussion) before the background images (i.e. the remaining images in the session) are restored. Thus, this chapter proposes a novel prioritized recovery policy in which the cross-linkage design of the ***TIH*** architecture is used to accomplish the restoration process free of the dependency constraints between the image contents and the image-affect commands. That is, the foreground image is restored as soon as the re-entrant / late user joins the session and the remaining images in the session are then restored in a transparent background mode. In this way, the user is able to observe the on-going session as the restoration of the background images proceeds. In this case, the perceived ***recovery-latency*** delay is significantly reduced. When the restoration process is performed, it is possible that the current foreground image may suddenly be replaced by one of the background images. In this event, it is necessary to suspend the current restoration process and to switch to the restoration of the new foreground image. To support this requirement, the proposed prioritized recovery policy maintains a set of resuming pointers for each re-entrant / late user to indicate the current restoration state of each image in the session and facilitate the process of suspending the current restoration process and switching to the restoration of the new foreground image in a timely and computationally-efficient manner.

The remainder of this chapter is organized as follows. Section 2 describes the basic indexing architecture used to facilitate the playback functions in Section 3 and the recovery mechanism in Section 4. Section 3 introduces the cross-linking mechanism used to relate the various data records within the teleconsultation session and explains the role of this mechanism in executing each of the proposed playback functions. Section 4 describes the prioritized recovery policy and discusses the use of the resuming pointers in resolving the foreground image substitution problem during the restoration process. Section 5 quantifies the performance of ***TIH*** in terms of the cut-in point determination time and the image content restoration time for the smart playback functions, and the performance of the proposed recovery mechanism when applied to typical teleconsultation sessions. Finally, Section 6 presents some brief concluding remarks.

2. Architecture of *TIH*

Typical medical teleconsultation sessions involve the exchange of multiple media data (e.g. audio, video, medical images, image processing commands, and so forth) between participating physicians. As described in Section 1, a dependency exists between the image contents of such sessions and the sequence and type of the image processing commands invoked during the course of the session. This chapter accounts for this dependency when implementing smart playback functions by utilizing the three-level indexing architecture shown in Fig. 1. Owing to that ***TIH*** is also adopted as the content-recording scheme for the recovery mechanism, the descriptions in this section focused on the smart playback functions are also suitable for the recovery mechanism. In ***TIH***, the *SessionNode* stores the high-level information required to identify the target *DataNode(s)*, while the *DataNodes* contain the detailed information describing all the session events invoked by a particular physician over a specific time period within the session. The details of each of the nodes within ***TIH*** are described in the following paragraphs.

2.1 Design of SessionNode

The *SessionNode* has two principal functions, namely to store general information relating to a particular session and to provide basic indexing information such that the target *DataNode(s)* for a particular playback function can be rapidly located. In designing and implementing the *SessionNode*, a number of issues arise. Firstly, it is possible that physicians may download additional medical images on-line during the course of a session to supplement the patient-related images. Irrespective of the playback function invoked by a user, these on-line images should be retrieved only once during the playback procedure in order to minimize the ***restart-latency time***. Thus, in ***TIH***, the information required to retrieve all of the on-line images associated with a particular session is stored in the form of an ***On-line_Index*** in the *SessionNode* such that all of the images can be retrieved in a one-shot process prior to commencing the playback routine. Secondly, a user may request the playback of only those periods of a session for which a certain medical image is discussed. To facilitate this requirement, the *SessionNode* maintains a ***Picture_Index*** to record the *DataNode* - *CommandNode* index pairs for every medical image discussed during the course of the session. Thirdly, a user may only be interested in viewing those parts of a session controlled by a particular physician. Thus, the *SessionNode* maintains a ***User_Index*** to record the indexes of all the *DataNodes* associated with each physician. Finally, the *SessionNode* also records general session information such as the Session ID and the total session time. Fig. 2 illustrates the typical contents of the *SessionNode*.

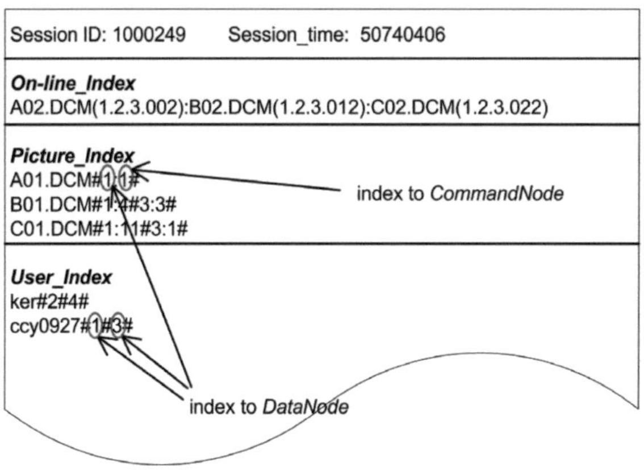

Fig. 2. Typical contents of *SessionNode* in ***TIH*** architecture.

2.2 Design of DataNode

The *DataNodes* in ***TIH*** store the index information relating to all the events which take place during the time period(s) within a session for which each particular physician has control. As discussed above, each *DataNode* comprises a *UserNode*, a *CommandNode* and a *PictureNode*. The details of each node are presented in the following.

2.2.1 UserNode

The *UserNode* records the ***Command-Record*** index of the first command performed in the *DataNode*, and maintains information regarding the ***Start_Time*** of the *DataNode* (i.e. the time at which the *DataNode* first became active in the session) and the identity of the physician in control of the *DataNode*. Fig. 3 presents the typical contents of a *UserNode*.

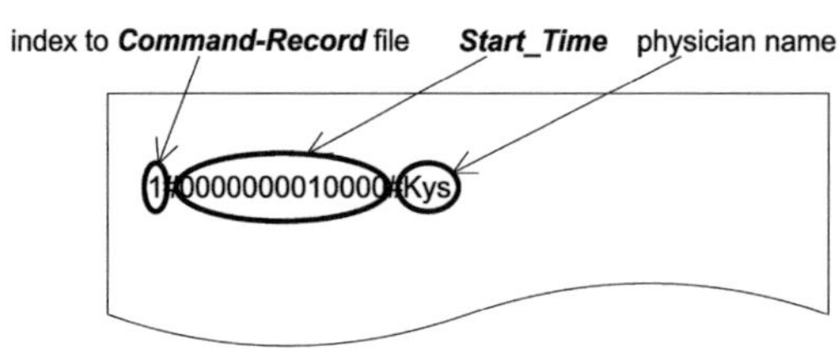

Fig. 3. Typical contents of *UserNode*.

2.2.2 CommandNode

The smart playback functions proposed in this chapter may commence at any point within the session. For example, if the user wishes to review the entire session, the cut-in point is located at the very beginning of the session. However, if he or she wishes to view only those segments concerning a particular medical image, the system must jump to the cut-in point corresponding to the first occurrence of this image in the session and then replay the session for so long as the image was discussed. Having done so, it should then jump to the next point in the session at which the image was discussed and replay the corresponding content. This process should be repeated until all of the relevant segments have been located and replayed. Having completed one playback function (e.g. view all segments associated with a particular medical image), the user may decide to replay all of the session segments controlled by a particular physician. In this case, the system is required to "fast forward" or "rewind" from the position at which the previous playback function terminated to the cut-in point associated with the new playback request. However, as described previously, the application of image-affect commands during the course of the session changes the image contents, and thus the current contents (i.e. those associated with the point in the session at which the previous playback function terminated) may well differ from those associated with the new cut-in point. As a result, it is necessary to record all the image-affect commands invoked during the course of the session such that an appropriate subset of these commands can be reapplied to modify the current image contents in such a way as to restore them to their condition at the time point corresponding to the new cut-in point. To support this requirement, all of the image-affect commands performed within each *DataNode* are recorded in the corresponding *CommandNode* together with the index of each command in the ***Command-Record*** file. Fig. 4 shows the typical contents of a *CommandNode*.

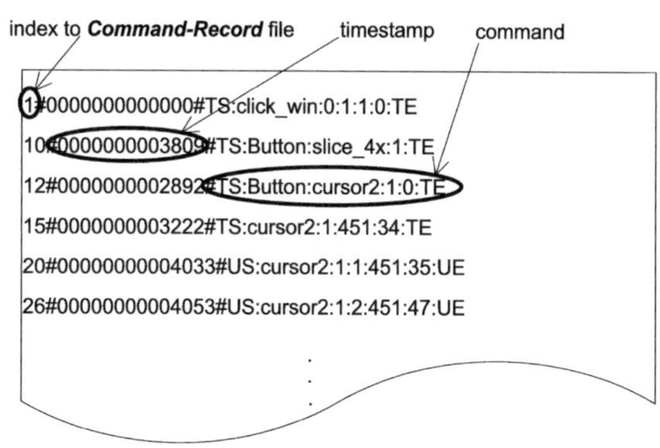

Fig. 4. Typical contents of *CommandNode*.

2.2.3 PictureNode

When a playback function is invoked, it is necessary to determine the particular medical image (defined as the ***target image***) associated with the corresponding cut-in point. In ***TIH***, this requirement is satisfied using the *PictureNode* within each *DataNode*. As shown in Fig. 5, the *PictureNode* contains a series of time-stamped records, each of which represents the introduction of a particular medical image during the course of the session. In addition, the *CommandNode* index of the command used to invoke the image is also recorded.

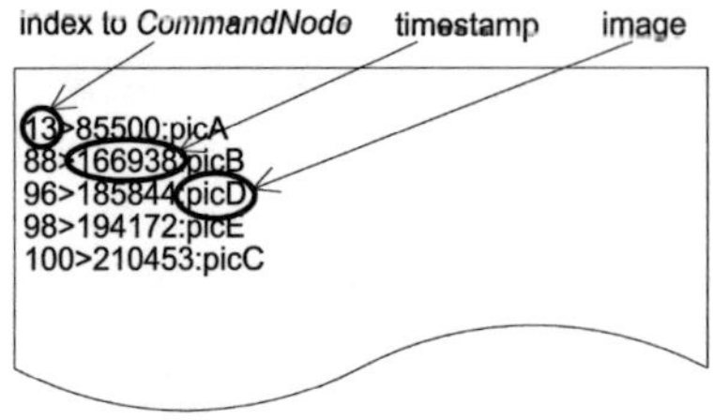

Fig. 5. Typical contents of *PictureNode*.

3. Use of *TIH* to facilitate smart playback functions

This section describes the use of the indexing mechanisms described above in locating the cut-in point and identifying the commands required to restore the contents of the target image to an appropriate condition when performing a variety of smart playback functions.

3.1 Playback from specified time point in a session

Assume that a particular playback function stops at a certain time point T_C in the session. Assume further that the user subsequently decides to replay the session from another time point, T. Upon receiving this user request, the system performs a binary search on the ***Start_Time*** information recorded at all the *UserNodes* in order to determine the *DataNode* corresponding to time T. Once the target *DataNode* has been located, the system initiates a search for the appropriate cut-in point within this *DataNode*. Fig. 6 presents an illustrative example of the search procedure performed for the case of a playback start time of T=20000. Having identified the target *DataNode*, the target image is determined by searching the corresponding *PictureNode* for the image associated with the timestamp immediately before T, i.e. "picA" in Step (1) of Fig. 6. Using the "index to *CommandNode*" field corresponding to this target image (i.e. "2" in the current example), the *CommandNode* is interrogated to determine the command used to select the target image (i.e. the second record in the

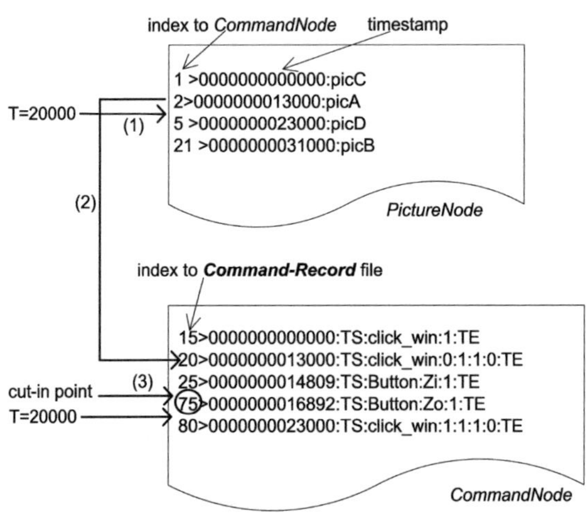

Fig. 6. Illustration of cut-in point determination procedure for specified time of T=20000. Note that labels (1), (2) and (3) indicate the three steps performed in locating the cut-in point.

CommandNode), as shown in Step (2). Starting from this command, the system then searches the contents of the *CommandNode* to identify the command with the timestamp closest to (but less than) the specified time T (i.e. the fourth record in the *CommandNode*). This command is then identified as the cut-in point for this particular playback request, as shown in Step (3). Having identified the cut-in point, the actions taken next to restore the image contents depend on the chronological relationship between T_C and T. In the event that $T_C < T$, the playback request prompts a high speed "forward winding" of the session sequence to the cut-in point. Once, it arrives at this point, the system starts to play the session sequence at the normal speed. To accomplish this fast forwarding effect, all of the image-affect commands recorded in the *CommandNode(s)* between T_C and T are sequentially applied to the related medical images in order to restore them to their corresponding states at time T. Conversely, if $T < T_C$, the medical image contents are restored by reapplying all of the image-affect commands invoked between the beginning of the session and time T.

3.2 Playback of session segments controlled by specified physician

As described in the following, two different playback functions may be invoked in this particular mode of user request.

3.2.1 Replay from time at which specified physician first takes control of a session

In this scenario, the system locates the first *DataNode* associated with the specified physician by searching the ***User_Index*** in the *SessionNode*. Having done so, the target image is identified from the first record in the *PictureNode* associated with this *DataNode*, while the cut-in point is specified as the first command in the *CommandNode* of the *DataNode*. The restoration mechanism described above is then applied to restore the contents of the medical images to the appropriate condition.

3.2.2 Replay all segments for which specified physician is in control of session

In this scenario, all the *DataNodes* associated with the specified physician are found by searching the ***User_Index*** in the *SessionNode* and these *DataNodes* are then replayed in chronological order. During the replay process, the image contents are restored by sequentially reapplying all the image-affect commands recorded between successive pairs of *DataNodes* during the original session.

3.3 Playback of all segments relating to particular medical image

When requested by a user to replay all the session segments relating to a particular medical image, the system interrogates the ***Picture_Index*** in the *SessionNode* of the ***TIH*** architecture to determine all the target *DataNodes* at which the particular medical image is selected and to identify the commands used within these *DataNodes* to select this image. In the illustrative example shown in Fig. 7, the index pair 2:1 indicates that picA was first selected in the second *DataNode* using the first command listed in the corresponding *CommandNode*. Having identified both the *DataNode* and the cut-in point (i.e. the first record in the *CommandNode* of *DataNode* 2), the restoration process described above is performed to restore the target image contents to their original state at the corresponding timestamp. Having performed the playback from the first index pair to the point at which a new image is selected for discussion purposes, the procedure described above is repeated to search for the cut-in point for the next index pair associated with picA.

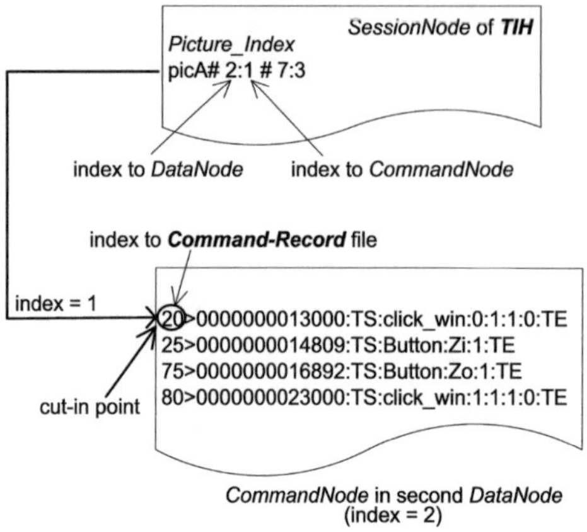

Fig. 7. Illustration of cut-in point determination procedure for specified image picA.

3.4 Montage playback - intro-scanning a session

In the movie world, the term "montage" refers to a string of shots extracted from a movie which are spliced together and played contiguously so as to provide the viewer with a brief overview of the entire movie. In compiling a montage of a commercial movie, the director carefully selects certain scenes from the movie to tantalize and intrigue potential moviegoers. By contrast, the montage of a teleconsultation session is generally produced by simply replaying a specified time interval ΔT within every time period T of the session. The parameter ΔT is conventionally referred to as the montage interval and is defined by a starting point and an ending point, respectively. As discussed above, the invocation of image-affect commands has a direct effect on the contents of a medical teleconsultation session. Thus, in the montage playback function proposed in this chapter, the occurrence of any image-affect command during the time period T is automatically taken as the starting point for the following montage interval ΔT (see Fig. 8) such that the montage contains all the most significant scenes within the session. Note that in the event that no image-affect commands are invoked during a particular time period T, the montage playback function simply selects a general command once the current time period expires. In order to implement the montage playback function, the system records the starting and ending points of each montage interval ΔT associated with a particular session in a ***Montage-Record*** file with the structure shown in Fig. 9. Note that in this figure, the M_point field contains

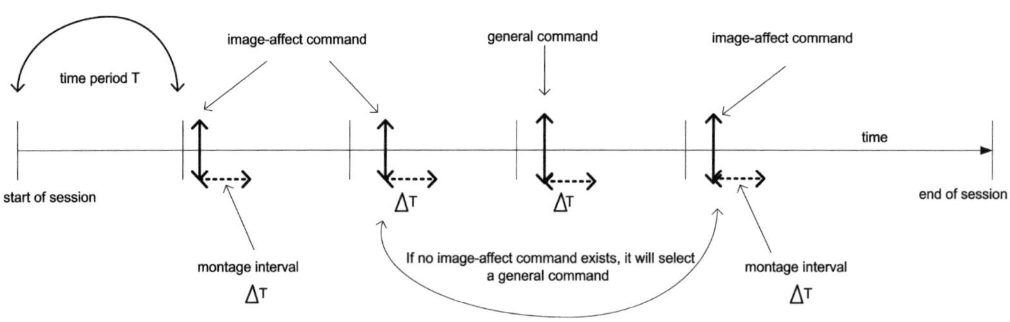

Fig. 8. Selection of montage playback points in each montage interval.

M_point	#	D_Node	#	Cmd_Node

Fig. 9. Structure of records in ***Montage-Record*** file.

either "montage_start" (indicating the starting point of the montage interval) or "montage_end" (indicating the ending point). In addition, the D_Node field specifies the *DataNode* containing each montage interval, while the Cmd_Node field indicates the index of the *CommandNode* associated with the corresponding starting or ending point. Finally, the hash symbol (#) simply denotes a field separator.

Fig. 10 presents an illustrative example of the ***Montage-Record*** file and the indexing procedure applied when executing the montage playback function. The first and second records in the ***Montage-Record*** file represent the starting and ending points of the first montage interval (M1), respectively. Similarly, the third and fourth records define the second montage interval (M2), the fifth and sixth records define the third montage interval (M3), and so on. The first record in the ***Montage-Record*** file, i.e. "montage_start#1#2", indicates that this particular montage interval starts from the second record listed in the *CommandNode* associated with the first *DataNode*. By examining the "index to ***Command-Record*** file" field associated with this record (value = 9), the system determines the starting

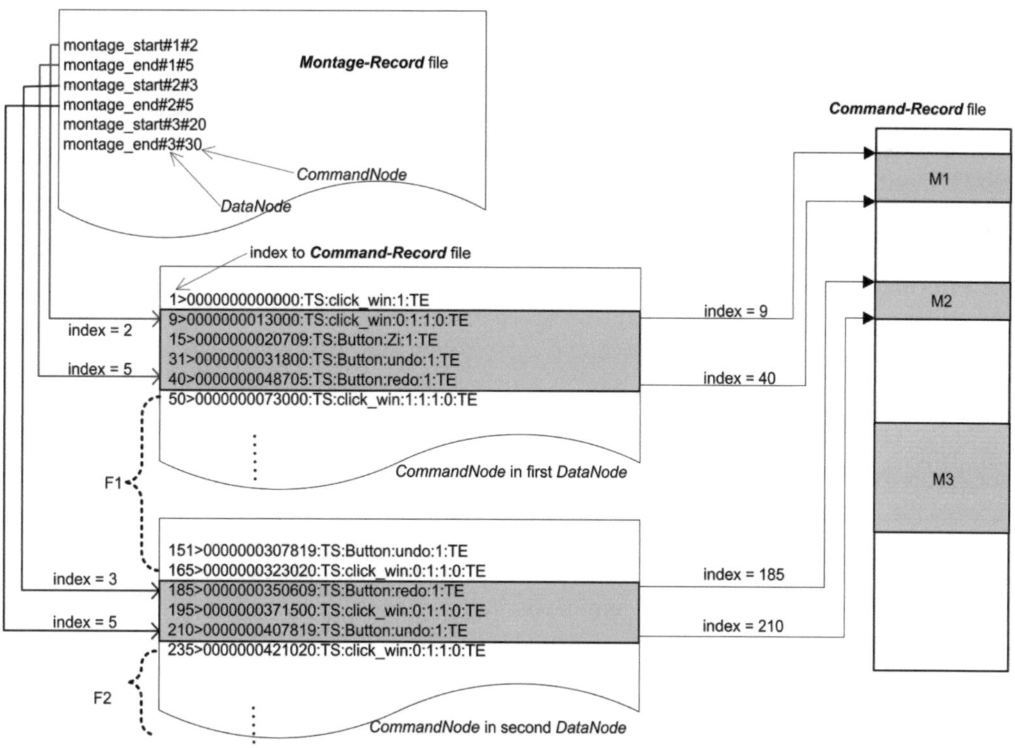

Fig. 10. Illustrative example of ***Montage-Record*** file showing determination of montage intervals M1, M2 and M3 in ***Command-Record*** file and restoration intervals F1 and F2 in *CommandNodes* of corresponding *DataNodes*.

point of the first montage interval in the ***Command-Record*** file. Meanwhile, the second record in the ***Montage-Record*** file, i.e. "montage_end#1#5", indicates that this particular montage interval ends with the fifth record listed in the *CommandNode* associated with the first *DataNode*. By examining the entry in the "index to ***Command-Record*** file" field associated with the fifth record in the *CommandNode* (value = 40), the system locates the ending point of the montage interval in the ***Command-Record*** file. Thus, the shaded area labeled M1 in the ***Command-Record*** file contains all the commands applied to the image contents during this particular montage interval. By repeating this process for all the montage intervals within the session, the system compiles all the commands applied during the intervals of interest in the session (indicated by the shaded areas M1, M2 and M3 in Fig. 10). During the montage playback procedure, the commands listed in the intervals F1 and F2 of the *CommandNode(s)* are used to fast forward the session sequence from the end of one montage interval to the beginning of the next, while the commands within the shaded areas of the ***Command-Record*** file in Fig. 10 are applied to the image contents at a normal speed in order to replay the session in its original form within each montage interval.

4. Use of *TIH* to facilitate recovery mechanism

As discussed in Section 1, it is necessary to perform the image content restoration process for two particular classes of participants, namely late and re-entrant participants. From the perspective of the session server, the mechanisms used to restore the session contents are identical for both types of participants. In both cases, the overriding requirement is to maintain the dependency between the image contents and the sequential order in which the image processing commands were used. As will be described in the following sub-sections, the cross-linkage design of the ***TIH*** architecture not only satisfies this dependency requirement, but also facilitates a prioritized recovery policy which enables re-entrant / late users to catch up with the on-going session with a minimal possible ***recovery-latency*** delay.

4.1 Prioritized recovery policy

In traditional message-logging based restoration systems, the server transmits every recorded command to the re-entrant / late user, and these commands are then re-executed in order to replicate the actions applied to the session contents before he / she joins the session. Whilst this approach results in an accurate reconstruction of the session contents, sequentially executing all of the commands transmitted from the session server is highly time consuming and forces the participant to wait before the participant can take an active part in the on-going discussions. Accordingly, the proposed ***TIH*** architecture is designed to accelerate the restoration process by using two key strategies, namely a selective transmission of the logged commands to the re-entrant / late user and a prioritized recovery policy.

As described in Section 2, all the commands invoked by each user during the session are recorded in the ***Command-Record*** file (Wang et al., 2005). However, of these commands, only those which change the image contents in some way are indexed at the *CommandNode* in each *DataNode*. In the restoration process, the session server transmits only the image-affect commands stored in the *CommandNodes* to re-entrant / late users. As a result, a significant reduction in the ***recovery-latency*** delay is gained compared to that used in a traditional message-logging scheme. The perceived ***recovery-latency*** delay is further reduced by using a prioritized recovery policy to preferentially restore the foreground image (i.e. the image under current discussion) before any of the background images (i.e. the other images in the session)

is restored. In other words, the image-affect commands related to the background images are not transmitted to the re-entrant / late user until the foreground image has been restored. As a result, the user is able to observe (but not participate in) the on-going session as the remaining images are restored transparently in the background.
The restoration process of a medical image in a session can be explained by means of the pseudo codes in Fig. 11. In Step 1 of Fig. 11, the name of the image that is to be restored is input. In Step 2, the session server initializes the restoration process by interrogating the ***Picture_Index*** in the *SessionNode* of ***TIH*** to retrieve the number of *DataNode* - *CommandNode* index pair associated with the specific image (designated as n). Also, the serial number of the *DataNode* - *CommandNode* index pair being processed (designated as i) is set to 0, representing the first index pair. In Step 3, in the event that $i < n$, Step 4 is performed; otherwise, Step 8 is performed. In Step 4, the *DataNode* at which the specific image was selected for discussion and the command used within the *DataNode* to select this image will be identified (the indexing process of Step 4 will be illustrated in the next paragraph). In Step 5, the *DataNode* and the command used to select another image for discussion will be identified (the indexing process of Step 5 will be illustrated in the next paragraph). In Step 6, the commands starting from the command found in Step 4 and ending with the one immediately prior to the command found in Step 5 will be re-executed, regarded as the restoration process of the ith *DataNode* - *CommandNode* index pair. In Step 7, the value of i is added with 1 and Step 3 is invoked again. Step 8 of Fig. 11 indicates that the whole restoration process for the specific image is completed.

Step 1: INPUT the name of the image to be restored.
Step 2: GET the number of *DataNode* – *CommandNode* index pair associated with the image (designated as n);
SET the serial number of the *DataNode* – *CommandNode* index pair being processed (designated as i) to 0.
Step 3: if $i < n$ then GOTO Step 4; otherwise, GOTO Step 8.
Step 4: INDEX the command used to select the image for discussion.
Step 5: INDEX the command used to select another image for discussion.
Step 6: RUN the commands starting from the command found in Step 4 and ending with the one immediately prior to the command found in Step 5.
Step 7: ADD 1 to i; GOTO Step 3.
Step 8: END

Fig. 11. The pseudo codes for the restoration process of certain medical image in a session.

To explain the indexing process in Steps 4 and 5 of Fig. 11, Fig. 7 presents an illustrative example in which picA is assumed to be restored for a re-entrant / late user entering the on-going session. The *DataNode* - *CommandNode* index pair 2:1 in the ***Picture_Index*** indicates that picA was selected for discussion in the second *DataNode* using the first command listed in the corresponding *CommandNode* (The command "TS:click_win" indicates the selection of a new image). Similarly, the index pair 7:3 shows that picA was later selected as the foreground image in the seventh *DataNode* using the third command in the corresponding *CommandNode*. Having identified all the *DataNodes* and commands used to select picA for discussion, the session server selects all the commands in the corresponding *CommandNodes* starting from the command used to select the image and ending with the command immediately prior to that used to select a new image as the foreground image, and then transmits these commands to the re-entrant / late user end, where they are re-executed. For example, taking the first index pair in Fig. 7 as an example, the restoration process commences with the first command in the *CommandNode* at *DataNode* 2 and terminates after the third command (since the fourth command, TS:click_win, is used to select a new image for discussion purposes). Having performed the restoration of the first index pair, the procedure is repeated for all the other index pairs associated with picA.

4.2 Resolving suspension / resumption issues when performing restoration process

Since the *CommandNode* indexes only those commands which directly affect the session contents, a parsing of the entire ***Command-Record*** file is not required. As a result, the time required to restore the foreground image is considerably shorter than that required when a traditional message-logging based system is used. Furthermore, since the restoration process commences with the foreground image, the participant is able to follow the on-going session as the remaining images in the session are restored in a transparent background mode. However, it is possible that another medical image may be selected as a new foreground image while the restoration process is still on going. In this situation, no matter whether the session server is currently performing the restoration of the foreground image or background images, it must suspend its restoration activities and resume (or start) the restoration of this new foreground image. To facilitate this suspension / resumption process, the session server creates a set of resuming pointers for each re-entrant / late user to indicate the current restoration state of each image in the session. In implementing this approach, a resuming pointer is appended to the next image-affect command associated with the restored image as soon as the previous image-affect command associated with the same image has been transmitted by the session server to the re-entrant / late user. If when processing the image-affect commands in the *CommandNode*, it is found that the resuming pointer points at the final image-affect command relating to the current image, the restoration of the image is completed as soon as this image-affect command has been transmitted to the user. Thus, the resuming pointer is removed from the set of resuming pointers to indicate that this particular image is now fully restored for this particular user. In addition, if the removed resuming pointer is associated with the foreground image, i.e. the foreground image has been fully restored, all of the image-affect and non-image-affect commands subsequently applied to this image by the other participants in the session are transmitted to the re-entrant / late user such that he / she can follow the on-going discussions in a passive mode as the background images are restored.

Upon completing the restoration of the foreground image the session server randomly picks a new resuming pointer from the set of resuming pointers and performs the restoration of the corresponding background image. The restoration process for a particular user is considered to be complete when the set of resuming pointers associated with that user is empty. Until then the re-entrant / late user can apply commands to the session contents in the same way as any other participant in the session. Note that this restriction is deliberately imposed in order to prevent re-entrant / late users from inadvertently selecting an image currently under restoration as the new foreground image, thereby resulting in an inconsistency between their versions of the image contents and that of the remaining participants in the session.

5. Evaluation results

5.1 Performance of *TIH* in facilitating smart playback functions

In this section, the feasibility of ***TIH*** was explored by performing a series of playback experiments using representative medical teleconsultation sessions. Fig. 12 presents a snapshot of the operational interface for the particular case in which the user requests the system to replay specific or all the session segments associated with a particular physician. In evaluating the performance of any indexing mechanism designed for playback purposes, the most important parameters include the ***target-setting time*** (i.e. the time spent by the user interacting with the system in specifying the target scene to be replayed) and the ***restart-latency time*** (i.e. the elapsed time between the moment at which the playback function is invoked and that at which the playback actually commences). The ***target-setting time*** of the *TIH*-based system proposed in this chapter was evaluated using the same experimental method as that used for ***PlayWatch*** (Tanaka et al., 2005). Specifically, eight medical staff with different levels of computer literacy were requested to perform four different playback tasks using the proposed playback system, namely: (1) playback from a specified time point in a session, (2) playback of all the session segments controlled by a specified physician, (3) playback of all the segments relating to a particular medical image, and (4) montage playback. The time spent by each user in specifying the target scene for each playback task was measured and taken as the corresponding ***target-setting time***. Meanwhile, the time between the moment at which the user invoked the playback function and the moment at which playback actually commenced was measured and taken as the ***restart-latency time***. In ***TIH***, the ***restart-latency time*** has two components, namely the ***search time***, i.e. the time required to locate the cut-in point, and the ***restoration time***, i.e. the time required to restore the image contents. Therefore, in quantifying the performance of the playback scheme, the search time and the restoration time were individually recorded for each of the playback tasks assigned to the eight users. The ***restart-latency time*** varies directly with the extent to which image-affect commands are invoked during the session. Thus, to evaluate the performance of the ***TIH***-based playback scheme under realistic conditions, three different session types, each with a different number of image-affect commands per minute, were designed, namely Type A with around 5 image-affect commands per minute, Type B with around 10 image-affect commands per minute, and Type C with around 20 image-affect commands per minute. Furthermore, to reflect the differing durations of typical real-world medical teleconsultation sessions, each type of session was run for both 10 and 30 minutes, respectively.

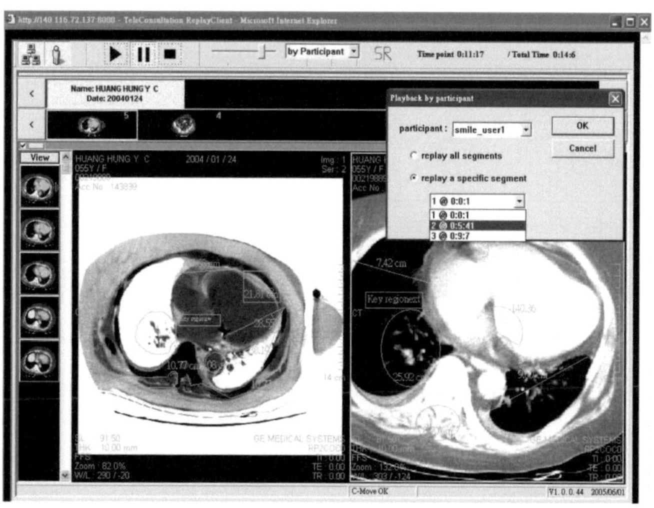

Fig. 12. Snapshot of operational interface for case where playback system is set to replay session segments associated with specified physician.

Fig. 13 and Fig. 14 present the evaluation results obtained for the ***target-setting time*** and the ***restart-latency time*** for each of the eight users when applying the playback functions to the 10-minute and 30-minute sessions, respectively. Note that all of the experiments were performed on a PC with a P4 2.4 GHz CPU and 1 GB of RAM. In both figures, it can be seen that the ***target-setting time*** varies notably from one user to the next due to their differing levels of computer literacy. However, no more than a slight variation is observed in the ***restart-latency time*** for each user. Tables 1 and 2 present a detailed breakdown of the ***restart-latency time*** for the 10-minute and 30-minute sessions, respectively. It can be seen that the search time required to locate the cut-in point varies in the range 7.4 ~ 17.4 ms for the three session types and two session durations considered in the evaluation trials. Comparing the search times associated with the different playback functions, it is found that playback from a specified time point in the session (designated as "Time" in Tables 1 and 2) induces the longest search time (i.e. 15.6 ~ 17.4ms), while the montage playback (Montage) induces the shortest search time (i.e. 7.4 ~ 9.6 ms). These findings are reasonable since playback from a specified time in the session contents requires the use of a binary search to locate the corresponding target *DataNode*, while in the montage playback function, the cut-in points are already pre-designated as the starting points of the montage intervals in the ***Montage-Record*** file. Furthermore, as shown in Tables 1 and 2, the search time accounts for only a very small proportion of the total ***restart-latency time***. In other words, the ***restart-latency time*** is dominated by the restoration time in every case. As implied above, it is reasonable to assume that the restoration time varies linearly with the number of image-affect commands applied during the restoration process. Fig. 15 confirms that this is indeed the case for both the 10-minute and 30-minute sessions. Tables 1 and 2 also reveal that for each session duration (i.e. 10 minutes or 30 minutes), the restoration time increases significantly as the density of the image-affect commands increases. Similarly, for each type of session (i.e. Type A, Type B or Type C), the restoration time increases dramatically as the length of the session is increased. By contrast, it can be seen that the search time component of the ***restart-latency time*** not only has a relatively small value compared to the restoration time (i.e. a mean value of just 11.8 ~ 12.65 ms), but also remains approximately constant for each of the different session durations and session types. In other words, the efficiency of the proposed ***TIH*** architecture in locating the cut-in point is confirmed.

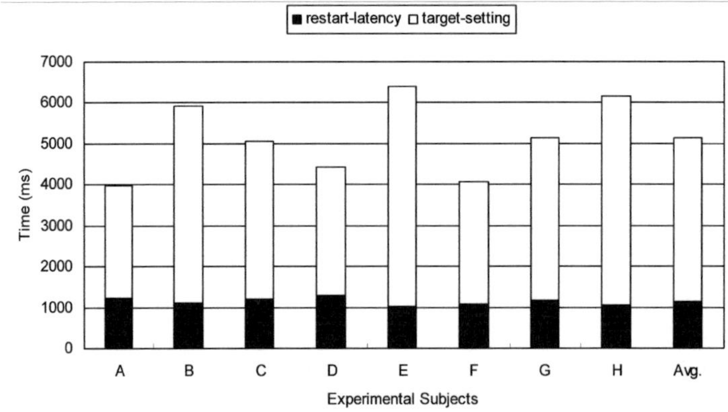

Fig. 13. Evaluation results for ***target-setting time*** and ***restart-latency time*** in 10-minute sessions.

In a recent study, a "scene-retrieval" system designated as ***PlayWatch*** was proposed, in which scene descriptors derived from the MPEG-7 standard were used to facilitate playback functions similar to those proposed in this chapter. However, the indexing mechanism proposed in this chapter is far more efficient than ***PlayWatch*** in terms of its storage capacity requirements. For example, in the proposed system, a typical 60-minute session generates a 6 Mbyte audio file, a 2 Mbyte ***Command-record*** file, and a 0.5 Mbyte ***TIH*** architecture. By contrast, ***PlayWatch*** requires a total of 88.9 Mbytes of storage capacity (with a CBR (compression bit rate) of 127.8 Kbytes/s) to store the scenes within a 12-minute video sequence. Moreover, ***PlayWatch*** requires an average of 20 seconds to retrieve a specified scene and spends around 50 seconds in locating a specific time position within the video sequence (Tanaka et al., 2005). By contrast, ***TIH*** has an average ***target-setting time*** of 4 seconds (see Figures 13 and 14), and most importantly, incurs an average ***restart-latency time*** of just 1 second for 10-minute sessions and 3 seconds for 30-minute sessions (see Tables

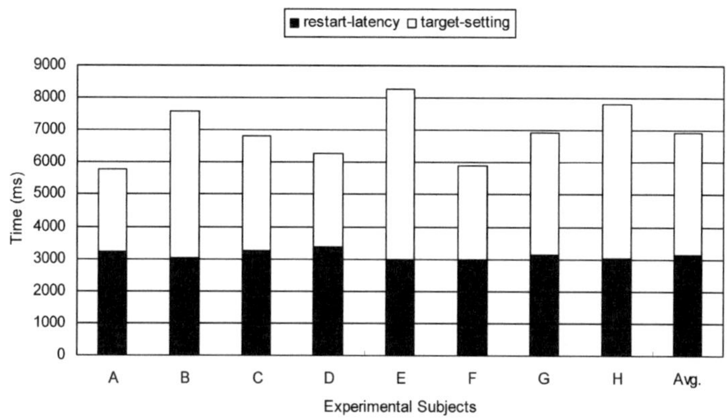

Fig. 14. Evaluation results for ***target-setting time*** and ***restart-latency time*** in 30-minute sessions.

Session type \ Playback functions \ Measure item		Search time (ms)	Restoration time (ms)	Number of restored image-affect commands	Restart-latency time (ms)
Type A	Time	15.9	387	27	402.9
	Physician	12.4	248	17	260.4
	Image	12.6	385	25	397.6
	Montage	8.7	368	20	376.7
	Average	12.4	347	22.25	359.4
Type B	Time	16.5	1035	67	1051.5
	Physician	12.8	1012	65	1024.8
	Image	12.2	1092	74	1104.2
	Montage	8.3	1020	60	1028.3
	Average	12.45	1039.75	66.5	1052.2
Type C	Time	16.2	2219	158	2235.2
	Physician	12.2	1425	98	1437.2
	Image	12.6	2422	166	2434.6
	Montage	9.6	1912	128	1921.6
	Average	12.65	1994.5	137.5	2007.15

Table 1. Performance evaluation results for playback functions in 10-minute sessions.

Session type	Playback functions / Measure item	Search time (ms)	Restoration time (ms)	Number of restored image-affect commands	Restart-latency time (ms)
Type A	Time	16.9	1195	81	1211.9
	Physician	13.2	1294	88	1307.2
	Image	12.2	1365	88	1377.2
	Montage	8.1	1570	98	1578.1
	Average	12.6	1356	88.75	1368.6
Type B	Time	15.6	2055	142	2070.6
	Physician	12.6	2797	188	2809.6
	Image	11.6	2130	145	2141.6
	Montage	7.4	2702	174	2709.4
	Average	11.8	2421	162.25	2432.8
Type C	Time	17.4	5054	323	5071.4
	Physician	12.6	4895	314	4907.6
	Image	12.5	6705	392	6717.5
	Montage	7.5	5580	345	5587.5
	Average	12.5	5558.5	343.5	5571

Table 2. Performance evaluation results for playback functions in 30-minute sessions.

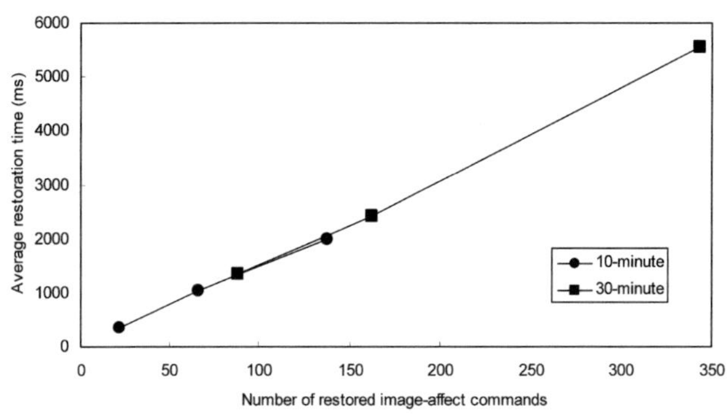

Fig. 15. Variation of restoration time with number of restored image-affect commands for sessions of two different durations.

1 and 2). In other words, the proposed ***TIH*** architecture yields a significant improvement in the cross-linking efficiency of the playback system, and therefore reduces the search time considerably compared to that of ***PlayWatch***.

5.2 Evaluation of proposed recovery mechanism

The performance of the proposed recovery mechanism was evaluated by performing a series of experiments in which disconnection failures were mimicked by intentionally unplugging the network connections of certain participants in a medical teleconsultation session and measuring the resulting ***recovery-latency***. Fig. 16 illustrates the experimental environment consisting of three clients and a server connected through the Internet. Here, Client_A is a PC with an Intel Pentium 4 2.4 GHz processor and 1 GB RAM; Client_B is a laptop with an Intel Pentium M 1.5 GHz processor and 768 MB RAM; Client_C is a PC with an Intel Pentium 4 2.8 GHz processor and 1 GB RAM; and the Session_Server is a PC with two Intel Xeon 2.4 GHz processors and 2 GB RAM. In evaluating the performance of any recovery mechanism (a conventional checkpoint or message-logging system or that proposed in this chapter), one of the most important performance parameters is that of the ***recovery-latency***, i.e. the elapsed time between the moment at which the re-entrant / late user joins the on-going session and the moment at which the restoration process is completed and the user can participate in the on-going discussions in a normal manner. In order to demonstrate the efficiency of the recovery mechanism proposed in this chapter, the ***recovery-latency*** is measured for two different recovery policies, namely a basic recovery policy and the prioritized recovery policy. The basic recovery policy simply re-executes every command invoked since the session begins, whereas the prioritized recovery policy uses ***TIH*** to identify and reapply only those commands which directly affect the image contents. In addition, the performance of the prioritized recovery policy is further evaluated by measuring the ***foreground sync-time***, i.e. the time for which the re-entrant / late user can watch the on-going session but can not take an active part in the discussions since the restoration of the background images is not yet fully completed.

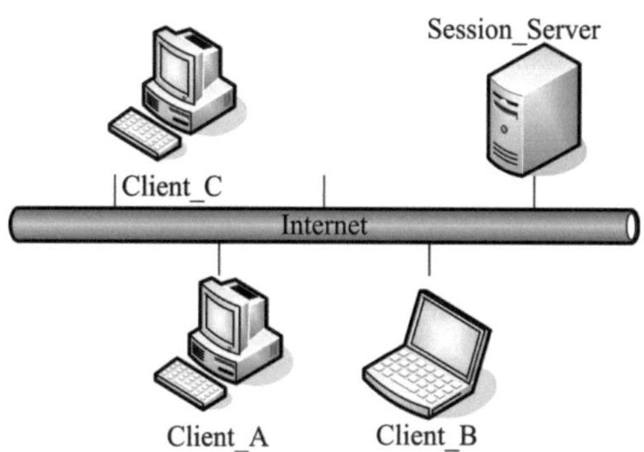

Fig. 16. Experimental environment.

In performing the evaluation experiments, the supported image-affect commands included the following: "black and white inversion", "90 degree rotation", "180 degree rotation", "270 degree rotation", "vertical flip", "horizontal flip", "zoom in", and "zoom out". The session included a total of 10 medical images, comprised 10 non-image-affect commands (i.e. "mouse move") per second, involved a total of 160 image-affect commands, and was run for 20 minutes. The probability density function describing the application of each image-affect command to each image was modeled by a normal distribution with mean of (μ) = 2 and a standard deviation of (σ) = 1. A total of five experimental patterns were obtained for evaluation purposes, as listed in Tables 3 to 7.
According to a series of experiments, the execution time of each image-affect command was evaluated at Client_A and Client_B, respectively. Table 8 presents the corresponding results obtained when averaging the execution time over 100 separate measurements of each image-affect command. Table 9 summarizes the ***recovery-latency*** at Client_A and Client_B for each of the five experimental patterns under the basic and prioritized recovery policies. It is observed that the average ***recovery-latency*** at Client_A was reduced from 58553 ms to 13206 ms when the basic recovery policy was replaced with the prioritized recovery policy. In other words, the ***recovery-latency*** at Client_A was reduced by around 77.45% when the proposed recovery mechanism was used. Similarly, the average ***recovery-latency*** at Client_B was reduced from 62909 ms of using the basic recovery policy to 15974 ms of using the

Image number	Black and white inversion	90° rotation	180° rotation	270° rotation	Vertical flip	Horizonta l flip	Zoom in	Zoom out
1	2	0	2	2	4	3	1	2
2	1	2	1	3	2	0	2	3
3	3	2	3	2	2	2	1	1
4	2	2	2	1	2	3	3	2
5	1	3	2	0	3	4	3	0
6	2	4	2	2	0	2	2	3
7	0	2	2	3	2	1	2	2
8	2	1	4	1	2	2	1	4
9	4	2	2	2	1	2	3	1
10	3	2	0	4	2	1	2	2

Table 3. Contents of experimental pattern 1

Image number	Black and white inversion	90° rotation	180° rotation	270° rotation	Vertical flip	Horizontal flip	Zoom in	Zoom out
1	1	2	1	2	2	4	2	2
2	2	3	2	1	1	2	3	2
3	3	2	3	2	2	0	1	3
4	2	1	2	3	2	1	2	3
5	1	2	2	1	3	3	2	2
6	2	3	3	0	1	2	2	2
7	2	4	3	2	2	1	2	0
8	3	1	2	3	2	2	3	1
9	2	2	0	2	2	2	2	3
10	2	0	2	4	3	3	1	2

Table 4. Contents of experimental pattern 2

Image number	Black and white inversion	90° rotation	180° rotation	270° rotation	Vertical flip	Horizontal flip	Zoom in	Zoom out
1	3	1	2	2	3	1	2	3
2	1	2	2	3	2	2	3	1
3	2	3	3	2	1	1	1	2
4	2	2	1	0	2	4	2	4
5	2	3	2	3	3	2	1	0
6	1	3	2	2	1	3	2	1
7	2	1	2	1	2	2	3	2
8	2	2	4	2	2	0	2	3
9	2	2	2	2	2	2	2	2
10	3	1	0	3	2	3	2	2

Table 5. Contents of experimental pattern 3

Image number	Black and white inversion	90° rotation	180° rotation	270° rotation	Vertical flip	Horizontal flip	Zoom in	Zoom out
1	2	1	3	2	2	3	2	2
2	2	4	1	2	3	2	1	2
3	3	2	2	1	2	1	2	3
4	2	0	2	3	1	2	4	1
5	1	2	3	2	2	2	2	2
6	2	2	1	1	2	4	2	2
7	3	1	2	2	1	2	3	1
8	2	2	4	2	2	1	2	2
9	1	3	2	3	2	2	0	3
10	2	3	0	2	3	1	2	2

Table 6. Contents of experimental pattern 4

prioritized recovery policy, corresponding to a performance improvement of 74.61%. The experimental results in Table 9 also shed light on the relative effects of the "image-affect" and "non-image-affect" commands on the performance of the restoration process. In the prioritized recovery policy, only the "image-affect" commands were reapplied during the restoration process, and thus the measured value of the ***recovery-latency*** provided an indication of the weight of the "image-affect" commands in the restoration process. By contrast, in the basic recovery policy, both the "image-affect" and the "non-image-affect" commands were re-executed during the restoration process. Consequently, the difference in the ***recovery-latency*** times of the basic and prioritized recovery policies provided an indication of the effect of the "non-image-affect" commands on the performance of the restoration process. In Table 9, when the additional weight of the "non-image-affect" commands was ignored, the ***TIH*** / prioritized recovery policy yielded a significant improvement in the restoration process. In practice, this performance improvement can be attributed to two main factors, namely (1) ***TIH*** facilitates the rapid identification of all the image-affect commands applied to the image of interest when performing the restoration process; and (2) the server transmits only those commands which directly affect the image contents, thereby reducing both the transmission time and the restoration time.

Image number	Black and white inversion	90° rotation	180° rotation	270° rotation	Vertical flip	Horizontal flip	Zoom in	Zoom out
1	2	1	3	2	3	2	1	2
2	1	2	2	3	2	2	3	1
3	1	3	2	1	2	3	3	2
4	2	2	4	2	3	1	1	2
5	2	2	0	2	1	2	3	3
6	2	2	1	4	3	0	0	3
7	3	1	2	1	2	3	2	2
8	2	3	2	3	1	2	2	1
9	2	1	2	2	2	3	1	2
10	3	3	2	0	1	2	4	2

Table 7. Contents of experimental pattern 5

	Black and white inversion	90° rotation	180° rotation	270° rotation	Vertical flip	Horizontal flip	Zoom in	Zoom out
Client_A	46.27	84.28	87.35	86.24	80.25	82.72	50.24	51.64
Client_B	56.25	106.45	109.65	107.15	97.75	96.24	58.85	59.55

Table 8. Average execution time for each image-affect command (unit: ms)

	Recovery policy	Pattern 1	Pattern 2	Pattern 3	Pattern 4	Pattern 5	Average	Improvement
Client_A	Prioritized	13117	13275	13463	12980	13195	13206	77.45%
	Basic	58625	58005	58755	59125	58255	58553	
Client_B	Prioritized	15817	16173	16281	15735	15864	15974	74.61%
	Basic	62755	63125	63015	62886	62764	62909	

Table 9. Experimental results: ***recovery-latency*** (unit: ms)

Table 10 summarizes the ***recovery-latency*** and ***foreground sync-time*** at Client_A and Client_B for each of the five experimental patterns when the prioritized recovery policy was implemented. It can be seen that the ***foreground sync-time*** is around 10.9~11.2 % (i.e. 1/10th) of the ***recovery-latency***. That is, the restoration time of the foreground image was just 1/N of the total ***recovery-latency*** time, where N is the number of medical images in the session. In other words, the prioritized recovery policy enabled the re-entrant / late users to join the on-going session in a passive capacity within a very short period of time following their entry to the session. As a result, the users perceived a significant reduction in the ***recovery-latency*** delay compared to that in a traditional message-logging based scheme.

	Time	Pattern 1	Pattern 2	Pattern 3	Pattern 4	Pattern 5	Average	Percentage
Client_A	***foreground sync-time***	1436	1452	1458	1412	1442	1440	10.9%
	recovery-latency	13117	13275	13463	12980	13195	13206	
Client_B	***foreground sync-time***	1780	1794	1809	1771	1786	1788	11.2%
	recovery-latency	15817	16173	16281	15735	15864	15974	

Table 10. Experimental results: ***foreground sync-time*** and ***recovery-latency*** (unit: ms)

In the following we evaluated the performance of the proposed recovery mechanism at Client_A in Fig. 16 for sessions characterized by different numbers of medical images, non-image-affect commands, and image-affect commands, respectively, and different session times. To evaluate the effect of the number of medical images on the ***recovery-latency*** and ***foreground sync-time***, three different sessions were designed, namely Session#1 with 5 medical images, Session#2 with 10 medical images, and Session#3 with 20 medical images. Note that the other experimental conditions for each session (i.e. the number of non-image-affect commands, the number of image-affect commands, and the session time) were assigned the same values as those used for the initial series of experiments. The corresponding results in Fig. 17 show that the ***recovery-latency*** remained approximately constant as the number of images in the session increased. However, the ***foreground sync-time*** decreased approximately linearly as the number of images is increased. In other words, an increasing number of images had no significant effect on the restoration process, but yielded a noticeable reduction in the ***foreground sync-time***.

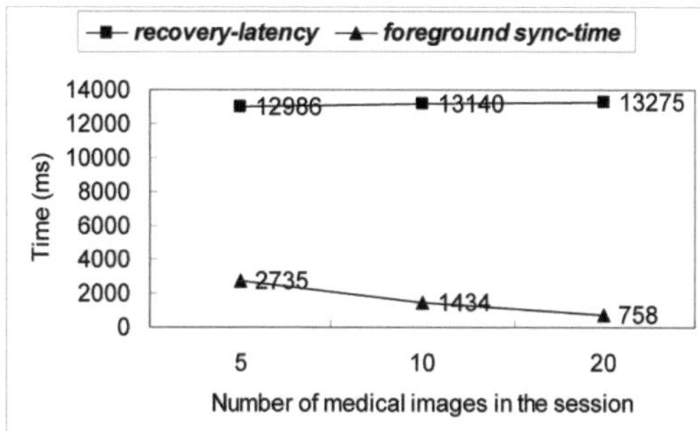

Fig. 17. Experimental results for ***recovery-latency*** and ***foreground sync-time*** in sessions with different numbers of medical images.

To evaluate the effect of the number of non-image-affect commands on the performance of the proposed recovery mechanism, three experimental sessions were designed with different "mouse move" command rates, i.e. 5 times per second (Session#1), 10 times per second (Session#2) and 20 times per second (Session#3). Note that the other experimental conditions (i.e. the number of medical images, the number of image-affect commands, and the session time) were specified in accordance with the values assigned in the original experiments. The experimental results are presented in Fig. 18. It was seen that both the ***recovery-latency*** and the ***foreground sync-time*** were insensitive to the number of non-image-affect commands.

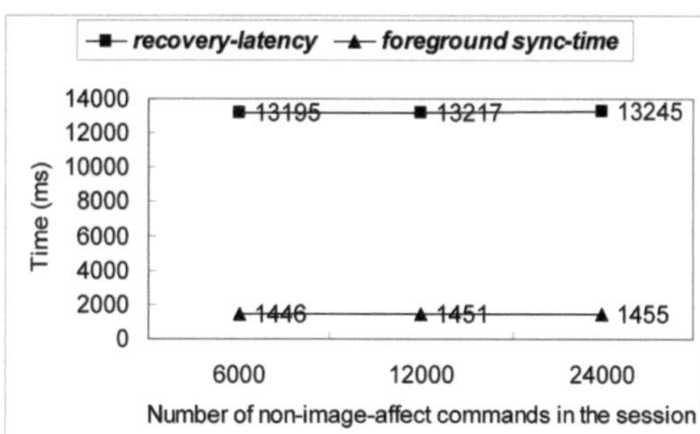

Fig. 18. Experimental results for ***recovery-latency*** and ***foreground sync-time*** in sessions with different numbers of non-image-affect commands.

The influence of the number of image-affect commands on the performance of the proposed recovery mechanism was evaluated using three different sessions, namely Session#1 with 80 image-affect commands, Session#2 with 160 image-affect commands, and Session#3 with 320 image-affect commands. Note that in each session, the image-affect commands were averagely distributed over the 10 medical images. The results presented in Fig. 19 show that the ***recovery-latency*** and the ***foreground sync-time*** both increased linearly with the number of image-affect commands. However, it can be seen that the number of image-affect commands had a greater effect on the ***recovery-latency*** time than on the ***foreground sync-time***. Since both the ***recovery-latency*** and the ***foreground sync-time*** were induced as a result of the re-execution of image-affect commands in the restoration process, the finding in Fig. 19 is expected since the ***recovery-latency*** and ***foreground sync-time*** both increased with an increasing number of image-affect commands. As discussed previously, the restoration of the foreground image accounted for approximately 1/N of the total restoration time, where N represents the number of medical images in the session and is equal to 10 in Fig. 19. Therefore, the rate at which the ***foreground sync-time*** increased with an increasing number of image-affect commands is around $1/10^{th}$ that of the increase in the ***recovery-latency*** time. For example, when the number of image-affect commands was increased from 160 to 320, Fig. 19 shows that the ***recovery-latency*** increased by about 12640 ms while the ***foreground sync-time*** increased by about 1313 ms.

Finally, the effect of the session duration on the performance of the proposed recovery mechanism was evaluated using three sessions of varying lengths, i.e. 10 minutes (Session#1), 20 minutes (Session#2) and 40 minutes (Session#3). The corresponding results are shown in Fig. 20. It can be seen that neither the ***recovery-latency*** nor the ***foreground sync-time*** was significantly affected by the session time. In general, the results presented in Fig. 17 ~ 20 show that the performance of the proposed recovery mechanism was insensitive to the number of medical images, the number of non-image-affect commands, and the session time. The ***recovery-latency*** inevitably increased with the number of image-affect commands. Nonetheless, the proposed prioritized recovery policy minimized the effect of an increasing number of image-affect commands on the ***foreground sync-time***, and thus

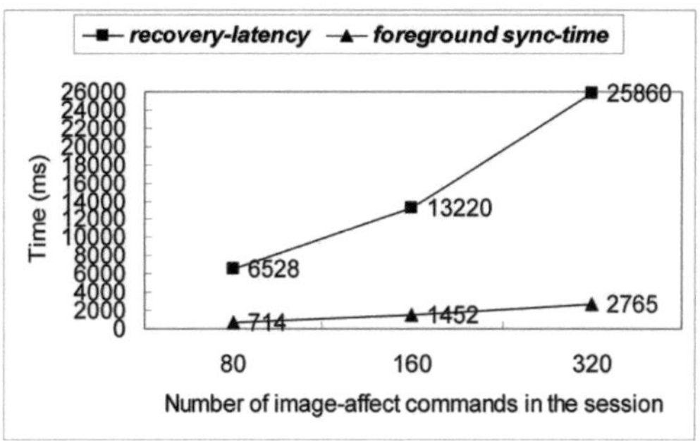

Fig. 19. Experimental results for ***recovery-latency*** and ***foreground sync-time*** in sessions with different numbers of image-affect commands.

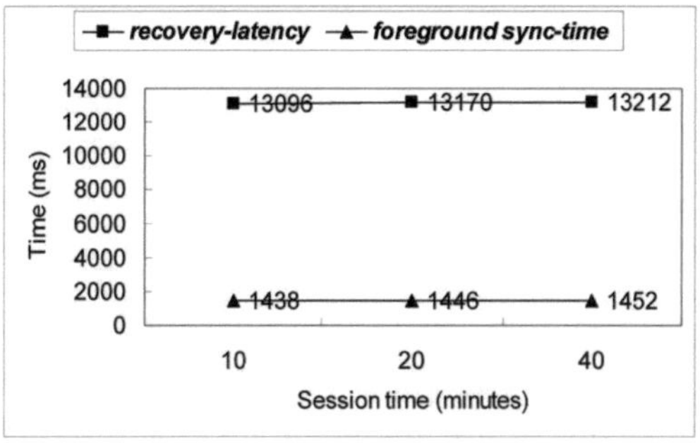

Fig. 20. Experimental results for sessions with different session times.

re-entrant / late users were able to rapidly join the session (albeit in a passive manner) even in sessions characterized by a large number of such commands.

6. Conclusion

This chapter has presented an indexing scheme designated as ***three-level indexing hierarchy*** (***TIH***) to support a range of smart playback functions and a novel recovery mechanism for teleconsultation sessions. Uniquely, the contents of such sessions are command dependent, i.e. the contents vary in accordance with the commands applied to them during the course of the session. Furthermore, when executing smart playback functions, the playback sequences invariably commence at different points within the session. As a result, it is necessary to "fast forward" or "fast rewind" the session contents to an appropriate cut-in point and to restore the contents to the corresponding condition before the playback procedure can commence. In this chapter, the content restoration process is achieved by reapplying an appropriate sub-set of the image-affect commands applied to the original image contents during the actual session. The efficiencies of the cut-in point determination process and the image content restoration procedure, respectively, are enhanced via the cross-linkage structure of ***TIH*** which records the time-based changes in the various types of multimedia content within the session and maintains a link between these changes and the commands which caused them. ***TIH*** makes possible a range of smart playback functions, including replaying from a specified time point within the session, replaying all the segments of a session controlled by a particular physician, replaying all the session segments for which a particular medical image is discussed, and playing a montage of the entire session. The evaluation results have shown that the proposed indexing mechanism yields a significant improvement in both the ***restart-latency time*** and the storage capacity requirements of the playback system compared to existing scene-based playback systems such as ***PlayWatch***. As for the recovery mechanism, a prioritized recovery policy is proposed to accomplish the preferential restoration of the foreground image (i.e. the medical image under current discussion) prior to the background images (i.e. all the other images in the session). The prioritized recovery policy enables re-entrant / late users to follow the on-going session in a passive capacity as the restoration of the remaining images is completed in a transparent background mode. Upon implementing the prioritized recovery policy for each re-entrant / late user, the suspension / resumption problem which arises when the foreground image is suddenly replaced by a new image before the restoration process is fully completed is managed by utilizing a set of resuming pointers to indicate the current restoration state of each medical image. The evaluation results have confirmed that the ***TIH*** / prioritized recovery policy yields a significant improvement in the ***recovery-latency*** delay compared to the traditional message-logging restoration scheme. In addition, the results have shown that the prioritized recovery policy enables re-entrant / late users to participate passively in the on-going session within 1/N of the total ***recovery-latency*** delay time, where N is the number of medical images in the session. Finally, it has been shown that the ***recovery-latency*** of the proposed recovery mechanism is insensitive to the number of medical images in the session, the number of non-image-affect commands, and the session time, respectively.

7. References

S.F. Chang; T. Sikora & A. Puri (2006). Overview of the MPEG-7 standard, *IEEE Transactions on Circuits and Systems for Video Technology*, Vol. 11, No. 6, June 2006, pp. 688-695.

E. N. Elnozahy; L. Alvisi; Y. M. Wang & D. B. Johnson (2002). A survey of rollback-recovery protocols in message-passing systems, *ACM Computing Surveys*, Vol. 34, No. 3, Sept. 2002, pp. 375-408.

William Gropp & Ewing Lusk (2004). Fault Tolerance in Message Passing Interface Programs, *The International Journal of High Performance Computing Applications*, Vol. 18, No. 3, Fall 2004, pp. 363-372.

J.C. Guerri; C.E. Palau; A. Pajares; A. Belda; J.J. Cermeno & M. Esteve (2003). A Multimedia Telemedicine System to Assess Musculoskeletal Disorders, *Proceedings of the 2003 International Conference on Multimedia and Expo*, Vol. 1, July 2003, pp. 1-701-4.

W. Huang; Y. Ai; Z. Chen; Q. Wu; H. Ouyang; P. Jiao; Z. Liu & C. Fang (2007). Computer Supported Cooperative Work (CSCW) for Telemedicine, *Computer Supported Cooperative Work in Design, 2007. CSCWD 2007. 11th International Conference on*, April 2007, pp. 1063-1065.

D. B. Johnson & W. Zwaenepoel (1987). Sender-based message logging, *17th international symposium on fault tolerant computing*, July 1987, pp. 14-18.

Kholief M.; Maly K. & Shen S. (2003). Event-Based Retrieval from a Digital Library Containing Medical Streams, *Proceedings of the 2003 Joint Conference on Digital Libraries*, May 2003, pp. 231-233.

Yeongho Kim; Jeong-Ho Choi; Jongki Lee; Myeng Ki Kim; Nam Kuk Kim; Jin Sup Yeom & Yong Oock Kim (2001). Collaborative surgical simulation over the Internet, *IEEE Internet Computing*, Vol. 5, No. 3, May-June 2001, pp. 65-73.

Chien-Cheng Lee; Pau-Choo Chung; Yunghsiang Sam Han; Dyi-Rong Duh & C. W. Lin (2004). A Practice of a Collaborative Multipoint Medical Teleconsultation System on Broadband Network, *Journal of High Speed Networks*, Vol. 13, No. 3, 2004, pp. 207-222.

J.J. Li; T. Li; Z. Lin; A. Mathur & K. Kanoun (2004). Computer supported cooperative work in software engineering, *Computer Software and Applications Conference, 2004. COMPSAC 2004. Proceedings of the 28th Annual International*, Sept. 2004, pp. 328.

Chien-Shun Lo; Ching-Wen Yang; Pau-Choo Chung; Yen-Chien Ouyang; San-Kan Lee & Ping-Song Liao (2000). A Mammography Tele-Consultation Pilot System in Taiwan, *Journal of High Speed Networks*, Vol. 9, 2000, pp. 31-46.

Marsh J.; Glencross M.; Pettifer S. & Hubbold R. (2006). A network architecture supporting consistent rich behavior in collaborative interactive applications, *Visualization and Computer Graphics, IEEE Transactions on*, Vol. 12, No. 3, May-June 2006, pp. 405-416.

Paul B.B. & Civanlar M.R. (1998). VTJukebox: implementation issues for RTP-based recording and on-demand multicast of multimedia conferences, *Multimedia Signal Processing, 1998 IEEE Second Workshop*, Dec. 1998, pp. 259-264.

P.J. Shah; R. Martinez & B.P. Zeigler (1997). Design, Analysis, and Implementation of a Telemedicine Remote Consultation and Diagnosis Session Playback Using Discrete Event System Specification, *IEEE Trans. on Information Technology in Biomedicine*, Vol. 1, No. 3, Sept. 1997, pp. 179-188.

K. Tanaka; T. Sasaki; Y. Tonomura; T. Nakanishi & N. Babaguchi (2005). PlayWatch: Chart-Style Video Playback Interface, in *Proc. ICME 2005*, 2005, pp. 731-734.

Jose Carlos Dafonte Vazquez; Alfonso Castro Martinez; Angel Gomez & Bernardino Arcay Varela (2007). Intelligent agents technology applied to tasks scheduling and communications management in a critical care telemonitoring system, *Computers in Biology and Medicine*, Vol. 37, No. 6, June 2007, pp. 760-773.

C.H. Wang; C.C. Lee; H.C. Jiau; P.C. Chung; T.L. Yang; K.F. Ssu & Y.S. Kuo (2005). Improving the Tele-consultation Services – Capabilities of Retro, in *Proceedings of the 3rd European Medical & Biological Engineering Conference*, 2005.

9

Statistics in Telemedicine

Anastasia N. Kastania[1,2] and Sophia Kossida[1]
[1]*Biomedical Research Foundation of the Academy of Athens*
[2]*Athens University of Economics and Business*
Greece

1. Introduction

All those concerned with the decision-making, they take better decisions when they use all the available information with practical and interpretable way. Statistics provide methods for data collection and analysis to support the decision-making.
Statistics is the Science of collection, analysis and interpretation of observed data reported in attributes of natural or social phenomena. Utilization of statistical methods included in the content of Statistical Science, allows the collection, classification, presentation and analysis of data. The statistical methods are objective and have mathematical background and formulation.
The term *population* in the Statistics (Dodge, 2008; Everitt & Howel, 2005; Salkind, 2007) implies enumerations or measurements reported in a collection of beings or objects. A *sample* is a limited number of units and is extracted from the population under study according to the rules placed by the theory of sampling. The term data collection involves the process of measurement or enumeration of attributes of units of the population.
In Statistics two sectors are included (Dodge, 2008; Everitt & Howel, 2005; Salkind, 2007), the Descriptive Statistics and the Inferential Statistics. *Descriptive Statistics* provides the systematic, quantitative description of natural, social and other phenomena. Descriptive statistics involves the study as well as the presentation, with more convenient way, of the data that exhibit features and behavior of these phenomena. *Inferential Statistics* has as subject the generalisation of conclusions that follow from the descriptive statistical data analyses performed in a representative sample, despite the existence of sampling errors, the margin of which is determined by the statistical induction at the generalisation.
This study attempts to provide answers regarding various questions. It presents the framework of statistical studies in Telemedicine and describes the statistical methods used in Telemedicine research and evaluation (diagnostic tests, quality control, reliability analysis, sensitivity analysis, multivariate analysis, statistical pattern recognition and meta-analysis). It also exploits the potential of statistical use in testing capacity/overall performance, reliability/endurance and scalability/benchmarking of a web based telemedicine platform with different numbers of simulated users for a user-defined time and presents vulnerability statistics available for testing the security of a web based Telemedicine platform. It also describes questionnaire based statistics for the evaluation of patient's satisfaction and the contribution of statistics in new bio-markers detection. Further, qualitative and quantitative statistical techniques, regarding the electronic medical records

and bio-banks are also presented together with application based data analysis techniques (primary care, teleradiology, telecardiology, telepathology, teleoncology, teledermatology and home-telecare). Finally, the use of statistics in the design, evaluation and re-engineering of public telemedicine strategies is discussed.

2. Organisation of statistical studies in Telemedicine

Various types of statistical studies in health exist which can improve the implementation of Telemedicine. The basic characteristics of studies and their ideas are summarized as follows:

- Need of understanding of *disease causation*
- Need of description of *disease occurrence*
- Utilization for creation and hypothesis testing and evaluation of *Telemedicine and e-Health interventions.*

Fundamental characteristics of designing studies for statistical data processing in Telemedicine are the creation of aims and objectives and the adoption of appropriate methodology. The Epidemiologist (Fig. 1) studies the models of diseases development and the factors that influence these models.

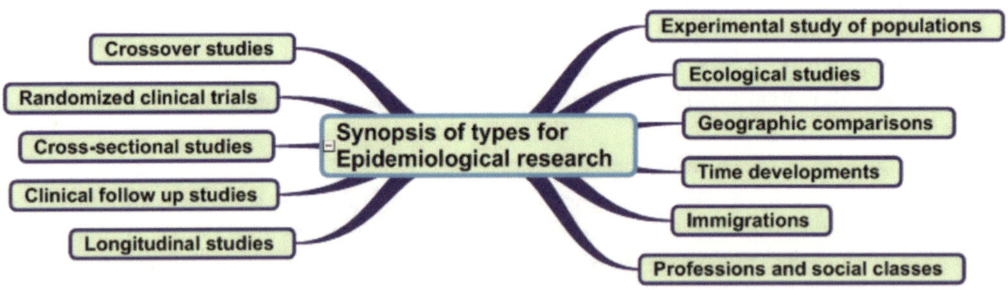

Fig. 1. Synopsis of types for Epidemiological research

The foundations of Epidemiology (Porta, 2008; Gordis, 2008; Rothman et al., 2008) are based on disease models, methods and approaches. Various epidemiological methods were developed at the pursuit of reasons of infectious diseases and epidemics. Epidemiology has also been proved effective in the localization of cross-correlations of cause-effect in non-infectious diseases as the use of narcotics, the suicide, the car accidents, the chemical poisonings, the cancer and the cardiopathies. Other advanced research sectors are Epidemiology of chronic diseases and behavioral Epidemiology.

As exploratory process, the Epidemiology constitutes the basis of public health and preventive medicine. It is used for the needs analysis for programs for diseases control, for the growth of prevention programs, for the planning of activities of health services and the identification of characteristics for *endemic diseases*, *epidemics* and *pandemics*.

Designs for epidemiologic research (Porta, 2008; Gordis, 2008; Rothman et al., 2008) are *Descriptive* and *Analytic*.

The aim of a descriptive design is the description of patterns and trends. These designs support the hypothesis formulation and the programme design. They determine the prevalence of a disease or the appearance of some other health outcome. They measure also risk factors and consequences in health outcomes. The risk factors and the consequences can be measured in connection (as a function) with the time.

The types of descriptive designs are (Abramson & Abramson, 2008; Abramson & Abramson, 2001; Porta, 2008; Gordis, 2008; Rothman et al., 2008):

- *Case Report:* the profile (model) of a patient is presented in detail from one or more clinical doctors.
- *Case Series:* a collection of cases is created by a case report that has been extended to include a number of patients with a given disease.
- *Surveillance Report:* The following stages are followed (i) data are collected with a standardized way for a disease as well as demographic elements, (ii) data collections are available (individual level) for a whole population, (iii) the appearance of a disease is examined per person, area and time. Systematic *(a-priori)* comparison of groups is not performed. The annual percentages or annual rates are many times attractive for the presentation of a tendency in connection with the time. Often the accumulative use of case reports is indicative of a new epidemic or a new disease.
- *Ecological Studies:* In these studies, all the population constitutes the object of analysis. The goal is to examine the ecological fallacy.
- *Correlation Studies:* They are comparable with ecological. The aim is to discover the power of the ecological cross-correlation.
- *Cross-sectional Studies:* Often, the interest of research is focused on the description of frequency and model or disease, or on a health-related outcome. The existing characteristics concern morbidity or some health related outcome and are measured simultaneously. Usually the collection of elements is realized via door-door visits, postal mail or with telephone interviews. There is no preselection of the cases or comparison groups (if they exist); post-hoc selection is realized.

The goal of an analytic design is to test the hypothesis of a relation existence between a risk factor and a disease or a health outcome. A measure of the association is selected, and the magnitude, the precision, and the statistical significance of the relationship are determined.

The types of analytical designs are (Abramson & Abramson, 2008; Abramson & Abramson, 2001; Porta, 2008; Gordis, 2008; Rothman et al., 2008):

- *Cross-sectional studies:* Apart from their descriptive use, sometimes are analytic. Preliminary selection of cases or comparison groups is not realized. Existing characteristics concern exposure or health outcome and are measured simultaneously. Consequently, the assessment of provisional result (temporality) in a relationship, which is revealed, is not possible.
- *Observational studies:* In this category, *longitudinal studies* are included. In a longitudinal study, the subjects are monitored in time with continuous or repeated follow-up of risk factors, health outcomes or both. The two types of longitudinal studies are (i) *Case-Control:* At this study, a population of cases and controls is selected that are comparable. The exposure or the risk factor between cases and controls is retrospectively measured. The exposure and the health outcomes are compared, between cases and controls, to test an *a-priori* hypothesis. (ii) *Cohort or Follow up:* The risk factor is measured to determine the exposed and non-exposed. This cohort is monitored in time, to find out the health outcome (morbidity). The *a-priori* hypothesis is tested at the end of the study period. (iii) *Intervention Studies:* In epidemiological research, the following designs can be applied: Clinical Trials, Field Trials and Intervention Trials.

There is software for epidemiological research design such as EPIINFO and WINPEPI (Abramson & Abramson, 2008; Abramson & Abramson, 2001) that are proposed to be used for the organization of statistical studies in Telemedicine.

3. Statistical methods used in Telemedicine research and evaluation

3.1 Power and sample size

An important issue in a statistical study is the determination of the appropriate sample size (Whitley & Ball, 2002d) needed to test a null hypothesis.

The effect size represents the magnitude of the effect and is usually known from previous research or specified from the researcher. Conventional values for effects have been suggested by Cohen (Borenstein et al., 2001). Alpha is the criterion required to establish statistical significance (usually set at 0.05).

The power (Whitley & Ball, 2002d) is the probability to detect and call significant the specified effect at the designated level of significance. As a general standard, power should be set to 80%. The higher the specified power (usually set between 80% and 95%), the larger the sample size.

Software is available to determine the sample size given the power, alpha and effect size and selecting the statistical analysis we want to apply. Note that when working with drugs and the study goal is to obtain FDA approval for use, then alpha should be set to 0.01, while keeping power at 95% (Borenstein et al. 2001).

Power and Precision, NQUERY Advisor, GPOWER, WINPEPI, SAS, NCSS-PASS can be used for the determination of power and sample size.

3.2 Diagnostic tests

Diagnostic tests or *Screening tests* are called the medical tests performed to detect and prevent diseases. These tests are the series of annual medical check-ups, blood tests, test Pap and various x-rays. Their goal is to detect diseases that cannot be detected with other way or for the discovery of a disease in premature stage (before the appearance of symptoms) to handle it in time and effectively. A characteristic of diagnostic tests is that if an individual has a positive outcome then it is probable to have the disease under investigation and consequently is submitted in more precise examinations or straight therapy (if the diagnostic test is extremely precise). In these cases, Bayes theorem is particularly beneficial. The *positive predictive value* of a diagnostic test is the probability of someone to be patient when the diagnostic test is found positive. The *negative predictive value* of a diagnostic test is the probability of someone not to be patient when the diagnostic test is found negative. *False negative case* is an individual who has the disease, but the diagnostic test is negative. When the individual does not have the disease, but the diagnostic test is positive we have a *false positive case*. In a study, we usually observe sensitivity and specificity. *Sensitivity* of a diagnostic test (or symptom) is the probability the test to be positive (or the symptom to appear) given that someone has the disease under investigation. *Specificity* of a diagnostic test (or symptom) is the probability the test to be negative (or the symptom not to appear) given that an individual does not have the disease under investigation. Both values should be high and close to one to have a suitable diagnostic test.

Usually, the measurements of diagnostic tests are performed using quantitative scale variables. In this case, we are interested in the *cutoff point* over which we consider that the test is positive (the point above which there is increased probability for the appearance of a disease). To select the cutoff point, we use ROC (Receiver Operating Characteristic) curve. A ROC curve (Bewick et al. 2004f) presents in a curve the combinations of false positive cases (1 – specificity) and sensitivity (in X and Y axes) for all the values observed in a

sample. Appropriate values as cutoff points are the values that are close to diagram's upper left corner (these have low count of false positive cases and high sensitivity).
Consequently ROC curves (Bewick et al. 2004f) are the graphical representation of the characteristics of a quantitative diagnostic test and help us to examine test performance for different points of a prognostic test. An important value in ROC curves is AUC (Area Under Curve). AUC measures the probability the value of a test for a patient to be higher from the value of a test for an individual without the under investigation disease. Of interest is the test of hypothesis H0: AUC = 0.5 with alternative H1: AUC > 0.5. The value AUC = 0.5 corresponds to a test that guesses randomly and has no prognostic ability.
WINPEPI, Stata, SPSS, NCSS, MedCalc, etc. can be used for the calculation of sensitivity and specificity and for ROC analysis.

3.3 Statistical quality control

Statistical quality control (Montgomery, 2004) is the collection of all methodologies that in collaboration with the management and marketing allows improving the productive process. A definition of quality with statistical meaning is: "a product or a service is of quality if it is adapted to the user requirements and is improved when its variability is minimized". Quality is also connected with a large number of characteristics that are related to whether the product will do the work for which it is intended, the reliability, etc. (Juran & Blanton Godfrey, 1999; Russel, 2000). Statistical quality control is constituted by three sectors: acceptance sampling, statistical process control and design of experiments.
Each productive process, independently of how well it is designed has a percentage of variability. This variability is the summation of variability of many small causes that are difficult to avoid. This variability is referred as a common form of variability, and a system that works with only the presence of this variability is considered to be under control. In a process also, other forms of variability may be present. These forms are mainly due to one of the following reasons: (i) erroneously regulated medical equipment, (ii) errors of medical equipment operator. These forms of variability are those that cause a process not to be under statistical control.
Telemedicine units should adopt the principles and administration of total quality management (Juran & Blanton Godfrey, 1999; Russel, 2000) and include the 5Qs: quality planning, quality laboratory process, quality control, quality assessment and quality improvement.
QI Analyst 3.5. by SPSS, SAS Quality Improvement, STATIT Quality Control First Aid Kit, STATISTICA, MINITAB 16, NCSS can be used for Statistical Quality Control.

3.4 Reliability statistics

The consistency of a collection of measurements is called reliability (Koran, 1975a; Koran, 1975b). Regarding its assurance in Telemedicine studies, four classes of reliability estimates exist (Dodge, 2008; Everitt & Howel, 2005; Salkind, 2007), all examining the variation of measurements.
Measurements can be taken, with the same method or instruments, by different observers (inter-rater reliability), or by a single observer under the same conditions (test-retest reliability including intra-rater reliability). Inter-method reliability deals with measurements derived using different methods or instruments on the same individual. Internal consistency reliability deals with the consistency of measurements across items within a test.
WINPEPI can be used for the calculation of reliability statistics (Fig. 2).

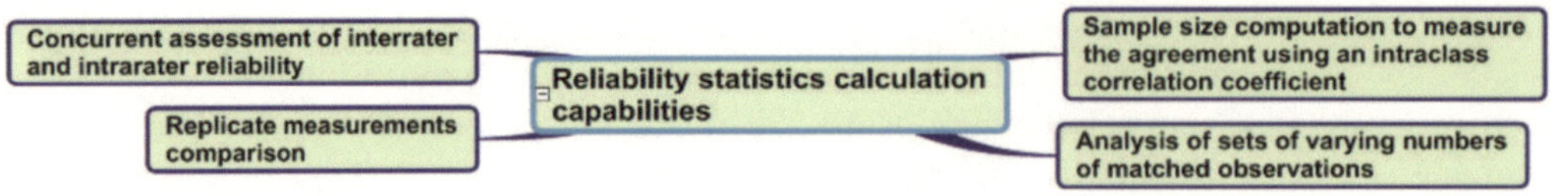

Fig. 2. Reliability statistics

3.5 Sensitivity analysis

Sensitivity analysis exploits the degree in which the conclusions can change if the values of the key variables or hypotheses statements change.

As examples, the following can be applied in Telemedicine:

The user may want to examine how power is affected changing the values of effect size, sample size and alpha. This analysis is provided using as software the GPower or Power and Precision.

Financial projections may show the effect of different hypotheses related to the expenses for telecommunications and other resources. A special problem in the evaluation of Telemedicine is the stability of the technology or the environment. With the technologies of data collection, communication and presentation aiming to improve healthcare quality simultaneously reducing cost, the evaluators may focus on (i) how sensitive the results may be in technological change, (ii) how to design the analysis to assess the impact of changes.

A cost-benefit analysis can include a sensitivity analysis that incorporates different hypotheses about the time and the cost of improvements or replacements in hardware or software (Briggs et al., 1994; Hamby, 1995).

3.6 Hypothesis testing

The Inferential Statistics are the sector of applied statistics that deals with the generalization of the descriptive statistics conclusions in the population.

Hypothesis testing is the effort of estimating unknown population parameters using samples, realizing the testing of concrete hypotheses about the under investigation population parameters. More analytically, the problem faced is how from the data of a sample, we can decide if a hypothesis must be rejected in the population. After the selection and the determination with clarity of the problem under investigation, what follows is the formulation of the hypothesis that is to be checked.

The hypotheses under consideration are not proved with testimonies, only they cannot be denied. In the hypotheses involved in a research study, some hierarchy can exist. Often, for the initial hypothesis the expression inquiring is used, while, for the one that results in the end, the term functional is used. The hypothesis should be solid and relatively easy in the testing. General hypotheses are not recommended. The hypotheses should not be incompatible with things that are already known and should be based on the existing knowledge.

The ways of a hypothesis formulation are an important point in the statistical analysis. We do not check the functional hypothesis, but the logic of the opposite one called the *null hypothesis*. In the case that the null hypothesis is rejected, then we accept the alternative hypothesis. The null hypothesis we usually denote it with H0 and its alternative with H1. The results of a decision that will be taken in significance level alpha in connection with what happens in the population are presented in the following Table 1.

Acceptance decision	Reality	
	True H0 (Null Hypothesis)	False H0 (Null Hypothesis)
H0 Null	Correct Decision	Error type II
H1 Alternative	Error type I	Correct Decision

Table 1. Correct decision and error types in statistical hypothesis testing process

As *error type I*, we define the probability to reject H0 while this is in effect. This error is also called significance level alpha of the test. As *error type II*, we define the probability to accept H0 while this is not in effect. In each test, what is of interest is to reduce error type I.
A decision tree for the statistical analysis of two variables is presented (Fig. 3).

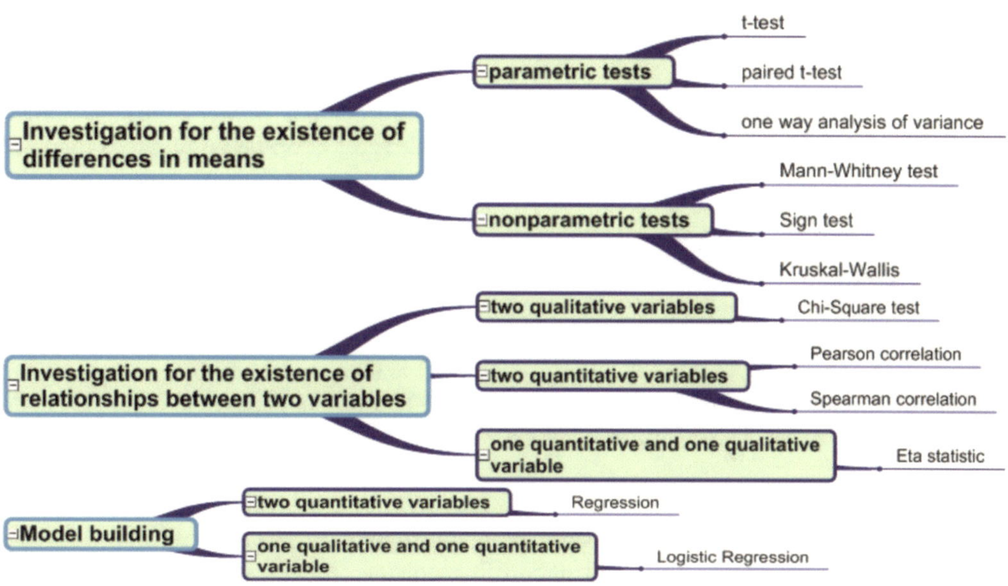

Fig. 3. Decision tree for the statistical analysis of two variables

Statistical data analysis principles (Matthews & Farewell, 2007; Bowers, 2008; Harris & Taylor 2003) are available in the form of reviews (Whitley & Ball, 2002a; Whitley & Ball, 2002b; Whitley & Ball, 2002c; Whitley & Ball, 2002e; Whitley & Ball, 2002f; Bewick et al., 2003; Bewick et al., 2004a, Bewick et al., 2004b; Bewick et al., 2004c; Bewick et al., 2005).
Various statistical packages are available to test a hypothesis involving two variables or for multivariate analysis: STATISTICA, SPSS, SAS, NCSS, MINITAB, StatView, Medcalc, Stata, BMDP and StatXact with Cytel Studio (non parametrics).

3.7 Multivariate analysis

In most cases, many variables are involved in the statistical analysis (Stevens, 2002; Rabe-Hesketh & Everitt, 2007; Landau & Everitt, 2004). Depending on the measurement scales of the data various data analysis options are available (Fig. 4).

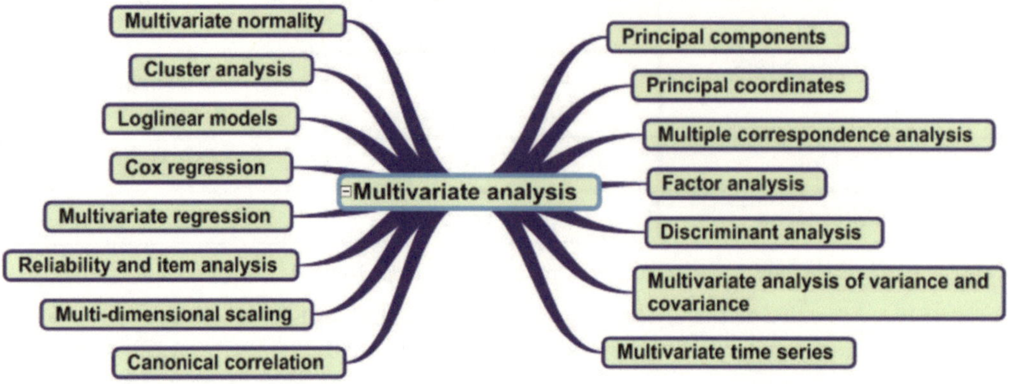

Fig. 4. Statistical techniques for multivariate data analysis

3.8 Statistical pattern recognition

Statistical pattern recognition is concerned with discrimination and classification both supervised and unsupervised (Webb, 2002). Two related approaches to supervised classification are the estimation of probability density functions and the construction of discriminant functions. There are also nonlinear models (projection-based methods) and the decision-tree approach to discrimination. Unsupervised classification or clustering is the process of grouping to discover the presence of structure. Statistical methods are also used in feature generation and feature selection (Theodoridis & Koutroumbas, 2009; Webb, 2002). Statistical pattern recognition has application in biosignal processing and medical image analysis.

Various statistical packages are available for discriminant analysis such as NCSS, SPSS, STATISTICA, and BMDP. For clustering, statistical packages are BMDP, Stata, NCSS, Statistica, SPSS, etc. A significant Statistical Pattern Recognition Toolbox (STPRTOOL) has been developed for MATLAB (Frank & Hlava, 2004).

3.9 Meta-analysis

Meta-analysis allows for general inspection of evidence for clinical problems and necessary with the exponential increase of information in medicine (Borenstein et al., 2009). Meta-analysis uses data from many different studies that deal with the same subject. This allows (i) the calculation of a total/ concise result from all the studies called *pooled effect*, (ii) extensive detection of systematic errors and calculation of differences (*heterogeneity*). Meta-analysis uses objective quantitative mathematical methods to summarize study data. Meta-analysis can be used in studies that are (i) empirical rather than theoretical, (ii) contain quantitative results, (iii) investigate the same relationships, (iv) results are presented with the same comparative statistical manner and (v) are comparable for the main question. Explicit criteria of studies choice and rejection are needed. Wide inquiring fields require detailed criteria. Strict criteria create a problem of generalization of results and relaxed criteria create a problem of results reliability. The study of *fixed effects* (results of different studies differ only from chance) is conducted using the Mantel-Haenszel method, and the study of *random effects* (results are not homogeneous) is conducted using DerSimonian & Laird method. Heterogeneity is tested using Cochran Q or the indicator of inconsistency (Higgins et al., 2003).

Statistical packages available are: RevMan (Cochrane), STATA (metan), SPSS (using macros), R (rmeta), Comprehensive meta-analysis and Meta-analyst.

4. Commonly used statistical methods in Telemedicine diagnosis

4.1 Analyzing validity

An ideal research technique is characterized from *validity* which means that it measures correctly what has to be measured (Dodge, 2008; Everitt & Howel, 2005; Salkind, 2007). Sometimes, an established framework is defined to determine the validity of a method. In the practice, therefore, the validity should be examined indirectly. Usually two ways are used. A technique, which has been simplified and standardised in order to be suitable for use in research, can be compared with the best conventional clinical examination. Alternative a measurement can be evaluated from its ability to predict a future disease. Examining validity through prediction ability may require the existence of many subjects in the study. When the purpose of a research or a test is based on the separation of subjects (e.g. as cases or controls, exposed or not exposed), validity is analyzed classifying the subjects with positive or negative outcomes, on the basis primarily of the research method and secondarily with the typical control test. A contingency table can be derived with the true positive, true negative, false positive and false negative outcomes. From this table sensitivity, specificity, *systematic error* and *predictive value* can be calculated.

4.2 Analyzing repeatability

Repeatability analysis (Salkind, 2007) can be organized as a separate study, for example, a sample of individuals with a second examination, or x-ray samples checked twice. Even a small sample can be reliable if (i) it is representative and (ii) duplicate tests are independent. If repeatability analysis is performed as a part of a pilot study, then care is needed to ensure that the subjects, the observers and the working conditions are representative of the main study. Repeatability is easy to be checked when the material can be transferred and stored (e.g. histologic samples and medical images). Repeatability analysis is useful when there is no acceptable standard to assess the validity of a measurement. Poor repeatability usually is related with poor validity or indicates that the measured characteristic is differentiated in time. In both cases, the results should be interpreted carefully. It is stressed that repeatable discoveries do not guarantee that the method that was used is valid. Repeatability can be checked from the same observer (realizes the measurement in two separate cases) and between observers (with comparison of measurements that became from different observers in the same subject). The repeatability of measurements for scale variables can be summarized with the standard deviation of the repeated measurements or with the coefficient of variation. The pairs of measurements from the same observer or different observers, the extent and the divergence can be presented in a scatterplot. For qualitative characteristics, such as clinical symptoms and indications, the results are initially presented in a contingency table (with the true positive, true negative, false positive and false negative outcomes) and then Kappa statistic is calculated. The minimal value of the Kappa statistic is less than zero (poor repeatability) and the highest is one (perfect repeatability).

4.3 Using statistics to serve clinical objectives

A Telemedicine program may have different outcomes that are proportional to the population under study and the health status of the specific group during the application time. The type and health status of the application group have direct repercussions both in quality and the access possibility of a patient. Proportional are also benefits from the reduction of patient cost of care.

The plan is to collect data regarding: (i) standard and variable program costs, (ii) use of services from the participating patients, (iii) demographic characteristics of patients and clinical history, (iv) presentation of symptoms and complaints, (v) health status, (vi) symptoms risk, (vii) operational capability, (viii) analysis of symptoms, and (viiii) characteristics of the teleconsultations.

In clinical level the following items should be recorded and evaluated:

- Demographic characteristics of patients and their clinical history.
- Symptoms of present disease.
- Evidence of reliable transmission and evaluation of data acquired from the physical examination of patients and the parameters acquired from telemedicine medical devices.
- Use of telemedicine services from the patients and recording of medical problems during program use.
- Changes in the ways of patient access (number of teleconsultations, teleconsultation type, and cost of diagnostic examinations).
- Changes in patient treatment with evaluation of the changes in the pharmaceutical treatment (change of drug, dose and the way of issuing of pharmaceutical substances, cost of these changes) and the therapeutic methods used (number, type and cost of chirurgical interventions).
- Changes in the medical or nursing visits, number of hospitalizations (morbidity) and mortality of patients.
- Improvement of quality of life and mental health of patients with the use of special questionnaires.

5. Statistics in testing the performance of a Web-based Telemedicine platform

There is the potential of statistics use (Fig. 5) in testing, capacity/overall performance, reliability/endurance and scalability/benchmarking of a web based telemedicine platform with different numbers of simulated users for a user-defined time.

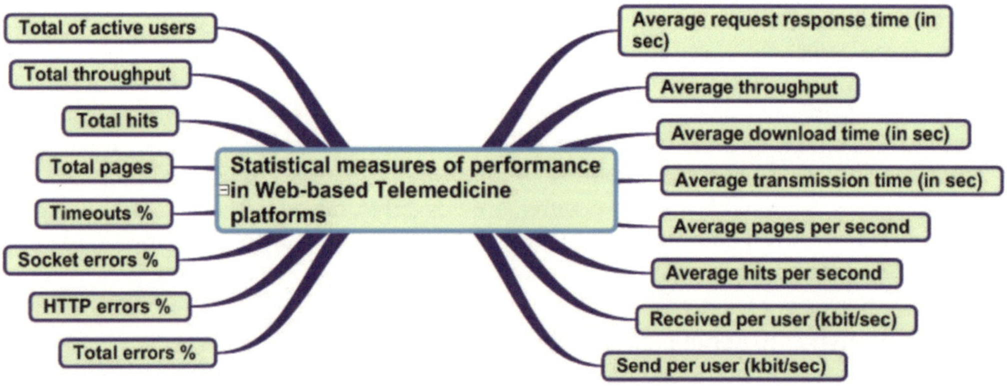

Fig. 5. Statistical measures of performance in Web-based Telemedicine platforms

Software that is proposed to be used is WAPT 6.0 and NEOLOAD.
Furthermore, in the Telemedicine network, each computer and medical device reliability and history should be continuously monitored regarding application failures, operating system failures, various other failures and warnings.

6. Statistics in testing the security of a Web-based Telemedicine platform

The percent of various security vulnerabilities (Web Application Security Consortium, 2008) in time (on a daily basis diagram) should be monitored for a web based telemedicine platform (Fig. 6).

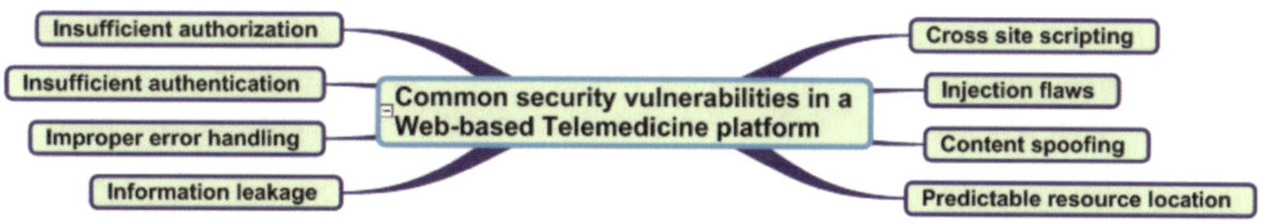

Fig. 6. Common security vulnerabilities in Web-based Telemedicine platforms

Software that can be used to produce security audits for Web based Telemedicine platforms is Acunetix.

7. Questionnaire based statistics for the evaluation of patient satisfaction

Herein, the strategy and the steps to get valid comparative data and analyze it, are presented.
Three types of questionnaires can be used: to the patient, to the provider and to the organization.
The questionnaires should be valid and reliable. In a questionnaire creation process, it is necessary to determine the reliability (internal consistency) of the new instrument. It is difficult to assess the quality of data collected during a research process. It is easier to evaluate the accuracy of the research tool used for data collection. This assessment is comprised by the analysis of validity and reliability. Each stakeholder class (patient, provider, organization) has expectations and satisfaction sentiments for the quality of information, services and operations which are offered. The goal is to identify the most significant factors that cause the highest level of dissatisfaction and have the bigger effect with respect to e-healthcare quality and the costs.
A method to test questionnaire validity: When the factors that produced the highest level of dissatisfaction are derived, using a questionnaire, a representative sample of each category stakeholder can be interviewed and asked to complete a new short questionnaire. This research will determine how appropriate, complete and comprehensive are the questions in a group of evaluators that have certain knowledge of the content. This process allows confirming questionnaire validity.
A method to test questionnaire reliability: To evaluate the reliability level of the questionnaires different methods can be used (test-retest method, split halves method). The reliability of internal consistency can be measured calculating Cronbach's coefficient alpha. An additional scale can be included to measure the questionnaire internal consistency. This scale can be defined with the characterization "satisfied/dissatisfied" and can be included in

the evaluation of each factor measuring quantitatively also the strength of the characterization (from poor to high). This "direct" evaluation should be related with each factor score measured from the strength of characterization. The same scale can be included at the end of the questionnaire, to provide an evaluation of the stakeholder overall satisfaction with aspects for the Telemedicine system, services and information. These scales allow the selection and the representitaviness of the factors and their characterizations to evaluate stakeholder satisfaction for a telemedicine system. These added scales can be used, during experimental research, to validate the internal consistency of the questionnaire.

Various multivariate statistical analyses can be performed on the questionnaires with focus on reliability analysis (for Cronbach's alpha coefficient calculation) and exploratory and confirmatory factor analysis.

Experimental processes to compare a Telemedicine treated group with an alternative, traditional care, group: During the pilot study to evaluate a Telemedicine program, patients with a known disease should be included that are exposed to health risk justifying the need of telemedicine and the highest benefit from it. The patients should be divided in two groups: the telemedicine group and the control group. The control group should be comprised from patients similar in age and sex and with the same disease and will receive regular traditional health monitoring (no telemedicine treatment).

Data Analysis: All the data (electronic recordings of medical signals, images and text) should be collected in the electronic medical record and the specialized questionnaires be collected and stored in a database.

The two groups of patients that participate in the study can be compared to find out if there are statistical significant differences in the following aspects:

- The diagnostic access, from the recording of the number, the type and the cost of diagnostic examinations needed during the study period.
- The therapeutic treatment from recording the changes in the pharmaceutical therapy using the drug type, the drug dose, the way of issuing the pharmaceutical substance, the cost of drug dose during the study period.
- The chirurgical therapeutic methods needed, recording the number, the type of surgery and the cost of surgery during the study period.
- The number and the cost of medical or/and other visits recorded during the study period.
- The number of hospital admissions (morbidity) during the study period and the cost of hospitalization.
- The number of patient deaths (mortality) during the study period.
- Quality of life and mental health, using analysis on appropriate questionnaires.

8. Exploit the use of statistics in new biomarkers detection

A biomarker is a measurable factor that is associated with a medical condition (a gene variant, a metabolite, a pattern of gene activity, etc.). Drug development process is most benefited from biomarkers that allow the early detection, diagnosis, and prognosis of diseases. It is an enormous challenge to analyze using statistics 'omics' data (genomics, transcriptomics, proteomics, metabolomics, interactomics, regulomics) (Lee, 2010).

A synthesis of available statistical techniques for new biomarkers detection is presented in Fig. 7.

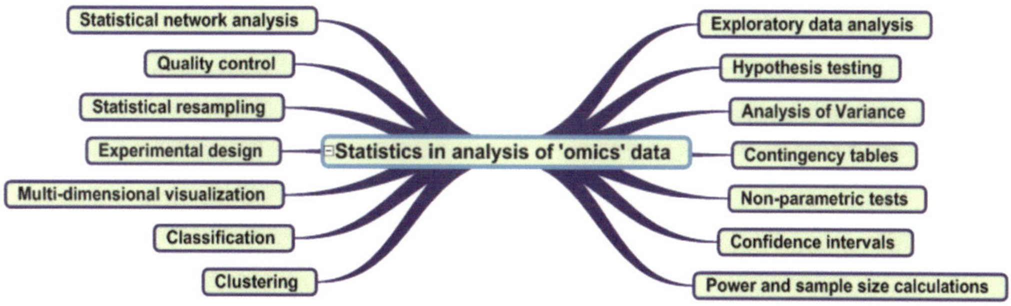

Fig. 7. Statistics in analysis of 'omics' data

Statistical packages in bioinformatics available are R and Bioconductor.

9. Qualitative and quantitative techniques regarding electronic medical records and biobanks

9.1 Statistics regarding the electronic medical records

Electronic medical records, apart from numerical measurements, also contain images, biosignals and text. Statistical analysis on numerical measurements (Fig. 3, Fig. 4), images (Fig. 8, Fig. 9), biosignals (Fig. 10), and text (Fig. 11), has already been applied.

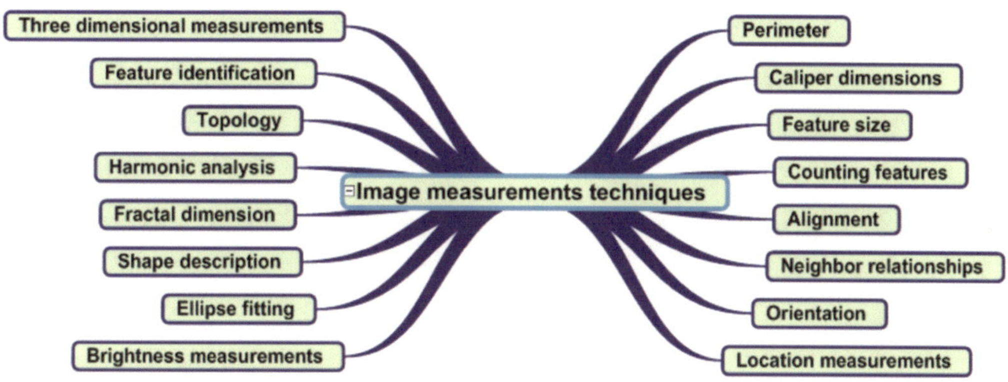

Fig. 8. Image measurements techniques (Russ, 1995)

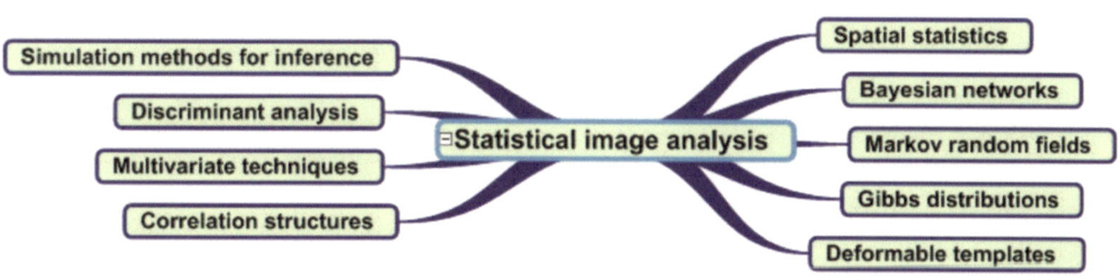

Fig. 9. Statistical image analysis techniques applied on image measurements

For spatial statistical image analysis SpatStat library is available in R as well as the Image Processing Toolbox in MATLAB.

Statistical packages that perform time series analysis on quantitative biosignal data are SPSS, NCSS, Statistica, SAS, Stata, BMDP, etc.

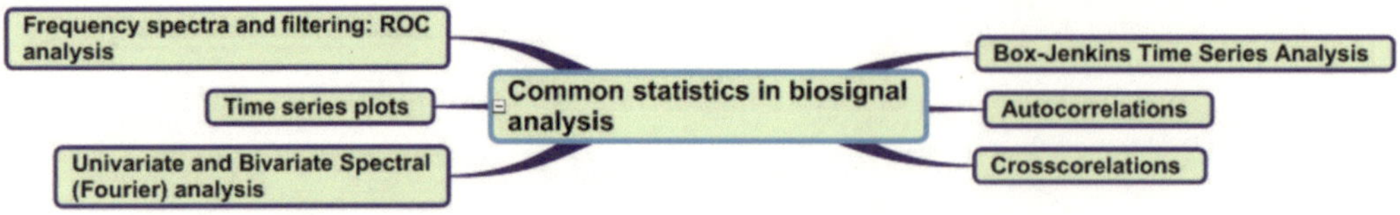

Fig. 10. Statistical analysis techniques applied on biosignals measurements

It also exists specialized software for biosignal analysis including statistics such as g.Bsanalyze and SIGVIEW.
For qualitative analysis of the texts included in the electronic patient records, NVIVO software can be used which allows after coding the extraction of relationships and the exploration of models produced. For mixed-model qualitative data analysis using coding, annotating, retrieving and analyzing small and large collections of documents and images in the electronic patient record, QDA Miner with WordStat & Simstat software can be used.

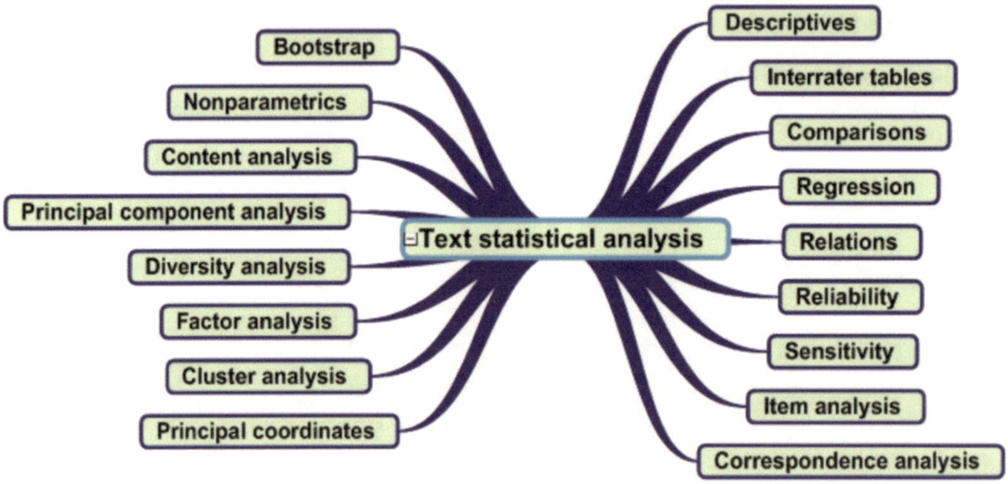

Fig. 11. Statistical analysis techniques applied on text data

9.2 Epidemiology using biobanks

Biobanks are repositories of human biological material linked to clinical data (medical and lifestyle data) for evaluation of interactions between the environment and genes. The ultimate goal is to understand the disease development process. Biobanks are categorized in (i) *prospective*: biological material is collected at study start and health status is monitored over subsequent years, and (ii) *retrospective*: biological material from people who have already developed a disease is collected, over subsequent years, to track down the association between environment, genes and the diseases.
The number of cases is essential for a reliable analysis. Other points of interest are the quantification of metatada acquired and biobanks security auditing. The ultimate goal is the creation of an *epidemiological meta-database* using regulations, standardized methodologies and coordination across biobanks. Ethical considerations involved are (i) the privacy of the donor and (ii) who owns the samples. Informed consent of the donor is a pre-requisite in storing data (in a biobank), as well as the established policies from biobanks.
There are various facilitations for epidemiology using biobanks (Fig. 12).

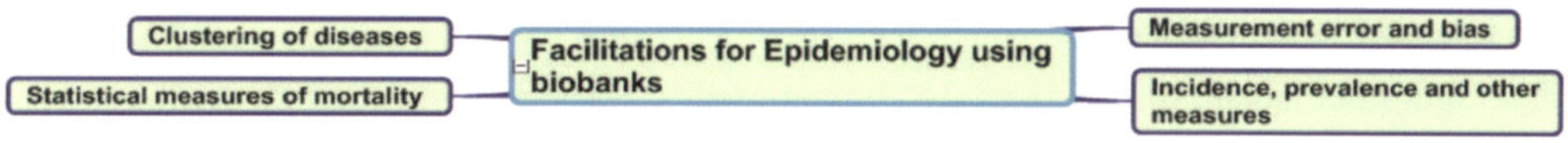

Fig. 12. Epidemiology using biobanks

Clustering of disease

Clustering of disease (Mantel, 1967; Manly, 1986) can be realized spatial, temporal and spatial temporal using data from electronic medical records. *Spatial* clustering of disease may be attributed to the population distribution, the relationship of disease with diet, the habits, the environment or the profession. Chi-square test can be used for statistical decision-making. *Temporal* clustering of disease may be attributed to seasonal variation, systematic trends or in rapid increases due to additional factors. Again, Chi-square test can be used for statistical decision-making. *Spatial temporal* clustering of disease concerns cases, where they are neighboring in the space (spatial) and simultaneously they are neighboring in the time (temporal) because of the existence of pestiferous factors, environmental episodes in regional scale or local immigrations. The main spatial temporal association in the appearance of a disease can involve the existence of certain infectious or environmental reasons. Mantel's test is used for the control of space-time interaction (Manly, 1986).

Quantification of disease frequency in populations

Disease frequency measurement in populations requires the careful formulation of diagnostic criteria. It has also been observed that the morbidity in populations is presented as development of severity. The two measures of disease frequency are *incidence* and (point or period) *prevalence*. Herein, we assume that the percentages in the exposed population are comparable with those of the unexposed individuals. Exposure can assess risk factors for which suspicions exist that they cause the disease (Bewick et al., 2004d). There are measures used to summarize the comparisons of morbidity percentages between populations: relative risk, attributable risk, population attributable risk, and attributable proportion. Most epidemiological studies are based on observation and compare persons that differ with a lot of ways, known and unknown. If the morbidity risk is determined by such differences varying from the exposure under consideration, then we can say that there is confounding of the classification factors (e.g. age and sex) in relation to morbidity. Confounding is handled using (i) (direct or indirect) standardization or (ii) mathematical modeling (e.g. logistic regression).

Statistical measures of mortality

Mortality is used to describe death as a disease outcome. Statistics are derived from data written in death certificates. In the published mortality tables, the actual numbers and the rates of death per sex, age and causality are presented. In clinical trials for diseases that lead to death the health outcome can be defined as case mortality or survival rate. Survival curves (Bewick et al., 2004e) can be drawn from the survival rates in different times.

Incidence, prevalence and other measures

The terms of incidence and prevalence have been defined concerning the presence of disease and can be extended to include other situations. Certain healthcare results do not necessarily describe incidence or prevalence. Alternatively, the following measures (related with a year) can be used: birth rate, fertility rate, infant mortality rate, stillbirth rate, and perinatal mortality rate.

Measurement errors and bias

The epidemiological studies measure characteristics of the populations. The parameter of interest may be the morbidity percentage of a disease, the prevalence of an exposure and more often a measure of association between the exposure and disease. Given that the studies are realised in human subjects and are conditioned by practical and ethical restrictions, the danger of bias exist. The possible cases of bias are (i) *Selection bias*: Selection bias is required to be examined when a sample is determined and in the cases the answers are not complete. (ii) *Information bias*: Bias also results from errors in the measurement of exposure or the severity of a disease. Bias can not be abolished entirely from epidemiological studies. The aim therefore is to ensure that it exists in a minimal degree, examining their possible impact and taking it into consideration when interpreting the results. The measurement errors in the exposure or the disease may be a valuable source of bias in epidemiological studies. Consequently at the implementation of research it is necessary to assess the quality of measurements.
Useful statistical packages for epidemiological research that can be used are EPIINFO and WINPEPI.

10. Telemedicine application based data analysis techniques

Exploiting the fundamental telemedicine applications (primary care, teleradiology, telecardiology, telepathology, teleoncology, teledermatology and home-telecare) it is obvious that text, biosignals and images are transferred. For these data types, various statistical data analysis techniques can be applied in the electronic medical records (Fig. 8, Fig. 9, Fig. 10, Fig. 11) collected using Telemedicine.
Furthermore, performance (Fig. 5) and security auditing statistics (Fig. 6) are required to be collected during monitoring of the telemedicine application and network.
Statistics can be extracted also using data from teleconsultations and telediagnosis (presented previously as statistics used to serve clinical objectives) as well as from evaluating the patient's and provider's satisfaction (presented as questionnaire based statistics) using questionnaires. Another important feature for Telemedicine diagnosis processes is careful statistical reliability analysis (Abramson & Abramson, 2008; Abramson & Abramson, 2001; Koran, 1975a; Koran, 1975b).

11. Statistics use in the design and re-engineering of public Telemedicine strategies

In the current era of Telemedicine and e-Health, all nations are interested in developing national strategies for the improvement of quality and reliability of Telemedicine. Material provided by WHO (World Health Organization, 2006a; World Health Organization, 2006b) can be used as effective assistance to this effort. Legal frameworks regarding the implementation of Telemedicine within a country as well as in trans-border care should be taken into account in this process accompanied with ethical issues, issues related to patient safety, patient empowerment and evaluation.
Statistical quality control can be used in the design and re-engineering of Public Telemedicine strategies. Statistical analysis of teleconsultations information and electronic

medical records (including genomic information) collected practising Telemedicine and e-Health provides enormous possibilities in decision-making (Fig. 13) and in facilitating epidemiological studies.

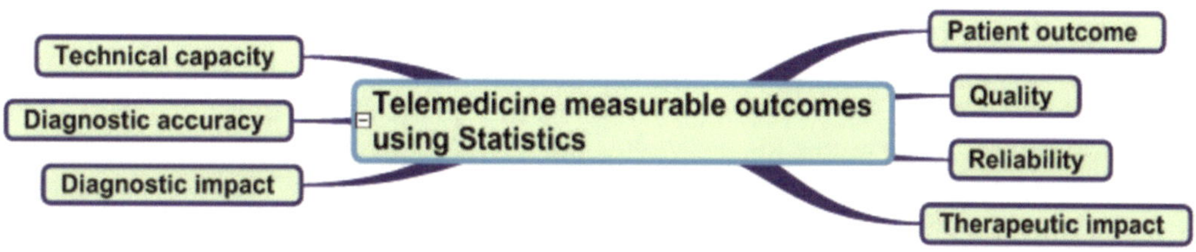

Fig. 13. The contribution of Statistics in Telemedicine

12. Conclusion

There was a lack in the scientific literature regarding a systematic presentation of statistical methods in Telemedicine. This work uncovered opportunities and challenges related to the contribution of statistical data processing in Telemedicine. It is our hope that the guidelines presented herein, in the form of concept maps, will serve as telemedicine assessment instruments for the improvement of Telemedicine systems and services. Future work will be focused on producing detailed statistics review frameworks for all Telemedicine applications accompanied with case studies.

13. References

Abramson, J. & Abramson, Z.H. (2008). *Research Methods in Community Medicine: Surveys, Epidemiological Research, Programme Evaluation, Clinical Trials*, 6th Edition, Wiley, ISBN: 978-0-470-98661-5

Abramson, J.H. & Abramson, Z.H. (2001). *Making Sense of Data: A Self-Instruction Manual on the Interpretation of Epidemiological Data, 3rd Edition*, Oxford University Press, ISBN: 978-0-19-514525-0

Bewick, V.; Cheek, L & Ball, J. (2003). Statistics review 7: Correlation and regression, *Critical Care*, Vol. 7, (November 2003), (451-459), ISSN 1364-8535

Bewick, V.; Cheek, L. & Ball, J. (2004a). Statistics review 8: Qualitative data - tests of association, *Critical Care*, Vol. 8, No. 1, (December 2003), (46-53), ISSN 1364-8535

Bewick, V.; Cheek, L. & Ball, J. (2004b). Statistics review 9: One-way analysis of variance, *Critical Care*, Vol. 8, No. 2, (April 2004), (130-136), ISSN 1364-8535

Bewick, V; Cheek, L. & Ball, J. (2004c). Statistics review 10: Further nonparametric methods, *Critical Care*, Vol. 8, No. 3, (June 2004), (196-199), ISSN 1364-8535

Bewick, V; Cheek, L. & Ball, J. (2004d). Statistics review 11: Assessing risk, *Critical Care*, Vol. 8, (June 2004), (287-291), ISSN 1364-8535

Bewick, V.; Cheek, L. & Ball, J. (2004e). Statistics review 12: Survival analysis, *Critical Care,* Vol. 8, (September 2004), (389-394), ISSN 1364-8535

Bewick, V.; Cheek, L & Ball, J. (2004f). Statistics review 13: Receiver operating characteristic curves, *Critical Care*, Vol. 8, No. 6, (December 2004) (508-512)

Bewick, V.; Cheek, L. & Ball, J. (2005). Statistics review 14: Logistic regression, *Critical Care,* Vol. 9, No. 1, (February 2005), (112-118), ISSN 1364-8535

Borenstein, M.; Rothstein, H. & Cohen, J. (2001). *Power And Precision™*, Biostat, Inc., ISBN 0-9709662-0-2, United States of America

Borenstein, M.; Hedges, L.V.; Higgins, J.P.T & Rothstein, H.R. (2009). Introduction to Meta-Analysis, Wiley online library, Online ISBN: 9780470743386

Briggs, A.; Sculpher, M., & Buxton, M. (1994). Uncertainty in the Economic Evaluation of Health Care Technologies: The Role of Sensitivity Analysis. *Health Economics* 3(2):95-104

Bowers, D. (2008). *Medical Statistics from Scratch: An introduction for Health Professionals,* Second Edition, JohnWiley & Sons Ltd, ISBN 978-0-470-51301-9, Great Britain

Dodge, Y. (2008). *The Concise Encyclopedia of Statistics*, Springer, ISBN: 978-0-387-32833-1

Everitt, B & Howel, D. (Eds) (2005). *Encyclopedia of Statistics in Behavioral Science,* John Wiley & Sons, Ltd, ISBN-13: 978-0-470-86080-9, Chichester

Frank, V. & Hlava V. (2004). *Statistical Pattern Recognition Toolbox for Matlab User's guide,* Research Reports of CMP, Czech Technical University in Prague, No. 8, Prague, Czech Republic

Gordis, L. (2008). *Epidemiology, Fourth Edition,* Saunders: An Imprint of Elsevier Inc., ISBN: 978-1-4160-4002-6, Philadelphia, Unites States of America

Hamby, D.M. (1995). A Comparison of Sensitivity Analysis Techniques. *Health Physicist* 68(2):195-204

Harris, M. & Taylor, G. (2003). Medical Statistics Made Easy, Martin Dunitz, an imprint of the Taylor & Francis Group, ISBN 0-203-59739-7, United States of America

Higgins, J.P.T.; Thompson, S.G.; Deeks, J.J. & Altman, D.G. (2003). Measuring inconsistency in meta-analyses. *BMJ, Vol* 327, (September 2003) (557-560)

Juran, J.M & Blanton Godfrey, A. (1999). *Juran's quality control handbook, Fifth Edition,* McGraw-Hill, ISBN 0-07-034003-X, United States of America

Koran, L.M. (1975a). The reliability of clinical methods, data and judgements. Part 1, *N Eng J Med,* 293: 642-648

Koran, L.M. (1975b). The reliability of clinical methods, data and judgements. Part 2, *N Eng J Med* 293: 695-701

Landau, S. & Everitt, B.S. (2004). *A Handbook of Statistical Analysis using SPSS*, Chapman & Hall/CRC Press LLC, ISBN 1-58488-369-3, United States of America

Lee, J.K. (Ed) (2010). *Statistical Bioinformatics: For Biomedical and Life Science Researchers,* Wiley-Blackwell, Hoboken, ISBN 978-0-471-69272-0 (cloth), New Jersey, United States of America

Manly, B.F.J.(1986). Randomization and regression methods for testing for associations with geographical, environmental and biological distances between populations. *Researches on Population Ecology*, Vol. 28, No.2 (201-218).

Mantel, N. (1967). The detection of disease clustering and a generalized regression approach. *Cancer Res*, Vol. 27, No.2, (February 1967) (209-220)

Matthews, D.E. & Farewell, V.T. (2007). *Using and understanding Medical Statistics*, S. Karger AG, ISBN-13: 978-3-8055-8189-9, Basel (Switzerland)

Montgomery, D.C. (2004). *Introduction to Statistical Quality Control*, Wiley, ISBN: 0471656313

Porta, M. (2008). *A Dictionary of Epidemiology, Fifth Edition*, Oxford University Press, ISBN 978-0-19-531450-2, New York, United States of America

Rabe-Hesketh, S. & Everitt, B.S. (2007). *A Handbook of Statistical Analysis using Stata*, Fourth Edition, Chapman & Hall/CRC Taylor & Francis Group, ISBN-13: 978-1-58488-756-0, United States of America

Rothman, K.J.; Greenland, S. & Lash, T.L. (2008). *Modern Epidemiology, 3rd Edition,* Lippincott Williams & Wilkins: a unit of Wolters Kluwer Health, ISBN: 978-0-7817-5564-1, Baltimore, United States of America

Russ, J.C. (1995). *The Image Processing Handbook, Second Edition,* CRC Press, Inc., ISBN: 0-8493-2516-1, United States of America

Russel, J.P. (Ed) (2000). *The Quality Audit Handbook, Second Edition,* American Society for Quality: Quality Press, ISBN 0-87389-460-X, Milwaukee, Wisconsin, United States of America

Salkind, N.J. (Ed) (2007). *Encyclopedia of Measurement and Statistics*, SAGE Publications, ISBN: 978-1-4129-1611-0, Thousand Oaks, California

Stevens, J. (2002). *Applied Multivariate Statistics for the social sciences, Fourth Edition,* Lawrence Erlbaum Associates, Inc., ISBN 0-8058-3776-0, New Jersey, United States of America

Theodoridis, S. & Koutroumbas, K. (2009). *Pattern Recognition, Fourth Edition*, Academic Press an imprint of Elsevier, ISBN: 978-1-59749-272-0, United States of America

Webb, A.R. (2002). *Statistical Pattern Recognition, Second Edition,* John Wiley & Sons, Ltd., ISBNs: 0-470-84513-9 (HB); 0-470-84514-7 (PB), West Sussex, England

Web Application Security Consortium (2008). *Web application Security Statistics 2008*, Available on line: http://projects.webappsec.org/f/WASS-SS-2008.pdf

Whitley, E. & Ball, J. (2002a). Statistics review 1: Presenting and summarizing data, *Critical Care,* Vol. 6, No. 1, (February 2002), (66-71), ISSN 1364-8535

Whitley, E. & Ball, J. (2002b). Statistics review 2: Samples and populations, *Critical Care,* Vol. 6, No. 1, (February 2002), (143-148), ISSN 1364-8535

Whitley, E. & Ball, J. (2002c). Statistics review 3: Hypothesis testing and P values, *Critical Care,* Vol. 6., No. 3., (March 2002), (222-225), ISSN 1364-8535

Whitley, E. & Ball, J (2002d). Statistics review 4: Sample size calculations, *Critical Care*, Vol. 6, (May 2002) (335-341), ISSN 1364-8535

Whitley, E. & Ball, J. (2002e). Statistics review 5: Comparison of means, *Critical Care,* Vol. 6, No. 5, (October 2002), (424-428), ISSN 1364-8535

Whitley, E. & Ball, J. (2002f). Statistics review 6: Nonparametric methods, *Critical Care,* Vol.6, (September 2002), (509-513), ISSN 1364-8535

World Health Organization (2006a). *eHealth Tools and Services - Needs of the Member States,* Report of the WHO Global Observatory for eHealth, WHO Press, Geneva, Switzerland

World Health Organization (2006b). *Building Foundations for e-health: Progress of Member States,* Report of the WHO Global Observatory for eHealth, WHO Press, Geneva, Switzerland

10

Video Communication in Telemedicine

Dejan Dinevski, Robi Kelc and Bogdan Dugonik
Faculty of Medicine and Faculty of Electrical Engineering and Computer Science, University of Maribor
Slovenia

1. Introduction

Since the emergence of telegraphy and telephone technologies in the 19th Century, doctors have been communicating and consulting with each other over long distances. Telemedicine, as distance healing was first highlighted in 1970, when Thomas Bird wrote about patient care in which physicians were able to examine their patients by using telecommunication technologies. In short, telemedicine can simply involve two health professionals discussing a case over the telephone, or be as sophisticated as using the satellite technology to broadcast a consultation between providers at facilities in two countries, using video conferencing equipment (Mishra & Mishra, 2006).

Telemedicine has the potential to reduce differences in the lives of people, especially those living in remote areas, away from hospitals and thus deprived of quality and timely medical care. The main role of telemedicine is to provide rapid access to experienced health care professionals at a distance using telecommunications and information technologies, no matter where the patient is located.

The spectrum of technology used in telemedicine is broad, ranging from simple phone, faxes and emails, to satellite-based relay transfers and state-of-the-art computer and videoconferencing facilities. We divide video communication in telemedicine into video-conferencing and telepresence.

Video-conferencing (VC) is defined as a real-time, live, interactive program in which one set of participants are at one or more locations and the other set of participants are at another location. VC permits interaction, including audio and/or video, and possibly other modalities, between at least two sites (S.A.G.E.S, 2009). Using VC, technical requirements regarding quality are not usually very demanding.

Telepresence, on the other hand, widens the purpose of practice beyond pure communication and has clear requirements, mainly concerning the quality and control of the picture as well as time latency.

Surgery has entered the computer age with the advent of video laparoscopy. Magnified and computer-enhanced video image provided surgeons with better exposure and visualization of the abdomen (Ballantyne, 2002). However, a decade after the launch of the new technology it is still poorly accepted. Most laparoscopic procedures are difficult to teach and learn, in addition, the learning curve is very flat. Obvious weaknesses of new technology are: unstable camera platforms, limited motion of straight laparoscopic instruments, two-dimensional imaging and poor ergonomics for the surgeon. Since the introduction of video laparoscopic cholecystectomy, surgeons have speculated that computers, 3-D imaging, and robotics could overcome these pitfalls of laparoscopy (Satava, 2001).

2. Video-conferencing

Video-conferencing (VC) is a specialized form of telemedicine that uses technology to provide real-time visual and audio patient assessment. (Kitamura et al., 2010) Originally, VC was developed to connect physicians with patients located in isolated areas at which climatic or geographical conditions render provider or patient transportation difficult and costly (Sezeur, 1998), resulting in inequalities in patient care (Woottoon, 1999). Examples of VC practice in telemedicine are: interdisciplinary team meetings, teleconsultation, and tele-education.

2.1 Interdisciplinary team communication

Interdisciplinary teams (IDTs) are an essential aspect of modern organizational work and are an important facilitator in achieving positive, cost-effective outcomes in various organizational settings (Procter & Currie, 2004). Nowhere is interdisciplinary team communication more important than in health care settings, as the complex nature and demands of the health care work environments require the expertise and knowledge of differing individuals or specialists who can work together to solve multifaceted and complex patient care problems (Heinmann & Zeis, 2002). Research has demonstrated that interdisciplinary teamwork can improve the diagnostic and prognostic abilities of health professionals, more than individual health professionals working alone, and is also essential for the prevention of medical errors (Coiera & Alvarez, 2006).

Over recent years, there have been significant advances in the development of technologies that support teamwork (Kuziemsky et al., 2009). VC, as a tool for improving communication between different levels of health care, has been described regarding a number of surgical subspecialties (Fleissig et al., 2006).

Norum and Jordhoy published a study demonstrating the feasibility of VC for clinical and educational support between specialists at the University Hospital of North Norway and colleagues at the oncology and palliative care unit of the Nordland Hospital in Bodø, 300 miles apart. VC was a success for education and clinical case discussions with the remote oncologists in Bodø. During a 12-month period, 32 VCs were performed and this study demonstrated that telemedicine can be used for incorporating a remote palliative care unit into a university department (Norum & Jordhoy, 2006).

Dickson-Witmer et al. recently published a study of a VC network to discuss prospective patient management issues. Information was shared on a weekly basis regarding the discussion of treatment decisions and diagnostic procedures. VC led to an increase in National Cancer Institute treatment and the accrual of cancer control clinical trials (Dickson-Witmer et al., 2008).

Three studies have been published on the experiences of breast cancer surgeons participating in IDTs. VC was compared to previous face-to-face clinical meetings through questionnaires, attendance, number of cases discussed, and anthropological analysis. Multidisciplinary case discussion can thus be facilitated by VC (Augestad & Lindsetmo, 2009).

Kunkler et al. proposed a comprehensive methodology to assess the clinical and economical effectiveness of VC in IDTs (Kunkler et al., 2005). This methodology was later tested in a randomized breast cancer trial (Kunkler et al., 2007), where 473 IDT patient discussions in two district general hospitals were cluster randomized to the intervention of telemedicine linkage to breast specialists in a cancer center, or to the control group of "in-person" meetings. VC was cost-effective, and breast cancer IDTs had clinical effectiveness similar to that of standard "in-person" meetings (Kunkler et al., 2007).

There is a shortage of thoracic surgeons in the United Kingdom, and IDT meetings by VC were therefore introduced. The telemedicine meetings saved more than three working weeks of thoracic surgical time during the year (Davison et al., 2004).

IDT meetings are used for establishing diagnoses; for tumor, node, and metastasis (TNM) classification; and for treating patients with head and neck tumors. In a Swedish study, telemedicine was introduced to link a regional hospital to two of the three district general hospitals. The conclusion was that costs could be saved by carrying out IDT meetings by means of telemedicine, instead of face-to-face meetings (Stalfors et al., 2005).

A recent report on cancer services in Wales recommended an integrated cancer service using VC as a clinical tool. Regular IDT meetings reduced the need for patients to travel. They also increased access to expert opinion and reduced any delay in implementing treatment (Axford et al., 2002).

2.2 Teleconsultation

Expert consultation has been a key element of medical knowledge development and decision making for ages. In modern times, consultation is frequently needed for interpretation of diagnostic images. This is particularly important when dealing with rare diseases (e.g., congenital anomalies) or complex multidisciplinary conditions that require special management (Gackowski et al., 2010). Teleconsulting or telementoring has been accepted as a possible answer to upcoming higher quality demands by utilizing expert knowledge in everyday clinical routines (Seemann et al., 2010). In the case of complicated surgical procedures with limited training capabilities, teleconsulting has opened up new perspectives in surgery. Furthermore, intraoperative teleconsultation can support continuous training and medical education, which is of great importance in minimally invasive procedures, which require very specific knowledge and expertise (Seemann et al., 2010).

Nowadays, many small cardiology units perform cardiac catheterization procedures or echocardiographic examinations far from referenced cardiosurgery centers. Experienced cardiologists can solve most hospitalized patients problems, locally. In particular cases, however, consultation with a cardiosurgeon is mandatory for optimal decision making (Gackowski et al., 2010). From a patient care perspective, medical patient consultations via video conferencing are now frequently used within the domains of dermatology, cardiology, wound-care, neurology, drug screening, diabetic training, and psychiatry (Krol, 1997).

Video Consultation is considered useful for the following reasons (Ibrahim & Fahim, 2009):

- e-doctors on health sites via video conference offer easy and almost immediate access.
- being unable to access an expert because of living in a rural area. It is often difficult for patients in rural areas to travel to large cities to seek medical advice in a tertiary hospital. As a result, it is quite common for serious medical conditions to be diagnosed at a later stage.
- Patients may require further counselling when the treatment given to them at their first visit has failed.

The technology used to perform teleconsultation can range from a simple telephone, fax, or email, to satellite-based relay transfers, up to state-of-the-art computer and videoconferencing facilities (Angood, 2001).

In Brisbane, Australia, home-based speech treatment for Parkinson's disease is delivered remotely (Constantinescu et al., 2010). The telerehabilitaion system is able to capture high quality video (640 x 480 pixel resolution) and audio, compressed at 384 kbit/s for later examination. A 128 kbit/s internet connection is being established between two videoconferencing systems using the public telecommunications network (ADSL). This connection enables videoconferencing at 320 x 240 pixel resolution between two systems.

According to study performed by Constantinescu et al., patients achieve substantial improvements in vocal sound pressure levels during sustained vowel phonation, reading, and conversational monologues. Improvements are also perceived in the degree of breathiness and roughness in the voice, and in overall speech intelligibility during conversation. Patient are very satisfied with the audio and video quality of conferencing, and with online treatment overall.

Telepsychiatry is becoming another specialty viewed as a reasonable alternative to office visits. Patients can be assessed, given psychological treatment, and prescribed medications from a distant site (Diamond & Bloch, 2010).

Hyler et al. (Hyler et al., 2005) carried out studies on a project included in their metanalysis, where 25 patients aged 4 - 16 years were interviewed, once in-person, and once via telepsychiatry. They concluded that telepsychiatric interviewing produced the same quantity and quality of diagnostic information as I-P interviews. There are, however, concerns about using telepsychiatry in emergencies (Diamond & Bloch, 2010).

To date, studies on telepsychiatric assessment have relied exclusively on superiority-design comparisons of diagnostic reliability and comparability with in-person assessments, and have accepted the null hypothesis that there are no differences between assessment methods (Diamond & Bloch, 2010).

In Vienna, Austria, Seeman et al. have been working on a tele-endoscopy project using UMTS cellphones where arthroscopic video streams with lengths of 60 s for each sequence, showing endoscopic arthroscopies of the temoporomandibular joint or endoscopic assisted open reductions in mandibular head fractures, are hosted on a server and analyzed on a UMTS cellphone. Each of the arthroscopic video sequences are independently evaluated by two consultants and a medical expert in temporomandibular joint (TMJ) surgery. UMTS, the third generation and most recent telecommunication standard was developed for a more efficient use of existing frequency resources and, on the other hand, the need for a higher data transfer rate, and can thus be used to transmit videos (Horn et al., 1999). In this project all video streams are encoded in the H.263 standard with resolution of 176 x 144 pixels and a selected bandwidth of 56 kbit/s. The experiences of the 20 arthroscopic video streams showed that use of UMTS technology permits the transmission of video streams in the field of craniomaxillofacial surgery. Recognition of corresponding diagnoses, anatomy or arthroscopic situations had been observed at a high level. With the development of new technologies such as highspeed downlink packet access (HSDPA), higher data transfer rates than UMTS technology (currently 384 kbit/s) become possible (see chapter 4.1. for technical details). Also, the higher quality of mobile phone displays may contribute to image quality (i.e., higher colour depth and higher resolution) (Seemann et al., 2010).

The digitization and transmission of real-time ultrasound images remains a major technical challenge. Bandwidths of about 70-100 Mbit/s are required to transmit ultrasound without compression. For this reason, teleultrasound has lagged behind other teleradiology applications. The vast majority of current teleultrasound systems rely on video compression, usually based on motion-compensated discrete cosine transforms (MC-DCT)(Chen et al., 1996).

Video compression predominantly causes a loss of high frequency data, distortion/displacement and alteration of pixel intensities/grey scale. There are currently no standards for teleultrasound image quality. The DICOM radiology image standard does not extend to video sequences apart from the storage of sequences as separate images, which is often impractical. There is, therefore little provision for the storage or transmission of ultrasound, ¯uoroscopy, angiography or cine MRI. An effective standard for storage and transmission of ultrasound images is required for ultrasound to follow the rest of imaging into the digital age (Burgul et al., 2000).

In Kuala Lumpur, Malaysia, a TeleUlstrasound was developed in response to the absence of a digital system, which enables the sharing of ultrasound images and data among radiologists, doctors, clinics, laboratories, and other medical officers who require this sort of data remotely, at any location in the country or the world. This system provides a Web interface with remotely accessed ".Net" Solution Imaging and Diagnostic, distributed application over the Internet for accessing and viewing information, while a Structured Query Language (SQL) database is deployed for data storage management. The ".Net" Solution technology enables a web-based distributed interface, which is server- and platform-independent across a network, without requiring preinstallation and tedious networking configuration. After log-in through a website this system determines the role specified by admin to the logged physician, and then directs the physician to his homepage, where he can view and examine the patient assigned to him and add his diagnosis. Patients can also log-in; however, this is limited to certain functions, such as viewing his diagnosis and updating his personal information (Hassan & Ibrahim, 2010).

In Krakow, Poland, Gackowski et al. developed Internet-based TeleDICOM software to make the teleconsultation of medical images possible. Interactive consultation between two or more centers offers real-time voice communication, visualization of synchronized Digital Imaging and Communications, and the use of interactive pointers and specific calculation tools. If direct interaction between physicians is not needed, the system can also be used in "offline" mode. This system is used for routine referral for cardiosurgical procedures (Gackowski et al., 2010).

According to Gackowski et al. an optimal teleconsultation system should fulfill the following theoretical requirements:

- Sending and receiving of high-resolution DICOM images, from all available medical imaging modalities
- Fast, real-time synchronized view of DICOM images and clips in 2 or more teleconsultation centers, avoiding delays during image loading
- Live voice interaction of all participants
- Availability of mouse-controlled pointers for real-tim e indication of a region of interest to other teleconsultation partners
- Integrated fully automatic calibration of the diagnostic images, measurement tools and calculations for all available imagistic modalities
- Secure and authorized access to medical data
- Compatibility with standard computers and networks
- Intuitive and easy to operate software
- 24-h availability and stability of the system
- Low cost

2.3 Tele-education

Telehealth applications are increasinlgy important for graduate and postgraduate education in the health professions, professional certification and recertification, contuniung medical eduacation, and health education for consumers and patients. Realizing telehealth's broad potential, for example, in telelearning, telemonitoring, telesurgical planning environments, telerobotic surgery, and teleconsultation, will allow forward-looking institutions to teach anything, anytime, anywhere with the same quality of curriculum and mentorship as delivered in traditional classroom settings, focusing on competence mastery rather than information mastery (Conde et al., 2010).

In India, the majority (70%) of medical experts live in the big cities. Thus, about 16% of the world's population, who reside in the rural areas of India, remain devoid of quality health care (Mahapatra et al., 2009). Therefore, telemedicine and tele-education in health science, is gradually becoming adopted by the Indian Health System after decade-long pilot studies across the country. Sanjay Gandhi Postgraduate Institute of Medical Sciences (SGPGIMS), a tertiary-level academic medical center, has been piloting distance medical education projects using telemedicine technology. The SGPGI Telemedicine Program uses various high-bandwidth communication networks, including satellite-based communication, leased lines through a terrestrial fiberoptic network, and ISDN, to connect district hospitals in rural and remote areas, medical colleges, and tertiary-level hospitals for medical knowledge exchange. From Spetember 2001 to March 2002, SGPGIMS conducted a distance medical education program for postgraduate students of the SCB Medical College, through ISDN. In March 2003, permanent satellite communication links for point-to-point connectivity were provided at three medical colleges in Orissa, along with an advanced video-conferencing platform (Singh et al., 2004). Tele-education activities were carried out by four departments (Endocrine Surgery, Gastrointestinal Surgery, Gastronenterology, and Endocrinology) with AIMS, Kochi, which is on the southern coast of India located 2.500 km away. The Department of Urology at SGPGIMS started a virtual clinical grand round with their peers in two premier institutions of the country, located 800 km away, and through point-to-multipoint connectivity. SGPGIMS also established a connection with Ranguel University, Toulouse, France, the Holy Family Hospital, Rawalpindi, Pakistan and the Oregon Health and Science University, Portland, Oregon, through high-bandwidth ISDN. Between September 2001 and April 2009, a total of 1.303 tele-educational sessions were carried out at SGPGIMS for the training and teaching of students, medical teachers, and practising doctors (Mishra et al., 2004).

During the process of establishing an effective national tele-educational system, Conde et al. give eight essential recommendations:

- Increase support for research in key areas including scalable, online, on-demand computional models for simulation that can be accessed from low-end computers; simplified software and hardware interfaces; software frameworks, artificial intelligence applications; remote 3-D visualization techniques.
- Support for collaboratory centers to disseminate the use of telehealth technologies in training, education, and research
- Creation of a Palpable Human Project.
- Establishment of national resource centers on virtual surgical trainers that focus on the development and testing of surgical simulations for training and education.
- Facilitation of bandwidth access to underserved areas and institutions through high-speed networks.

- Implementation and provision of access to dynamic circuit networks technology.
- Collaboration with professional societies in setting standard guidelines for the simulation of medical procedures.
- Accelerating the development of telehealth tools for biomedical, translational, and clinical research

3. Telepresence

Telepresence in general means projecting virtual images of the operative field to remote sites (Satava, 1998). By using a telerobot to telecast their hand-motions to a remote operating room, surgeons perform operations without actually being with their patients (Ballantyne, 2002). Telerobotics was first developed with grants from the US Department of Defense to allow surgeons at remote locations to operate on wounded soldiers on the battlefield (Satava, 1995). Telepresence surgery offers a technological solution to surgical manpower shortages in remote and underserved areas. Moreover, it offers a means of improving outcomes for infrequently performed and technically-demanding operations.(Ballantyne, 2002).
Examples of telepresence practice in telemedicine are: surgical telementoring, teledermatology, teleophtalmology, teletrauma, and emergency telemedicine.

3.1 Surgical telemonitoring

Telemonitoring is is an active process and comprises the ability to guide, direct, and interact with another health care professional (in this case, a surgeon) in a different location during an operation or clinical episode. The level of interaction from the mentor can be as simple as verbal guidance while watching a transmitted real-time video of the operation (Challacombe, 2010).
Surgery is, most of all, a visual specialty. Live pictures provide detailed information about anatomic landmarks, giving the mentor instant information about the patient's normal anatomy and pathological structures. Based on this instant information, the mentor can give advice to the operating surgeon and immediately correct his or her surgical actions (Augestad & Lindestmo, 2009).
Telementoring requires a secure high-speed connection with sufficient bandwidth to transmit a good picture and audio quality to the mentor's station. It has been shown that surgeons are generally able to compensate for delays of up to 700 ms, but delays over 500 ms are quite noticeable (Fabrizio et al., 2000). If using an ISDN connection, a bandwidth of 384 kB per second is needed to give sufficient picture quality for accurate interpretation by the mentor, although clinical work has been carried out using bandwidths as low as 128 Kb per second (Rosser et al., 1999).
There is a knowledge gap between central and local hospitals, which is even more problematic in mainly rural countries, with community surgeons dispersed in remote corners of a large country (Anvari, 2007). The introduction of VC as an educational tool has led to a decrease in this knowledge gap. Until recently, the only proven technique for teaching surgeons new skills was one-site mentoring completed with hands-on course training and conferences. However, because of an overwhelming need for mentors/proctors and supporting evidence in the literature, telementoring is an application whose time has come (Augestad & Lindsetmo, 2009).
In order to illustrate the potential of telementoring in remote environments, a laparoscopic cholecystectomy was telementored from Yale University to a mobile surgery unit in Ecuador

(Rosser et al., 1999), and in urology the Johns Hopkins team, in collaboration with an Italian group, successfully telementored remote surgeons in laparoscopic nephrectomy (Micali et al., 2000).

More recently, a renal transplant surgeon who was a relative novice at laparoscopy was able to initiate independent hand-assisted laparoscopic donor nephrectomy by means of telementoring from an expert. Early results appeared to show that telementoring can significantly shorten the learning curve (Challacombe et al., 2005).

The Johns Hopkins group successfully telementored a laparoscopic varicocelectomy and a percutaneous renal access for percutaneous nephrolithotomy between Baltimore and Sao Paulo, Brazil (Rodrigues et al., 2003). The remote surgeon controlled the laparoscope via an Automated Endoscopic System for Optimal Positioning (AESOP 3000, Intuitive Surgical, Inc., Sunnyvale, CA). This group has now carried out telesurgical telementoring in more than 17 cases using AESOP or the Percutaneous Access to the Kidney robot (PAKY, Johns Hopkins University, Baltimore, MD) (Bove et al., 2003).

Besides the postgraduate tele-education mentioned in the Video-conferencing section, SGPGIMS also focuses on the training of medical professionals, and skill transfers by telemonitoring. The first successful experiment was carried out in 2004 when parathyroid surgery was done under expert guidance from SGPGIMS (Pradeep, 2006).

3.2 Teledermatology

The use of telemedicine has been described regarding many medical specialties, mainly for those in which imaging interpretation is a key step for diagnostic purposes. Dermatology is a specialty with a significant visual component, in a particularly favorable field for using of telemedicine. The application of teledermatology (as the use of telemedicine in dermatology is named) has been studied mainly as a form of distance medical care, modality known as teleconsultation. The use of teledermatology for distance consultation may be classified into two main groups. In the modality store-and-forward-system data referring to distance consultation, once sent, are stored in a database and are accessed after a variable time interval. In this modality, communication between the agents involved in the process occurs in a synchronic way. Digital photos of cutaneous lesions are usualy acquired under artificial light (fluorescent light). Images are then transferred from the camera to the computer using a USB cable, and stored in JPEG format (*Joint Photographic Experts Group*).

On this issue, Seidenari *et al.* demonstrated that there was no significant difference in diagnostic accuracy between uncompressed images (tagged image file format, TIFF) and compressed ones (JPEG), showing that a factor 30 for compressed videomicroscopic images enables a good diagnostic accuracy (Seidernari et al., 2004). Files are then transmitted over telecommunication networks via e-mail or a specific web application.

In 2003 a pilot study of the dermoscopicpathological approach using telediagnosis for melanocytic skin neoplasms revealed that the diagnostic accuracy reached 83% *versus* gold standard (conventional histopathological diagnosis by experts) (Ferrara et al., 2004). In a prospective analysis, where 60 patients were included in evaluating the role of teledermatology within a primary care system, the total agreement rate between live diagnosis and distant diagnosis was considered high, ranging from 86. 6% to 91.6%. When considering partial agreement, the figures went up to 98.3% - 100% (Silva et al., 2009).

Sharing images and comments on a given case together with other colleagues has been an incredible new tool and available for a few years on the net (www.telederm.org). This project is based on an Open Access Philosophy and a freely available teleconsultation service. On-line registration and password-protected log-in are needed. Once logged-in, users are immediately guided to the forum, which is characterized by high usability. Two moderators check the properties of the requests and contents. Dermatologists from all over the world can both see cases posted by other colleagues and express on-line their opinions on given cases or they can seek advice on their own patients. Cases are directly submitted to the discussion forum, and world class experts in that field answer the requests. To date, several hundred users have subscribed and over 2300 requests have been processed, each request received being on average, about 4 comments. Each day new cases are submitted and commented on (Massone et al., 2010).

In some countries (i.e., New Zealand, Great Britain, the USA) a striking disparity between the dermatology workforce and the demand for melanoma screening has led to the commercialization of "teledennoscopy" by different companies. A patient arrives at a center to have pictures taken by a nurse or medical photographer who is trained by a dermatologist on how to capture the best images. This procedure obtains a detailed description of each lesion at both the clinical and dennoscopic levels. The nurse is trained to ask the patient a series of questions about his/ber skin and uses a low imaging threshold to avoid missing important lesions. Images and data are sent electronically to expert dennoscopists (teleconsultant) in a STF fashion. The dermoscopist's report, with provisional diagnosis and recommendations, is returned to the patient for self-monitoring purposes or to the patient's primary care providers, or both, for referral for excision (Psaty & Halpern, 2009).

Modem PDAs and 3G mobile phones revolutionize the dimensions of data transmission, network coverage, and the number of pixels. As a result, technical limitations can be reduced to a minimum (Massone et al., 2008).

A preliminary study demonstrates the feasibility and the potentiality of mobile teledermoscopy as a triage system for pigmented skin lesions (Meystre, 2005).

Mobile teledermoscopy brings advantages for both physicians and patients. The former easy-to-use and lightweight tools that allow the rapid acquisition of suspected pigmented skin lesions images. These can be stored in a digital archive for follow-up control or dermoscopic-pathologic correlation, or sent to expert colleagues for a second opinion. This methodology only needs a new-generation cellular phone with a built-in camera, a dem1atoscope suited for image acquisition, and a personal computer (Massone et al., 2010).

In fact, one of the cardinal points of the e-Health program of the European Commission Information Society and Media is the prevention and management of diseases through research on "Personal Health Systems". The hallmark of this concept is to empower citizens to adopt an active role in managing their own health status and, in addition, to facilitate early diagnoses of diseases (Massone et al., 2007).

In this context, mobile teledermatology and mobile teledermoscopy have the potential to become practical tools for everyone and may open the door for a new flexible triage system for the detection of skin cancer in general, and melanoma in particular. A high risk melanoma patient could be given a suitable modern cellular phone with an in-built digital camera and dermatoscope. In this way, suspected lesions could easily be followed-up using digital mobile teledermoscopy. Patients could be alerted *via-SMS,* reminding them of their mole-check e-visit (Massone et al., 2009).

3.3 Teleophtalmology

Teleophtalmology is an entity of telemedicine mostly used for screening retinopathy in diabetic patients. Throughout Canada, for example, diabetic retinopathy is common, with a prevalence up to 40% in people with diabetes (Ross et al., 2007). Up to a third of patients with diabetes do not receive an annual dilated eye examination by an ophthalmologist, despite universal access to health care (Tennant et al., 2007). In an effort to improve access, a teleophtalmology program was developed to overcome these barriers to eye care.

In the teleophtalmology program, Alberta patients undergo stereoscopic digital retinal photographs following pupillary dilation. Digital images are then packaged into an encrypted password-protected compressed file for uploading onto a secure server. Images are digitally unpackaged for review as a stereoscopic digital slide show, and graded with a modified Early Treatment Diabetic Retinopathy Study (ETDRS) algorithm. Reports are then generated automatically as a PDF file and sent back to the referring physician (Ng et al., 2009).

Teleophthalmology programs in Alberta have assessed more than 5500 patients (9016 visits) to date. Nine hundred and thirty patients have been referred for additional testing or treatment. Approximately 2% of teleophthalmology assessments have required referral for in-person examination due to ungradable image sets.

Eye assessment by teleophthalmology, when compared to a screening examination, is according to NG et al. beneficial for three reasons (Ng et al., 2009):

- *Unnecessary referrals are reduced or eliminated.* As an example, diabetes patients with diabetic retinopathy need only be referred once they develop proliferative diabetic retinopathy (PDR) with high-risk characteristics or clinically significant macular edema (CSME).
- *Following treatment, patients can be followed up at a distance without the need for further travel.* For example, having undergone focal laser treatment for CSME, a patient can be followed up by teleophthalmology and only requires an in-person clinical evaluation should they need re-treatment.
- A comprehensive teleophthalmology examination enables the consultant to plan for necessary testing and treatment at the time of a patient's first visit. As an example, if a patient is found to have elevated intraocular pressure and enlarged cup-to-disc ratio, a visual field and diurnal tension curve can be ordered for the day of the patient's clinical referral. The teleophthalmology visit becomes the first contact visit with the patient, while the second "office" visit enables the ophthalmologist to review the findings of diagnostic testing and make expedient management decisions.

3.4 Teletrauma and emergency care telemedicine

When applied to trauma, surgery and emergency care medicine, telepresence makes it possible for an experienced trauma surgeon or other specialist to assist or direct another less-experienced physician and/or surgeon who is operating or attending a patient at a distance. In order for true telepresence to be perceived by all participants, and thus have successful telepresence, it should have technology that creates an environment that mimics flawless motion, audio and video transmission (Latifi et al., 2007). In its nature, trauma requires fast, definitive and precise care, as well as major resources and continuous expertise. Trauma systems and major trauma centers have been shown to reduce mortality and morbidity (Trunkey, 2003), however, most trauma specialists and trauma centers around the world are concentrated within urban settings (Branas et al., 2005). Subsequently, most of the population of the world is not covered by specialized trauma systems. Advanced technologies such as computers, diagnostic imaging, robotics, voice-activating machines, and remote controls have changed operating theatres in hospitals around the Western world (Latifi et al., 2007).

The first published example of true telesurgery was a transrectal ultrasound (TRUS)-guided prostate biopsy performed by Rovetta in Italy but due to the costs and complexity of the robotic procedure the benefits of telesurgery were outweighted (Rovetta & Sala, 1995).
The Arizona Telemedicine Program which uses broadband T1 line allows trauma surgeons to have video, audio and vital signs access to events unfolding in trauma and emergency rooms in remote emergency sites. This helps to guide physicians or nurses taking care of patients by being »virtually« present at the remote location (McNeill et al., 1998).
In 2002, a collaboration between Johns Hopkins (Baltimore, MD) and Guy's Hospital (London, England) resulted in the first randomized controlled trial of telerobotic surgery (Challacombe et al., 2003) The group compared human with robotic and trans-Atlantic telerobotic percutaneous needle access using a validated kidney model into which a Kellet needle (Rocket Medical, Washington, England) was inserted 304 times. Half the insertions were performed by a robotic arm and the other half by urological surgeons. Order was decided randomly except for a subgroup of 30 Trans-Atlantic robotic procedures that were controlled by a team at Johns Hopkins via four ISDN lines. The robot was slower than the human but was more accurate both locally and remotely compared with human operators, as it needed less attempts for successful needle insertions (Challacombe et al., 2010).
The possibility of true telesurgery arrived in the late 1990s with the introduction of the da Vinci and Zeus master–slave robotic systems. The surgical telerobot, which is positioned by the side of the patient, holds the camera and manipulates two or more surgical instruments. The surgeon and computer console can be positioned at the remote site. The surgeon acts as the »master« and the robot as the »slave« (Challacombe et al., 2010).
In 2005, Colonel Noah Schenkman of the Walter Reed Army Medical Center performed live telesurgery (nephrectomy on two pigs) at the American Telemedicine Association, Washington, DC. (Hanley et al., 2005). This was the first telesurgery using the da Vinci surgical system, the first procedure to use stereoscopic surgical video streaming, and the first telesurgery over the Internet (Challacombe & Wheatstone, 2010).
Anvari et al. (Anvari et al., 2005) established a remote surgical service between Hamilton, Ontario, Canada, and North Bay General Hospital (North Bay, Ontario, Canada), some 400 km away. Using the Zeus system communicating through a redundant Internet protocol virtual private network (VPN) at a bandwidth of up to 15 MB per second, the authors reported on 21 cases, including Nissen fundoplications and anterior resections. The transmission latency was 140 ms, and the surgeon adapted to this easily. More recently, the da Vinci system has been modified and enabled for use over the Internet as well (Challacombe & Wheatstone, 2010).
The Level I trauma center of the City of Tucson, Arizona, the University Medical Center, in collaboration with Tucson Fire Department and Tucson Transportation Department launched Wireless Mobile Telemedicine and Telepresence in a prehospital setting by having video, audio, and data access from 17 Advance Life Support (ALS) ambulances of Tucson the Fire Department (TFD) since August of 2007. The City of Tucson Emergency Room Link or "ER-Link Tucson" project allows physicians to be virtually present at the scene and/or in the ambulance, while the patient is being transported to the trauma centre (Latifi et al., 2007). Through ER-Link, medical doctors at Tucson's University Medical Centre can use video and vital information telemetry to gain a sense of the severity of a patient's condition. This is achieved by viewing and in some cases speaking, to patients in real time from Tucson Fire Department ambulances en route to the hospital. All of the Department's 17 ambulances have been equipped with the ER-Link system. This system allows for constant

two-way audio-video and near-constant medical data transmissions between ambulance personnel and the trauma and emergency room personnel. The communications are provided via regional traffic control and city communications infrastructure and wireless technology. Telepresence at the scene of an event is made possible from cameras mounted externally to the emergency vehicle. These cameras, in conjunction with the existing highway cameras (operating along the freeways or at intersections) provide command and control video to the regional 911 centres and emergency departments (Latifi et al., 2007).

The clinical accuracy of telemedicine in evaluating trauma patients was assessed, when telemedicine was used for minor trauma consultation and compared with face-to-face consultations in two hundred patients. Skin-colour changes were accurately defined in 97%, the presence of swelling or deformity in 98%, diminished joint movement in 95%, presence of tenderness in 97%, weight bearing and gait 99%, and radiological diagnosis was made correctly in 98% of cases (Tachakra et al., 2000). This application of telemedicine can make expert trauma care available to patients in hospitals and emergency rooms without advanced trauma systems, and potentially reduce costs, prevent unnecessary transfers, and promote early transfer when indicated.

Telemedicine tools have also been applied to the field of wound care management where the sensitivity of remote diagnosis ranges from 78% for gangrene to 98% for identification of problem wound-healing respectively, whereas specificity ranges from 27% for erythema to 100% for ischemia (Wirthlin et al., 1998).

Telemedicine will become a major tool in trauma care and trauma education. Trauma resuscitation can be performed successfully and safely using telemedicine principles, when guided by and under direct supervision of a trauma surgeon (Latifi et al., 2007).

4. The technology aspects of telemedicine

Using up-to-date technology is of crucial importance for telemedicine. This can be divided into two main elements (Austerberry, 2005):

- *Peripherals,* digital video cameras, microphones, speakers, monitors or even special equipment such as digital microscopes with built-in digital cameras, video endoscopes, ultrasound imaging devices.
- *Transmission of voice and video signals,* where transmission is regarded as a process of sending, propagating and receiving an analogue or digital information signal over a physical point-to-point or point-to-multipoint transmission medium, either wired, optical fibre or wireless. The core technology used in transmission systems, especially audio and video signals, is the digital compression of audio and video streams in real-time.

4.1 Peripherals

In order to transfer images over a distance, a digital video or still camera is needed for capturing, and for visualisation on a screen. There are several different industrial standards for such devices depending on the purpose and image quality required by such a device. The quality of the image the camera is able to capture and transfer to another device, such as the monitor, depends on the components from which it is built. The digital camera generally consists of three elements: lens, image sensor, and electronics for the image processing, encoding, and transmission of the image. It is important that the individual elements are properly aligned. The industry is able to produce high-quality cameras of extremely small sizes. They are used for example, in installed endoscopic devices. Cheap or simple camera models can be used in simple application devices for teleconferencing. It is important that the camera has the option to focus on an image automatically in the case of moving objects or entities in space. Autofocus systems rely on one or more sensors to determine correct focus. Simple camera models have a built-in single sensor to capture images. The brightness of the image is automatically adjusted by the electronic circuit. Such cameras are often used for remotely controlling a patient during surgery, for teleconsulting (as mentioned in 2.2.), and to transfer images from the operating room to the classroom for students.

Camera image quality depends on the size and resolution of the image sensor (a device that converts an optical image to an electrical signal). The image sensor consists of millions of special type transistors sensitive into light integrated on one chip. Today, the industry uses two types of image sensors for cameras: CCD (charge coupled device) or CMOS (complementary oxide semiconductor). Both technologies have advantages and disadvantages regarding image quality. Image quality is usually delivered by a resolution image, which is expressed in pixels. Examples of standard image sizes are: 320x240, 640x480, 720x576, 720x480, 1440x720, and 1920x1080. Some high-end still-camera models can capture at a resolution of 8984x6732 pixels.

The quality of the integrated lens is of great importance. They are divided into fixed focal length lenses and zoom lenses, where the focal length of the lens is changeable. In general, fixed focal length lenses overall give better image quality and they allow for capturing images under critical low-light conditions. Additional lighting is provided under low-light conditions.

A 3-CCD camera is used instead of single chip CCD for better picture quality. 3-CCD imaging system uses three separate charge-coupled devices, each one taking separate captures of red, green, or light blue. Light coming into the lens is split by a prism, into the separate wavelength lights (R-red, G-green, B-blue) which are then directed in CCD sensors. The captured image is next processed in the electronic camera module and occupies a certain memory space. A video clip includes a sequence of successive 25p (progressive) or 50i (interlaced) captured images, the quantities of data being measured in Mbs. The volume of data transfer (and storage space) affects the number of pixels in the individual image frame, and the number of captured images in each second. Normally, the non-compressed data amount from a CCD sensor is too high for transmission. Compression reduces the number of bits used to represent each pixel in the image. Codec's (compression/ decompression algorithm) is used for the compression process. Some of the more frequently used video codec's today are DV, MPEG1, MPEG2, MPEG4, DIVIX, and others. The goal of compression is clear: how to reduce the data amount as much as possible in order to keep the image/sound quality as high as possible.

Telephone lines are one of the media through which we can transmit video signals, but with some limitations. Data transfer is limited by the so-called bandwidth. The transfer of video via telephone links initially allowed a theoretical bandwidth rate of 56 kbit/s, and 128 kbit/s later for ISDN. Video transmission was limited to low-resolution image. The standard defines the screen sizes of the Common Intermediate Format (CIF) 352x288, and Quarter CIF (QCIF) to be of 176x144 pixels. The number of progressively-scanned frames transmitted each second was limited to 8 fps. After applying sophisticated DSP technology and by using a wider bandwidth, it was possible to achieve transmission data rated from 1.5 to 8 Mbit/s. Today technology allows for the transferring of high-quality video and audio data over extremely short delay times (latency). If there is no guaranteed fixed bandwidth, the latency can be extended. The problem of packet loss arises if there is no guaranteed fixed bandwidth. The video and audio become disjointed. This problem is solved by adaptive streaming technology. In the case of network saturation, the ratio of video compression increases and vice versa. Once the network is re-released, the volume of data transferred can be increased again. The alternative to a copper or fibre connection is a microwave connection. This could be a satellite. Very small aperture satellite antenna offer one or two-way connection links to the internet. In Europe this service is offered by the Astra satellites. This service includes point-to-point (fixed or portable stations), point-to-multipoint (star configuration), and meshed networks.

The next alternative to fixed lines is to use wireless communication, through cellular networks covering large territories. Mobile networks have a long way to go before achieving a fixed wired transmission capacity, but they have two advantages mobility, and availability. The second-generation digital phones were limited to about 14 kbit/s data rate. The third-generation (3G) offers a theoretical data rate up to 2.4 Mbit/s. In both Europe and the wider world these is great anticipation about the introduction next-generation networks (NGN), including the important place occupied by the next-generation of mobile networks (NGMN).

In Europe there is already intense transition from analogue to digital TV. The switchover from analogue to digital terrestrial TV will free-up an unprecedented amount of spectrum in the 800 MHz field - the Digital Dividend. Allocating some of the Digital Dividend spectrum to mobile broadband will allow mobile operators to provide broadband services to everyone, even in rural areas.

International Mobile Telecommunications (IMT) includes a set of standards for a variety of multimedia mobile networks (EDGE, UMTS, DECT, WiMAX). Different standards (HSDPA, HSUPA, HSP+, LTE) allowing for transfer speeds up to 50 Mbs. For the fourth-generation network, ITU requires download transmission speeds of up to 1 Gbit/s.

How will all this technology help telemedicine?

Not long ago, mobile phones only had small screens with extremely low resolution. Today's cell phones already have a much larger screen with high-resolution, and development trends are moving in this direction continuously. Many of these mobile devices - also known as smart mobile devices (smart phones) also have touch screens and the ability to increase a certain part of the picture. Smart mobile phones with touch screen web browsers have a built-in big, high resolution screen, giving access to the Internet. This phone can also be used as a camcorder, because of the built-in camera. The qualities of built-in mobile phone cameras are constantly being improved, but they still lag behind traditional digital cameras.

4.1.1 Digital video camera

A digital camera (still or video) is a camera that digitally takes either video or still images or both, by capturing images via an electronic image sensor. Commercial digital cameras recording of a sound is standard. Digital cameras are incorporated into many devices ranging from PDAs to mobile phones. A digital camera can be divided into two segments, compact cameras and DSLR cameras. Both of them can be used for still image and/or video capturing. Both types of camera can be used for documentation and be directly connected via cable for the immediate transfer of stills or video to distance locations.

Images (stills) can be stored using lossy compression JPEG format. Many DSLR cameras, especially professional, support a RAW image format which is an unprocessed set of pixel data directly from the camera's sensor. The formats for movies are AVI, MPEG, MOV, and

WMV. The video resolution extends from 640x480 pixels to HD 1920x1080 pixels, with a frame rate from 15 to 50 fps. There are some commercially-available models with capturing speeds up to 1000 fps.
Many cameras store the pictures into memory cards. The more-widely used are SD memory cards having storage capacity from 128 MB, and up to 32 GB. Some DSLRs use SD and Compact Flash (CF) with storage capacities up to 128 GB of memory.
Digital still or video cameras use either a CCD image sensor or a CMOS sensor. The task of a sensor is the capturing of light and converting it into electrical signals. It is difficult to give advantage to either CCD or CMOS types of sensor. Some professional DSLR cameras with built-in CMOS image sensors are also widely used in professional video production. Cameras can capture video in HD resolution of 1920x1080 pixels by 25 fps, but they suffer against the rolling-shutter effect.
Professional video cameras are focused in order to provide high-quality video images. They can have either one single sensor or a triple sensor. Most of triple-sensor designed cameras utilize an optical prism block directly behind the lens. This prism block divides incoming light into the three primary colours, red (R), green (G), and blue (B), directing each colour into a separate CCD or CMOS image sensor mounted on each face of the prism (Austerberry, 2005). The cameras are able to produce a higher-resolution image, with better colour fidelity than is normally possible with just a single video pickup.
In both single-sensor and triple-sensor designs, the weak signal created by the sensors is amplified before being encoded into analogue signals for use by the viewfinder and monitor outputs, and also encoded into digital signals for transmission and recording. The analogue outputs are normally in the form of either a composite video signal, which combines the colour and luminance information into a single output; or an R-Y, B-Y, Y component video output through three separate connectors. Some special camera models for industry or medical use are very compact but also use 3-chip Full HDTV Camera head with various available outputs: 720p, 1080i and 1080p. The last sign i-interlace or p-progressive denotes either interlaced (the odd then even lines of image frame are scanned alternately) and progressive, where an image frame is scanned top-to-bottom over a pass. This interlaced manner is used for the reducing the amount of data. It was first designed for display on CRT televisions. Each picture is separated into two fields: the "top field," which has the odd numbered horizontal lines, and the "bottom field," which has the even-numbered lines. After reception/decoding, the two fields are displayed alternately with the lines of one field interlacing between the lines of the previous field. This format is called interlaced video; two successive fields are called a frame. The typical field rate is then 50 (Europe/PAL) or 59.94 (US/NTSC) fields per second (Austerberry, 2005). If the video is not interlaced, then it is called progressive video and each picture is a frame.

4.1.2 Displays
High-definition video displays are needed for medical applications when delivering accurate colour reproduction (dermatology). The monitor should display natural images with minimal ghosting. The screen format ranging from 15 ins up to 40 ins. It should deliver a 1929x1200 pixels HDTV quality with full colour (16.7 million) graduated reproduction. The brightness performance must be as high as possible. The ingoing signals to the monitor can be analogue or digital. It is useful to have robust interface connectors. Today's standard for input signals are composite signals, RGB signals, HDTV 1080 HD signal, and digitals HD-SDI or SD-SDI signals.

4.2 Transmission of voice and video signals

4.2.1 Video compression

Audio, video, and image signals require a vast amount of data for their representation. There are many reasons why the data must be compressed, such as large storage requirements, slow storage (playback in real time), and because of the network bandwidth (bottleneck) .

Compression reduces the number of bits used to represent each pixel in the image. The compression system exploits the mechanisms of human visual perception to remove redundant information, but still produces a compelling viewing experience. A video is a sequence of picture frames, usually 24 fps (film industry), 25 pfs (PAL video system) or 30 fps (NTSC video system). The most used compressing format for stills is JPEG, it is a lossy format based on technique called the discrete cosine transform (DCT) (Furht et al., 1995). A restoration procedure does not exist to present an original picture back from a JPEG. The standard supports different levels of compression. The compression of a single frame in video is called intraframe - compression within the frame. In a sequence of video images there is a little change from one picture to the next. Transmitting only the differences between successive pictures can produce a large reduction in video data. This procedure is called temporal or inerframe compression. It allows for 3:1 reduction over a interframe compression. Compression can be lossless or lossy. In lossless compression all original data can be retrieved. In video compression, where a higher level of compression is used, the lossless codec's would be insufficient. Most video compression is lossy. Video compression is a trade-off between disk space, video quality, and the cost of hardware required to decompress the video in a reasonable time. The human visual system has psycho-visual redundancy - not all visual information is treated with the same relevance. An example is lower accuracy to colour detail than luminance. A common practice for reducing the data rate is to "thin out" or sub-sample the two chrominance planes. In effect, the remaining chrominance values represent the nearby values that are deleted. This works because the eye better resolves brightness details than chrominance details. The 4:2:2 chrominance format indicates that half the chrominance values have been deleted, while the 4:2:0 chrominance format indicates that three quarters of the chrominance values have been deleted (Austerberry, 2005):. If no chrominance values have been deleted, the chrominance format is 4:4:4. The compressing codecs must be used for compressing the video. These codecs belong either to the international standards, open standards or proprietary standards. Some the most frequently used codecs are (Austerberry, 2005):

- *H.261 - videoconferencing codecs* formulated under the ITU for videophones and videoconferencing over ISDN lines. One of the demands of H.261 is the real-time operation. The standard defines screen size of CIF 352x 288 and QCIF of 176x144 pixels. It uses progressive scan and 4:2:0 sampling. Data rates from 64 kbit/s up to 2 Mbit/as are supported by the standard.
- *MPEG-1,* is the first standard by the multimedia community and is a standard for lossy compression of video and audio. This standard has long been used for audio and video presentations on CD-ROMs. It is designed for storage based applications at data rates of 1.5 Mbit/s. It does not support streaming.
- *H.263* - is developed from H.261 for low-bit rate applications. It solves the problem of operating at 28 kbit/s and can be used for videophone applications.
- *MPEG*-2 is a standard aimed at higher resolution (up to 40 Mbits/sec), a high-quality system for broadcasting television and intended to replace analog composite systems for digital transmission systems. It is also used for DVD recording systems.

- *MPEG-4* is a patented collection of methods defining the compression of audio and visual digital data. It is the first MPEG system to support streaming. The format is designed to support a wide range of bit dates, from 5 Kbit/s up to 50 Mbit/s. This allows it to low-bit rate wireless data through to HDTV applications.

4.2.2 Streaming the video over internet

The first task of the internet was delivering only data. The first audio and video applications used the Internet only as media for file transfer. A computer needed to download the complete file to the disk before it could play them. As soon as the slow analog telephone connections were replaced with xDSL, and with higher data transfer speeds, the delivery of multimedia files (especially video) in real-time over IP became a reality (Skalar, 2000). Streaming technology now allows playing of audio and video files immediately after being transmitted on the internet, in real-time. The User Database Protocol (UDP) instead of Transmission Control Protocol (TCP) is used for streaming technologies. The difference between the two protocols is how they check for errors. Streaming needs a transmission protocol that can ignore data errors.

One of the first applications used the real-time was video-conferencing. Video conferencing codecs started with H.261 followed by H.263 codecs and the latest advanced video codecs H.264. The time latency (propagation delay of audio and video signals) is an important factor in video-conferencing, especially in telemedicine. A webcasting system uses the same real-time protocols, where the latency of some seconds doesn't play a role. Another way to distribute audio and video files over IP is on-demand. The audio and video content is streamed on-demand whenever a client seeks for the content. This service is very popular in advertising, product and sales training, entertainment, Tele-education and medicine (as already mentioned in 2.3).

The streaming procedure can be realized in four steps:

- Microphone, Video camera: audio and video capture and encoding (compression)
- Server: storage and streaming
- IP Network: distribution
- Computer on site: Media player plays the content

Video cameras and microphones are used for capturing the audio/video. Most commercial models of video cameras already have built-in microphones. The microphone or surrounding noise level is too high for special occasions where the sound quality is of higher importance. In that case we need to set the microphones close to the speakers as much as possible; this eliminates the reception of disturbing surrounding noise. If there are more speakers in a larger room, we need one microphone, a lavaliere type, for each speaker. Lavalieres are small and lightweight microphones which do not disturb the speaker. The microphones are connected by wire, or are wireless, where the digital audio signal is radio transferred to the mixer station.

Many cameras are usually installed in typical surgical theatres. The outgoing signals from the camera (video/audio) can be analog or digital. It is preferable to use robust interfaces that use coaxial cable and connectors. Analog composite uses 75 Ohms coaxial with BNC connectors, but industry uses RCA connectors for consumer cameras. Many low-cost video monitors are only equipped with composite inputs, but professional monitors provide BNC connectors. The next analog video signal is S-Video or Y/C, which uses a small 4-pin connector. The IEEE 1394 (FireWire) is a IEEE Standard, and now widely used by many manufacturers to transfer digital video/audio (and remote control signals) data up to 800 Mbit/s. There are two versions of these connectors, a six-pin and a four-pin.

HDMI (High-Definition Multimedia Interface) is a compact audio/video interface for transmitting non-compressed digital data. HDMI connects digital audio/video sources such as video cameras, digital still cameras, computer monitors, and graphic computer interfaces. A video capture card installed in the computer converts analog or digital video and audio into the AVI format. Next, the video/audio file in AVI format is compressed with codec. Different codecs use several methods to compress the video. The result of this compression is smaller amounts of video/audio data, which reduces the need for the network bandwidth. The original audio/video data rate of a DV camcorder (where video in compressed 5:1) is 25 Mbit/s, and the data rate for studio video cameras can reach 350 Mbit/s.

4.3 3D Imaging technologies in medicine

Three-dimensional (3D) visualisation adds a new dimension to presenting video content. 3D has the ability to visualize human internal organs in their true form and shape (White, 2006). 3D Imaging technologies not only make is possible to visualize, but also to analyze and manipulate 3D structures from the captured 3D image. This is significant for a number of diagnostic and therapeutic applications. The importance of 3D technology is obvious. At the end of 2009, at the Radiological Society of North America's Scientific Assembly and Annual Meeting (NVIDIA and Siemens Healthcare) a new, 3D ultrasound viewing experience was demonstrated that enables expectant parents and their medical caregivers to view the fetus in incredible detail using 3D Vision-ready LCD, and NVIDIA 3D Vision glasses to demonstrate how patients and their doctors can view remarkable, high-resolution, three-dimensional sonograms in true 3D. Results of recent developments in three-dimensional screens give the possibility to presenting 3D video content, where special 3d glasses are no longer required. Efficient 3D content creation and media technology, such as VoD (Video on Demand), could all be in place within the next few years. We need new technologies for capturing or presenting images in 3D. Although stereoscopic vision was first presented in the 18th century, digital technologies have brought new extensions. In traditional stereo vision, two cameras, displaced horizontally from one another were used to obtain differing views of a scene, in a manner similar to human binocular vision. Although most image capturing cameras are based on a twin-lens system, the latest achievements of industry show a new professional camera which allows the recording of 3D images using just a single lens. We need double memory and special 3D camera/3D vision screens or glasses for 3D image visualisation. Glasses have always been seen as a major drawback to 3D on televisions. In order to visualise 3D images on 2D monitors, there are different technologies, such as anaglyph technology (anaglyph images are used to provide a stereoscopic 3D effect), polarisation technology, or auto stereoscopy technology.

5. References

Angood, PB. (2001). Telemedicine, the Internet, and world wide web: overview, current status, and relevance to surgeons. *World J Surg,* 25, 11, (Nov 2001) 1449–1457

Austerberry, D., (2005). *The Technology of Video&Audio Streaming,* Focal Press, ISBN-13: 978-0240805801, Burlinghton

Anvari, M., McKinley, C., Stein, H. (2005). Establishment of the world's first telerobotic remote surgical service for provision of advanced laparoscopic surgery in a rural community. *Ann Surg,* 241, 3, (Mar 2005), 241:460–464.

Anvari, M. (2007). Telesurgery: remote knowledge translation in clinical surgery. *World J Surg,* 31, 8, (Aug 2007) 1545-1550

Augestad, KM., Lindsetmo, RO. (2009). Overcoming distance: video-conferencing as a clinical and educational tool among surgeons. *World J Surg,* 33, 7, (Jul 2009) 1356-65

Axford, AT., Askill, C., Jones, AJ. (2002). Virtual multidisciplinary teams for cancer care. *J Telemed Telecare,* 8, Suppl 2, (2002) 3-4

Ballantyne, GH. (2002). Robotic surgery, telerobotic surgery, telepresence, and telementoring. Review of early clinical results. Surg Endosc, 16, 10, (Oct 2002) 1389-402

Bove, P., Stoianovici, D., Micali, S., et al. (2003). Is telesurgery a new reality? Our experience with laparoscopic and percutaneous procedures. *J Endourol.* 17, 3, (Apr 2003) 137-142.

Branas, CC., MacKenzie, EJ., Williams, JC., et al (2005). Access to trauma centers in the United States. *JAMA,* 293, 1, (Jun 2005) 2626- 2633

Burgul, R., Gilbert, FJ., Undrill, PE. (2000). Methods of measurement of image quality in teleultrasound. Br J Radiol, 2000 Dec;73(876):1306-12.

Challacombe, BJ., Kavoussi, LR., Dasgupta, R. (2003). Trans-oceanic telerobotic surgery. *BJU Int,* 92, 7, (Nov 2003) 678-680

Challacombe, B., Kandaswamy, R., Dasgupta, P., Mamode, N. (2005). Telementoring facilitates independent hand-assisted laparoscopic living donor nephrectomy. *Transplant Proc,* 37, 2, (Mar 2005) 613-616.

Challacombe, B., Patriciu, A., Glass, J., et al. (2005). A randomized controlled trial of human versus robotic and telerobotic access to the kidney as the first step in percutaneous nephrolithotomy. *Comput Aided Surg,* 10, 3, (May 2005) 165-171.

Challacombe, B., Wheatstone, S. (2010). Telemonitoring and Telerobotics in Urological Surgery. *Curr Urol Rep,* 11, 1, (Feb 2010) 22-28

Chen, W., Gupta, S., Turner, J. (1996). Motion-compensated discrete-cosine transform as the enabling technology for video conferencing and telemedicine. *Telemed J,* 2, 4, (Winter 1996) 313-7.

Chen, W., Turner, J., Crawford, C. (1996). The process of elimination: video compression in telemedicine. *Telemed, J* 2, 1, (Spring 1996) 36-41

Coiera, E., Alvarez, G. (2006). Interdisciplinary communication: An uncharted source of medical error?*Journal of Critical Care,* 21, 3, (Sep 2006) 236-242.

Conde, JG., De, S., Hall, RW., Johansen, E., Meglan, D., Peng, GC. (2010). Telehealth innovations in health education and training. *Telemed J E Health.* 16, 1, Jan 2010) 103-6.

Constantinescu, GA., Theodoros, DG., Russell, TG., Ward, EC., Wilson, SJ., Wootton, R. (2010). Home-based speech treatment for Parkinson's disease delivered remotely: a case report. *J Telemed Telecare.* 16, 2, (Dec 2010) 100-4.

Davison, AG., Eraut, CD., Haque, AS. et al. (2004). Telemedicine for multidisciplinary lung cancer meetings. *J Telemed Telecare,* 10, 3, (2004) 140-143

Diamond, JM., Bloch, RM. (2010). Telepsychiatry Assessments of Child or Adolescent Behavior Disorders: A Review of Evidence and Issues. *Telemed J E Health,* 16, 6, (Jun 2010) 1-5

Dickson-Witmer, D., Petrelli, NJ., Witmer, DR. et al. (2008). A statewide community cancer center videoconferencing program. *Ann Surg Oncol,* 15, 11, (Nov 2008) 3058-3064

Fabrizio, MD., Lee, BR., Chan, DY., et al. (2000). Effect of time delay on surgical performance during telesurgical manipulation. *J Endourol,* 14, 2, (Mar 2000) 133-138.

Ferrara, G., Argenziano, G., Cerroni, L. (2004). Cusano F, Di Blasi A, Ursa C *el* til. A pilot stUdy of a combined dermoscopic-pathological approach to the telediagnosis of melanocytic skin neoplasms. *J Telemed Telecare, 10, 1,* (2004) 34-8.

Fleissig, A., Jenkins, V., Catt, S., Followfield, L. (2006). Multidisciplinary teams in cancer care: are they effective in the UK? *Lancet Oncol,* 7, 11, (Nov 2006) 935–943

Furht, B., Smoliar S., W., HongJiang Z., (1995). *Video Image Processing in Multimedia Systems,* Kluwer Academic Publishersr, ISBN-13: 978-0792396048, Norwell

Gackowski, A., Czekierda, L., Chrustowicz, A., Cała, J., Nowak, M., Sadowski, J., Podolec, P., Pasowicz, M., Zieliński, K. (2010). Development, Implementation, and Multicenter Clinical Validation of the TeleDICOM-Advanced, Interactive Teleconsultation System. *J Digit Imaging,* (May 2010).

Hanley, EJ., Miller, BE., Herman, BC., et al. (2005). Stereoscopic robotic surgical telementoring: feasibility and future applications. 10th Annual Meeting and Exposition of the American Telemedicine Association, Denver, CO, April 2005. *Telemed and E Health,* 11, 2, (Apr 2005) 247

Hassan, A., Ibrahim, F. (2010). Development of a Kidney TeleUltrasound Consultation System. *J Digit Imaging.* (Apr 2010)

Heinmann, GD. & Zeiss, AM. (2002). *Team performance in health care: Assessment and development.* Heinmann, GD. & Zeiss, AM. (Ed.), Springer, ISBN: 978-0306467073, Kluwer

Horn, U., Stuhlmuller, K., Link, M., Girod, B. (1999). Robust Internet video transmission based on scalable coding and unequal error protection. *Signal Process,* 15, (Jul 1999) 77–94

Hyler, SE., Gangure, DP., Batchelder, ST. (2005). Can telepsychiatry replace in-person osychiatric assessmnets? A review and meta-analysis of comparison studies. *CNS Spectrums,* 10, 5, (May 2005) 403-413

Ibrahim, K., Fahim, S. (2009). Cooperative Remote Video Consultation on Demand for e-Patients. *J Med Syst,* 33, 6, (Dec 2009) 475-483

Kitamura, C., Zurawel-Balaura, L., Wong, RKS. (2010). How effective is video consultation in clinical oncology? A systematic review. *Curr Oncol,* 17, 3, (June 2010) 17-27

Krol,M. (1997). Telemedicine. *IEEE Potentials, 16*(4), 29–31, October/November. 1997

Kunkler, IH., Fielding, RG., Brebner, J. et al. (2005). A comprehensive approach for evaluating telemedicine-delivered multidisciplinary breast cancer meetings in southern Scotland. *J Telemed Telecare.* 11(Suppl 1), (2005) 71–73

Kunkler, IH., Prescott, RJ., Lee, RJ. et al. (2007). TELEMAM: a cluster randomised trial to assess the use of telemedicine in multi-disciplinary breast cancer decision making. *Eur J Cancer,* 43, 17, (Nov 2007) 2506–2514

Kuziemsky, CE., Borycki, EM., Purkis, ME., Black, F., Boyle, M., Cloutier-Fisher, D., Fox, LA., MacKenzie, P., Syme, A., Tschanz, C., Wainwright, W., Wong, H. (2009). Interprofessional Practices Team. An interdisciplinary team communication framework and its application to healthcare 'e-teams' systems design. *BMC Med Inform Decis Mak,* 15, 9, (Sep 2009) 43.

Latifi, R., Weinstein, RS., Porter, JM., Ziemba, M., Judkins, D., Ridings, D., Nassi, R., Valenzuela, T., Holcomb, M., Leyva, F. (2007). Telemedicine and telepresence for trauma and emergency care management. *Scand J Surg,* 96, 4, (2007) 281-9.

Mahapatra, AK., Mishra, SK., Kapoor, L., Singh, IP. (2009). Critical issues in medical education and the implications for telemedicine technology. *Telemed J E Health*, 15, 6, (Jul 2009) 592-6.

Massone, C., Hofmann-Wellenhof, R., Ahlgrim-Siess, V., Gabler, G., Ebner, C., Soyer, HP. (2007). Melanoma screening with cellular phones. *PLoS One*, 2, 5, (May 2007) e483

Massone, C., Wurm, EMT., Hofmalln-Wellenhof, R. (2008). Soyer HP. Teledemmtology: an update. *Sem Cut Med Surg*, 27, 1, (Mar 2008) 101-5.

Massone, C., Brunasso, AM. (2009). Campbell TM. Soyer HP. Mobile teledermoscopy-melanoma diagnosis by one click? *Semin Cutan Med Surg*, 28, 3, (Sep 2009) 203-5.

Massone, C., Brunasso, AM., Hofmann-Wellenhof, R., Gulia, A., Soyer, HP. (2010). Teledermoscopy: education, discussion forums, teleconsulting and mobile teledermoscopy. *G Ital Dermatol Venereol*, 145, 1, (Feb 2010) 127-32.

McNeill, KM., Weinstein, RS., Holcomb, MJ. (1998). Arizona Telemedicine Program. *J Am Med Inform Assoc*, 5, 5, (Sep 1998) 441–447.

Meystre, S. (2005). The current state of telemonitoring: a comment on the literatme. *Telemed J E Health*, 11, 1, (Feb 2005) 63-9.

Micali, S., Virgili, G., Vannozzi, E., et al. (2000). Feasibility of telementoring between Baltimore (USA) and Rome (Italy): the first five cases. *J Endourol, 14, 6, (Aug* 2000) 493–496.

Mishra, UK., Kalita, J., Mishra, SK., Yadav, RK. (2004). Telemedicine for distance education in neurology: Preliminary experience in India. *J Telemed Telecare*, 10, 6, (2004) 363-365

Mishra, S., Mishra, KC. (2006). Medical Informatics: An Exploration. Mishra, S., Mishra, KC. (Ed.), pp 4, ICFAI Books, ISBN: 81-314-0378-5, Hyderabad

Ng, M., Nathoo, N., Rudnisky, CJ., Tennant, MT. (2009). Improving access to eye care: teleophthalmology in Alberta, Canada. *J Diabetes Sci Technol*, 3, 2, (Mar 2009) 289-96.

Norum, J., Jordhoy, MS. (2006). A university oncology department and a remote palliative care unit linked together by email and videoconferencing. *J Telemed Telecare*, 12, 2, (2006) 92–96

Pradeep, PV., Mishra, A., Mohanty, BN., Mohapatra, KC., Agarwal, G., Mishra, SK. (2006). Reinforcement of endocrine surgery training: Impact of telemedicine technology in a developing country context. *World J Surg*, 31, 8, (Aug 2006) 1665-71

Pradeep, PV., Mishra, SK., Vaidyanathan, S et al. (2006). Telemonitoring in endocrine surgery: Preliminary Indian Experience. *Telemed J E Health*, 12, (2006) 73-77

Procter, S., Currie, G. (2004). Target-based teamworking: groups, work and interdependence in the UK civil service. *Human Relations*, 57, (2004) 1547–1572

Psaty, EL., Halpern, AC. (2009). Current and emerging technologies in melanoma diagnosis: the state of the art. *Clin Dermatol*, 27, 1, (Jan 2009) 35-45

Rodrigues Netto, N. Jr., Mitre, AI., Lima, SV., et al. (2003). Telementoring between Brazil and the United States: initial experience. *J Endourol*, 17, 4, (May 2003) 217–220.

Ross, SA., McKenna, A., Mozejko, S., Fick, GH. (2007). Diabetic retinopathy in native and nonnative Canadians.*Exp Diabetes Res*, 2007, (2007) 76271.

Rosser, JC. Jr., Bell, RL., Harnett, B., et al.(1999). Use of mobile lowbandwidth telemedical techniques for extreme telemedicine applications. *J Am Coll Surg*, 189, 4, (Oct 1999) 397–404.

Rovetta, A., Sala, R. (1995). Execution of robot assisted biopsies within the clinical context. *J Image Guid Surg,* 1, 5, (1995) 280–287.

S.A.G.E.S (2009). The Society of American Gastrointestinal and Endoscopic Surgeons (January 2009) Guidelines for the surgical practice of telemedicine; practice/clinical guidelines. http://www.sages.org/publication/id/21.

Satava, RM. (1995). Virtual reality, telesurgery, and the new world order of medicine. *J Image Guid Surg.* 1, 1, (1995) 12-16

Satava, RM. (1998). Transitionin to the future. *J Am Coll Surg,* 186, (1998) 691-692

Satava, RM. (2001). Surgery 2001: a technologic framework for the future. *Surg Endosc,* 7, 2, (Mar 2001) 111-113

Seemann, R., Guevara, G., Undt, G., Ewers, R., Schicho, K. (2010). Clinical evaluation of tele-endoscopy using UMTS cellphones. *Surg Endosc,* (May 2010).

Seidenari, S., Pellacani, G., Righi, E., Oi, NA. (2004. Is JPEG compression of videomicroscopic images ('Compatible with telediagnosis'? Comparison between diagnostic performance and pattern recognition on uncompressed TIFF images and JPEG compressed ones. *Telemed J E Health,* 10, 3, (Fall 2004) 294-303.

Sezeur, A. (1998). Telemedicine applied to surgery. *Ann Chir, 52, 5, (*1998) 403–11.

Sklar, B., (2000). *Digital Communications,* Prentice-Hall, Inc. , ISBN 0-13-084788-7, New Jersey

Silva, CS., Souza, MB., Duque, IA., de Medeiros, LM., Melo, NR., Araujo, CA., Criado, PR. (2009). Teledermatology: diagnostic correlation in a primary care service. *An Bas Dermatol,* 84, 5, (Oct 2009) 489-493

Singh, K., Mishra, R., Gujral, RB., Guptaq, RK., Misra, UK., Ayygari, A., Basnet, R., Mohanty, BN. (2004). Strenghtening postgraduate medical education in preipheral medical colleges through telemedicine. *Telemed E Health,* 10, (2004) S55-S56

Stalfors, J., Bjorholt, I., Westin, T. (2005). A cost analysis of participation via personal attendance versus telemedicine at a head and neck oncology multidisciplinary team meeting. *J Telemed Telecare,* 11, 4, (2005) 205–10

Tachakra, S., Lynch, M., Newsom, R. et al. (2000). A comparison of telemedicine with face-to faces consultations for trauma management. *J Telemed Telecarem,* 6, Suppl 1, (2000) Diabetes and eye disease in Alberta S178–181

Tennant, MT., Rudnisky, CJ., Johnson, JA. (2007). Diabetes and eye disease in Alberta. In: *Alberta diabetes atlas.* Johnson JA (Ed.), 95-113, Alberta Health and Wellness, ISBN: 978-0-9780024-4-2, Edmonton

Trunkey, DD. (2003). Trauma centers and trauma systems. *JAMA,* 289, 12, (2003) 1566–1567

White, R., (2008). *How Computer Work,* QUE Publishing , ISBN-13: 978-0-789-73613-0, Indianapolis

Wirthlin, DJ., Buradagunta, S., Edwards, RA., Brewster, DC. et al. (1998). Telemedicine in vascular surgery: feasibility of digital imaging for remote management of wounds. *J Vasc Surg,* 27, 6, (Jun 1998) 1089–1099

Wootton, R. (1999). Telemedicine and isolated communities: a U.K. perspective. *J Telemed Telecar,.* 5, Suppl 1, *(*1999) S27–34.

11

Telemedicine & Broadband

Annarita Tedesco[1], Donatella Di Lieto[2], Leopoldo Angrisani[3], Marta Campanile[4], Marianna De Falco[5] and Andrea Di Lieto[6]

[1]Telecommunications Engineer, Critical Infrastructure Expert, Scientific Collaborator, Dept of Computer Science and Control Systems, University of Naples Federico II
[2]Lawyer - Specialist in Legal Professions - Law of New Technologies and Communications
[3]Full Professor of Electrical and Electronic Measurements, Communication Systems and Networks Test and Measurement Expert, Dept of Computer Science and Control Systems, University of Naples Federico II
[4]Specialist in Obstetrics and Gynaecology - University High Professional Physician Operation Center of Conventional and Computerized Telecardiotocography – Medical School University Federico II of Naples.
[5]Specialist in Obstetrics and Gynaecology- PhD in Reproduction, Growth and Human Development - Head Physician - University Hospital Federico II of Naples.
[6]Full Professor of Obstetrics and Gynaecology - Director of Prenatal Unit - Responsible of Project of Telecardiotocography in Campania region - Responsible of European Project Conventional and Computerized Telecardiotocography - Medical School University Federico II of Naples.
Italy

1. Introduction

Advances in telecommunications and internet technology have greatly contributed to practically every aspect of our life. Medicine has taken a cue from this growing trend by combining telecommunications technology and medicine to create telehealth and telemedicine. Telehealth is "the practice of healthcare delivery using telecommunications technology including but not limited to diagnosis, consultation, treatment, transfer of medical data, education, dissemination of public health alerts and/or emergency updates". Telemedicine is "the use of telecommunications technology to deliver clinical diagnosis, services and patient consultation". Although different, for the purposes of this chapter telehealth and telemedicine are treated as one, and in the following referred simply to as "telemedicine" (Di Lieto et al., 2006), (Di Lieto et al., 2002), (Di Lieto et al., 2008).
There are two common types of telemedicine applications: "store-and-forward" and "real-time". Store-and-forward applications exploit the transmission of digital images from one location to another. A healthcare professional takes a picture of a subject or an area of concern with a digital camera. The information on the digital camera is "stored" and then "forwarded" by computer to another computer at a different location. This type of applications are utilized for non-emergent situations, when there's time for a diagnosis or consultation to be made, usually within 24 to 48 hours, with the findings then sent back.

Real-time applications come into play when the patient, along with his healthcare provider (a doctor or a nurse practitioner) and a telemedicine coordinator (or a combination of the three), gather at one site (the originating site), and a specialist is at another site (the referral site) which is usually at a large, metropolitan medical center. Videoconferencing equipment is placed at both locations allowing for a consultation to take place in "real-time". Almost all areas of medicine can benefit from this type of applications, including psychiatry, internal medicine, rehabilitation, cardiology, pediatrics, obstetrics, neurology and gynecology. Also, many different peripheral devices like otoscopes and stethoscopes can be attached to computers, aiding with an interactive examination (Khoumbati et al., 2010), (Hahm et al., 2009).

In Italy, the first application of telemedicine to prenatal medicine is represented by the TOCOMAT system of conventional and computerised cardiotocography and tele-ultrasonography. Cardiotocography (that is the simultaneous recording of the fetal heart rate pattern and of the uterine contractions during the second half of pregnancy) and ultrasonography are crucial for the assessment of fetal well-being, as expected by the modern prenatal medicine.

In its first version, born in 1998 at the University Federico II of Naples, the TOCOMAT network (Di Lieto et al., 2006), (Di Lieto et al., 2002) connected nine peripheral units located in small hospitals and consulting rooms in Campania, a region of Southern Italy, and two foreign units located at the Department of Obstetrics and Gynaecology of the Semmelweis University of Budapest (Hungary) and at the Hospital of Tripoli (Greece) [3]. The network Operation Centre is located in Naples, the regional capital, at the University Federico II. Peripheral units are equipped with a traditional cardiotocograph able to transmit via modem both fetal heart rate traces and data about patients to the Operation Centre. Transmission takes 40-60 seconds. At the Operation Centre, data are analysed by a software which provides the computerized analysis of the traces. Within few minutes, the computerized trace, together with the analysis and medical reports, is sent back to the peripheral unit by fax or by e-mail. Until December 2009, 3194 patients have been monitored with the TOCOMAT system, and about 10000 traces have been recorded and analysed. Admissions were efficiently planned, as a consequence of a continuous interaction between peripheral units and the Operation Centre.

Currently the main applications of Telemedicine fall within the conventional Telemedicine, which consists of connecting two different locations using a wired connection. This means that the conventional Telemedicine is not suitable for mobility, flexibility and portability. These three aspects encourage the use of wireless connections. When the Telemedicine equipment become mobile, flexible and portable, the chances of delivering a health consultation increase and are especially useful in case of emergencies. The availability of new technologies for the organization of wireless Telemedicine networks represents the ground of the recent updating of the TOCOMAT system, in order to allow intensive cardiotocographic monitoring of fetuses at risk independently from the mother and doctor location. In this way, the remaining space limitations related to the TOCOMAT network can be overcome.

In the updated version of the TOCOMAT network (Fig.1), each remote unit is equipped with a last generation, small, user-friendly cardiotocograph, able to transmit the traces and the data related to the patient and her pregnancy to a T-Mobile MDA GPRS Smart Phone using a Bluetooth wireless port. The Smart Phone is equipped with the software which allows receiving all signals coming from the cardiotocograph and sending them in real time to the Operation Centre. Moreover, the Smart Phone receives via e-mail the medical report and the report of the computerized analysis from the Operation Centre. This new system does not use a traditional telephone line for data transmission. So, it overcomes the considerable space limit of the old system, and could allow trace recording and transmission also of patients at home.

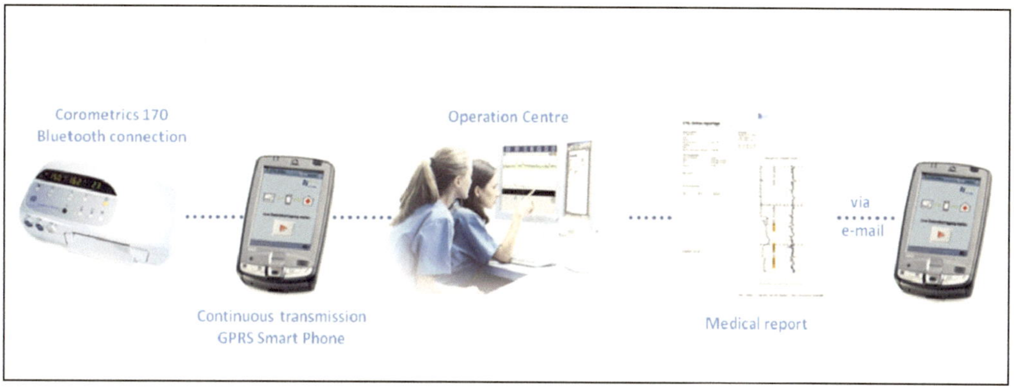

Fig. 1. Organization of the new TOCOMAT network for Telecardiotocography.

The new version of the TOCOMAT network also includes a Tele-Ultrasonography application (Fig.2). It is configured as a Mini-PACS system, able to manage ultrasound images, independently by the site where the patients have been examined (main hospital, remote hospital, patient's home, patient's bed, etc.). The Tele-Ultrasonography application of the TOCOMAT system consists of two workstations able to share ultrasound clinical data and images via Internet to the hospital network using a secure connection via VPN. Ultrasound scans are recorded using a portable last-generation scanner able to transmit the scans to the Operation Centre through a T-Mobile MDA GPRS Smart Phone using a Bluetooth wireless port. The availability of a portable scanner allows performing the examination independently from the location of the remote unit. Also for the Tele-Ultrasonography application of the TOCOMAT system, wireless networking is the milestone of the project.

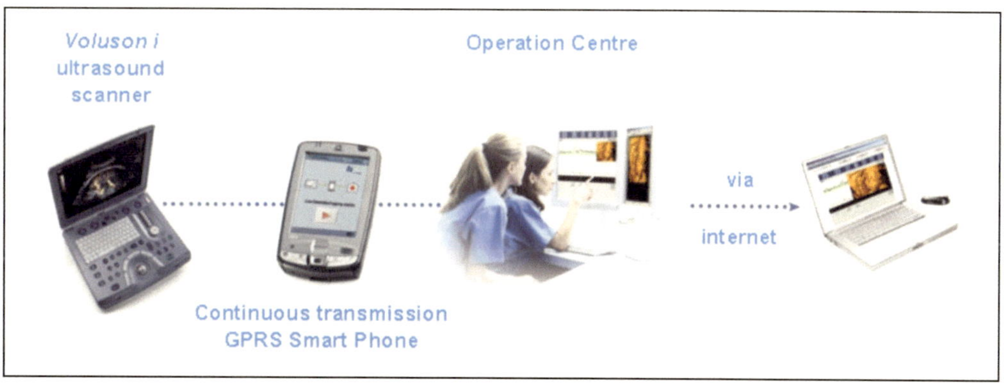

Fig. 2. Organization of the new TOCOMAT network for Tele-Ultrasonography.

Telemedicine has been a matter of research and convulsive generation of pilot networks and trials in all the world, all aiming to find the most appropriate solution and draw the economic model that could be of reference to define directives and guidelines which may help to provide remote medical cares. The aim of this chapter is to focus on some of the most significant broadband technologies, which can be of help to identify solutions addressing sustainable telemedicine service networks. The reader is given some highlights on the enormous growth and development that have characterized the telecommunication industry in this last decade, which has seen the domination of Internet, the IP protocols along with the new and much more economic broadband approach, allowing end users to access advanced network services in a much easier, faster and economic way, than some years ago. These events have opened new frontiers of interactive applications, related to data transmission, video and IP voice, originating new services, which one can find useful and comfortable for itself, but in a more general contest, are essential tools to improve social benefits and communities quality of life.

2. Benefits of telemedicine

The growing use of telemedicine is giving rise to a great number of benefits, which are in the following summarized from three different points of view: 1) Economic development and quality of life, 2) Patients, and 3) Providers (*Benefits of Telemedicine*, 2004), (Darkins & Cary, 2000).

2.1 Economic development and quality of life

- *Advancements in delivery of services*
  Certain health services can be greatly enhanced via telemedicine. For example, home health services are receiving a great deal of attention and investment in some states. Telemedicine technologies enable home health providers to redefine patient treatment plans, as they are able to increase patient visits due to elimination of a significant percentage of travel to patients' homes. Rural patients can now have access to specialists.
- *Keeping money in the local economy*
  Telemedicine helps provide service locally so people don't have to travel out of the community for care. Spending on health care is an especially significant portion of any economy, especially rural economies. The more the money that can be kept locally the better off the local economy will be. Standard economic multiplier effects also apply here; any money spent locally ripples through the local economy.
- *Aiding business recruitment and retention*
  Telemedicine provides the capability to deliver clinical services in the community. Locally available quality health care and quality schools are two important factors in the recruitment of new businesses, especially for businesses in rural communities. So there is a potential business recruitment and retention factor to consider.
- *Workforce development/jobs*
  There is a severe shortage of medical staff, particularly nurses, in rural hospitals. At the same time there is high poverty and unemployment in rural communities. One way to address that problem is to equip local healthcare facilities with advanced telecommunications services for telemedicine purposes and then to appropriately share the videoconferencing capability in a partnership with educational institutions to train

more local people for the jobs in health care that are available locally. Local jobs for local people could be a significant economic impact particularly for people who could not afford to travel outside the community for training.

- *Quality of life and longevity gains are worth a lot*
  Use of telemedicine can have a significant impact on individual health and can therefore favorably impact longevity. The value to the economy of improvements in life expectancy is about as large as the value of all other consumption goods and services put together. It is an intriguing thought to contemplate that the social productivity of health-care spending might be many times that of other spending.

2.2 Patient's perspective

- *Access to healthcare*
  Access to quality, state of the art health care in underserved areas, such as rural communities, is one of the most important promised benefits of telemedicine. Rural residents are not second-class citizens; they deserve access to health care services that those in metropolitan areas enjoy.
- *Saving time, travel, and other expenses*
  Telemedicine entails moving from a service delivery system in which patients (and often parent or guardian) physically travel from a rural area where they reside to an urban area to consult with a medical specialist, to a system in which the specialist consults with the patient and rural primary care provider using telecommunications facilities. An obvious opportunity is the potential for transportation cost savings.
- *Healthcare at home*
  Home care and community based health services are becoming an increasingly important part of the healthcare service continuum. There are many reasons for this including: patients are leaving hospital sooner and need some additional care at home while they recover, treating patients at home is less expensive than treating them in the hospital, many patients prefer to stay in their homes as long as possible before moving onto a higher level of healthcare service, e.g. nursing home, hospice.
- *Health provider integration*
  Improved collaboration between providers (e.g., shared access to electronic medical records and provider to provider consultations) provides patients with enhanced confidence that all that can be done is being done.

2.3 Provider's perspective

- *Emergency Room "front line" support*
  Instant access to information, whether it be about a certain patient or a certain topic, can be essential or even life saving.
- *Accuracy of diagnosis: reduction of medical errors*
  Reduction of medical errors is a huge concern for the medical community. Getting it right on the first try is obviously the preferred way of doing things. With "tele-assistance" (e.g., communication with specialists), it is hoped that it will be easier for a doctor to get a "second opinion" on their diagnosis of a patient. With greater access to help, more patients will be treated correctly, the first time. This leads to even more benefits, such as quicker average recovery time, less use of unneeded medicines, and reduced costs to patients and hospitals.

- *A multifold increase in efficiency*
  Travel times for patients and doctors could be significantly reduced as well as research time and "paper handling" of medical records (which can be unbearably slow). It has already been seen that telemedicine on foreign military bases has sped up the whole process of treatment for soldiers abroad. Consultations from major medical centers to the military bases make diagnosis quicker and more accurate. Telemedicine saves time over traditional "paper-based" data transfer.
- *Continuing Medical Education / Lifelong learning*
  Telemedicine can enhance educational opportunities for health care providers, patients, and families, improving clinical outcomes and reducing hospitalizations. The opportunity to participate in continuing education on the latest in medical advances without having to travel long distances saves providers time, money and minimizes air pollution.

3. Benefits of broadband

Governments around the world increasingly view broadband as the "fourth utility" alongside water, heating and electricity. The power of broadband has been confirmed by recent research, which shows that broadband fosters GDP growth, creates jobs and stimulates innovation, while also enabling improvements in education, health care and other social services. In particular "Broadband is not just an infrastructure. It is a general-purpose technology that can fundamentally restructure an economy" (*World Bank*, 2009).

To realize the many benefits of broadband, governments around the world are implementing comprehensive nationwide plans, as well as more tightly focused broadband programs. When combined with strategies that ensure the availability and affordability of ICT, these efforts help countries reap the benefits of broadband more quickly and provide broadband services to more citizens at an affordable price (*Realizing the Benefits of Broadband*, 2010).

3.1 Defining broadband

Broadband can be defined in many ways, but is generally understood to be a service that enables reliable, high-speed transfer of data, voice and video over the Internet. The connectivity afforded by broadband is an essential element in a larger effort to make ICT resources available, affordable and reliable for individuals and businesses worldwide.

Broadband speeds vary greatly depending on technology, location, applications and other factors. Because of this, it may be more helpful to focus on "acceptable broadband" speeds, which are the speeds necessary to meet the particular demands of any given market segment, such as schools, homes, businesses or medical centers. In emerging markets, download speeds during peak hours of at least 1 to 3 megabits per second (Mbps) should be granted to most citizens. Although this is currently an acceptable minimum, by 2012, developing countries should aim for much higher speeds of 3 to 6 Mbps, and up to 15 Mbps soon after 2012.

Broadband networks can be accessed through a variety of wired and wireless services, each of which offers unique advantages in speed, reliability and affordability. Wired, or fixed, broadband services (ADSL, cable, etc.) tend to be faster than wireless alternatives, but often cannot reach geographically remote areas. Wireless broadband networks, which can be accessed via cell phones, satellite, WiMAX and Wi-Fi signals, provide advantages in mobility and convenience. Users can access broadband services through a range of equipment, including desktop computers, notebooks, netbooks, tablets, cell phones and smartphones. The access speeds for these devices vary greatly, with download speeds as low as 200 Kbps for wireless, entry-level 3G cell-phone services. Other wireless broadband options such as WiMAX can deliver higher speeds, less latency, and in many cases, lower costs.

3.2 Why broadband?

Compared to narrowband connections, broadband networks provide unique benefits that enable emerging economies to enter and compete in world markets. When combined with other ICT resources, broadband delivers benefits including:

- *Ubiquitous access*
  Broadband networks are always on and always available for usage.
- *Enhanced multimedia applications*
  Broadband speeds enable ready access to online video content, interactive applications, gaming and other multimedia resources.
- *Cost reductions*
  Web browsing, e-mail and other online activities can increase labor productivity and lower the cost of gathering market intelligence.
- *Improved communication*
  Broadband networks enable real-time communication through e-mail, instant messaging, Voice-over-Internet Protocol (VoIP) and more, enabling businesses to communicate more frequently and at a lower cost with suppliers, customers and business partners worldwide.
- *Energy efficiencies*
  Broadband reduces travel demands and leads to lower carbon emissions and greater overall energy efficiency.

3.3 Economic benefits of broadband

For more than a decade, a variety of case studies, anecdotes and qualitative studies have detailed the economic benefits of broadband networks in developed economies. More recently, quantitative research and empirical analyses have gone further, firmly establishing the fact that broadband networks support GDP (Gross Domestic Product) growth and many other economic benefits in both developed and developing economies.

- *GDP growth*
  An analysis by the World Bank found that in developing economies, every 10 percent increase in broadband penetration accelerates economic growth by about 1.38 percentage points – more than the increase of 1.21 percentage points for developed economies, and more than the increases seen for other telecommunications services (Fig.3). Moreover, countries in the top tier of broadband penetration have exhibited 2 percent higher GDP growth than countries in the bottom tier.
- *Job growth*
  Along with its direct and positive impact on GDP, research has repeatedly shown that increased broadband penetration leads to significant job growth. In the United States, the Information Technology and Innovation Foundation estimates that a stimulus package spurring or supporting $10 billion of investment in broadband networks would support nearly 500.000 new or retained jobs.

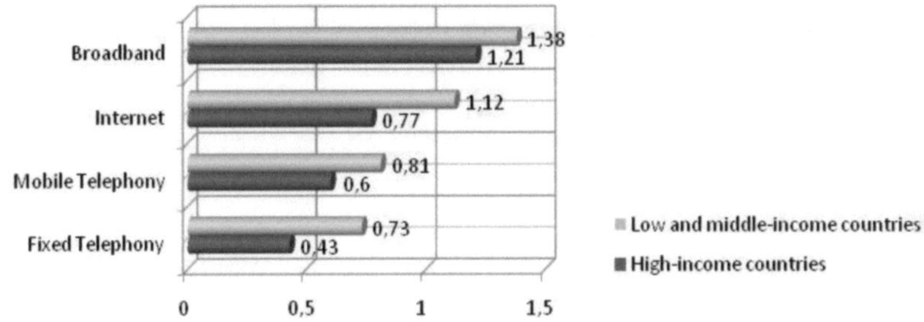

	Fixed Telephony	Mobile Telephony	Internet	Broadband
Low and middle-income countries	0,73	0,81	1,12	1,38
High-income countries	0,43	0,6	0,77	1,21

Fig. 3. Growth impact of telecommunications. (GDP percentage point increase due to 10 percentage-point increase in penetration).

- *Other economic benefits*
  Other proven economic effects of broadband include trade creation and facilitation, lower costs for international communications and greater access to foreign markets. Broadband can also help countries attract, train and retain a valuable "creative class" of workers, and the presence of broadband leads to new business models and new business opportunities to employ those and other workers.
  Mobile communications in general, and broadband in particular, have an especially strong impact on the economies of rural areas, which are home to nearly three out of four of the world's poor. Expanding broadband networks to rural areas leads to new opportunities for nonagricultural employment, better-paying agricultural jobs and greater overall productivity. Access to broadband also fosters small-business growth, allows citizens in remote areas to work from home, provides greater access to crop market prices and enables rural businesses to compete more effectively in world markets.

3.4 Social benefits of broadband

The social benefits of broadband are difficult to quantify, but they are nonetheless an essential part of the overall value of broadband. By connecting citizens to each other, as well as to businesses, governments and social services, broadband helps people become more informed and more active in their communities, leading to a better quality of life, and richer personal and business opportunities.

The benefits and opportunities broadband creates for all people, regardless of location, lifestyle or income, can help nations cross the digital divide. As broadband access becomes more available and less expensive, citizens and businesses in rural and remote areas can engage more directly in the national economy. Broadband is a cultural equalizer with the potential to allow all citizens to access essential government services and take advantage of new economic opportunities such as working from home.

Broadband networks also provide a more efficient and less expensive way to deliver essential public services such as health care, education, public safety and emergency services. Broadband-enabled telemedicine provides better access to specialized care, reduces unnecessary travel, and facilitates rapid diagnosis and treatment.16 Mobile health workers, who deliver health care to remote regions around the globe, often rely on mobile broadband to communicate their findings and patient concerns with regional clinics.

Although not broadband-specific, studies have shown that household Internet access is also associated with better educational performance. Numerous examples demonstrate that broadband-specific education creates valuable educational opportunities that can help countries develop a competitive, technology-literate workforce. Students with access to broadband connectivity become entrepreneurs, employers and employees with the skills and experience necessary to compete and succeed in the 21st-century global economy.

3.5 Telemedicine benefits of broadband

Broadband is entitled to play an increasingly important role in healthcare by enabling a universe of telemedicine services that, in turn, can provide a number of life-enhancing, and potentially lifesaving, benefits. The wide range of impacts that broadband is capable of producing on telemedicine can be summarized as follows:

- *Increase of range of healthcare*
  Broadband-enabled telemedicine tools can extend the range of healthcare to rural and unserved parts of a country, thus assisting in leveling the quality of care across all demographics and geographies. These tools can, for example, help to compensate for a lack of physicians in some rural areas.
- *In-home care made easier*
  The wide availability and increasing affordability of broadband can enable the use of effective in-home diagnostic, monitoring, and treatment services. Seniors in particular can benefit from these tools by having the ability to receive more care at home.
- *Streamlining of administration of healthcare*
  Health information technology (HIT) systems, especially electronic health records (EHRs), can create efficiencies in back-office operations and enable a number of cost-savings.
- *Enhancement of care for children, seniors and people with disabilities*
  Broadband-enabled telemedicine can provide effective and affordable care to rural and low-income children. Tools and services can be crafted for use by senior citizens and people with disabilities, leading to vast savings.

With healthcare costs soaring, broadband-enabled telemedicine offers policymakers, healthcare providers, and patients a set of tools that have the potential to drastically cut costs and enhance the quality of care. Moreover, broadband-enabled telemedicine services are expected to provide enormous benefits to rural users and to user groups that require more acute care. With the senior population expected to largely increase by 2050, and with senior care accounting for an extremely high percent of healthcare spending, broadband-enabled telemedicine holds much immediate and long-term promise for this user group in particular. However, intensive and efficient adoption and usage of broadband-enabled telemedicine services is poised to increase rapidly as the many barriers discussed in the last part of the chapter are eliminated by policy and cultural changes.

4. Broadband technologies

As the bandwidth revolution continues, the ever increasing completion in the broadband service market is forcing broadband service suppliers to plan their strategies for delivery of "triple play" services, with voice, data and video provided by a single connection. Over recent years, as the internet and intranets have evolved, increasing requirements for bandwidth intensive applications such as peer-to-peer file sharing and tele-working have resulted in relentlessly increasing demands for higher broadband bandwidth provisioning. However, it is the bandwidth required by next generation television and video services, such as video-on-demand (VoD) and, more significantly, high definition television (HDTV), which have recently begun to place the most pressure on bandwidth provisioning in broadband networks. Even with the latest data compression techniques, HDTV requires in the order of 15 to 20 Mpbs of downstream downlink and this is testing the capabilities of a number of broadband technologies (Solymar, 1999), (Huurdeman, 2003), (Angrisani et al., 2006), (Angrisani & Narduzzi, 2008), (*Broadband Technology Overview*, 2005).

There are a myriad of competing broadband technologies potentially capable of providing the bandwidth necessary to efficiently support telemedicine applications, but each technology has its limits in terms of reliability, cost or coverage. Optical fiber offers almost limitless bandwidth capabilities, has excellent reliability and is becoming increasingly economical to install. Consequently, fiber seems to be unsurpassed in its superiority over the other broadband technologies. However, many competitive copper and wireless technologies are developing at a significant pace and some technologies have so far managed to definitively meet the bandwidth requirements of typical telemedicine services.

In general, broadband solutions can be classified by two groups: fixed line technologies or wireless technologies. The fixed line solutions communicate via a physical network that provides a direct "wired" connection from the user to the service supplier. The best example is the plain old telephone systems (POTS), where the user is physically connected to the operator by a pair of twisted copper cables. Wireless solutions use radio or microwave frequencies to provide a connection between the user and the service supplier; mobile phone connectivity is a prime example (Bates, 2002), (Sauter, 2006).

4.1 Fixed line technologies

Fixed line broadband technologies rely o a direct physical connection to the user's (subscriber's) residence or business. Many broadband technologies such as cable modem, xDSL (digital subscriber line) and broadband powerline have evolved to use an existing form of subscriber connection as the medium for communication. Cable modem systems use existing hybrid fiber-coaxial Cable TV networks. xDSL systems use the twisted copper pair traditionally used for voice services by the POTS. Broadband powerline technology uses the power lines feeding into the subscriber's home to carry broadband signals. In general, all three aforementioned technologies strive to avoid any upgrades to the existing network due to the inherent implications for capital expenditure (*Broadband Technology Overview*, 2005).

By contrast, fiber to the home (FTTH) or fiber to the curb (FTTC) networks require the installation of a new (fiber) link from the local exchange (central office) directly to or closer to the user. Consequently, although fiber is known to offer the ultimate in broadband bandwidth capability, the installation costs of such networks have, up until recently, been prohibitively high.

The fixed line technologies described here include:

- *Hybrid Fiber Coax*: Cable TV – Cable Modems;
- *Digital Subscriber Line* (xDSL);
- *Broadband Power Line* (BPL);
- *Fiber to the Home/Curb.*

- *Hybrid Fiber Coax*: Cable TV - Cable Modems
  Digital cable TV networks are able to offer bi-directional data transfer bandwidth in addition to voice and digital TV services. Using a cable modem in the user premise and a Cable Modem Termination System (CMTS) at the network's head-end, the well established HFC standard, DOCSIS 1.1, provides for a data transmission service with speeds of up to a 30 Mbps on one 8 MHz channel (6 MHz is used in USA) using quadrature amplitude modulation (QAM) techniques. The successive HFC standard, DOCSIS 3.0, is nowadays capable of 100 Mbps of bandwidth per channel. Data transmission over Cable TV networks has the advantage that where the coaxial cable is in good condition and radiofrequency (RF) amplifiers exist (or can be installed) to extend the network reach, relatively high bandwidths can be provided to the end user without distance limitations. However, a cable TV broadband service relies on a shared network architecture (Fig.4); this results in the limitation that the amount of bandwidth delivered to the user is dependent on how many people share the connection back to the head-end. Typically, a service of 1 Mbps downstream and 128 kpbs upstream is offered (more recently a 3-5 Mbps downstream service has become available), but up to 1000 users may share the connection to the head-end and so the actual bandwidth obtained can be lower due to excessive loading of the system by other users.

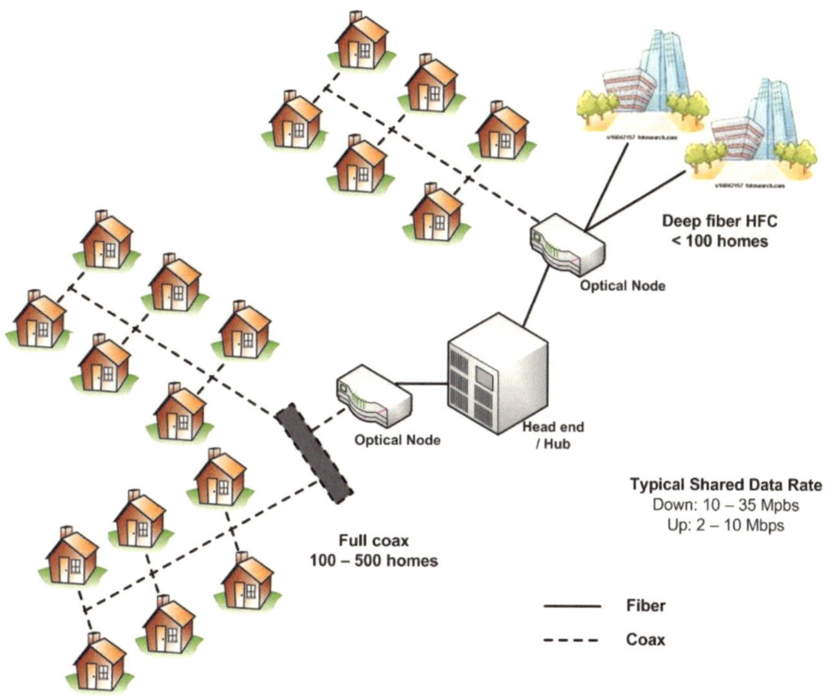

Fig. 4. Cable TV, Hybrid Fiber Coax (HFC) architectures.

- *Digital Subscriber Line (xDSL)*
  DSL delivers broadband to more people today than any other technology. Roughly two-thirds of all broadband subscribers are DSL subscribers, and there are more new DSL subscribers each month than new subscribers for all other broadband access technologies combined.

DSL is a technology that delivers broadband speeds over distances of miles or kilometers via copper wiring. DSL was originally delivered over the same wires that are used to provide traditional voice telephony services. These wires run from a telephone company's central office, the location where voice switching and other traditional telephony functions are performed, to the user's home or business. Increasingly, DSL is delivered from a device situated closer to the user's home or business that is connected to a central office via an optical fiber link, and then to the user's premises via copper wires. In all cases, however, DSL delivers broadband over the copper connections that exist already in almost every residence and business in the developing and developed worlds.

This architecture is depicted in Fig.5. At the central office, or at a remote location typically connected to the CO via fiber optics, there is a DSL Access Multiplexer (DSLAM) that sends and receives broadband data to many users via DSL technology. At each user's location, there is a modem (modulator-demodulator) that communicates with the DSLAM to send and receive that user's broadband data to and from the Internet and other networks. A DSLAM communicates with many individual modems. Each user's modem is dedicated to that subscriber's broadband connection.

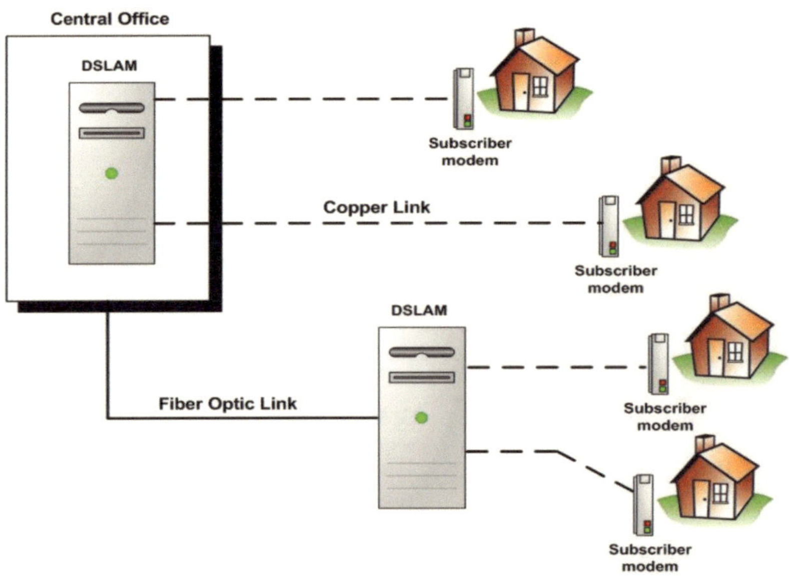

Fig. 5. DSL architecture

Voice services utilize only a small fraction of the total information carrying capacity of copper connections. In an analogous manner to Ethernet technology, which can transmit a Gigabit per second of data over copper connections or the equivalent of tens of thousands of simultaneous phone conversations, DSL exploits the information carrying capacity of copper lines to deliver broadband services over long distances.

To engineers, "DSL" means a set of formal standards for communicating broadband signals over copper lines. It also means equipment that complies with those standards. The principal DSL standards are published by the International Telecommunications Union (ITU), a standards body based in Geneva, Switzerland, that establishes standards for communications systems. Within the ITU, there is a division responsible for communications over copper, named the ITU-T, and a division responsible for communications using radio technology, known as the ITU-R. The ITU has several other divisions including one devoted to telecommunications in the developing world, known as the ITU-D.

DSL standards have evolved significantly since the first DSL standards were established in the early 1990's. The DSL standards have evolved to support higher data rates, to take advantage of advances in equipment technologies, and to ensure that DSL can coexist on copper lines with other communications standards such as Integrated Services Digital Network (ISDN), an early digital voice and data service that is still in use in many countries. Table I lists some of the principal DSL standards in use today (*ADSL Technology – Overview*).

Common Name	*Peak Speed*	*Standard*	*Deployment Status*
ADSL1	8 Mbps	ITU-T G.992.1	Pervasive
ADSL2+	24 Mbps	ITU-T G.992.5	Pervasive
VDSL2	50-75 Mbps	ITU-T G.993.2	Pervasive
Vectored VDSL2	120+ Mbps	ITU-T G.993.5	Standard complete, field use by 2011

1. "Mbps" means Megabits per second. A Megabit is a million of bits.
2. DSLAMs and Subscriber modems are capable of the peak speeds listed in the Table. Lower speeds may be delivered depending on the service packages offered by a subscriber's DSL provider, and also on the provider's network design and management practices.
3. There are several variants of the VDSL2 standard. The peak speed is dependent on the particular VDSL2 variant implemented by the DSL service provider.

Table I. Main DSL standards

With few exceptions, DSL technology is unique among broadband access technologies in that subscribers do not compete with one another for broadband access. Because each subscriber has their own copper connection to the DSLAM, all subscribers can achieve the peak speeds listed in the table above so long as the connection from the DSLAM to the Internet or other networks has adequate capacity. This is a significant advantage of DSL relative to other broadband access technologies where subscribers share a single physical connection, such as in a cable network, or a limited allocation of radio frequencies, such as in a 3G or 4G wireless network (*DSL Technology Tutorial*, 2010).

- *Broadband Powerline (BPL)*

BPL systems allow for high speed data transmission over existing power lines, and do not need a network overlay as they have direct access to the ubiquitous power utility service coverage areas. BPL systems are being promoted as a cost-effective way to service a large number of subscribers with broadband. In a BPL system, the data is transmitted over the existing power line as a low voltage, high frequency signal, which is coupled to the high voltage, low frequency power signal. The frequency transmission band has been chosen to ensure minimum interference with the existing power signal. Typical data rates in actual tests are 2 to 3 Mbps. Most BPL systems at present are limited to a range of 1 km within the low voltage grid, but some operators are extending this reach in to the medium voltage grid. Experience has shown that BPL requires a high investment cost, to upgrade the power transmission network and bypass transformers, to support high speed and reliable broadband services, like those peculiar to telemedicine. In addition, the frequencies used for BPL often interfere with amateur radio transmission, and some BPL experiments have consequently suffered considerable opposition. At present, given the cost and the lack of an upgrade path, it seems unlikely that BPL will emerge as a leading broadband technology, but will remain as a nice fixed-line broadband option (*Broadband Technology Overview*, 2005).

- *Fiber to the Home/Curb*

  FTTx is a generic term for those technologies that bring fiber a step closer to the user. However, not all fiber solutions in access networks bring the fiber directly to the home/subscriber. Some technologies in the access that rely on fiber, like VDSL, bring fiber from the local exchange (central office) down to a node in the access network or to the curb, where equipment is housed in a street cabinet to convert signals from optical to electronic, ready for the final hop to the subscriber over twisted copper pair. This level of fiber provision in the network would be called FTTC (fiber to the curb) or FTTN (fiber to the node). Other architectures include FTTB (fiber to the building) and FTTP (fiber to the premises), where the fiber is brought as far as the building and then distributed amongst the resident subscribers over twisted copper pair or using wireless technology. FTTH is the ultimate fiber access solution where each subscriber is connected to the optical fiber.

  As FTTH has matured, applications have converged on to two consensus solutions. Th first is the Passive Optical Network (PON).PONs have been described for FTTH as early as 1986. In this architecture, th main signal from the local exchange is passively split in such a way that it is shared by several subscribers (Fig.6). Privacy is ensured by time shifting, and personal encryption of each subscriber's traffic. Upstream traffic is enabled by Time Division Multiple Access (TDMA) synchronization. Fixed network and exchange costs are shared among all subscribers. The PON solution benefits from having no outside-plant electronics. This reduces network complexity and life-cycle costs, while simultaneously improving reliability.

  The second common FTTH architecture is a point-to-point (P2P) network, which is often referred to as an All Optical Ethernet Network (AOEN). In this solution, each home is directly connected by an optical fiber to the local exchange. This provides a dedicated line of connection to the operator for each subscriber, which is the main advantage of P2P networks over PONs. The dedicated connection lines of a P2P network facilitate subscriber specific service supply, higher subscriber bandwidth with improved traffic security, and simple provision of symmetric services. The P2P network architecture is similar to the common enterprise Local Area Network (LAN) design, and so has the advantage of being able to use existing components and equipment, which helps to reduce system cost. However, P2P networks require activities in the field, which can increase installation, operating and life-cycle costs and also reduce reliability.

Standards are established for both PON and P2P networks, and suppliers exist for both PON and P2P systems, offering either Asynchronous Transfer Mode (ATM) or IP/Ethernet transmission on either architecture type.
Current Ethernet PON (EPON) systems can operate at up to 2.5 Gbps over distances of up to 20 km. Even with the EPON bandwidth shared amongst 64 users, the bandwidth offered to the FTTH consumer can grealy outstrip anything achievable by cable services or ADSL2+ over a radial coverage area of 20 km. In addition, Wavelength Division Multiplexed PON (WDM PON) is being explored. This technology, by bringing a single optical channel to each subscriber (eliminating bandwidth sharing), will furher increase the bandwidth offered by PON systems (*Broadband Technology Overview*, 2005).

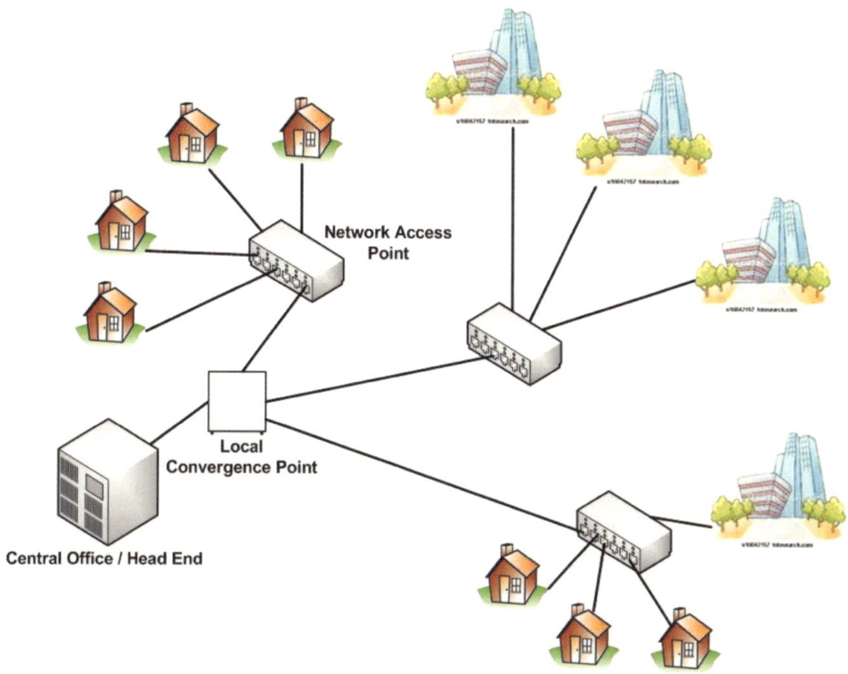

Fig. 6. Passive Optical Network (PON) architecture.

4.2 Wireless technologies

Wireless broadband generally refers to technologies that use point-to-point or point-to-multipoint microwave in various frequencies within 2.5 - 43 GHz to transmit signals between hub sites and an end-user receiver. While on the network level, they are suitable for both access and backbone infrastructure, it is in the access network where wireless broadband technology is proliferating. As a consequence, the terms "wireless broadband" and "wireless broadband access" are used interchangeably.
There is a wide range of frequencies within which wireless broadband technologies can operate, with a choice of licensed and unlicensed band. Generally speaking, higher frequencies are advantaged relative to lower frequencies a more spectrum is available at high frequencies and smaller antennas can be used, enabling ease of installation. Most higher bandwidth systems use frequencies above 10 GHz. However, high frequency systems are severely attenuated by poor weather conditions, and suffer from distance limitations.

Wireless technologies can be broadly categorized into those requiring line-of-sight (LOS) and those that do not. Point-to-point microwave and broadband satellite require line-of-sight for reliable signal transmission, while cellular technologies like UMTS, WiFi, WiMax require no line-of-sight between the transmission hub and receiving equipment. Clearly, the non line-of-sight technologies provide advantages in terms of case of deployment and wider network coverage (*Surfing into the Future*, 2007), (Webb, 1999), (Pahlavan & Levesque, 2005), (Arslan et al. 2006), (Schwartz, 2005).
The wireless technologies described here include:

- *Microwave links;*
- *Broadband satellite;*
- *UMTS-TDD* (Universal Mobile Telecommunication Access-Time Division Duplexing);
- *HSPA* (High Speed Packet Access);
- *Wi-Fi* (Wireless Fidelity);
- *WiMAX* (Worldwide Interoperability for Microwave Access).

- *Microwave links*
  Microwave links are the traditional workhorse of fixed-wireless broadband systems and were around long before the term wireless broadband was coined. It is the point-to-point LOS wireless transmission method for up to 155 Mbps, with a range of up to 5 km. Single channel microwave links are relatively inexpensive and simple to install. This is particularly true in areas of difficult (e.g. mountainous) terrain or of high population density where the installation costs of a traditional buried cabled network are prohibitively high. However, microwave networks have the great disadvantage of being limited by a very low data rate and are therefore of little use for high capacity links or for networks where it is essential to ensure that bandwidth capability is never outstripped by user bandwidth demand. Microwave capacity can be enhanced by installing more links, but deployment of additional links will soon push the overall cost of a microwave network to the point where it outstrips the cost of a much higher bandwidth traditional buried cables system. For networks with a low predicted capacity, microwave can be the lowest cost solution, but microwave will inhibit significant capacity expansion and in the longer term may result in lost business opportunity [20].
- *Direct Broadcast Satellite (DBS)*
  Primarily a direct-to-home digital TV broadcasting wireless solution, newer Direct Broadcast Satellite (DBS) services also provide two-way high-speed data transmission services. DBS uses geostationary satellites operating in the Ku band with a 12 GHz downlink and a 14 GHz uplink. Fig.7 shows the architecture of a DBS wireless broadband network, where the satellite relays the composite signal of digitized video and data services from a headend via an earth station and then broadcasts that signal to an area of targeted subscribers. Data rates within 16 – 155 Mbps can be obtained, but the major drawback is that geostationary satellites being 22300 km from the earth's surface introduce a 250 ms delay into the network. For most broadband services this latency is unacceptable. The use of a network of low-earth-orbit or LEOS satellites orbiting at only 1000 km will reduce this latency to 50 ms, but such systems are not widely available as yet. However, satellites, like all other systems using the radio spectrum, are limited in capacity by the bandwidth available. For satellites operating in the Ku band, there is a limit of 2 GHz of available bandwidth (*Surfing into the Future*, 2007).

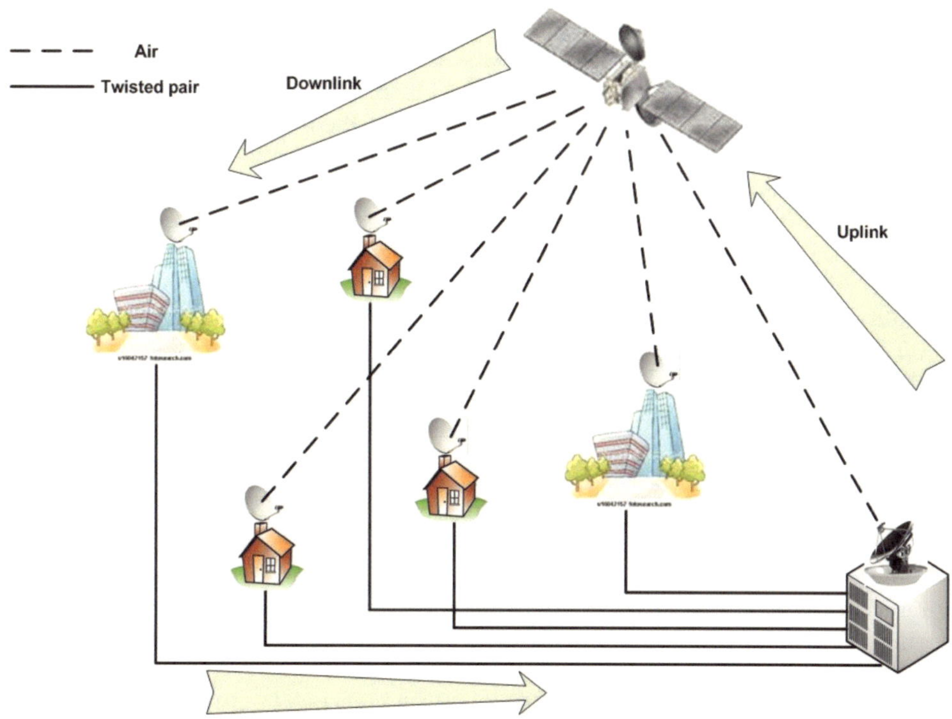

Fig. 7. Direct Broadcast Satellite (DBS) network architecture.

- *UMTS TDD*
  UMTS TDD uses Time Division Duplexing (TDD) and is a packet data based technology of the 3G (Third Generation) UMTS standard. It is being supported by the 3GPP alliance and is also known as Time Division-Code Domain Multiple Access (TD-CDMA). The technology has the advantage of having a larger user base, which includes the numerous operators across Europe and Asia, who use the IMT-2000 TDD frequencies of 1900-1920 MHz and 2010-2025 MHz. There is also the provision of operating in the 3.6 GHz licensed band.
  The peak downlink speeds are around 12 Mbps. UMTS TDD is one of three standards supported by UMTS that share the same higher layer protocol stacks (*Surfing into the Future*, 2007), (Holma & Toskala, 2006).
- *HSPA*
  HSPA (High Speed Packet Access) is the UMTS Forum's generic term for improvements in the UMTS Radio Interface in Releases 5 and 6 of the 3rd Generation Partnership Project (3GPP) standards, and represents the packet data service for the Wideband CDMA (WCDMA) standard. This means both improvements in the downlink allowing operators to increase throughput, often referred to as High Speed Downlink Packet Access (HSDPA), and in the uplink, often called High Speed Uplink Packet Access (HSUPA) but also called Enhanced Dedicated Channel (E-DCH).
  3GPP Release 5 (announced in 2003 and initially rolled out in 2005) introduced HSDPA. With HSDPA, WCDMA has been extended with additional transport and control channels, such as the high-speed downlink shared channel (HS-DSCH), which provides improved support for interactive, background and, to some extent, streaming services.

HSDPA enables speeds of up to a maximum of 14.4 Mbps, subject to network conditions. HSDPA is a software upgrade that doubles the air interface capacity of WCDMA networks and provides a 5 – 10 fold increase in downlink speeds of standard GSM/WCMDA networks. It enables users to access the Internet on mobile phones and PC notebooks, at speeds previously reserved for DSL. Release 5 also introduced the IP Multimedia Subsystem (IMS) architecture to enhance integrated multimedia applications and offer mobile operators a more efficient way of offering these services.

3GPP Release 6 provides for High Speed Uplink Packet Access (HSUPA) with increased speed up to 5.8 Mbps via a dedicated uplink channel, the second phase of IP Multimedia Subsystem (IMS), inter-working with Wireless Local Area Networks (WLAN), Multimedia Broadcast Multicast Service (MBMS), and Enablers for Push-to-talk (PoC).

The next phase of HSDPA is specified in 3GPP Release 7 and enhances Release 6 HSPA performance. Release 7's main priority is improved support and performance for conversational and interactive services such as Push-to-talk, picture and video sharing, and Voice and Video over IP (*Surfing into the Future*, 2007), (Holma & Toskala, 2006).

However, there is also a 3GPP vision of Long Term Evolution (LTE). The overall aim is to improve the capacity of the 3GPP system to cope with ever-increasing volumes of traffic in the longer term - over 10 years. The system needs to continually evolve to remain competitive in cost and performance versus the other mobile data technologies. LTE goals include:

- downlink peak data rates up to 100 Mbps with 20 MHz bandwidth;
- uplink peak data rates up to 50 Mbps with 20 MHz bandwidth;
- operation in both TDD and FDD modes;
- increased spectral efficiency over Release 6 HSPA by a factor of two to four;
- reduced latency.

- *Wi-Fi*

Wireless local area networks (WLANs) compliant with the family of IEEE 802.11 standards (also known as Wi-Fi standards) are nowadays one of the most successful emerging network technologies in the wireless communication scenario. They are commonly used to provide wireless access to the Internet and network connectivity for personal digital assistants, laptops, and modern consumer electronics. In particular, they are widely available worldwide, through thousands of public hotspots located anywhere, in millions of homes, factories, and university campuses.

A great interest in Wi-Fi technology is also rapidly growing in the field of real-time multimedia, for audio/voice and video streaming applications over a wireless link, like those peculiar to telemedicine. With regard to video streaming, although new applications are very likely to appear soon with upcoming WiMAX or DVB-H enabled devices, the research community is in-depth studying new protocols, able to make Wi-Fi apparatuses overcome some notable drawbacks, thus allowing them to satisfy the stringent real-time unicast and multicast requirements.

The family of IEEE 802.11 standards concerns wireless connectivity for fixed, portable, and moving stations within a local area. It applies at the lowest two layers of the Open System Interconnection (OSI) protocol stack, namely, the physical layer and the data link layer. The physical layer (PHY) essentially provides three functions. First, it interfaces the upper media access control (MAC) sublayer for transmission and reception of data. Second, it provides signal modulation through direct sequence spread spectrum (DSSS) techniques or orthogonal frequency division multiplexing (OFDM) schemes. Third, it sends a carrier sense indication back to the upper MAC sublayer, to verify activity in the wireless bandwidth. The data link layer includes the MAC sublayer, which allows the reliable transmission of data from the upper layers over the PHY media. To this aim, it provides for a controlled access to the shared wireless media, called carrier-sense multiple access with collision avoidance (CSMA/CA). It also protects the data being delivered through proper security policies.

The 802.11 family currently includes multiple extensions to the original standard, based on the same basic protocol and essentially different in terms of modulation techniques. The most popular extensions are those defined by the IEEE 802.11a/b/g amendments (also referred to as standards), on which most of the today's manufactured devices are based. Nowadays, IEEE 802.11g is becoming the WLAN standard more widely accepted worldwide. It involves the license-free 2.4GHz ISM band (2.4–2.4845 GHz), like the IEEE 802.11b standard, and supports a maximum data rate of 54 Mbps, like the IEEE 802.11a. IEEE 802.11g devices are backwards compatible with IEEE 802.11b ones. They use the OFDM modulation scheme for the data rates of 6, 9, 12, 18, 24, 36, 48, and 54Mbps and revert to complementary code keying (CCK, as in the case of the IEEE 802.11b standard) for 5.5 and 11Mbps and differential binary phase shift keying (DBPSK)/differential quadrature phase shift keying (DQPSK) + DSSS for 1 and 2 Mbps.

In the 2.4GHz ISM band, the IEEE 802.11g standard defines a total of 14 frequency channels, each of which is characterized by 22MHz bandwidth. In USA, channels 1 through 11 are allowed, in Europe channels 1 through 13 can be used, and in Japan only channel 14 is accessible. Due to the available bandwidth, channels are partially overlapped, and the number of nonoverlapping usable channels is only 3 in USA and Europe (e.g., channels 1, 6, and 11) (*Surfing into the Future*, 2007), (IEEE Standard 802.11, 1999), (Angrisani et al., 2010).

- *WiMAX*

  Worldwide interoperability for microwave access (WiMAX) is the latest wireless broadband technology that is designed to deliver Wi-Fi type connectivity over a much greater range, and thereby compete as a point-to-multipoint last-mile broadband wireless access solution. There are two types of WiMAX : line of sight (LOS) and non-line of sight (NLOS). The LOS WiMAX systems are point-to-point only, while the NLOS WiMAX are point to multi-point.

  Although the LOS systems have much better reach capabilities, they will not facilitate a large consumer service coverage area, and so it is the much shorter reach. Conversely, NLOS systems are being developed to offer an alternative large-scale consumer broadband service technology. WiMAX is based on the IEEE 802.16 standard and refers both to fixed-wireless and mobile broadband technology. WiMAX equipment suppliers aim to provide fixed, nomadic, portable and, eventually, mobile wireless broadband connectivity without the need for direct line-of-sight with a base station within a given sector cell. In a typical cell radius deployment of 3 to 9 km, WiMAX Forum Certified™ systems aim to ultimately deliver capacity of up to 75 Mbps per channel, for fixed and portable access applications. Mobile network deployments are aiming to provide up to 15 Mbps of capacity within a typical cell radius deployment of up to 3 km.

WiMAX System Type	Reach Capability	Max Downlink Bandwidth per Sector	Max Uplink Bandwidth per Sector	Downlink Bandwidth per CPE at Cell Edge	Uplink Bandwidth per CPE at Cell Edge
Standard					
LOS	10 - 16 km	8 - 11.3 Mbps	8 - 11.3 Mbps	2.8 - 11.3 Mbps	2.8 - 11.3 Mbps
NLOS	1 - 2 km 0.3 - 0.5 km (indoor self-install)	8 - 11.3 Mbps	8 - 11.3 Mbps	2.8 - 11.3 Mbps	2.8 - 11.3 Mbps
Full-Featured					
LOS	30 - 50 km	8 - 11.3 Mbps	8 - 11.3 Mbps	2.8 - 11.3 Mbps	2.8 - 11.3 Mbps
NLOS	4 - 9 km 1 - 2 km (indoor self-install)	8 - 11.3 Mbps	8 - 11.3 Mbps	2.8 - 11.3 Mbps	0.7 - 0.175 Mbps (assumes only one subchannel is used to extend to edge of sector cell)

Table II. Typical performance of current WiMAX systems

For NLOS systems, there is a further choice between indoor self-install or outdoor consumer premise equipment (CPE). The indoor self-install equipment will be favoured by the consumer market as it has the distinct advantages of simplicity of installation, but the reach is severely reduced as the signal is attenuated by the infrastructure of the building. There are also two grades of WiMAX network installations: standard and full-featured. Table II shows that the performance of WiMAX varies greatly and is a very complex function of the type of WiMAX deployed, be it NLOS or LOS, the user friendly indoor self-install or the outdoor equipment, a standard or a full-featured installation.

Table II shows that standard WiMAX equipment aims at delivering an upstream and downstream bandwidth per channel within 8 - 11 Mbps, but only over a range of 1 -2 km for NLOS operations. Equivalent indoor self-install WiMAX solutions aim to achieve similar bandwidths, but only over 0.3 – 0.5 km of range. The latest generation of full-featured WiMAX equipment aims at delivering a bidirectional bandwidth of up to 11 Mbp over 3 - 9 km with NLOS capability and the same bandwidth over a range within 1 - 2 km for NLOS indoor self-install applications (*Surfing into the Future*, 2007), (Angrisani & Napolitano, 2010).

5. Open challenges for broadband adoption in telemedicine

This part outlines the wide array of still open, policy and non-policy challenges to further adoption and usage of broadband in the telemedicine sector (*Barriers to Broadband Adoption*, 2009). As an overview, these challenges involve:

- *Outdated and fragmented privacy policies for the electronic transmission of health data;*
- *Lack of security standards for data generated from telemedicine services;*
- *Lack of standards to guide the interoperability of new telemedicine services;*
- *Negative perceptions and inadequate value propositions for using telemedicine services by patients;*
- *Costs/Evaluation/Outcomes.*

5.1 Outdated and fragmented privacy policies for the electronic transmission of health data

An outdated set of privacy policies that may not provide adequate protection to sensitive medical information is a challenge to more robust adoption and use of telemedicine services. Indeed, the security of personal health information is paramount to doctors and patients as more advanced telemedicine services and devices collect and transmit an increasingly large volume of medical data over the Internet. Although transferring personal health information electronically via e-mail or an EHR may be efficient, it raises important issues regarding the confidentiality of patient data and the possibility of private medical information being illegally viewed or stolen by a third-party. Privacy laws, however, have largely failed to keep pace with technological change and afford suboptimal protections for patients.

Patient medical data is generally protected by state law. To this end, most states have enacted laws of general applicability regarding the electronic transmission of health information. However, these were crafted in response to the mostly intrastate nature of many modern telemedicine services that have been launched and may be inadequate in a world where broadband-enabled telemedicine services allow for the transmission of health data in real-time manner across state lines and international borders.

5.2 Lack of security standards for data generated from telemedicine services

In addition to privacy challenges, there is a general lack of standards to ensure the security of medical data being transferred via the Internet.

The amount of data generated from telemedicine services is substantial. Indeed, telemedicine enables the use of devices such as video, audio, sensors, and various health meters to send patient information over a broadband network in real time. At a time when harmful content like spam and malware continues to threaten the general user experience, more robust policies that protect sensitive medical data are especially needed.

In addition, enhancing the security of networks could increase more regular usage of these services. Issues continue to arise when data is sent over an unencrypted network or is accessed by unauthorized personnel. A string of cyber-attacks against epileptic patients in 2008 is illustrative of how certain parts of the Web remain vulnerable to criminals who use networks to inflict harm. In one case, a group of hackers "descended on an epilepsy support message board used JavaScript code and flashing computer animation to trigger migraine headaches and seizures in some users." At first, the hackers "used a script to post hundreds of messages embedded with flashing animated gifs." However, subsequent attacks used a similar tactic to "redirect users' browsers to a page with a more complex image designed to trigger seizures in both photosensitive and pattern-sensitive epileptics." Other such attacks have targeted visually impaired users.

Other security concerns arise from the increased use of Wi-Fi networks for in-home monitoring. These types of networks tend to be less secure than wire-based ones, but their relative affordability and ability to interact with other wireless technologies (e.g., wireless sensors) have made them very attractive to researchers and patients.331 As one article recently observed, "If patients are not confident that their information is acquired, transmitted and stored in a secure and confidential way, they will probably not be keen to reveal accurate and complete information." Consequently, the overall quality of telemedicine care may diminish as a result of improper data security controls.

The Civic Research Institute in USA has found that four key factors determine electronic data security. These include: (1) the authentication of users requesting access to data, (2) the authorization of users before providing access, (3) the confidentiality of data while it is sent over the network, and (4) the integrity of the sent data. These factors protect the network from service disruptions (denial of service), the destruction or changing of data (viruses or worms), and the theft of data (copying from the network or server). Passwords, cryptography, and biometrics are used for the authentication and authorization of users, and log files track user access to data files. Unauthorized communications can be filtered out through the use of firewalls, and secure networks, such as Virtual Private Networks, are utilized to protect data confidentiality and integrity. While such technologies provide enhanced network security from external threats, the risks arising from internal negligence are another critical concern.

Internal threats resulting from employee and patient activity may also compromise network security. The American Computer Security Institute and the FBI recently found that half of all security breaches are the result of internal errors. Employees may unintentionally expose networks to attack by misplacing passwords, leaving confidential files open, failing to update the list of authorized employees, opening unsafe email attachments, and losing critical data.

Training of personnel is an often neglected aspect of system implementation, and may result in complications if employees are unprepared to properly operate the network and secure patient data. A 2005 survey of computer security practitioners found that the vast majority of participants believed security awareness training was important. However, respondents from all industry sectors believed that their organization failed to invest enough resources in it. When security measures are overly complicated and difficult to use, both employees and patients may have difficulty complying with the system requirements. For example, if safety alerts are provided too frequently, users may ignore the warnings and become unresponsive. Older adults in particular may experience difficulty when operating complicated interfaces and may abandon the system all together.

Security threats vary significantly by type of network and the requirements of users. However, a lack of data security standards for telemedicine services, for telemedicine practitioners, and for other stakeholders creates an important barrier towards further usage of these services.

5.3 Lack of standards to guide the interoperability of new telemedicine services

Telecommunications systems often operate on networks that do not facilitate the interoperability of telemedicine services. In particular, interoperability is a significant issue for EHRs, the vast majority of which do not interoperate well with other applications. If advanced telemedicine applications (e.g., various proprietary HER programs) are unable to work with one another, then their value will be limited.

A variety of standards-setting bodies have been established to help ensure interoperability. HHS, for example, launched the Healthcare IT Standards Panel (HITSP) in 2005. This panel "serve[s] as a cooperative partnership between the public and private sectors for the purpose of achieving a widely accepted and useful set of standards specifically to enable and support widespread interoperability among healthcare software applications, as they will interact in a local, regional, and national health information network for the United States." A number of other such efforts have been launched in recent years, including the Nationwide Health Information Network, the National Institute for Standards & Technology, and the Certification Commission for Health IT, among others. As doctors and hospitals across the country migrate from paper-based medical records to EHRs, and as innovative new broadband-enabled telemedicine tools continue to be deployed, these efforts will be essential to ensuring that these new services are interoperable and thus of value to all stakeholders.

However, until robust and widely accepted standards are developed and adopted by the vast array of service providers, innovators, and other stakeholders in the market, broadband-enabled telemedicine tools may remain fragmented in nature and unable to leverage true economies of scale to provide efficient and effectives services.

5.4 Negative perceptions and inadequate value propositions for using telemedicine services by patients

A significant number of patients, many of whom are older adults, remain wary of telemedicine services generally. This skepticism often stems from an unawareness of the true value of using these types of tools or a preference to continue using traditional healthcare methods (e.g., face-to-face consultations).

Studies have shown that, while patient satisfaction with telemedicine services is generally positive, patients express negative concerns both before and after receiving treatment. A recent study of remote monitoring patients found that "[a]lthough the response to the home telehealth service [for congestive heart failure] was overwhelmingly positive, respondents remained undecided regarding the perceived benefits of telehealth versus in-person care." Though the majority of patients advocated its future use, most still favored the in-person visit over the tele-visit. Moreover, while significant advantages were identified by patients, the most common disadvantages cited include confusion with the technology, the monotony of repetitive processes, and disruption of activities. In addition, research suggests that patients are more willing to use telemedicine services as a supplement to, rather than a replacement for, traditional face-to-face consultations "as long as privacy safeguards are maintained."

The current baby boomer and senior populations are especially wary of one type of telemedicine application: in-home health monitoring services. Two-thirds of both groups currently see little to no value in such technologies. According to AARP (American Association of Retired Persons), "Older adults often find little of interest to convince them of the value of making the change, and very frequently, poor design makes technology products very hard to learn or use." More specifically, many older adults fear that remote home health monitoring will reduce the personal relationships they have built with their doctors and their social interaction overall. Indeed, many older patients see "aging in place" with the help of home health monitors as a negative aspect of telemedicine and would rather "age in community" without losing social interaction. Sufficient interpersonal contact is not only beneficial to an older patient's health, but also a critical aspect to an older adult's quality of life. In addition, a perceived stigma towards aging and disease may cause seniors to resent the monitoring devices and view them as a constant reminder of their poor physical condition. Wearing a health monitor in public may cause older adults to feel old and weak in the eyes of others. Anecdotal evidence also supports the observation that many older adults may resent the lack of privacy afforded by in-home monitoring technologies, and they may dislike ceding authority over their medical state to their children, who often assume control over the monitoring system.

Thus, a primary barrier to further adoption and utilization of these services by all patients, especially older adults, is overcoming initial negative perceptions associated with telemedicine, shifting preferences away from traditional medical care, and providing adequate value propositions to spur use.

5.5 Costs/Evaluation/Outcomes

Although much anecdotal evidence exists, there is scant hard evidence that the communications technology will provide appropriate health care at a reasonable cost, despite the fact that in certain situations the cost-effectiveness of telemedicine appears obvious. Therefore, before payers and providers are willing to move on the issue, they want to know the likely economic effects of the use of telemedicine. Reimbursement policy issues are further complicated by rapid changes in equipment technology and faster communications networks that are making telemedicine capability more mobile, available for more applications, and with lower equipment costs and operational expenses. Metrics for telemedicine outcomes should be developed to demonstrate sufficient evidence of socio-economic benefit to indicate ongoing investment is appropriate. Evaluations should include examination of the social, cultural, organizational, and policy aspects of telemedicine. Suitable frameworks for economic analysis should capture non-monetary and unintended consequences, as well as monetary measures. Full integration of telemedicine will increase its use and decrease the per contact episode cost. Investment in information and communications technology infrastructure should be considered as an investment not only in health, but also in business, education, and other e-sectors. Sustainable telemedicine 'programs' and not 'projects' should be targeted.

6. Conclusions

Recent research firmly establishes broadband as an essential part of the global information society. Broadband fosters GDP growth, can create new jobs, spur innovation and improve public services, like telemedicine. Delivering affordable, reliable and accessible broadband to more citizens will help countries become stronger, more competitive and more prepared for continued growth in the years and decades to come.

More specifically, the notes hereby given have made the point on how consolidated broadband technologies, properly assembled and merged with well-defined medical needs, can successfully be exploited in many countries as a suitable aid to provide better cares to elderly and weak persons, as well as a compelling support to healthcare and telemedicine applications and services. Broadband-enabled telemedicine has the potential to transform healthcare by connecting more institutions and allowing for the faster transmission of vital information. It is pushing healthcare into homes with the consequent decrease of reliance on hospitals and nursing homes, and it is empowering individual patients by providing them with access to personal health and medical information.

It is essential, however, to bear in mind that technology suitability and availability are not the only issues to make a feasible solution replicable and widely deployed in a sustainable manner. Successfulness is still cost related, and a more critical factor is the identification of the most appropriate telemedicine business model. As a matter of fact, telemedicine applications addressed a few years ago would have a cost impact higher than 30-40% or even more compared to today's solutions and broadband cost benefits. Policymakers should thus implement (or continue to implement) policies that support investment and encourage innovation while also reforming and updating a variety of healthcare-related laws in order to spur the adoption and use of telemedicine services. To this end, stimulus funding should be allocated to support broadband deployment and adoption, to spur use of cutting-edge services like electronic health records, and to support innovative pilot programs

7. References

ADSL Technology - Overview, Line Qualification and Service Turn-up. JDSU White Paper, (available at http://www.jdsu.com/product-literature/ADSL_Technology_White_Paper.pdf).

Angrisani, L.; Napolitano, A. & Sona, A. (2010). Cross-layer measurements on an IEEE 802.11g wireless network supporting MPEG-2 video streaming applications in the presence of interference, *EURASIP Journal on Wireless Communications and Networking*, Hindawi Publishing Corporation, Vol.2010, Article ID 620832, April 2010, pp.1-11.

Angrisani, L. & Napolitano, A. (2010). Modulation quality measurement in WiMAX systems through a fully digital signal processing approach, *IEEE Trans. on Instr. and Meas.*, vol.59, No.9, September 2010, pp.2286-2302.

Angrisani, L. & Narduzzi, C. (2008). Testing communication and computer networks: an overview, *IEEE Instrumentation & Measurement Magazine*, October 2008, pp.12 24.

Angrisani, L.; Peluso, L.; Tedesco, A. & Ventre, G. (2006). Measurement of processing and queuing delays introduced by an open-source router in a single-hop network, *IEEE Trans. on Instr. and Meas.*, Vol.55, No.4, August 2006, pp.1065 1076.

Arslan, H.; Chen, Z.N. & Di Benedetto, M.G. (2006). *Ultra Wideband Wireless Communication*, John Wiley & Sons Inc., ISBN 0-471-71521-2, New Jersey, USA.

Barriers to Broadband Adoption: A Report to the Federal Communications Commission (2009). The Advanced Communications Law&Policy Institute Literature, New York Law School, (available at http://www.law.northwestern.edu/searlecenter/uploads/ACLP%20Report%20to%20the%20FCC%20-%20Barriers%20to%20BB%20Adoption.pdf).

Bates, R.J. (2002). *Broadband Telecommunications Handbook*, The McGraw-Hill Companies Inc., ISBN 0-07-139851-1, USA.

Benefits of Telemedicine (2004). Telemedicine Association of Oregon Literature, January 2004, (available at http://www.ortcc.org/PDF/BenefitsofTelemedicine.pdf).

Broadband Technology Overview, (2005). CORNING - Discovering Beyond Imagination, June 2005, (available at http://www.corning.com/docs/opticalfiber/wp6321.pdf).

Darkins, A.W.& Cary, M.A. (2000). *Telemedicine and Telehealth - Principles, Policies, Performance, and Pitfalls*, Springer Publishing Company Inc., ISBN 0-8261-1302-8, New York, USA.

Di Lieto, A.; De Falco, M.; Campanile, M.; Papa, R.; Torok, M.; Scaramellino, M.; Pontillo, M.; Pollio, F.; Spanik, G.; Schiraldi & P.; Bibbò, G. (2006). Four years' experience with antepartum cardiotocography using telemedicine, *J Telemed Telecare*, Vol.12, No.5, pp.228-33.

Di Lieto, A.; De Falco, M.; Campanile, M.; Török, M.; Gábor, S.; Scaramellino, M.; Schiraldi, P. & Ciociola, F. (2008). Regional and international prenatal telemedicine network for computerized antepartum cardiotocography, *Telemed J E Health*, Vol.14, No.1, (Jan-Feb 2008), pp.49-54.

Di Lieto, A.; Scaramellino, M.; Campanile, M.; Iannotti, F.; De Falco, M.; Pontillo, M. & Pollio, F. (2002). Prenatal telemedicine and teledidactic networking. A report on the TOCOMAT project, *Minerva Ginecol*, Vol.54, No.5, pp.447-51.

DSL Technology Tutorial (2010). ASSIA Literature, (available at http://www.assia-inc.com/DSL-technology/DSL-knowledge-center/tutorials/DSL-technology-tutorial.php).

Hahm, J.S.; Lee, H.L.; Choi, H.S. & Shimizu, S. (2009). Telemedicine System Using a High-Speed Network: Past, Present, and Future, *Gut and Liver*, Vol.3, No.4, December 2009, pp.247-251 (available at http://www.ncbi.nlm.nih.gov/pmc/articles/PMC2852732/pdf/gnl-3-247.pdf).

Holma, H. & Toskala, A. (2006). *HSDPA/HSUPA for UMTS - High Speed Radio Access for Mobile Communications*, John Wiley & Sons Ltd, ISBN-13 978-0-470-01884-2, England, UK.

Huurdeman, A.A. (2003). *The Worldwide History of Telecommunications*, John Wiley & Sons, Inc., ISBN 0-471-20505-2, Hoboken, New Jersey, USA.

IEEE Standard 802.11-1999 (1999).Wireless LAN Medium Access Control (MAC) and Physical Layer (PHY) Specifications.

Khoumbati, K.; Dwivedi, Y.K.; Srivastava, A. & Lal, B. (2010). *Handbook of Research on Advances in Health Informatics and Electronic Healthcare Applications: Global Adoption and Impact of Information Communication Technologies*, Medical Information Science Reference, ISBN 978-1-60566-030-1, Hershey, New York, USA.

Pahlavan, K. & Levesque, A.H. (2005). *Wireless Information Networks*, John Wiley & Sons Inc., ISBN-13 978-0-471-72542-8, New Jersey, USA.

Realizing the Benefits of Broadband (2010). Intel Corporation White Paper, (available at http://www.intel.org/Assets/PDF/Article/WA-323857001.pdf).

Sauter, M. (2006). *Communication Systems for the Mobile Information Society*, John Wiley & Sons Ltd, ISBN-13 978-0-470-02676-2, England, UK.

Schwartz, M. (2005). *Mobile Wireless Communications*, Cambridge University Press, ISBN 0-521-84347-2, Cambridge, UK.

Solymar, L. (1999). *Getting the Message - A History of Communications*, Oxford University Press Inc., ISBN-019 850333-4, New York, USA.

Surfing into the Future: Mobile Broadband Technologies (2007). Juniper Research Limited White Paper, (available at **Error! Hyperlink reference not valid.**).

Webb, W. (1999). *The Complete Wireless Communications Professional: A Guide for Engineers and Managers*, Artech House Inc., ISBN 0-89006-338-9, Norwood, Massachusetts, USA.

Part 3

Enabling Factors

12

Quality Control in Telemedicine - "CE" Label

Prof. Dr. O. Ferrer-Roca MD. PhD.
UNESCO Chair of Telemedicine. Faculty of Medicine. University of La Laguna. 38075 La Laguna. Tenerife. Canary Islands Spain

1. Introduction

As explained previously [1], the European Directive for Medical Devices (MDs) and equipment, the DIR 2007/47/EC [2], aims at achieving the goal of quality of medical delivery at a distance, providing comparable demands in telemedicine or distance support as in face-to-face healthcare.
The transposition into Spanish law of the EU directive was the Royal Decree RD-1591/2009, dated 16 October 2009 [3], which regulates the use of medical devices called "PRODUCTOS SANITARIOS (PS)" (= health-care products) in Spanish, which came into force on the 21st of March 2010. As from that date, the **CE-Label** is always required in all "MDDS or Medical Device Data Systems" according to the FDA.
In this article, we will explain the philosophy behind the EU-Directive and the Spanish RD with respect to quality in medical assistance. We will also try to demonstrate that the same norms apply to Telemedicine, and we will finally underline the importance of training medical and health-care workers in those aspects linked to the Body of Knowledge of Telemedicine as well as in the essential safety aspects linked to medical assistance. These professionals may indeed be guilty of infringing the law and liable if the law is not applied. As is well known, ignorance of the law is no excuse. This has indirect consequences on the training and licensing of health-workers. •

2. Medical device- definitions

According to the EU directive and the transposed RD:
The definition of an MD in the RD (in Spanish) is based on the European Commission Directive 2007/47/ec which defines a medical device as <<any instrument, apparatus, appliance, software, material or other article, whether used alone or in combination, including the software intended by its manufacturer to be used specifically for diagnostic and/or therapeutic purposes and necessary for its proper application, intended by the manufacturer to be used for human beings. Devices are to be used for the purpose of:

- Diagnosis, prevention, monitoring, treatment or alleviation of disease.
- Diagnosis, monitoring, treatment, alleviation of or compensation for an injury or handicap.
- Investigation, replacement or modification of the anatomy or of a physiological process.
- Control of conception.

This includes devices that do not achieve its principal intended action in or on the human body by pharmacological, immunological or metabolic means, but which may be assisted in its function by such means.>>

An MD is not a medicine in the sense that it does not produce its principal effect inside or on the surface of the body by pharmacological, immunological, or metabolically active substances, but whose function may contribute to them.

The so-called "in vitro" diagnostic systems are not covered by the 1591/2009 decree; they are regulated by the RD-1662/2000 decree.

The goal of the EU directive as well as that of the RD is to guarantee a quality system for MDs with periodic inspection and control by means of 5 distinct procedures:

1. **EXAMINATION of the CE type** is defined as the procedure by which a **NOTIFIED BODY** **tests** a representative sample of the product and **certifies** that it is in accordance with the RD demands. The result is the CERTIFICATION of the MD-type.
2. **CE-VERIFICATION** is defined as the procedure by which the **MANUFACTURER** or its authorized representative **guarantees and declares** that the products are in **conformity** with the **MD-Type described** in the certification of the CE-examination, and that **they fulfill all the requirements** set out in the RD. The conformity declaration includes a statement according to which the manufacturer agrees to guarantee the product after its sale and installation and to correct any defect that could occur.

> *This means that the manufacturer must implement all required controls and tests linked to the MD-type.*

3. & 4. **CE DECLARATION OF CONFORMITY** for the **PRODUCTION** and the **PRODUCT** is defined as the procedure by which the MANUFACTURER puts into practice all warranty requirements **and declares** that all the products are **in conformity with the MD-type** described in the Certificate of the CE-examination, and that they fulfill all the requirements set up in the RD.

> *This means that the manufacturer must implement the whole quality system to assure conformity not only of the final product but of the whole production.*

Part of this task is to guarantee the organizational structures and the responsibility of the directives, the methods of efficacy in the function, and the control to third parties, whenever applicable.

Furthermore, a **VALIDATION REPORT** should accompany those MDs whose **function is "measurements".**

> *This is the case of Telemetry and distance measurement that require a VALIDATION REPORT before being authorized for use in real world situations. This is an important qualitative difference from the previous situation in which software systems had to be validated by the users and hospital before being used. Now, the software as an MD requires a previous Validation Report by the manufacturer.*

Similarly, the manufacturer whose products require "**connection with other products"** to work must provide proof that their products fulfill the essential requirements once connected to other products according to the manufacturer's goal or to those specified as **a special purpose** (custom made[1], research[2], etc.).

> *This means that for any product connected to another to send information, the manufacturer must guarantee that this information is not altered in any way (manipulation, lost information, lossy compression, encryption, etc…), and must not be integrated without a Validation Report.*
> *In other words, the manufacturer is responsible for the integration processes, whether added functions are included or not.*

5. **CE-LABEL.** Only those products with a CE-Label will be authorized to appear on the **market and to be used in medical practice**. The CE-label will always be accompanied by the identification of the Notified Organ responsible for the evaluation procedures. Exceptions for the CE-Label are:
   a. As an exception, products or devices built for one person or for clinical research do not require CE-Label.
   b. For medical devices and products for which the Certificate of Conformity **does not require the intervention of the NOTIFIED BODY (these are the Type I devices),** the CE-Label will not carry an identification number assigned by the Notified Body.

> *This means that the CE-label is mandatory for all MDs or Health Products, but that those included in the **Type I group** will not carry an identification number.*

   c. According to the RD, CE-Label conformity is not required for those MDs that are not included in article 2, paragraph 1, points a) and b)-

> *Therefore, the CE-Label only applies to MDs together with their ACCESSORIES.*

To ensure the product guarantee, the manufacturer must be able to demonstrate CE-Label conformity during a period of 5 years, but for implantable MDs or products, the period is 15 years. This information must be available to the authorities in charge of quality control.

> *Therefore, in order to claim for any malfunctioning or defect of the product, we should understand the terms defined in the law, particularly the term MANUFACTURER.*

Custom-made devices are intended for the sole use by a particular patient and produced in accordance with specifications prescribed by a qualified practitioner. A mass-produced MD that only needs adaptation is not a custom made device. Custom- made devices do not carry a visible CE mark, but remain subject to the Medical Device Directive (MDD) requirements.

---

[1] 'Custom made' means that the device is for one patient only and should carry his/her name as well as the name of the medical doctor who authorized it (encrypted or not) along with the medical prescription.

[2] Guarantee for patients in the trial, permission from the ethical committee as well as the medical doctor and center authorization must be provided.

The manufacturer must issue a statement of conformity for each device stating the patient's name, device identification, and responsible medical practitioners.

2.1 Definitions

In the RD the following terms of importance are defined:

Manufacturer: the person or legal entity responsible for the design, manufacture, packaging and labeling of the MD to be **introduced on the market** in his own name, regardless of whether any of these operations are carried out by the same person/entity or by a third party.

Introduction on the market: this term refers to the first time an MD or Health product, **not designed for clinical research**, arrives on the market with or **without economic transaction** (i.e., for free), for its **distribution and/or use** in the EU market, regardless of whether it is a new or a totally refurbished product.

This means that a manufacturer is a person or legal entity who produces an MD whether it is for financial profit or not, whether it is produced voluntarily or by contract or even by mandate within an organization in a public or a private system, provided that the medical device is used in the real world (i.e., not only for research) in a country member state of the EU.

Commercialization: any **provision**, with or without economic transaction (i.e., **for free)**, for its **distribution or use** in the EU market during a commercial activity.

This means the real use of the product coming from a manufacturer to a final user for its real use, regardless of whether the transaction involves financial gain or not.

Deployment: refers to the phase in which a product, **prepared to be marketed in the EU** for the first time **according to the manufacturer's intended goal, is given to the final user.**

Goal assignation: The use for which the MD is built according to the indications of the manufacturer in the labeling of the product, user's instructions and/or marketing material or flyers.

This means that, although the manufacturer does the product either by contact, for free o by obligation, the device should have, before any use, a label with user's instructions and a detailed specification explaining why the system was built and validated for according to the manufacturer.

Medical specialist: a medical doctor or any other person with accredited professional qualifications who is **legally authorized** to issue a medical prescription or **to perform biomedical research**.

This means that the validation of a system must be performed, tested and supervised by a specialized medical doctor.
Obviously, a medical specialist must supervise medical assistance from the very start, whether this assistance is provided for research or for regular assistance.

Promoter: manufacturer, legal representative or any other **person or organization** that becomes **responsible for the indications** and/or deployment of a **clinical research.**

This means that a promoter is a person who indicates an MD "deployment" by giving it to the final user for free or after payment. This activity is usually performed by the local health-care authorities with MDs and products of the software and telemetry types, specifically designed at a regional or "in house" level for local healthcare use.

Chapter II of the RD specifies that the manufacturers should be registered and should possess a previous license to operate in order to make sure that they have an **organizational structure capable of guaranteeing the quality of their products** and the performance **of the procedures and controls** mentioned above. They have to have a **technical responsible** personnel, with an **university-licensure (title)** that assure an **ad-hoc qualification** to control and supervise the product in charge; furthermore, his availability for this task must be demonstrated devoting a sufficient **labor time-schedule**. Finally he should carry out a series of documents to collect all information produced during product-manufacture. These documents should include the **design, production and capabilities** of the product so as to check the conformity of the product to the essential requirements (*i.e in a software application to encrypt clinical information in order to send it at distance, documents should demonstrate that the application fulfill the data-protection law. This could avoid for example the case to steal and disseminate sensitive information located in the memory chip of the printers once those are replaced or even when those are repaired…*)

If this is the case, local health-authorities that produce their own software for medical-clinical-assistance should be registered and required to fulfill the same demands as any other manufacturer. And of course, once in public call for tender, it should be mandatory to include those requisites for enterprises applying the call to build "regional" or "in house" assistant systems.

However, the RD also mentions that the Spanish Agency of Medications and Health Products could **authorize, in an individualized and specific manner** and based on health care considerations, the marketing and deployment of products that **have not satisfied all the validation procedures** indicated in article 13.

We hope that, for the final users' safety, there will be few such exceptions to the norm, and that this provision for exceptions will never become a repetitive practice. An example of the use of this exceptional authorization put into practice in the case of medication was the vaccination campaign against influenza A (H1N1): the vaccine did not fulfill all the requirements to be on the market.

3. Essential information & definitions relevant for health care workers

The RD starts a procedure to understand the design, manufacture and applications of the product together with the design, risk analysis, investigation and clinical trials etc., with respect to product safety, including **electromagnetic compatibility** and radiation protection, as well as ergonomic **design** and the **level of training** of future users[3].

[3] Training should also involve the medical doctors as users.

That means that the manufacturer must train users to assure that they will use the device in a proper manner, without risk for patients and health care workers, and to make sure that they know their liability when using it. Therefore, the liability for the products and devices introduced on the market is the manufacturers.
This also clearly applies to local healthcare authorities if they act as manufacturers.

As specified above, based on the level of potential risk to the human body, MDs are classified as one of four types: types I, IIa, IIb y III.
The higher the number, the greater the risk. In the lowest risk class (type I MD), the evaluation is the exclusive responsibility of the manufacturer. For the other types, the evaluation is performed by a "NOTIFIED BODY" appointed by national authorities to issue a **Certificate of Conformity.**

As we will see, most Telemedicine systems are classified as type I MDs because they are not invasive. Thus, they do not require a number or a Certificate of Conformity from the "Notified Body". Nevertheless, it is mandatory for them to carry the CE-label. This means that, under the responsibility of the manufacturer, the device must meet the requirements for quality and safety demanded for any MD and be supported by documents proving that verification and manufacture control etc., have been carried out. These documents must be available to the competent authorities in case of any legal demand or claim.
A problem arises when the so-called "competent authority" coincides with the manufacturer or is the entity that establishes the system requirements in the call for tenders.

This is why all MDs require initial classification by the manufacturer as one of four types for the CE-label, as follows:
Type I- NON INVASIVE PRODUCTS[4], with the exception of those connected to higher type numbers or in contact with human body substances, fluids or tissues. These comprise all PSANI-**P**roducto **S**anitario **A**ctivo **N**o **I**nvasivo (in English: non-invasive Active Medical Device) with the exception of the cases that we will study further on.
INVASIVE PRODUCTS FOR A SHORT PERIOD OF TIME (less than 60 min) and those used in the natural orifices (oral cavity up to the pharynx, external ear conduct up to the tympanic membrane, nasal cavity).
Type II-ALL INVASIVE PRODUCTS, including the PSA-**P**roductos **S**anitarios **A**ctivos (In English: Active Medical Devices). These exclude invasive surgical devices connected to a type I MD. This group is divided into two sub-groups, as follows:
IIa- MDs USED for A LIMITED PERIOD OF TIME (up to 30 days). This includes those used in wounds or around micro-wounds and surgical invasive devices, except those used for monitoring, diagnosis, surveillance, and cardio-circulatory correction. Those invasive to natural orifices that are connected to a PSA type IIa (active device type IIa). Dental implants. All products for diagnosis or surveillance of non-critical vital signs[5] and those involved with the introduction of non-harmful substances in the body. Products used for disinfection.
IIb- MDs USED FOR LONG PERIODS OF TIME (more than 30 days). Those MDs or products carrying ionizing radiation, having a biologic effect, capable of being absorbed by

[4] All active software and telemedicine devices belong to this group.
[5] Among these are all telemetry systems (including vital sign telemetry if the patient is not in a critical condition. It therefore refers to the classical home-care), tele-ultrasonography, etc.

the human body or capable of being modified by it. Any active MD connected to a type IIb[6] or PSAI -**P**roducto **S**anitario **A**ctivo **I**nvasivo (In English: Invasive Active Medical Device). This includes all MDs for the surveillance of critical vital signs[7] and those that are potentially harmful[8] because they introduce substances into the body. Blood bags. Contraceptives. Contact lenses, disinfection products.

Type IIb also include all implantable products, with the exception of dental implants, cardio-vascular or central nervous system implants, and those that produce chemical or biological changes in the human body.

Type III- Surgical instruments which are in contact with the Central Nervous System and cardio-vascular system, or MDs that are absorbed or produce a biological or chemical modification in the human body. Products containing human blood or derived products (hemo-derivatives). Contraceptive devices used for long periods of time. All products that contain animal tissue or their derivatives.

The RD specifies that any substantial changes in an MD or Health product must be notified to the "Notified Body". The RD specifies that all MDs, health care products and their ACCESSORIES must carry the CE-label, numbered by the Notified Organism, except for Type I MDs which must exhibit the CE-label, but which are not numbered.

Type I-MDs, despite carrying a non-numbered CE-Label (which means that the product is not certified by a "Notified Body"), must be supported by documents demonstrating that the product has been subjected to the same quality control process. These documents will be required any time by the authorities when claims or civil and penal liability arise.

The Royal Decree, which is complex to understand, aims at implementing international standards on quality control in the production, design and vital cycle of the product, such as the UNE EN 60601-1:2008, IEC 60601-1/2005, ISO 14971:2007, IEC 62304:2006, etc.

*This means that those devices showing the CE-label must provide a guarantee of information (there will be no secret products); of security (required to be tested in clinical trials); of functionality (they require a previous validation before marketing and real functioning); of quality design (they should have a quality design ISO-13485). If not, the device or product can only be considered as **a demonstrator[6].***

3.1 Definitions

In the previous paragraphs, we defined what is considered a MEDICAL DEVICE or a HEALTH CARE PRODUCT. Here we introduce definitions relevant for health-care workers, such as:

An MD or PRODUCT FOR CLINICAL INVESTIGATION: **this** is an MD or product devoted **to a medical specialist[9] to carry out the research** in an adequate clinical human environment.

---

[6] i.e: more than 30 days Home-care.

[7] Vital sign telemetry including EEG y EEC.

[8] Harmful for the organ or due to the type of substance.

[9] This means that a telemetry system or a telemedicine device cannot be in the hands of an engineer (Take into consideration that innovation units, tele-ictus units and so on… are leader by engineers) nor the i+D+D projects that involve clinical research or clinical trials.

A RE-USABLE SURGICAL INSTRUMENT is one that is not connected to an active MD or PSA.

An **ACTIVE-MD** or PSA (*implantable-PSAI or non- implantable-PSANI*) is any MD that requires electrical power or any other energy source different from the one coming from the human body, or that is due to gravity, and that transforms this energy (i.e., *telemetry systems*). All **SOFWARE PROGRAMES** are considered **Active-MDs**. Excluded from this group are those MDs used for transmitting provided that there is no significant modification, energy, substances or other elements from an active-MD to the patient.

The criteria of Software programs are those that allow diagnosis, treatment, follow up, prevention, whether or not they include artificial intelligence. The latter could be as a completely autonomous or when those results are taken by healthcare workers to make decisions with respect to a local or distant patient (at home; tele-ictus; anti-cloth treatment; telemedicine in general). And although administrative computer programs (HIS-Hospital information system) will probably be excluded from future regulation, the EMR or Electronic Medical Record is directly linked to them. The EMR contains essential elements for patients' treatment or follow up that involve liability of medical doctors, such as medical orders, or electronic prescription requiring a legally recognized digital signature, and that in any case requires strict QUALITY CONTROL and therefore should be included in the RD. Many EMR and applications for e-prescriptions contain decision rules on treatment protocols, assistance to the diagnosis, prescription, patient surveillance or follow up that transform them into an Active-MD that requires active quality control [7].

The problem arises when those computer programs without quality control are developed and updated by the health-care authorities either at the national or regional or local level as "in house" "custom" products for health-care. In private healthcare entities, quality control could be easy to provide since the company responsible for marketing and supplying those products for real use is in effect the manufacturer and is subject to control by the local authorities. However, in local public authorities the manufacturer and the controller may be the same entity. This is so even if the manufacturer is an outside company contracted through a call for tenders, since the requirements for the design are established by the local authority and in many cases this is limited to compatibility with other in-house applications and not to manufacturing quality control. Being aware that manufacturing quality control items are titles and preparation of the developers, legal-preparation, time devoted for the technical personnel in the design, who is responsible for the life cycle of the product, who is responsible for the necessary technical migration in 3-5 years time to update technology and security (i.e. electronic signature, cipher according to law, to adapt to registration and certification organisms, management of new parameters and medical devices, etc….). And more specifically in wireless active-MD (telemetry) or not (WIFI hospitals) the degree of interaction of their magnetic fields with other monitoring or measurement systems are not verified or tested properly because the assembly is done "in house" without verification of the quality control.

This is regardless of the requirements of **CONFORMITY** which are defined as an MD following national norms taken to **implement harmonized standards to fulfill essential requirements** and officially published in the Government bulletins.

Thus, software manufacturers will be responsible during the whole active-life of the product. Being Type I or low risk MDs, the products will not require auditing by law, except if there is a claim, but as medical software, they will be regulated by the IEC 62304:2006 standard.

The European Commission stresses the need to use standards in order to ensure connectivity that should include semantic and technical norms, and physics of connectors and cables. However, national standards that determine the connectivity of telemetry and telemedicine systems are still to be established.
With respect to telemedicine, the minimum connectivity specified by the WHO is the IEEE 11073 [8]. Following the guide for validation of automatic systems (GAMP- Good Automated Manufacturing Practice)[9], bioengineering hospital services should control the operative systems, the hardware and the software embedded in the systems, as well as COTS (Commercial-off-the-shelf) software, configurable systems and any modification of PIMS (Personal Information Manager Software).
Furthermore the CMM or Capability Maturity Model for software[10] in their version 1.3 established VALIDATION and VERIFICATION at level 3, requiring thereafter level 4 or the quantization of processes and level 5 of Optimization. And it should be kept in mind that in many software health-care applications, even level 3 is missing[11].

4. USA ahead

As predicted elsewhere [12], the Obama health reform has forced the adoption of medicine at a distance (telemedicine) in order to optimize resources and reduce costs in the system.
The USA are very concerned about quality control and have created several government organizations to guarantee the quality control of medical assistance, standardization and connectivity, establishing minimum requirements to obtain a quality label. One of the most interesting bills passed by the US Congress is the ARRA (the American Recovery and Reinvestment Act of 2009) aimed at stimulating the use of IT (Information Technology), but what is surprising is the provision for penalties after 2015 for those professionals and organizations that do not use connective solutions. [13].
We will therefore see the time when those responsible for education and health-care will accept that all these technologies have to be integrated into the professional training. This implies that telemedicine and bioengineering applied to telemedicine will become core subject matters in the university degree of Medicine [14].

5. Summary

The transposition of the EU Directive DIR 2007/47/EC into European countries will improve the quality of the Telemedicine software and devices [15][16]. Nevertheless, health-care authorities have not yet understood the important requirements and the level of changes they will have to introduce. This is in part due to the fact that this information is not taken into consideration in the training of health care professionals.
The discipline of Telemedicine and e-health is mature if we take into consideration the level of standards existing nowadays. In contrast, maturity of the IT applications in health care is far from being optimal. This is in part because we associate maturity with penetration and not with quality, and mechanisms to ensure a quality control of the applications are still to be built.

Abbreviations

AIQ Analytical Instrument Qualification | **CFR** Code of Federal Regulations | **CSV** Computer System Validation | **EMEA** European Medicine Evaluation Agency | **EU**

European Union | **FDA** U.S. Food and Drug Administration | **GAMP** Good Automated Manufacturing Practice | **GLP** Good Laboratory Practice | **GMP** Good Manufacturing Practice | **ISMS** Information Security Management System | **ISO** International Organization for Standardization | **USP** United States Pharmacopeia

6. References

[1] Ferrer-Roca O (2009). Departamento de Anatomia Patologica a Tenor de la Legislacion vigente en Rev.Esp.Pat. 42(1):17-23

[2] DIR 2007/47/EC Nueva directiva sobre equipos médicos. Disponible en http://en.wikipedia.org/wiki/Medical_device

[3] MINISTERIO DE SANIDAD Y POLÍTICA SOCIAL Productos sanitarios. Real Decreto 1591/2009, de 16 de octubre, por el que se regulan los productos sanitarios. BOE 268 de 6 Noviembre 2009. pp: 92708 a 92778. Disponible en http://www.boe.es/boe/dias/2009/11/06/

[4] IEC 60601-1: 2006. Seguridad en los equipos electromédicos incluyendo los PESS o subsistemas electrónicos programables. Disponible en http://www.tecno-med.es/boletin/60601-1aprobacion-cenelec.pdf

[5] ISO 14971:2007 specifies a process for a manufacturer to identify the hazards associated with medical devices. Disponible en http://www.iso.org/iso/iso_catalogue/catalogue_tc/catalogye_detail.htm?csnumber=38193

[6] Ferrer-Roca O., Marcano F (2009). "Anatomía Patológica Digital. Control de calidad y pato-informática." Rev. Esp. Patol 42(2): 85-95 http://www.patologia.es/volumen42/vol42-num2/42-2n02.htm

[7] Ferrer-Roca O., Marcano F., Diaz Cardama A (2008). Quality Labels for e-Health. IET Communications 2(2): 202-207. doi:10.1049/iet-com:20060596

[8] ISO/IEEE 11073 o estándar plug & play. Disponible en www.ieee1073.org

[9] Ferrer Roca O. September 2010: http://catai.net/blog//2010/09/criterio-calidad-sofware/

[10] Ferrer Roca O. May 2010: http://catai.net/blog//2010/05/cmm-sw-en-aparatos-medicos/

[11] Pearson S, Balis UJ, Fuller J, Kowalski B, Locke AP, Tillman D, Vantu QH. Managing and validating laboratory information systems; approved guideline. Clinical and Laboratory Standards Insititute document AUTO8-A 2006; 26 (36)

[12] Ferrer Roca O. Julio 2009: http://catai.net/blog//2009/07/2009-el-ano-de-la-reforma-sanitaria-usando-tics-en-usa/

[13] Blumenthal D (2009). Stimulating the Adoption of Health Information Technology. N Engl J Med 360 (15): 1477-1479.

[14] O Ferrer-Roca. J A Abreu Reyes. R Abreu González. M Suárez Delgado. E Sola-Reche (2001). Capacitación médica en la sociedad de la información. Rev Clin Esp. 201:315-21.

[15] Ferrer Roca O.Junio 2009: http://catai.net/blog//2009/06/control-calidad-aparatos-medicos/

[16] Ferrer-Roca O. Abril 2010: http://catai.net/blog//2010/04/sanidad-sin-espacio-para-amateurs/

13

Innovative Healthcare Delivery: the Quest for Effective Telemedicine-based Services

Laura Bartoli, Emanuele Lettieri and Cristina Masella
Department of Management, Economics and Industrial Engineering,
Politecnico di Milano, Milan,
Italy

1. Introduction

Healthcare is a complex industry that is facing great changes in its structure, organization, service delivery and operations. One of the most impactful trends for healthcare is probably the progressive ageing of population. It creates pressures in many ways, such as reducing the pool of economically active population, posing growing problems of compliance to medication and lifestyle guidance, and increasing the number of elderly people in need of long-term care and assistance. This entails increasing costs for healthcare, in a time when the availability of both economic and human resources is decreasing (Whitten et al., 2010). Within this context, the development of new paradigms of healthcare delivery that may be sustainable over time has become an imperative (Forbes & While, 2009).

With this regard, technology has drawn increasing attention as one of the emerging service delivery vehicles running on the information highway (Zajtchuk, 1996). In fact, also a cursory review of literature would identify that Information and Communication Technology (ICT) is commonly considered a major enabler for the innovation of healthcare delivery. Despite this enthusiasm, less is understood about how to make these changes factual. Technology alone, in fact, is not enough, but is the interplay of technical and organizational factors in designing and implementing technologies that lead to improved outcomes (Obstfelder et al., 2007). In this view, a sustainable technology-based healthcare service, which entails the effective introduction of the innovation into the routine processes, is mainly underpinned by human and organizational issues, and their deep interrelation with technical aspects (Gagnon et al., 2005; Aas, 2001).

To this extent, and within the care innovation context, the use of ICT to support delivery of healthcare over a distance, namely "telemedicine" (Lehoux et al., 2002), was often mentioned as a shift in paradigms, which impacts on task design and delivery processes (de Bont & Bal, 2008; Gagnon et al., 2005). The assessment of telemedicine-based services has often highlighted the effects of these new technologies on quality, accessibility and service costs (Gagnon et al., 2008). However, although many demonstration projects have presented evidence about clinical benefits, cost effectiveness and high levels of patient satisfaction (Whitten et al., 2010), some of them yet failed to become part of everyday clinical routine (de Bont & Bal, 2008). This is because telemedicine-based services have been mainly considered

as a "black box", which moves on a linear trajectory from design to diffusion (Timmermans, 2003), rather than a system in which human participants and/or machines perform work using information, technology, and other resources (namely "work systems"). Handling these latter complex, heterogeneous factors, which are expressed in controversies and solved through social negotiation, are keys to draw on effective telemedicine-based services, i.e. "sustainable work systems" (Obstfelder et al., 2007).
This challenge grounds into the largely acknowledged literature of Socio Technical Systems, which assumes that scientific knowledge and technology do not evolve in a vacuum. Rather, they should be seen as parts of the social world, being shaped by it, and simultaneously shaping it (Obstfelder et al., 2007). According to this research stream, a work system can be assumed as sustainable when it is able to function in its environment and achieve economic or operational goals over time (Docherty et al., 2002). Indeed, not only it preserves the resources it utilizes, but actually supports their growth and development.
This approach is particularly meaningful as lens of analysis because it allows to get insights that may be hard to acquire through other approaches. Despite the recognized general impact of telemedicine in healthcare delivery and the political willingness to promote it in public healthcare, in fact, previous telemedicine projects did not communicate the whole story about what is needed to make telemedicine-based services effective (Obstfelder et al., 2007). On the contrary, they mainly focused on the outcomes of clinical trials, while a limited attention was posed on the conditions, operating within the work system, which are important for the enhancement of these outcomes. Because of this gap in the literature, particularly interesting are those projects which draw on the characteristics a telemedicine-based service needs to nurture to be a sustainable work system. These projects, in particular, leaned on the belief that decisions about the care of individual patients within single structures should be based on the conscientious, explicit, and judicious use of current best evidence. This means that individual expertise should be integrated with the best information from scientifically-based and systematic research, and applied in light of each patient's values and circumstances. This approach leverages on an international political consensus. Recently, in fact, the US Congress too highlighted the need to establish standards and processes "that yield credible, unbiased, and understandable syntheses of the available evidence" about clinical practices effectiveness (IOM, 2008).
Within this context, the Italian Ministry of Health promoted a National Research Project which deepened the characteristics of telemedicine-based services for patients affected by Chronic Obstructive Pulmonary Disease (COPD).This disease, according to the data provided by the Global Initiative for Chronic Obstructive Lung Disease (www.goldcopd.it), is the 5th cause of death in the world. Symptoms increases with the age, and the prevalence of the pathology enhances the 50% in male smokers older than 60. In 2002, cost related to COPD enhanced 32 billion of dollars in US. This pathology is still widely under-estimated, even if its incidence keeps increasing from the 80s'.
On the basis of the findings gathered through this National Research Project, the chapter is organized as follows. The next section will illustrate the specific objectives of this study and the methodology adopted to enhance them. Then, the conceptual framework and the results will be reported to show the solutions adopted in terms of sustainable work system within telemedicine-based services in the Italian context. The last section presents a discussion, the conclusions and the main directions for future research.

2. Research objective and methodology

The research adopted an explanatory approach that aimed at knowing what works in telemedicine. In particular, the design principles that an effective telemedicine-based service needs to entail to introduce a sustainable work system are deepened. We focused the attention on the Italian context, considering health policy as a contextual factor. The healthcare context, in fact, is widely impacted by regulations. Moreover, when the research moves from the clinical outcomes to the organizational impact, international benchmarking and comparison become more difficult. For clarity, the main characteristics or the Italian National Healthcare System are reported in Fig. 1.
The potential generalization of our findings will be presented in the "Discussion" section.

The Italian National Healthcare System (NHS) is characterized by an universal tax-based coverage with free access to all Italian citizens and legal immigrants. Patients' co-payment is limited, despite it is increasing year after year. The NHS is organized at three levels: national, regional and local. The national level is responsible for ensuring the strategic objectives and the fundamental operating principles. The Regional Governments with their regional health departments are responsible for ensuring the delivery of a package of services through a network of Local Health Agencies, General Practitioners (GPs) and public or private accredited hospitals. Prices are based on Diagnostic Related Groups.

Fig. 1. Characteristics or the Italian National Healthcare System

In order to investigate the Italian telemedicine-based services for patients affected by COPD nationwide, an effort has gone into including the active and constant involvement of both the practitioners and the researchers in framing the research agenda, selecting and pursuing methods, and developing the implications for action. In particular, the continue attempt to learn from experience and the accumulation of knowledge over time resulted in the development of theoretical evidence for researchers and practical wisdom for practitioners (Pasmore et al., 2008).
Following this research approach, results were achieved in two sequential steps. First, the researchers, coached by expert practitioners, conducted a review of the literature and a survey throughout the Italian Pulmonary Hospital Departments in order to identify the most relevant experiences of Italian telemedicine-based services for COPD patients. In contrast to quantitative research, which often makes use of random samples, our sampling for qualitative research had to be purposive (Lijphart, 1971). Second, an analysis of the selected telemedicine-based services was conducted. The sampling was empirical (Yin, 1984), and selected cases were both the most relevant and most paradigmatic. The analysis these cases were conducted by means of a holistic multiple cases-design (Yin, 1984) in order to develop rich and accurate insights that may be hard to acquire through other research designs (Lijphart, 1971).

2.1 Data collection

Because of the explanatory nature of the research, and according to the limited number of professionals usually employed in the delivery of the service, the key informants have been carefully individuated for face-to-face interviews. In particular, 11 physicians and 5 nurses were selected with respect to six relevant cases. They were all responsible of developing the

service, and thus they had been more widely exposed to the change rather than colleagues. Key informants were asked to discuss about the main design principles the telemedicine-based service entails, and which organizational levers have been introduced to render the work system sustainable. Questions concerning the service backsides and the weaknesses have been asked too. Finally, information about the interviewee background were collected to better illuminate her/his perspective.
Interviews were semi-structured grounding on the research framework, and they lasted 150 minutes as average. Information gathered through face-to-face interviews were integrated with secondary-sources data. In particular, business process documentations, performance data reports, technical information system documentation, unpublished management reports, administrative guidelines, jurisdictional papers and fields' notes were analyzed to gather an overview of the processes. In fact, data triangulation from multiple informants and data sources enhances objectivity (Mitroff, 1972), mitigates potential bias (Miller et al., 1997; Huber & Power, 1985) and helps developing converging lines of enquiry (Patton, 2002).

2.2 Data analysis

Every interview was transcript and sent back to the interviewee for validation. Afterward, validated information and supplementary data were utilized to build individual case studies. Follow up information was used to clarify events and resolve discrepancies. Next, the cross-cases analysis began. It aimed at developing consistent patterns of the theoretical relationships across the cases (e.g., Gilbert, 2005; Eisenhardt, 1989). Once the cross-cases analysis was underway, researchers cycled among theory, data and the literature to adjust emerging construct definitions, abstraction levels, construct measures and theoretical relationships. This cycling process continued until a strong match between the case data and theory was achieved across most (sometimes all) of the cases.

3. Conceptual framework

The research adopts the notion of *work system* to capture the essence of a telemedicine-based service. In particular, a "work system" has been defined as *"a system in which human participants and/or machines perform a business process using information, technology, and other resources to produce products and/or services for internal or external customers"* (Alter, 2004: 321). This perspective represents a particularly meaningful lens of analysis to study telemedicine-based services because it digs into the relationships between technology, work context and organizational activities from a social and organizational perspective (Niccolini, 2005). In particular, this perspective is precious to analyze the controversies which always arise when a new technology is implemented (Obstfelder et al., 2007). To highlight the design principles an effective telemedicine-based service needs to entail, the concept of sustainable work system has been introduced. In particular, a sustainable work system is a system where human and social resources are regenerated through the process of work while still maintaining productive and competitive forms (Docherty et al., 2002). That is, the ability of a system to regenerate the resources that employs and the incentives that change behaviors and goals.
The analysis of sustainable work systems requires a comprehensive guiding framework for action (Docherty et al., 2008). Acknowledging the increased pace and complexity of change, and reconciling some of the conundrums and criticisms of the traditional organizational and

change management research streams, we referred to organizational agility principles (de Bont & Bal, 2008) to investigate the design characteristics a telemedicine-based service should entail in order to be sustainable. Frameworks based on agility are in fact a suitable guidance to analyze sustainable work systems (Worley & Lawler, 2009). In particular, instead of trying to specify the criteria of effectiveness, agility models describe the design features that are necessary to deliver on a sustainable work system, which are (1) a maximum surface area structure; (2) transparent information and decision-making processes; (3) flexible performance management systems; and (4) clear human capital strategies (Worley & Lawler, 2009).

These principles have been conceptualized in order to gather evidence with respect to our specific work system (i.e. a telemedicine-based service).

First, work systems adopt structures that maximize the "surface area" of the firm by connecting as many employees as possible with the external environment. Organizations that accomplish this increase the external focus of their members. A variety of companies have increased their surface area by adopting process-based or network structures, which increase the centrality of customer (Galbraith, 2005). Drawing on telemedicine-based services, this aspect highlights the need to develop work systems based on services networks. Any tensions between goals in primary and secondary care need to be handled with care, and patient-centric approach needs to be developed (Obstfelder et al., 2007; Aas, 2001).

Second, work systems need to adopt transparent information systems and decision-making processes. This widely available information allows everyone throughout the work system to make customer-related decisions, moving decision-making to wherever decisions can best be made and implemented. Adopting this principle within telemedicine-based services, this renders nurses more autonomous in decision-making, producing the redistribution of tasks and workload within the clinical team. The adoption of transparent information systems, in fact, might empower nurses able to handle most cases autonomously, asking for doctors' consult only in exceptional cases. This not only underpins the delegation of medical tasks to non-medical personnel (Niccolini et al., 2005), but it even allows patients to improve their self monitoring attitude, rendering them and caregivers active partners in the disease management.

Third, work systems need to adopt flexible talent management and reward systems. Accordingly, a focus on human capital strategies is incentivized, and people are encouraged to find out what needs to be done instead of waiting for someone who tells them about their tasks. In this context, the need to invest in the development of operators' skills and competencies is mandatory. The concerns that arise from the interplay of new technology with existing professional practices, in fact, go beyond simple training issues. The literature about telemedicine-based services, for example, remarks that a critical issue that healthcare professionals encounter when new technologies need to be integrated into routine service delivery is that the technology often undermines the previous professional security and credibility, and arises some concern about the possibility to replace professionals with technologies. This issue is particularly severe for nurses, since their previous consolidated relationships with doctors and healthcare assistants have to change (Hibbert et al., 2004). Work system designers need to deal with these challenges, investing in a strengthening of competences which will reassure professionals.

Finally, work system needs to invest to nurture a highly motivated and satisfied workforce. Organizations utilize a variety of reward practices, including bonuses, stocks, and "person based pay". However, interventions based on extrinsic motivation are often problematic and

ineffective, because it is difficult to link performances and financial incentives (Kohn, 1993). These findings suggest the need to adopt "softer" approaches that work through intrinsic motivations. In particular, it is widely accepted that healthcare professionals should be motivated by larger themes of social responsibility, public trust, teamwork and civic virtue (Wynia, 2009).
The conceptualization of our framework is reported in Table 1.

Agility models design principles (Worley and Lawler, 2009)	Sustainable work system design principles for an effective telemedicine-based service
Maximize the surface area structure: Work systems adopt structures that maximize the "surface area" of the firm by connecting as many employees as possible with the external environment. It entails the adoption of network structures and customer-based processes.	**Coordination:** The maximization of the "surface area" aims at weakening tensions between goals and practices in primary and secondary care, developing and diffusing a patient-centric approach.
Transparent information and decision-making processes: Work systems need to adopt transparent information systems and decision-making processes to allow everyone to make customer-related decisions, moving decision-making to wherever decisions can best be made and implemented.	**Workload distribution:** The adoption of transparent information systems allows the delegation of medical tasks to non-medical personnel. The easier access to information, in fact, renders nurses more autonomous in decision making, and patients more aware in self-monitoring. It entails the redistribution of tasks and workload.
Flexible performance management systems: Work systems need to adopt flexible talent management and reward systems, focusing on human capital strategies.	**Competences:** Investments and actions aimed at strengthening competences are needed, especially for reassuring professionals about their role in service delivery.
Clear human capital strategies: Work system needs to invest to nurture a highly motivated and satisfied workforce.	**Satisfaction:** Softer approaches should be preferred to financial incentives to enhance operators' satisfaction.

Table 1. The conceptual framework

4. Results from the survey: the selection of the most relevant experiences

A survey throughout the Italian Respiratory Hospital Departments has been conducted to identify the relevant Italian telemedicine-based services for patients affected by COPD. 240 questionnaires were sent, with a satisfactory answer rate about 44%. 26 telemedicine-based services were identified. The 50% (n=13) of them were conducted within non-teaching hospitals, the 19% (n=5) in territorial hospitals, the 19% (n=5) in a Scientific Institutes for Research, Hospitalization and Health Care (namely IRCCS), and the 12% (n=3) in teaching hospitals (Fig. 2). This variety highlights that experiences are very heterogeneous among them. Moreover, eleven were ongoing (42%), eight (31%) were concluded and seven were on the initial stage (27%) (Fig. 3). Collected data highlight telemedicine-based services are wide spreading, and although several projects started, only some of them were introduced into a routine. It confirms that discussions concerning telemedicine-based services are getting pivotal, and both the description of the state of art and arguments about what does really works are getting mandatory. This information, in fact, is key for policy makers, who are asked to take decisions concerning the topic.

Since we aimed at deepening how to get telemedicine-based services effective, referring to the design principle a work system need to entail for a sustainable introduction of the innovation into the routine processes, we will focus on ongoing projects. Accordingly, additional information was retrieved with respect to the stage of maturity enhanced by the ongoing experimentations. Results are reported in Fig. 4.

The six institutionalized telemedicine-based services were selected for a further and deeper analysis. More mature services, in fact, have more to say concerning the design principles a work system needs to entail to be sustainable over time. The reason is twofold. First, these projects officially entered into the routine of organizations. Accordingly, they express processes and work systems which have been accurately thought, shared, designed and

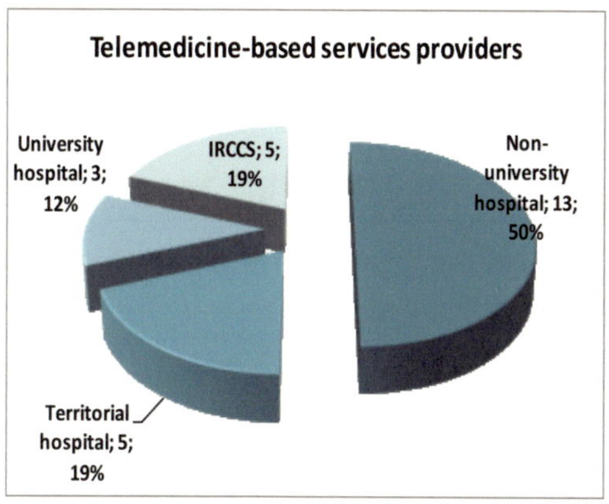

Fig. 2. The services providers

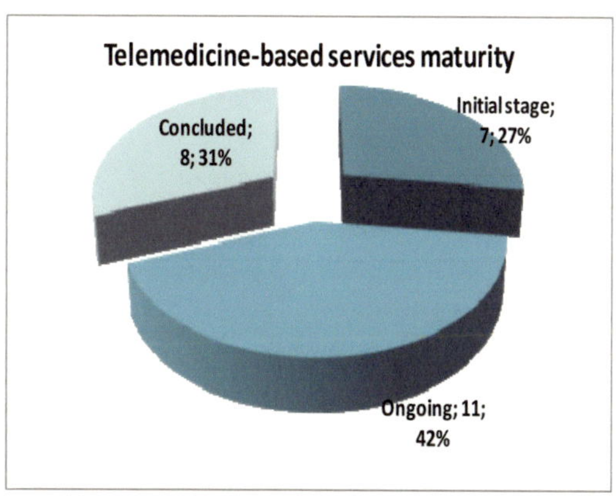

Fig. 3. The services maturity

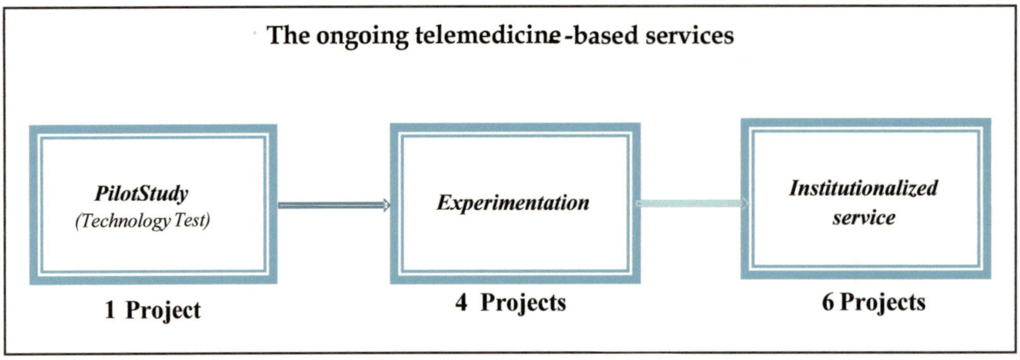

Fig. 4. The services state of art

organized by operators and management, before being introduced. Second, these services, have been running for a number of years, often being pilot projects or experimentations before than institutionalized services. Accordingly, they have had the possibility to pass trough incremental improvements pathways before being institutionalized.

These two arguments characterize institutionalized services as a richer and more complete empirical setting for the scope of our analysis. Accordingly, they have been preferred to others for a deeper analysis.

5. Results from the case studies

An in-depth analysis of the six institutionalized telemedicine-based services has been conducted. Results gathered through the six explanatory case studies are reported. In particular, first a brief characterization of the healthcare organization which hosted the telemedicine-based service is highlighted. Second, a description of the services provided is conducted. Third, a short picture of the evolution of the service and a report of the main characteristics of the enrolled patients is stated to offer a wider overview concerning the results. Finally, a discussion on the lever adopted to enhance a sustainable work system, and indeed an effective telemedicine-based service, is shown, following the principle designs highlighted in the framework.

A synthesis of the main characteristics of the projects are reported in Tab. 2

5.1 Case 1

The first project is provided by the Respiratory Department of a non-university hospital of the Northern Italy (30 beds, 9 physicians).

The organization design: which services are provided and how

The telemedicine-based services provided are the following:

Telemonitoring: a technologic device records the patients' main vital parameters during the night (blood pressure, pulse and saturation). The outline is then automatically sent via-telephone to the referential hospital physician. Routinely, the specialist examines the parameters and sends the medical report back to the patient via e-mail. The frequency of the transmission of data is scheduled patient by patient, according to his/her clinical conditions. In case of out-of range parameters, the physician can (i) go with his/her staff to the patients' home, (ii) contact the LHA staff for a domiciliary visit or (iii) alert the Hospital Emergency Department service.

Case	Telemedicine-based services provided	Telemedicine-based Services Main Goals	Patients		Main Actors involved
			Number (as yearly average)	Typology	
1	Telemonitoring; Teleconsulting	Home hospitalization.	20	Seriously severe	Hospital physicians; LHA staff
2	Telemonitoring	Follow up of ambulatory patients.	15-60	Quite severe	Hospital physicians; Call Center operators
3	Telemonitoring; Telenursing	Follow up of ambulatory patients; Overcoming of geographical barriers.	30	Severe	Hospital Nurses
4	Telemonitoring; Teleconsulting	Follow up of ambulatory patients; Overcoming of geographical barriers.	100	Severe	Hospital nurses
5	Telemonitoring; Teleconsulting	Home hospitalization.	160	Severe/ seriously severe	Hospital nurses; LHA staff
6	Telemonitoring; Teleconsulting	Home hospitalization.	240	Severe/ seriously severe	Hospital team; GPs

Legend: LHA: Local Health Agency, GP: General Practitioner

Table 2. The cases

Teleconsulting: the home-assisted patients have the possibility to contact directly the referring specialist in case of a perceived worsening of symptoms. The specialist knows personally each patient and his/her clinical conditions. Accordingly, the physician can understand more easily the situation, and intervene in a more effective and quick way.
Since the service is not available out of the service hours, potential emergency interventions remain under the responsibility of the Hospital Emergency Department.

Evolution of the service and patients enrolled

An institutionalized telemedicine-based service has been running since 2006. Nine clinicians and two nurses are involved in the service delivery. The number of patients enrolled in the program is 20 as average. This number is not destined to grow. Each specialist is the referent for from 1 to 3 patients. To this concern, the responsible of the service believes that following a limited number of patients preserves a correct relationship patient-clinician, which represents a crucial element in the care of chronic illnesses, because the awareness and knowledge of the clinical situation of every patient increases the effectiveness of the interventions.
Patients are enrolled within the hospital district. Since it has an extension of 30 kilometers as averages, the possibility for the hospital staff to suddenly intervene when required is guaranteed.

Enrolled patients are in extremely serious clinical conditions: they are in a severe stage of COPD, ventilated or tracheostomized, interested by highly weakening co-morbidities (i.e. Amyotrophic Lateral Sclerosis -ALS-). Given these severe patients' conditions, the service aims at giving them the opportunity to be de-hospitalized and live in their own houses with the same level of safety that a hospitalization would assure.

The organizational levers adopted to enhance a sustainable work system

The major lever utilized to render the work system sustainable is the definition of an inter-organizational business model, which coordinates the hospital team and the Local Health Agency (LHA) operators in the conjunct provision of the telemedicine-based service.

The definition of an inter-organizational business model

An inter-organizational business model, which coordinates the hospital team and the Local Health Agency operators, underpins the provision of the service. In particular, the hospital team, mainly physicians, tele-monitors patients' conditions and is responsible for handling acute events. The Local Health Agency (LHA) staff, instead, manages the technology supply and the delivery of general home care assistance. The coordination between hospitals and LHAs came out being an enabling factor to enhance a sustainable service: it allows an easier definition of shared strategies between secondary and territorial healthcare facilities, and a more coherent human resources management.

The actual organization of the service is perceived as positive from the physicians' point of views because it allows them to follow up patients even if they are not hospitalized. Caregivers are satisfied too, because they become more aware with respect to how to handle the patients' clinical conditions. On the contrary, nurses reported they are not satisfied with the provision of the service. This latter represents the real backside of this service delivery. This un-satisfaction is related to the fact that they do not play an active role in the management of the service. In particular, they intervene only when the specialist asks them to perform a specific intervention at domicile. Moreover, they do not receive any additional remuneration for the service provision. The scarce involvement of nurses is endurable only because the service is dedicated, on purpose, to a limited number of patients.

A summary of how the utilized lever impacts on the sustainable work system design principles to enhance an effective telemedicine-based service is reported above (Tab. 3).

Coordination	(+) the structured coordination between LHA and hospital enables a wider contact between the clinical team and the territory.
Workload distribution	(+) the structured business model between LHA and hospital enables a better distribution of tasks and responsibilities; (-) the enrollment of a limited number of patients is key to maintain the work system sustainable.
Competences	(+) thanks to the direct and constant relationship with the physicians, caregivers become more aware with respect to how to handle patients' conditions.
Satisfaction	(+) caregivers are satisfied because they acquire a better and more aware knowledge of how to handle the pathology; (+) the clinical staff has the chance to better follow up chronic patients, without hospitalize them; (-) nurses are not satisfied because no new incentives have been introduced, even if they partly participate to the new service delivery.

Table 3. Synthesis of the Case 1.

5.2 Case 2

The second project is provided by the Respiratory Department of a territorial hospital of the Northern Italy (5 physicians, 3 nurses and 2 socio-assistant operators).

The organization design: which services are provided and how

The service provided is described above.

Telemonitoring: a technologic device records the patients' main vital parameters during the night (blood pressure, pulse and saturation). At predefined cadence, an operator of the Call Center of the Technologic Service Provider calls the patient to both (i) asks some defined questions regarding his/her general conditions; (ii) allows the transmission of data previously recorded. Afterward, the caller uploads the file resulting from the interview in a server, and sends it to the physician. The clinician examines the outline (both clinical data and answers to a questionnaire), being helped by a meaningful interface in detecting potential suspicious values. In case of out-of-range parameters, the physician contacts the patient and defines the interventions required, which may imply the intervention of the GP, the physician's visit at the domicile or a predating of the ambulatory visit.

Evolution of the service and patients enrolled

The project started two years ago (2008), and nowadays it counts 15 enrolled patients. Because of the success of the initiative, in 2011 the number of patients enrolled will grow to 60.

Patients live within the district, are personally known by the two involved physician, and are in quite severe but stable clinical conditions.

The organizational levers adopted to enhance a sustainable work system

The major lever utilized to render the work system sustainable is the definition of the direct involvement of the Call Center of the Technologic Service Provider in the provision of the service.

Involvement of the Call Center of the Technologic Service Provider

The Call Center of the Technologic Service Provider plays a key role in the delivery of the service. It allows the two physicians involved to have a higher visibility on patients' progression of the pathology, keeping the workload burden affordable. Accordingly, physicians consider themselves satisfied with the service. Patients are satisfied too, because they acquire a better knowledge and awareness concerning their pathology and its evolution. However, some of them expressed discomfort about the intrusiveness of the operator of the Call Center, and others decided to abandon the service since they felt that the personal relationship with the specialists was diminishing.

According to these service delivery models, it has to be highlighted that nurses are not involved at all, while the coordination with the territory is facilitated by the fact that the hospital is a presidium of the LHA.

To sum up, a scheme of how the utilized lever impact on the sustainable work system design principles to enhance an effective telemedicine-based service is reported above (Tab. 4).

5.3 Case 3

The third project is provided by the Respiratory Department of a territorial hospital of the Central Italy (5 physicians, 6 nurses, 2 socio-assistant operators, 1 bed for day-hospital treatments). The territory under discussion is particularly suited for home care delivery through telemedicine, since it is mountainous, with little towns scarcely populated. Accordingly, travelling is difficult and public transportations insufficient.

Coordination	(+) the coordination with the territory (i.e. GPs) is facilitated by the fact that the hospital is a presidium of the LHA.
Workload distribution	(+) the involvement of the Call Center keeps the workload burden affordable.
Competences	(+) thanks to the direct and constant relationship with the physician, patients and caregivers acquire a better and more aware knowledge of how to handle the pathology.
Satisfaction	(+) the clinical staff has the chance to better follow up chronic patients, without hospitalize them; (+) thanks to the direct and constant relationship with the physician, patients and caregivers acquire a better and more aware knowledge of how to handle the pathology; (-) the involvement of Call Center makes some patients uncomfortable since they perceive the personal relationship with the specialist was diminishing.

Table 4. Synthesis of the Case 2.

The organization design: which services are provided and how

The main telemedicine-based services provided are two.

Telemonitoring: a technologic device records the patients' main vital parameters, and sends them to the hospital. The schedule of transmissions is defined through an accordance between the hospital nurses and the patients. When data are received, the nurse, aided by a meaningful interface, controls the outlines and, in case out-of-range parameters, contacts the domicile of the patient to understand if a specific intervention is needed. After this preliminary analysis, the nurses decided whether to alert the specialist, the GP or the emergency service.

Telenursing: following a predefined schedule, the nurses call the domicile of the patients, even if the vital parameters are regular, in order to get sure that the situation is under control. The nurses are interested in analyzing the situation under every point of view (family troubles, need for psychological help etc). Moreover, the patient/caregiver himself/herself may call a special number to talk directly with the nurses and to ask some specific questions, when needed.

Evolution of the service and patients enrolled

The service has been running since the end of the 1990s. Different organizational and institutional solutions came one after the other thus far. In the latest years, the service acquired the characteristics and functionalities above described.

Nowadays, 29 patients affected by chronic respiratory insufficiency are enrolled in the service. Patients live in the hospital district, and are in severe clinical conditions. Each of them is univocally followed by an assigned tutor nurse. Tempts to increase the number of patients enrolled are ongoing. However barriers, mainly cultural, still hinder the wide spreading of the service.

The organizational levers adopted to enhance a sustainable work system

The major lever utilized to render the work system sustainable is the empowerment of nurses.

The empowerment of nurses

The nurses of the Respiratory Nursing Ambulatory (PNA), which is a unit hosted by the hospital, play a pivotal role in patients' assistance, as they provide the tele-nursing service, autonomously define the patients' care plans and are responsible for the education and training of patients and/or caregivers. Because of this, nurses express great satisfaction, as their professionalism is emphasized and taken in higher consideration. This satisfaction is measured not only by the general positive mood of the professionals involved, but through quantitative data gathered through a satisfaction survey too. To nurture this sense of satisfaction, a process of continuous innovation is entailed. In particular, a budget for nurses' permanent training has been allocated by the strategic administration, and specific courses are organized every year to keep nurses and personnel updated about the treatment of the chronic illnesses.

Patients are satisfied too concerning this delivery model. In particular, they are very reassured by the fact they have a unique and dedicated interface with the hospital, i.e. their tutor nurse. Moreover, they appreciate the possibility to take advantage of the clinical assistance from their home, since for some of them it is hard to move away from home because of both their severe clinical conditions and the territorial geographical barriers.

Finally, the coordination with the territory should be assured by the fact that the hospital is a presidium of the LHA. However, the collaboration with GPs is particularly scarce. In facts, while some of them understand the importance of the service and turn out to be highly collaborative in its delivery, others mistrust the initiative and spread an unjustified skepticism among potential patients.

A synthesis of how the empowerment of nurses impacted on the enhancement of a sustainable work system is reported above (Tab. 5).

Coordination	(+) the coordination with the territory is facilitated by the fact that the hospital is a presidium of the LHA; (-) GPs are not always collaborative.
Workload distribution	(+) the involvement of the nurses keeps the workload burden affordable; (+) patients acquire a more aware access to hospitals.
Competences	(+) thanks to the direct and constant relationship with the nurses, patients and caregivers acquire a better and more aware knowledge of how to handle the pathology; (+) nurses competences have been empowered through continuous training programs.
Satisfaction	(+) the clinical staff has the chance to better follow up chronic patients, without hospitalize them; (+) nurses are satisfied because their professionalism has been enhanced; (+) patients and caregivers are satisfied because they are a unique interface within the hospital, and they avoid unnecessary trips to hospitals.

Table 5. Synthesis of the Case 3.

5.4 Case 4

The fourth project is provided by the Respiratory Departments of a network of hospitals of the Northern Italy. The service in rooted in an experimentation which aimed at increasing the access to care of low populated areas. Among the structures involved, the one with the highest number of patients enrolled has been selected for a deeper analysis. In particular, the analysis focuses on the telemedicine-based service provided by the Respiratory Department of a teaching hospital of the Northern Italy (14 physicians, 50 nurses, 62 beds, among which 25 for rehabilitative activities and 2 beds for day-hospital).

The organization design: which services are provided and how

The main telemedicine-based services provided are two.
Telemonitoring: Patients are weekly contacted by their tutor nurse, who tells them to perform the measures of blood pressure, oxygen content and cardiac frequency. These parameters are then automatically sent to the hospital, via the Service Center Provider. Afterward, nurses ask patients a predefined questionnaire, posing questions concerning health conditions and perceptions. In case of out-of-range parameters, or critical scenario highlighted through the questionnaire, the nurse intervenes through a modify of the therapy. When the situation is considered particularly critical, the nurse contacts the specialist for a second opinion. The specialist, on his/her hand, may decide to (i) contact the GP and ask him/her to perform a visit at domicile, (ii) contact the emergency service for an immediate intervention or (iii) hospitalize the patient.
Teleconsulting: In case of perceived worsening of symptoms, patients have the possibility to directly contact their hospital tutor nurse, who, when needed, forwards the call to the physician. Hospital nurses are available for teleconsultations from Monday to Friday during the working hours. During the night and on week-ends, indeed, these teleconsultation are handled by the nurses operating in the Call Center of the Service Center Provider. Every nurse, both hospitals' and Call Center's, has access to the patients' online medical record.

Evolution of the service and patients enrolled

The first experience of domiciliary assistance for patients affected by chronic respiratory illness dates back to the beginning of the 2000s. In 2006, a more structured experimentation has been instituted, in collaboration with the Regional Government. The service has been institutionalized in 2010.
Patients involved in the experimentation belong to the hospital district and Province; access criteria are related to their dependency on oxygen and ventilator and to the severity stadium of the illness. The structure enrolls one hundred patients as average. Each of them is assigned to a specific tutor nurse.

The organizational levers adopted to enhance a sustainable work system

Two major levers have been utilized to render the telemedicine-based service work system sustainable: (i) the empowerment of nurses and (ii) the involvement of the Call Center of the Technologic Service Provider for the provision of the service.

The empowerment of nurse

The nurses of the Hospital Respiratory Department play a pivotal role in patients' assistance, since they represent (i) the hospital interface for patients, (ii) the filter for hospital specialists in handling/signaling the emergency situations and (iii) the responsible for educating and training patients and/or caregivers. Within this scenario, nurses are very satisfied because they perceive that the telemedicine-based service would enhance their professionalism. This positive mood is witnessed by the increased number of applications received from other nurses who would like to join the service. The stricter relationship established between the nurse and the patient increases this latter satisfaction too. Patients, in fact, feel more safety, increase their quality of life and, most importantly, have the chance to comprehend their pathology better, assuming major autonomy in dealing with it.
Though the service is particularly appreciated, its organizational burden is high, since it requires that 3 nurses work on it full time, and that at least a specialist of the Hospital Respiratory Department is available to perform a second opinion when needed.

Involvement of the Call Center of the Technologic Service Provider

The direct involvement of the Call Center allows the provision of a 24h service, without asking the hospital team for an all-day-availability. Moreover, since data and phone calls always transit through the Technologic Service Provider network, every information is recorded and backed up, relieving hospitals by medic-legal responsibilities.
However, the possibility for patients to be connected with the personnel of the call center is considered a very delicate aspect. The possibility of harmful interferences (though limited by the presence of the online clinical record) and the uncertainties about the legal responsibilities of actions are, in facts, matters of concern.
Finally, the territorial facilities are rarely involved, and seldom GPs intervene.
A summary of how the utilized levers impact on the sustainable work system design principles to enhance an effective telemedicine-based service is reported above (Tab. 6).

Coordination	(-) GPs are seldom involved	
Workload distribution	(+) the involvement of the nurses introduces a filter in the service delivery processes; (-) the organizational burden for nurses is high.	(+) the involvement of the Call Center guarantees a 24h service without asking hospital personnel for an all-day-availability
Competences	(+) thanks to the direct and constant relationship with the nurses, patients and caregivers acquire a better and more aware knowledge of how to handle the pathology; (+) nurses competences have been empowered.	
Satisfaction	(+) nurses are satisfied because their professionalism has been enhanced; (+) patients and caregivers are satisfied because they have a direct and constant hospital interface available.	(+) the clinical staff has the chance to monitor patients for 24h, without hospitalize them.
	(+) the clinical staff has the chance to better follow up chronic patients, without hospitalize them.	

Table 6. Synthesis of the Case 4.

5.5 Case 5

The fifth project is provided by the Respiratory Department of a non teaching hospital of the Northern Italy (11 physicians, 3 therapists and 26 nurses; 20 beds).

The organization design: which services are provided and how

The main telemedicine-based services provided are two.
Telemonitoring: The staff of the LHA reaches the domicile of the patient and proceeds in recording a list of predefined parameters. The frequency of the visits depends on the health conditions of the patient (from once a week to once a day). Once data have been gathered, the LHA staff sends them via fax to the hospital unit of Domiciliary Respiratory Assistance (DRA), where the patient's tutor nurse verifies the patient's clinical conditions. In case of out-of-range parameters, or critical scenario highlighted by the LHA staff, the DRA nurse

has the chance to contact the hospital physician for a second opinion. The specialist, on his/her hand, may decide to (i) contact the GP and ask him/her to perform a visit at domicile, (ii) contact the emergency service for an immediate intervention or (iii) hospitalize the patient.

Periodically, a nurse of the DRA and a hospital physician visit the patient at domicile to perform activities that go beyond the competencies of the staff of the LHA.

Teleconsulting: Each patient has the possibility to directly contact his/her DRA tutor nurse to receive an immediate consultation. The service is available from Monday to Friday, from 7.30 to 19.30 and on Saturday from 7.30 to 13.30. On holy-days and during the night, the staff of the Respiratory Intensive Care Department of the hospital is available to handle patients' requests for teleconsultations.

Evolution of the service and patients enrolled

A first phase of the experimentation started in 1994; from the beginning of 1995, the service required the involvement of a lung specialist and a part-time nurse. In 2001, the service enhanced an extent of 175 patients per year. Since 2008, 4 nurses have been completely staffed on the service and they manage the whole service delivery autonomously. The patients involved in the service are now 160, and they are resident of the hospital district. Access criteria are related to the dependency of patients on the ventilator, being it partial (8 hours minimum) or continuous.

The organizational levers adopted to enhance a sustainable work system

Two major levers have been utilized to render the telemedicine-based service work system sustainable: (i) the empowerment of nurses and (ii) the definition of an inter-organizational business model.

The empowerment of nurses

The nurses of the Domiciliary Hospital Assistance have been delegated to be responsible for the provision of the telemedicine-based service. This decision has turned out being particularly effective, as it has been calculated that more than 80% of the requests posed by patients have been faced and solved without involving physicians. Because of this, nurses are satisfied with the service since they perceive their professionalism has been enhanced. The stricter relationship established between the nurse and the patient, moreover, increases this latter satisfaction too.

Though the service is particularly appreciated, nurses highlighted ulterior personnel should be involved in its provision, especially if a wider amount of patients will be enrolled. Thus far, in fact, the organizational burden is high: the 4 nurses receive an average of 50 calls per day, while busy with the training activities too.

The definition of an inter-organizational business model

The continuity of care assured by the service is one of its main critical success factors, since it involves in a very effective way specialists, hospital and LHA staff, i.e. nurses, psychologists, social operators and technicians. In particular, the hospital team is responsible for tele-monitoring the patients' clinical conditions, and to intervene in case of out-of-range parameters. The LHA staff, on its hand, visits the patients' domicile, monitors the effective suitability of the caregiver, and identifies eventual conflicting situations within the patient's family.

Patients widely appreciate the possibility to interact with a complete clinical team, composed not only by hospital specialists, but also by LHA staff, dedicated for example to psychological care.

Coordination		(+) the structured coordination between territorial services and hospital enables a wider contact between the clinical team and the territory
Workload distribution	(+) nurses demonstrated their potentialities for being autonomous in taking most of the decisions; (-) the organizational burden for nurses is high.	(+) the structured business model between LHA and hospital enables a better distribution of tasks and responsibilities
Competences	(+) thanks to the direct and constant relationship with the nurses, patients and caregivers acquire a better and more aware knowledge of how to handle the pathology (+) nurses competences have been empowered	
Satisfaction	(+) nurses are satisfied because their professionalism has been enhanced; (+) patients and caregivers are satisfied because they have a direct and constant hospital interface available	(+) patients widely appreciated the various and completed competences rendered available from the heterogeneous clinical team
	(+) the clinical staff has the chance to better follow up chronic patients, without hospitalize them.	

Table 7. Synthesis of the Case 5.

Moreover, great coordination is contemplated among the DRA and the Hospital Emergency Department. Each patient, in facts, is provided with an informative outline which sums up the main clinical conditions of the patients. In this way the emergency intervention is facilitated since information on the plan of care in progress are available for operators. To further increase the degree of collaboration with the emergency service, the nurses prepare and update periodically an informative prospect with a list of the most precarious patients in mechanical ventilation: next to the name and address of every patient, it is indicated the pathology from which it suffers, the model of ventilator employed, the maximum autonomy of batteries, while a colored light (green, yellow, red) indicates the priority of intervention in case of prolonged electric black out. In this way, in case of request of emergency intervention or electric black out that causes the deactivation of the respiratory and of other electrical devices, the emergency operators are able to plan the order of intervention effectively, according to the specific patients' needs.

This high level of coordination is very helpful to face the main sources of risks of care at distance, which are prolonged electrical blackouts, caregiver's stress, infections, scarce ethical and welfare continuity. The possibility to create shared and well managed plans and the presence of common guidelines is very helpful in keeping all these aspects under control.

To sum up, a synthesis of how the above explained levers contributed to the enhancement of a sustainable work system is reported above (Tab. 7).

5.6 Case 6

The sixth project is provided by the Respiratory Department of a non teaching hospital of the Northern Italy (6 physicians, 6 technicians of physiopathology, 1 molecular biologists, 1 technician biologist, 25 nurses, 2 psychologists; 16 beds of ordinary hospitalization, 2 beds for monitoring in breath therapy).

The organization design: which services are provided and how

The main provided telemedicine-based services are two.
Telemonitoring: a technologic device records the patients' main vital parameters, and sends them to the hospital. Daily the physicians or the nurses read the outlines and evaluate the patients' health conditions. If they detect out-of-range parameters, the clinician contacts the patient to evaluate a potential necessity to perform an emergency intervention. In some cases the specialist contacts the GP, asking him to perform a domicile visit.
Teleconsulting: the hospital Unit is equipped with an alarm that is activated when (i) the software detects an out-of-range parameter, or (ii) the patient contacts the Unit because of a perceived worsening of his/her clinical conditions. When the alarm rings, a nurse or a specialist reaches the office where computers are located and checks the outlines. If necessary, a telephone call to the patient is performed. The service is active during the weekdays, on working hours.

Evolution of the service and patients enrolled

The service is ongoing since 1994, when it was institutionalized as Home Hospitalization (HH). The patients enrolled are 240 as average, 70 of which in intensive or continuous ventilation. Access criteria deal with a serious respiratory insufficiency and, with it, oxygen therapy in continuous/partial ventilation.
Enrolled patients live within the hospital district.

The organizational levers adopted to enhance a sustainable work system

The major lever utilized to render the work system sustainable is the empowerment of nurses.

The empowerment of nurses

Nurses play a pivotal role in the service delivery, since they manage, in accordance with the physicians, the patients care plan, are in charge of the training of patients and, most importantly, are responsible to make patients able to enhance a satisfactory level of comprehensiveness and awareness with respect to their pathology. This task increases nurses' responsibilities and professionalism, and it is source of great satisfaction for them.
Not only medical professionalisms, but even patients are very satisfied with this service. In particular, a survey distributed among patients highlighted that the perceived quality of life widely increased after the enrollment: 17% of them said to have feelings about having made progress toward recovery after three years from their enrollment into the service. It represents a strong signal of the satisfaction of patients.
Finally, the level of coordination with the GPs is considerable, since they play an active role in the service by performing interventions at domicile when needed.

A summary of how the utilized lever impacts on the sustainable work system design principles to enhance an effective telemedicine-based service is reported above (Tab 8).

Coordination	(+) GPs are actively involved in the service delivery
Workload distribution	(+) patients has a more aware and appropriate access to care; (+) the involvement of the nurses keeps the workload burden affordable.
Competences	(+) nurses competences are enhanced; (+) thanks to the direct and constant relationship with the nurses and physicians, patients and caregivers acquire a better and more aware knowledge of how to handle the pathology patients and caregivers acquire a better and more aware knowledge about how to handle the pathology.
Satisfaction	(+) the clinical staff has the chance to better follow up chronic patients without hospitalize them; (+) nurses are satisfied because their professionalism has been enhanced; (+) patients and caregivers are satisfied because acquire a better and more aware knowledge of how to handle the pathology.

Table 8. Synthesis of the Case 6.

6. Discussion and conclusions

The discussion and conclusions are organized as follows. First, evidence gathered through the analysis of the sample of selected telemedicine-based services is shown. Second, remarks concerning the applicability and the meaningfulness of the adopted conceptual framework are reported. Finally, the managerial implications and the directions for future researches are proposed.

The explanatory results

Drawing on our results, three main levers emerge as keys for enhancing the sustainability of the peculiar work system "telemedicine-based service". They are (i) the formalization of a clear and agreed business model between the hospital unit and the Local Health Agency (LHA); (ii) the involvement of a call center for the provision of the service and (iii) the empowerment of nurses. In other terms, three distinct enabling levers have been identified for the enhancement of sustainable work system's design principles (see Tab. 9).

Some of these retrieved levers have a specific impact on one of the design principle. The definition of a business model between the hospital unit and the LHA (see case 1 e case 5), for example, enables a coordination between the clinical team and the territory which is much tighter than the one enhanced through other levers.

Drawing on the retrieved levers, moreover, it is highlighted that the empowerment of nurses is the most effective for the enhancement of a sustainable work system. This latter, in fact, maximizes the positive impacts on sustainable work system's design principles. In particular, it underpins the institution of new professionals' boundaries and of new team practices, rendering the team the key organizational structure. Although the need to re-shape the professionals' boundaries (mainly physicians' and nurses') has been highlighted in all the analyzed studies, however, it impacts differently on the specific professionals' workload: in some cases (case 3 and case 6) the division of work is considered sustainable, while in others (case 4 and case 5) nurses denounced to have been working to a too tight schedule.

The main levers:	Definition of a business model between the hospital unit and the LHA	Involvement of a Call Center for the provision of the service	Empowerment of nurses
Coordination	(+) the structured coordination between the LHA staff and the hospital team enables a wider collaboration between the clinical team and the territory (case 1 e case 5).		
Workload distribution	(+) the definition of a structured business model between LHA and hospital enables a better distribution of tasks and responsibilities (case 1 and 5); (-) the enrollment of a limited number of patients is key to maintain the work system sustainable (case 1).	(+) the involvement of the Call Center keeps the workload burden affordable (case 2); (+) the involvement of the Call Center guarantees a 24h service without asking hospital personnel for an all-day-availability (case 4).	(+) the involvement of the nurses keeps the workload burden affordable (case 3 and case 6); (+) patients acquire a more aware access to hospitals (case 3 and case 6). (+) the involvement of the nurses introduces a filter in the service delivery processes (case 4); (+) nurses demonstrated their potentialities for being autonomous in taking most of the decisions (case 5). (-) the organizational burden for nurses is high (case 4 and case 5).
Competences			(+) nurses widely widened their competences (case 3, case 4, case 5 and case 6);
Satisfaction	(-) nurses are not satisfied because no new incentives have been introduced, although they are partly involved in the service delivery (case 1); (+) patients widely appreciated the various and completed competences rendered available from the heterogeneous clinical team (case 5).	(+) the clinical staff has the chance to monitor patients for 24h, without hospitalize them (case 4); (-) the involvement of Call Center makes some patients uncomfortable since they perceive the personal relationship with the specialist was diminishing (case 2).	(+) patients and caregivers are satisfied because they avoid unnecessary trips to hospitals (case 3); (+) nurses are satisfied because their professionalism has been enhanced (case 3, case 4, case 5 and case 6).

Table 9. Synthesis of data

Theoretical implications

This study confirms that both the agility model framework and the concept of sustainable work system are useful bases to support policy makers to design and introduce effective telemedicine-based services. The conceptualisation of this model to the specific context of telemedicine-based services allowed us to analyze the innovation of previous practice as a whole, and helped us to identify and discuss a list of critical success factors that are usually overlooked or underestimated.

Managerial implications and directions for future researches

Two major managerial implications about the introduction of telemedicine-based services can be remarked. First, the relationships and the balances both within the hospital team and between hospitals and the territorial healthcare facilities potentially change. Accordingly, not only intra-hospital but even inter- healthcare-providers processes get modified. Second, non-clinical members (i.e. patients and suppliers) become part of the clinical team, and start playing an active role within routine healthcare delivery processes. Accordingly, a strong, not only operational, but even cultural challenge needs to be enhanced to introduce an effective telemedicine-based service. Professionals and professionals' associations need to be aware of it. However, since healthcare is a highly-regulated context, these organizational and cultural changes need to be accompanied by a regulator's intervention.

Because of these implications, we believe that the identification of the design principles that might promote the sustainability over time of a telemedicine-based service is a relevant field of research and there is need for further investigation by both academicians and healthcare practitioners. In particular, we believe that three main directions for future researchers might be relevant.

First, our analysis of the six experiences formalizes three main leverages that might help the design of effective telemedicine-based services. The role and relevance of these leverages should be deepened and verified by means of further research. The understanding of their factual contribution to sustainability would have significant impacts on policy makers and healthcare professionals. For instance, the empowerment of nurses obliges wide and severe debates about how to reshape the command (and responsibility) chain in healthcare. The institutionalization of regional public vs. private call centers is a controversial issue. On the one hand, there is a need for efficiency and thus a large-scale provider should be preferred, on the other hand, physicians and nurses arise concerns about the externalization beyond the hospital walls of such a delicate service. An in-depth investigation of pros and cons should be thus recommended.

Second, the ways by means of which the command (and responsibility) chain is reshaped among doctors, nurses, healthcare assistants and technicians should be investigated in order to enhance our current understanding of how promoting changes in healthcare. Two useful perspectives for this research stream might be, on the one hand, the one provided by Abbott (1988) with respect to the clash among different professions, or, on the other hand, the one provided by Carroll and Edmondson (2002) about the relevance of a context of psychological safety to facilitate change and improve organizational learning.

Finally, our study and results refer to the specific context of telemedicine-based services for patients affected by COPD in Italy. Thus there are at least two contingencies that should be explored by further research to understand the generalizability of our results. On the one hand, telemedicine-based services for patients affected by other pathologies (e.g. chronic heart disease) should be investigated to collect evidence about how the peculiarities of a specific pathology could affect the design of the service. On the other hand, we know that healthcare delivery is largely affected by institutional contingencies. In this view, it would be value adding to explore to what extent our results (and successful experiences) could be translated in other Countries, such as US or UK.

7. Acknowledgements

This research was supported by grants from the Italian Minister of Health Care and the Health Care Counsellorship of the Lombardy region within the project "Progetto Strategico BPCO". The authors gratefully acknowledge the interviewees, Federica Segato for her fundamental support and the authors of comments on previous versions of this manuscript.

8. References

Aas, M. (2001). A qualitative study of the organizational consequences of telemedicine. *Telemedicine journal and e-Health*, 14, 9, (February 2001), 18-26.

Abbott, A. (1988). *A system of professions.*The university of Chicago Press. London.

Alter S. (2004). A work system view of DSS in its fourth decade. *Decision Support Systems*, 38, 3, (December 2004), 319- 327.

de Bont, A. & Bal, R. (2008). Telemedicine in interdisciplinary work practices: on an IT system that met the criteria for success set out by its sponsors, yet failed to become part of every-day clinical routine. *BMC Medical Informatics and Decision Making*, 8, 47, (October 2008).

Carroll, J.S. & Edmonson, A.C. (2002). Leading organizational learning in Health Care. *Qualitaty and Safety in Healthcare*, 11, (January 2002), 51-56.

Docherty, P.; Forslin, J. & Shani A.B. (2002). *Creating sustainable work systems.* Routledge, London.

Docherty, P. & Shani A.B. (2008). Learning mechanisms as means and ends in collaborative management research. In *Handbook of collaborative management research* Shani ,A. B.; Mohrman, S. A.; Pasmore, W. A.; Stymne, B. N. & Adler, (163-182), Sage, Thousand Oaks, CA.

Eisenhardt, K. M. (1989). Building theories from case study research. *Academy of Management Review*, 14, 4, (October 1989), 532–550.

Forbes, A. & While, A. (2009). The nursing contribution to chronic disease management: a discussion paper. *International Journal of Nursing Studies*. 46, 1, (January 2009), 120-131.

Gagnon, M.; Legare, F.; Fortin, J.; Lamothe, L.; Labrecque, M. & Duplantie, J. (2008). An integrated strategy of knowledge application for optimal e-health implementation: a multi-method study protocol. *BMC Medical Informatics and Decision Making*, 8, 17, (April 2008).

Galbraith, J.R. (2005). *Designing the customer-centric organization: A guide to strategy structure, and processes.*Jossey-Bass, San Francisco, CA.

Gilbert, C. G. (2005). Unbundling the structure of inertia: Resource versus routine rigidity. *Academy of Management Journal*, 48, 5, 741–763.

Hibbert, D.; Mair, FS.; May, CR.; Boland, A.; O'Connor, J.; Capewell, S. & Angus, RM. (2004). Health professionals' responses to the introduction of a home telehealth service. *Journal of Telemedicine and Telecare*, 10. 4, (August 2004), 226–230.

Huber, G. P. & Power D. J. (1985). Retrospective reports of strategic-level managers: Guidelines for increasing their accuracy. *Strategic Management Journal*, 6, 2, (April/June, 1985), 171–180.

Institute of Medicine (IOM) (2008). Knowing what works: a roadmap for the nation. (January 2008).

Kohn A. (1993). Why Incentive Plans Cannot Work. *Harvard Business Review.* (September-October 1993), 54-63.

Lehoux, P.; Sicotte, C.; Denis, JL.; Berg, M. & Lacroix, A. (2002), The theory of use behind telemedicine: how compatible with physicians' clinical routines?". *Social Science & Medicine*, 54, 6, (March 2002), 889-904.

Lijphart, A. (1971). Comparative politics and comparative methods. *The American Political Science review*, 65, 3, 682-693.

Miller, C. C.; Cardinal, L. B. & Glick W. H. (1997). Retrospective reports in organizational research: A reexamination of recent evidence. *Academia of Management Journal*, 40, 1, (February 1997), 189–204.

Mitroff, I. I. (1972). The myth of objectivity or why science needs a new psychology of science. *Management Science*, 18, 10, (June 1972), 613–618.

Nicolini, D. (2006). The work to make telemedicine work: A social and articulative view. *Social Science & Medicine*,. 62, 11, (June 2006), 2754–2767.

Obstfelder, A.; Engeseth, K.H. & Wynn, R. (2007). Characteristics of successfully implemented telemedical applications. *Implementation Science*, 2, 25, (July 2007).

Pasmore, W. A.; Woodman, R. W. & Simmons, A. L. (2008). Toward a more rigorous, reflective, and relevant science of collaborative management research. In *Handbook of collaborative management research* Shani, A. B.; Mohrman, S. A.; Pasmore, W. A.; Stymne, B. N. & Adler, (567-582), Sage, Thousand Oaks, CA.

Patton, M. Q. (2002). *Qualitative Research and Evaluation Methods*, 3rd ed.Sage Publications, Thousand Oaks, CA.

Timmermans, S. & Berg, M. (2003). The practice of medical technology. *Sociology of Health & Illness*, 25, 3, (April 2003), 97–114.

Whitten, P.; Holtz, B. & Nguyen, L. (2010) Keys to a successful and sustainable telemedicine program. *International Journal of Technology Assessment in Health Care*, 26, 2, (April 2010), 211-216.

Worley, C. & Lawler, E. (2010). Built to Change Organizations and Responsible Progress: Twin Pillars of Sustainable Success, in *Research in Organizational Change and Development (Volume 18)*, Woodman, R.; Pasmore, W. & Shani, A.B. Emerald Group Publishing Limited.

Wynia M.K. (2009). The Risks of Rewards in Health Care: how pay-for-performance could threaten, or bolster, medical professionalism. *Journal of General Internal Medicine,* 24, 7, (July 2009), 884-887.

Yin, R. (1984) *Case Study research: design and method,* Sage, Thousand Oaks, California.

Zajtchuk, J.T. & Zajtchuk, R. (1996). Strategy for Medical Readiness: Transition to the Digital Age. *Telemedicine Journal*, 2, 3, (Fall 1996), 179-186.

www.goldcopd.it

Part 4

Scenarios

14

Real-time Interactive Telemedicine for Ubiquitous Healthcare: Networks, Services and Scenarios

Georgi Graschew, Theo A. Roelofs
Stefan Rakowsky and Peter M. Schlag
Surgical Research Unit OP 2000,
Experimental and Clinical Research Center ECRC,
Max-Delbrück-Center for Molecular Medicine and
Charité – University Medicine Berlin,
Charité Campus Berlin-Buch, Lindenberger Weg 80,
D-13125 Berlin
Germany

1. Introduction

Ubiquitous access to high-level healthcare (u-Health) requires increasing use of Information and Communication Technology (ICT) solutions. Telemedicine describes the use of ICT for the delivery of medical services. It aims at equal access to medical expertise irrespective of the geographical location of the person in need. New developments in ICT have enabled the transmission of medical images in sufficiently high quality that allows for a reliable diagnosis to be determined by the expert at the receiving site (Pande et al., 2003; Lacroix et al., 2002). Through Telemedicine patients can get access to medical expertise that may not be available at the patients' site. Networks for Telemedicine enable the integration of distributed medical competence and contribute to the improvement of the quality of medical care, to the cost-effective use of medical resources and to quick and reliable decisions.

For optimal performance of telemedical applications, the networks and communication tools used must be optimised for medical applications, both with respect to the Quality-of-Service (QoS, a set of parameters characterising the performance of the communication channel per se, such as transmission bandwidth, delay, jitter, data loss, etc.) as well as to the Class-of-Service (CoS; a set of terms specifying the medical services offered in the network, like Telesurgery, Telepathology, Telesonography, Tele-Teaching, -Training & -Education, etc.).

Using the specially-developed high-end interactive video communication system WinVicos for real-time interactive telemedical applications at a moderate transmission bandwidth of 0.5-1 Mbps OP 2000 has designed and implemented various satellite-based networks for telemedicine. To serve the specific requirements for management of disaster emergencies, the system developed in the framework of the DELTASS project provides logistic and telemedical services for disaster emergencies. OP 2000 has designed and validated various satellite-based interactive telemedical services that support the medical staff of a mobile field hospital within the disaster area by medical experts from a designated Reference

Hospital outside of the disaster area. In MEDASHIP a system for telemedical support on-board of cruise ships and ferries has been set-up and evaluated. The EMISPHER project provides an equal access for most of the Euro-Mediterranean countries to online services for healthcare in expedient quality. Most of these services use WinVicos and combine high quality live video transmission with remote control of medical equipment.

The use of specifically designed networks for telemedicine contributes to the continuous improvement of patient care. Combined with the implementation of various enabling ICT tools to support distributed collaborative medical scenarios, such as high immersive visualisation, haptic feedback and stereoscopic and high-resolution visualisation, it can really contribute to the realisation of ubiquitous healthcare.

At the same time, however, these innovative developments in ICT bear the risk of creating and amplifying a digital divide in the world, creating a disparity in the quality of life, as this new ICT-based era leads to an increasingly dominant role of access to ICT resources in securing the quality of performance in many aspects of society (Graschew et al., 2003a; Dario et al., 2005; Graschew et al., 2004a). In recent years different projects have demonstrated how the digital divide is only one part of a more complex problem: the need for integration. (Wootton et al., 2005; Rheuban & Sullivan, 2005; Graschew et al., 2003b; Graschew et al., 2002a).

In order to progress from e-Health and Telemedicine towards u-Health (i.e. ubiquitous access to high-level healthcare for everyone, anytime, anywhere) a real integration of both the various technology platforms (Quality of Service) and the various medical services (Class of Services) is needed. A virtual combination of interactive telemedical services to support medical telepresence serves as a basic concept for the development of Virtual Hospitals (VH). One key element within VH will be the medical workplace of the future, which is to provide each of the various user groups with tailored access to all relevant information at the right place and time and in an optimised form.

2. Methodology

During the last years OP 2000 (Operating Room of the future) has designed, developed and validated various modules for interactive telemedicine services (Schlag et al., 1999; Graschew et al., 2000). One of the key elements is the interactive telecommunication module WoTeSa / WinVicos: WoTeSa, a dedicated Workstation for Telemedical applications via Satellite that uses the communication software WinVicos (Wavelet-based interactive Video communication system).

WoTeSa is a PC with sufficient processing capacity (≥ 3 GHz Pentium IV, ≥ 512 MB RAM), one or more Osprey video capture boards (Osprey 100 or Osprey 500), a camera with composite and s-video outputs as live source (e. g. Canon VC-C4); a second camera as document camera for transmission of non-digital images; standard headset or microphone with small loudspeakers. The different video inputs of the Osprey video capture card can be used for direct connection to various medical video sources. WoTeSa thus serves quasi as a medical video hub. It is noteworthy that WoTeSa is a dedicated workstation and yet it can be realised with off-the-shelf components, thus making it readily available and at the same time very flexible and adaptive.

WinVicos is an all-software high-quality interactive video communication system, supplying real-time video, still-image and audio-transmission. WinVicos is especially designed for telemedical applications (e.g. telesurgery, teleradiology, telepathology) using a hybrid speed-optimised wavelet-codec that is based on the concepts of Partition, Aggregation and Conditional Coding (PACC; Patent DE 197 34 542 A1 from "Deutsche Telekom", Darmstadt, Germany). In contrast to most mainstream video coding systems that are mostly optimised for cinema and home entertainment, the PACC codec does not employ motion estimation but maximises the frame resolution to allow for maximal details to be visualised. WinVicos communicates IP-based and allows for online scaling of the transmission parameters (bit rate, frame rate and frame size from 128x96 up to 640x480 pixel). It supports both point-to-point and multipoint communication scenarios. Besides high quality live video transmission using moderate bandwidths (0.5–1 Mbit/s) it also allows for still-image transmission. WinVicos is very easy to use: there is a main user interface that is sufficient for the standard actions of the user. This includes calling the video conference partner via a telephone book, adjustment of both local and remote transmission parameters, as well as speaker and microphone volume control (see Fig. 1).

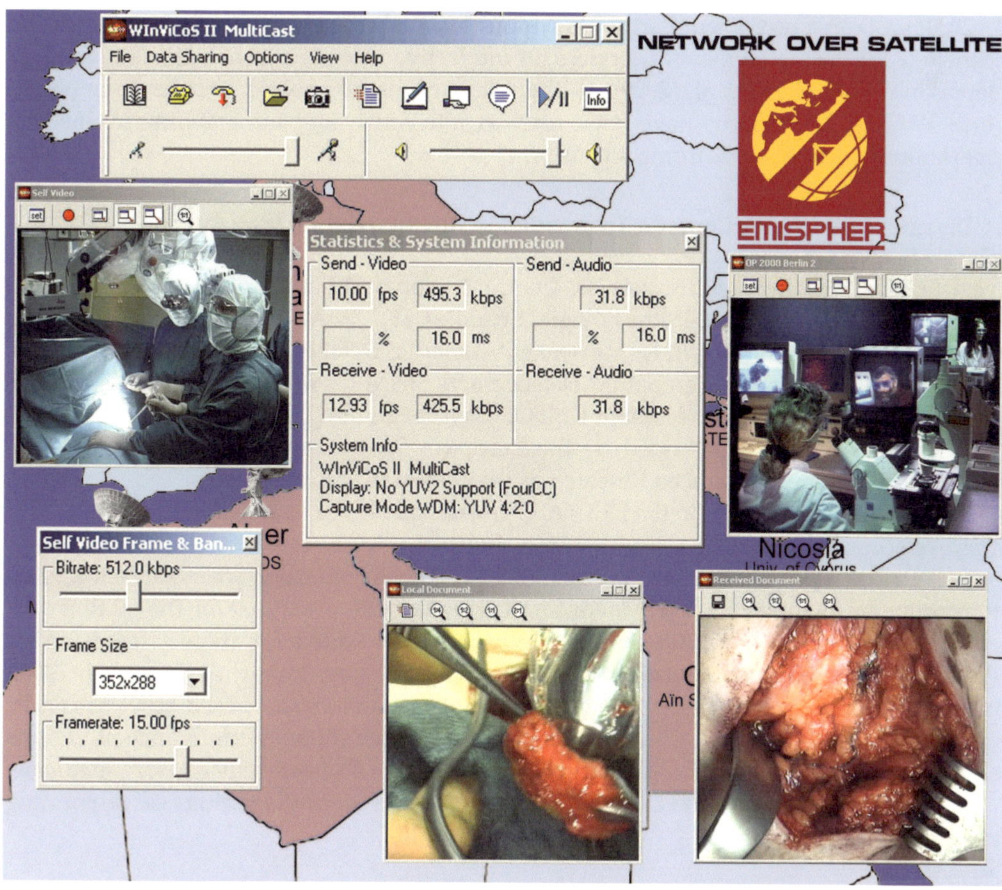

Fig. 1. WinVicos main user interface (top): two live video windows (top) and two still-image windows (bottom), online flexible adjustment of transmission parameters (bottom left), transmission performance can be monitored online (center).

In both the video windows and the still-image windows WinVicos supports the use of common cursors shared by the conference partners. As WinVicos is an all-software system

not only the implementation of other video codecs can be readily realised, but also a continuous performance improvement is supported to keep up with recent developments in the field. The most recent version of WinVicos also supports the transmission of video streams in full high definition (HD) resolution.
Other telemedicine systems are used e.g. for tele-ultrasound in rural areas where telementoring by live videoconferencing allowed to guide the ultrasound technician to record additional images of the patient (O'Neill et al., 2000) for clinical assessment of pediatric burns which showed a good agreement between the face-to-face consultation and seeing the patient via videoconference (Smith et al., 2004) and for home telecare services likely to improve quality of health services (Guillen et al., 2002). Other systems are described in Sable 2002; Latifi et al., 2004; Eadie et al., 2003.

3. Networks and services

OP 2000 has been a prominent partner in various telemedical networks using satellite-based technology for the deployment of services for interactive video communication and medical telepresence (Graschew et al., 2009). In the following, three projects will be described in which WoTeSa / WinVicos have been used as interactive tool for real-time telemedical application services and e-learning scenarios.

3.1 Disaster Emergency Logistic Telemedicine Advanced Satellites System - DELTASS

The DELTASS Consortium consists of: Centre National D'Etudes Spatiales (F), MEDES (Institut de Médecine et de Physiologie Spatiales (F), SPACEBEL (B), Alcatel Space Industries (F), EADS - DORNIER (European Aeronautic Defence and Space Company (D), EADS - MS&I (European Aeronautic Defence and Space Company - Matra Systémes & Information (F), and Surgical Research Unit OP 2000 at Charité (D).
The DELTASS project was funded by the European Space Agency (ESA) as part of the ARTES-5 programme (Advanced Research in Telecommunications Systems).
Further general information on the DELTASS project can also be found at:
http://telecom.esa.int/telecom/www/object/index.cfm?fobjectid=750.
In the DELTASS-project (Graschew et al., 2008) a disaster scenario was analysed and an appropriate telecommunication system for effective rescue measures for the victims was set up and evaluated. Satellite-based systems are well suited for these circumstances, where generally ground infrastructures are partly or even totally destroyed. In such situations, even on a large geographic area or isolated area, space-based services can be easily and quickly deployed. DELTASS demonstrates operational performance of various services, covering the different aspects/phases of disaster emergency medicine. According to these phases, the DELTASS system is made up of the various corresponding subsystems (Fig. 2):

Mobile Teams

Mobile teams are deployed on the disaster site for search, identification, triage and evacuation of victims. They communicate with the coordination- and medical- teams located in Permanent Center or Mobile Field Hospital via low-rate (Globalstar, 9.6 kbps) and medium-rate (Inmarsat, 64 kbps) satellite telecommunication systems. Their positions are tracked via the established Global Positioning System (GPS satellite system).

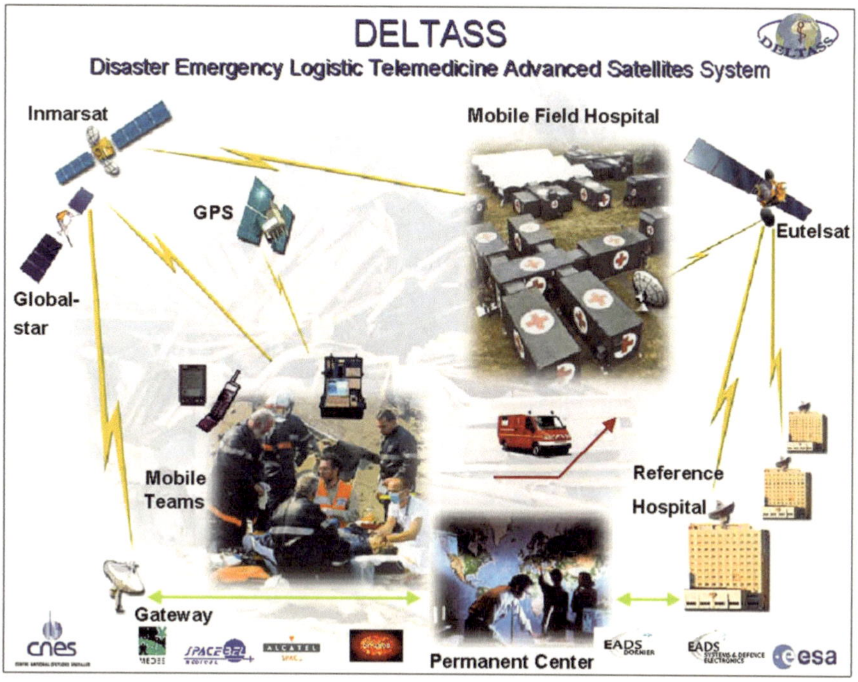

Fig. 2. DELTASS System Architecture: Mobile Teams, Permanent Center (PC), Mobile Field Hospital (MFH) and Reference Hospital (RH) are interconnected via several satellite systems with different bandwidths. Additionally terrestrial communication channels support the data exchange between the PC and the RH.

Permanent Center

The Permanent Center is located outside the disaster area. The Permanent Center constitutes a new element in the architecture of support systems for disaster emergencies and is unique to the DELTASS system. In conventional set-ups the mobile teams at the disaster site are coordinated and supported by the staff of a Mobile Field Hospital deployed at or close to the disaster site. However, complete deployment of such a Mobile Field Hospital takes at least ~6 hours, usually ~12 hours, and consequently the activities of mobile teams in these first, highly critical hours, are ill-coordinated and far from optimal. To improve this bottleneck, DELTASS has a designated Permanent Center that is in control of coordination and medical support to the mobile teams from time zero on. The Permanent Center is equipped with terrestrial gateways to the Globalstar and Inmarsat satellite systems through which it receives all data from the mobile teams. It coordinates all actions of the mobile teams and manages all medical and logistic data, thus assuring efficient operation during the first critical phase. All data received at the Permanent Center are processed, appropriate Reference Hospitals (RH; see below) are identified and the logistic and medical data are transferred to these RH via terrestrial telecommunication links.

Mobile Field Hospital (MFH)

A Mobile Field Hospital (MFH), which will be deployed at or close to the disaster site, provides all activities related to the co-ordination of the mobile teams on the disaster site, the victims medical triage, reception, first aid treatment, conditioning for transportation, further medical expertise for some patients by teleconsultations between MFH and Reference Hospital(s).

Reference Hospital (RH)

The Reference Hospital(s) (RH), located outside of the disaster area, acts as an expert center by providing telemedical services to the MFH using the high-bandwidth satellite link (VSAT, 2 Mbps). These services consist of off-line and on-line telediagnosis, access to external medical databases, as well as real-time interactive telemedical services such as live teleconsultations, live telesonography, intraoperative virtual reality simulation and interactive telemicrobiology (see Fig. 3).

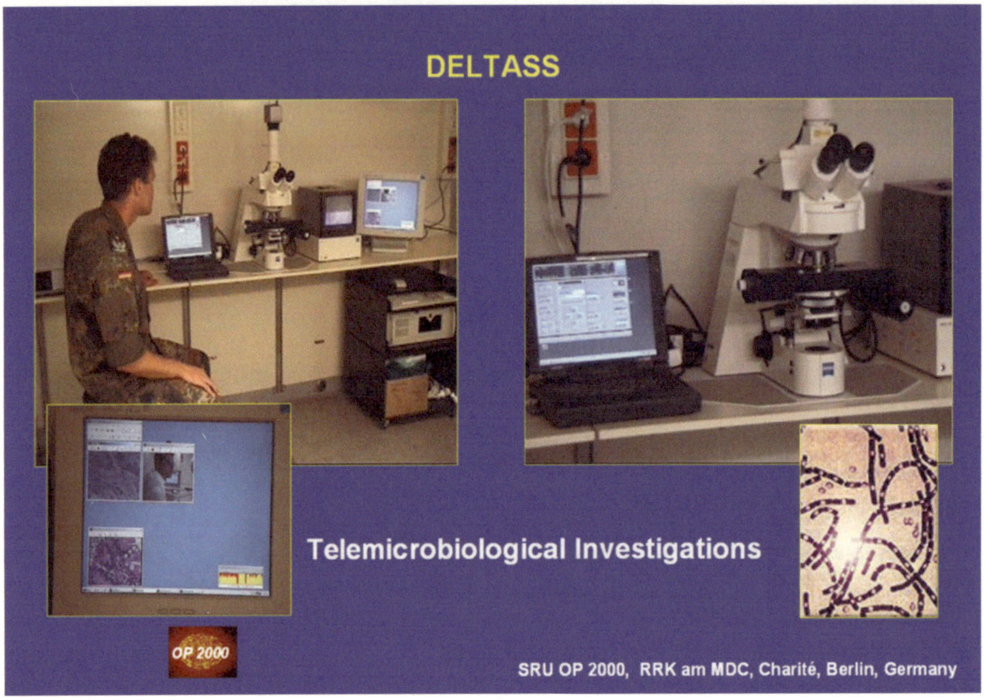

Fig. 3. Interactive Telemicrobiology: The microscope in the MFH can be completely controlled by an expert in the RH. The video data stream of the microscope camera is transmitted live to the RH using WoTeSa / WinVicos (insert left). In this way the expert in the RH can perform the investigation of the microbiological sample in the MFH (insert right) completely and interactively.

Statistics show that in cases of disaster emergency medicine, approx. 40% more amputations are performed, as compared to normal situation. One of the aims of providing live second opinion by remote experts is to reduce this number of unneeded amputations, manipulations and subsequent complications substantially, by expert support during triage, diagnosis and medical treatment.

These interactive telemedical services between the MFH and the RH are realised using the dedicated WoTeSa/WinVicos system. WoTeSa/WinVicos combines the user-friendliness and flexibility of IP-based communication protocols with the security and sufficiently-high quality of the live video transmission at a satellite bandwidth of only up to 2 Mbps. Medical experts at

the RH support the medical treatments in the MFH and enable a quick and reliable decision concerning treatment and/or evacuation of the patient/victim. In this way, the quality of the provided medical service during and after disaster emergencies is strongly improved.
The performance of the DELTASS system has been shown during various full-size live demonstrations (http://telecom.esa.int/telecom/www/object/index.cfm?fobjectid=6324).

3.2 Medical Assistance for Ships - MEDASHIP

Cooperating partners: D'Appolonia (I), AVIENDA (UK), Eutelsat (F), NCSR Demokritos (GR); co-funded by the European Union (EU) under the eTEN programme.
The main objective of the service developed by the MEDASHIP project is to supply integrated solutions for medical consultations on-board of ships (Graschew et al., 2004b). The satellite-based telemedicine services address both passenger ships and merchant vessels and are intended to provide passengers and crew members with an effective medical assistance in cases of emergency and in all those cases where the on board medical staff requires second opinion. During the validation phase the service was tested on board of three ships with the possibility to have it connected to three land medical centers (Fig. 4).
In addition to the standard medical equipment aboard the ships, two video cameras, an electrocardiograph (ECG) and an ultrasound (US) equipment are used. With this equipment the following telemedical services have been realised using satellite transmission at a bandwidth of 512 kbps up to 1 Mbps offering the required high quality of images and video transmission:

Teleconsultation

The live camera on-board of the ship can be used to transmit the image of the doctor who is leading the examination on-board of the ship or the image of the patient when being questioned by the land-based expert. It can also be used to show the land-based expert an injured part of the patient's body which he needs to see for his consultation. Thus a very realistic and effective live communication is possible.

Electrocardiography

The ECG system is connected to WoTeSa on board the ship and can be controlled by the physician from this workstation. Via application sharing software also the expert can control the ECG system from the land-based workstation. The main menu that includes all the functions of the ECG as well as the patient's ECG is transmitted to the expert. Thus the expert and the physician on board can jointly acquire and analyse the ECG report.

Telesonography

The S-video output of the US equipment is directly connected to the Osprey video capture board. Satellite transmission tests have shown that not only still images can be transferred but also live ultrasound investigations can be transmitted at 500-700 kbps (see Fig. 5).
With a document camera analogous patient data can be captured and digitised by WinVicos as a document. For example X-ray or CT-images can be captured from an illumination board and displayed locally and transmitted using this document camera function.

Reduction of cost

The costs for emergency interventions for removing a passenger from the ship and hospitalisation abroad are not to be undervalued. The removal of a passenger in the

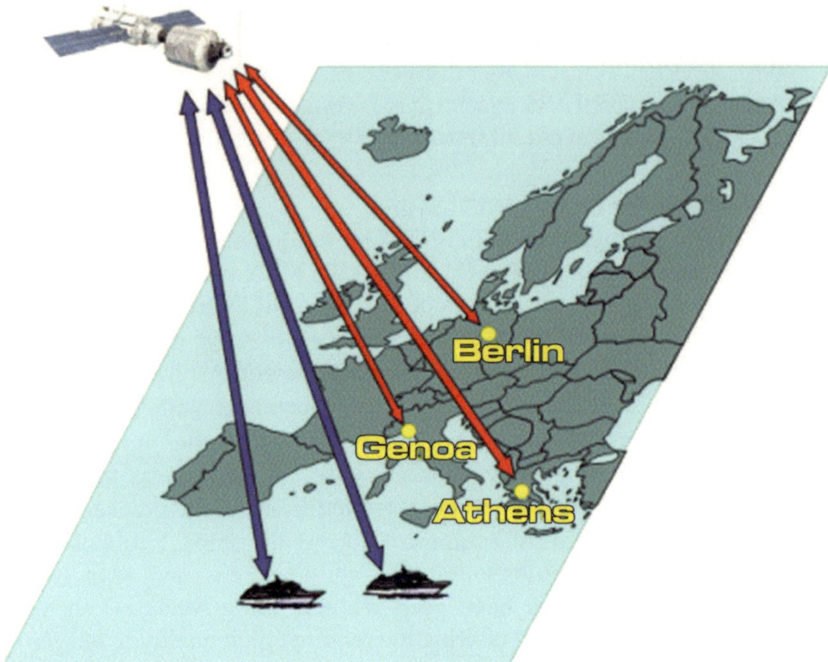

Fig. 4. MEDASHIP network connecting specially equipped ships in the Mediterranean Sea with three Reference Hospitals in Athens, Genoa and Berlin.

Carribean can cost up to $ 11.000 and the cost for hospitalisation can range from 500-1000 € per day. Consequently, market trends force passenger shipping lines to offer services that help to improve the response to on-board clinical emergencies, improve the customer satisfaction and the companies' image.

3.3 Euro-Mediterranean Internet-Satellite Platform for Health, medical Education and Research - EMISPHER

In cooperation with: FMPC - Faculty of Medicine and Pharmacy of Casablanca, Morocco; ANDS - Agence National de Documentation de la Santé (Ministère de la Santé), Algiers, Algeria; Tunis - Faculty of Medicine of Tunis, Tunisia; ASU - Aïn Shams University, Cairo, Egypt; NIFRT - Nasser Institute for Research and Treatment (Ministry of Health and Population, MOHP), Cairo, Egypt; UCY – University of Cyprus, Nicosia, Cyprus; ISTEM - Continuing Medical Education and Research Center, University of Istanbul, Turkey; NCSR Demokritos, Athens, Greece; IsMeTT - Istituto Mediterraneo per i Trapianti e Terapie ad Alta Specializzazione, Palermo, Italy; CICE - Centre International de Chirurgie Endoscopique, Clermont-Ferrand, France; and Charité University Medicine Berlin, Germany; co-funded by the European Union (EU) under the EUMEDIS / MEDA programme.

EMISPHER is dedicated to establish an equal access for most of the countries of the Euro-Mediterranean area to real-time and on-line services for healthcare in the required quality of service (see www.emispher.org). In the project an integrated Internet-Satellite platform has been set up on which three main areas of work have been realised: Virtual Medical University, Real-Time Telemedicine, and Medical Assistance (Graschew et al., 2005a). The

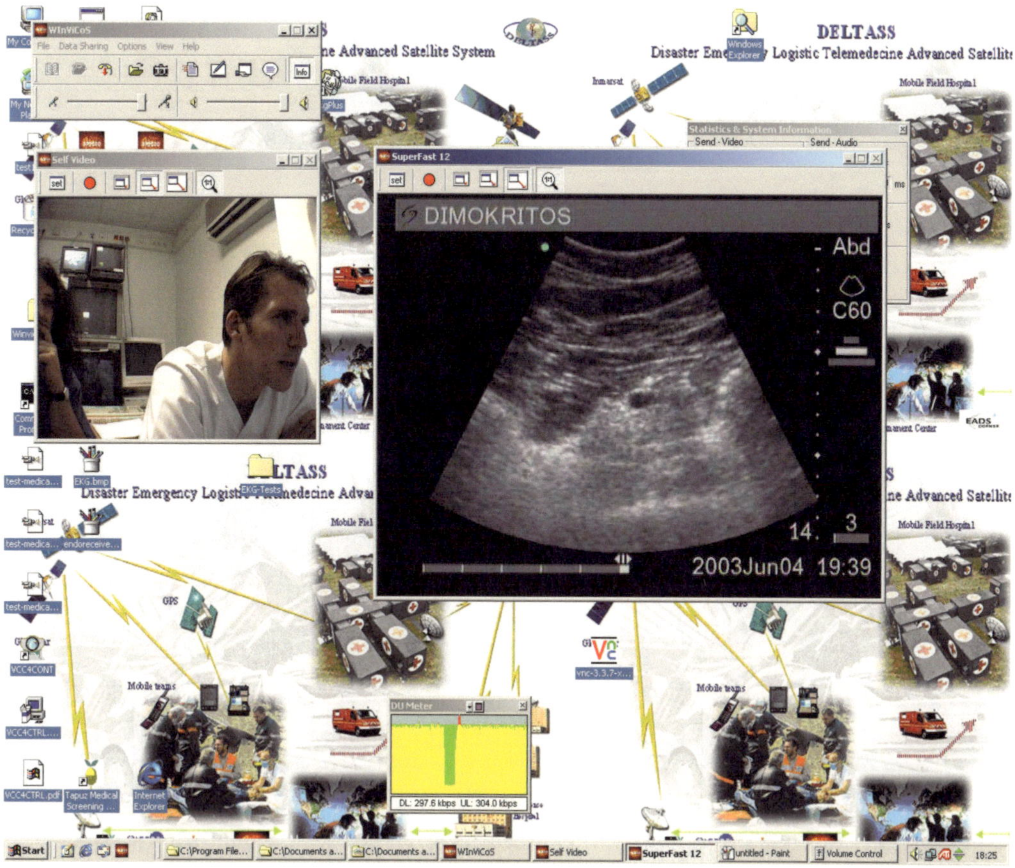

Fig. 5. Telesonography: Tehe live signals of the ultrasound equipment on-board of the ship are transmitted to the reference hospital. A physician at Charité is consulting the ultrasound examination of a patient on board of the cruise ship.

platform includes a bi-directional satellite network (up to 2 Mbps) between 10 Centers of Excellence in the Euro-Mediterranean region (Morocco, Algeria, Tunisia, Egypt, Cyprus, Turkey, Greece, Italy, France and Germany; see Fig. 6). For dissemination of the achieved results and for maximising its impact, EMISPHER has organised international conferences at each of the Mediterranean partner sites.

The EMISPHER Virtual Medical University

The formation and operation of the EMISPHER Virtual Medical University (EVMU) for e-learning (teleteaching) is one of the main efforts in the project. The EVMU uses real-time broadcast of lectures, live surgical operations and pre-recorded video sequences etc., as well as web-based e-learning applications. The target population of the EVMU is comprised of medical students (both undergraduate and postgraduate) hospital staff, general practitioners and specialists, health officers and citizens.

Each of the leading medical centers provides didactical material and modules for synchronous and asynchronous e-learning in their medical specialties. The central gateway to EVMU is the project's website: www.emispher.org.

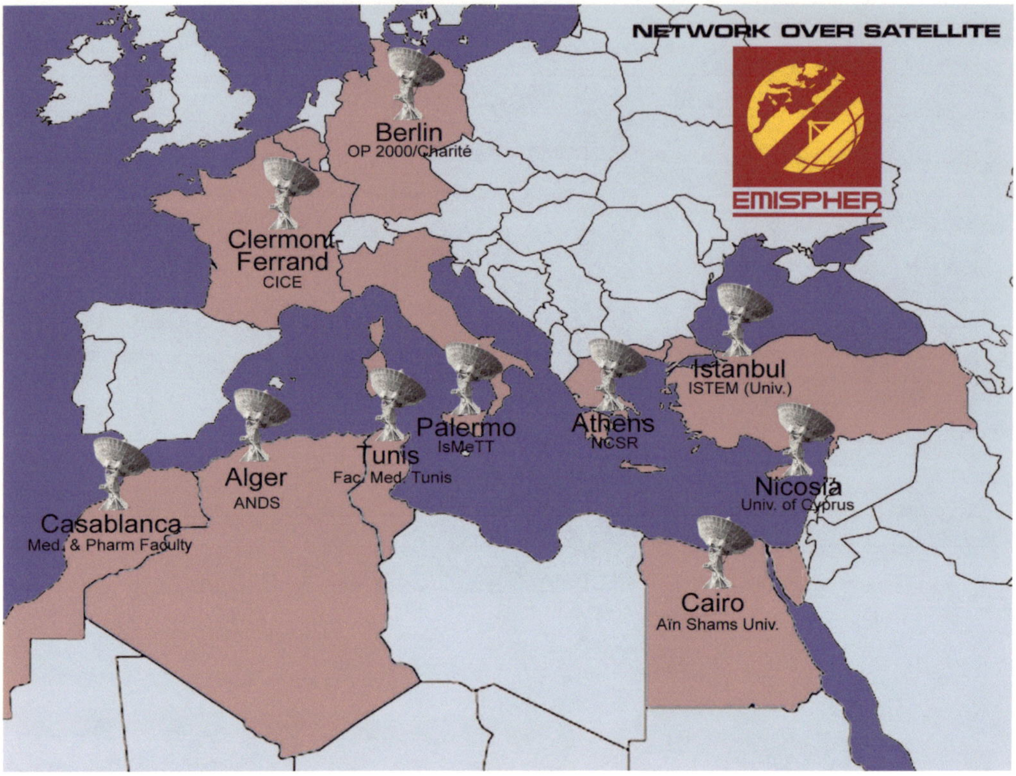

Fig. 6. Medical Centers in the EMISPHER Network

Some of the multimedia teaching material needs to be presented in real-time. Live transmission of surgical operations from operating theatres, lectures, etc. from one site to one or several sites simultaneously (point-to-point or multipoint) are possible in the network between the 10 partners.

Real-Time Telemedicine

EMISPHER has set up a satellite-based network using the combined WoTeSa and WinVicos modules for real-time telemedicine. In the field of real-time telemedicine the following categories of applications are offered: second opinion (Fig. 7), teleteaching & teletraining (demonstration and spread of new techniques), telementoring (enhancement of staff qualification), and undergraduate teaching courses and optimisation of the learning curve. The leading medical centers in the project provide expertise in the following medical fields: open and minimally-invasive surgery, multi-organ transplantation, endoscopy, pathology, radiology, interventional imaging, neurology, infectious diseases, oncology, gynaecology and obstetrics, reproductive medicine, etc. These real-time telemedical applications contribute to improved quality of patient care and to accelerated qualification of medical doctors in their respective specialty. The main target audience are specialist doctors.

Medical Assistance

The third field of service operated in EMISPHER is medical assistance. As tourism constitutes a substantial economical factor in the Mediterranean region and because of the increasing mobility of the population, continuity of care through improved medical

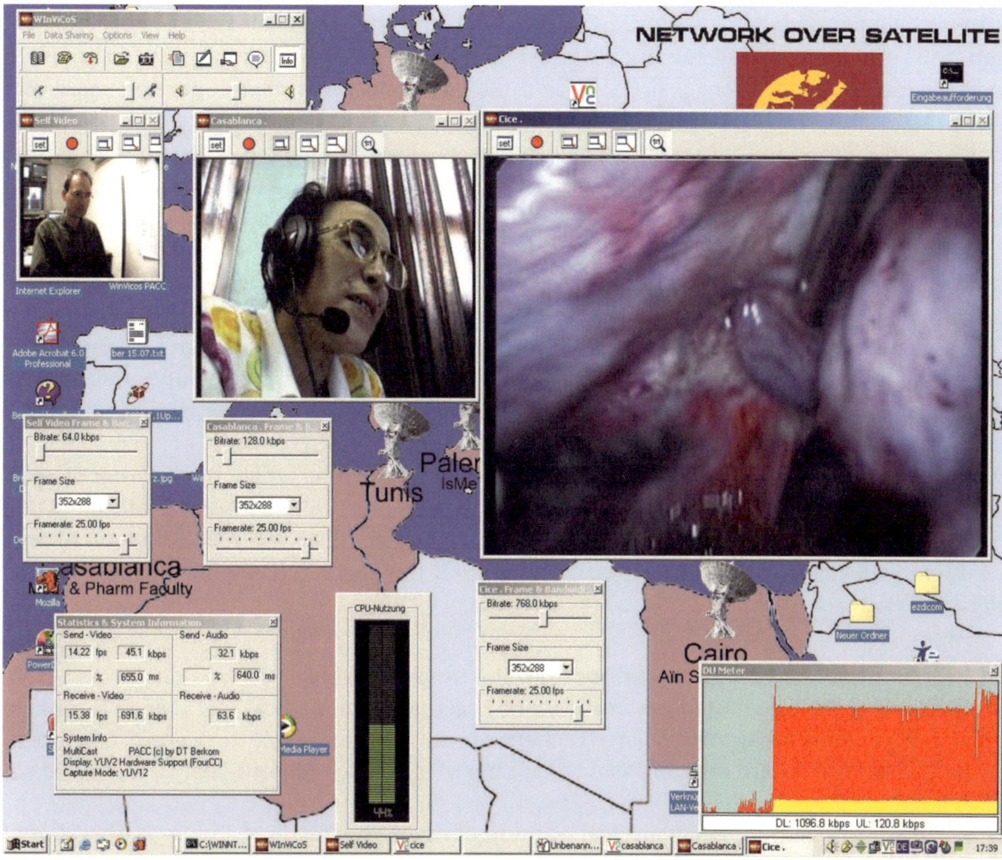

Fig. 7. Interactive multipoint teleconsultation during laparoscopy between OP 2000 (Berlin), Faculté de Médecine et de Pharmacie (FMPC, Casablanca) and Centre International de Chirurgie Endoscopique (CICE, France)

assistance is of major importance for improved healthcare in the Euro-Mediterranean region. Introduction of standardised procedures, integration of the platform with the various local communication systems and training of the medical and non-medical staff involved in the medical assistance chain allow for shared management of files related to medical assistance (medical images, diagnosis, workflow, financial management, etc.) and thus for improved care for travellers and expatriates.

4. Advanced scenarios for ubiquitous healthcare

Besides the implementation of telemedicine networks and services OP 2000 also designs, and develops modules for the operating room of the future by combined use of computer-, video-, communication- and laser technology in the clinical routine of surgery and surgical oncology. Its goal is to achieve more precise, optimised tumour diagnosis and therapy.
OP 2000 is a concept for the operating room of the future by the combined application of computer-, video- and communication-technology in the clinical routine. Its goal is to optimise user interfaces for intraoperative tasks and to introduce virtual reality simulation, haptic feedback, stereoscopic visualisation and interactive real-time video communication to

support telemanipulation, teletraining and telementoring, thus achieving more precise, optimised and personalised tumour diagnosis and therapy.

In medicine the acquisition, processing and display of medical data is gaining more and more importance with increasing processing capacity. The advantages of the computer-assisted simulation of surgical procedures in a high-immersive, distributed, virtual environment are that one can gain a precise and intuitive image of an individual organ for diagnostic purposes or operation planning. The more senses are addressed by the display the quicker, more intuitive and more exact details are conveyed to the medical doctor. One approach is the implementation of a haptic device to enable to feel the shape and surface structure of the organ with simultaneous stereoscopic visualisation and tracking of the user.

For patient-specific pre-operative planning stereoscopic high-resolution imaging and collaboration are important (Montgomery, 2005). The use of a virtual reality environment e.g. for pre-operative planning of total hip replacement yields a high accuracy and steep learning curve even for first-time users (Testi, 2006).

Different haptic feedback systems have been applied and evaluated for the training of open surgery (Hu, 2006), minimally-invasive procedures or colonoscopy (Hellier, 2008), neurosurgery (Lemole, 2007), cataract eye surgery (Doyle, 2008). Virtual reality simulators need haptic devices with force feedback capability if tissue consistency information is to be delivered (Lamata, 2006).

4.1 High immersive workbench projection: the surgical table

On the basis of the distributed environment of a cooperative medical workbench (Fröhlich, 1995) a high immersive virtual environment called Surgical Table has been developed, specially designed for the simulation and training of surgical interventions (Graschew et al., 2002b).

Briefly: a surgeon supervises a surgical training of one of his medical students. Therefore a three-dimensional reconstruction of radiological patient data is being projected onto the workbench. The student manipulates the model, rotates and moves it on the workbench. He may touch bones or cut through some skin or tissue with a virtual tool. While doing so he watches his actions in 3D and feels matching haptic sensations. At the same time the surgeon is able to observe his student's actions and he can give guidance as he is able to point at structures (e.g. a tumour), to talk to the student or to demonstrate an intervention (telementoring). During such a training session it is also possible to have virtual windows showing additional information, movies, or video conferences with other experts or participants. The Surgical Table consists of two high-resolution HDTV-projectors (1600x1200 pixels) integrated in a mobile unit, where virtual objects and control tools are projected on a real workbench (Fig. 8). Collaborative simulations for two users positioned on opposite sides of the Surgical Table are possible, as is the case during real surgery.

The projective display system frees the user from the heavy load and inconvenience related to head mounted displays and enables virtual reality for routine applications. Due to the combined application of two HDTV-projectors, polarisation technique and shutter glasses the Surgical Table allows for several working modes:

- *Double-tracked mode:*

  Simultaneous projection (in broadcast quality) of two different stereoscopic views of a virtual scenario by combination of shutter and linear polarisation techniques. Both users are individually tracked with the electromagnetic multi-channel Polhemus Fastrak sytem (sensors on the glasses and the stylus) and wear polarised glasses that only allow visibility of their corresponding projector. For stereoscopic imaging active shutter glasses are used. Both users can work on the common data set, each using their own toolbar. In this mode, collaborative simulations for two users positioned on opposite sides of the surgical table are possible, as is the situation during real surgery (see Fig. 9).

- *Double mode:*
  This mode enables two users to work simultaneously on the Surgical Table, each on their distinct data set. Each user has an additional monitor for medical second opinioning.
- *Stereoscopic HDTV-mode:*
  Projection of stereoscopic, full resolution HDTV. Sources for the displayed scenarios are computer-generated, three-dimensional models, computer-based movies, as well live pictures from stereoscopic HDTV cameras. In the SRU OP2000 these are various 3D HDTV camera systems available: 3D HDTV camera for open surgery, a 3D HDTV surgical microscope and a HDTV pathological microscope.

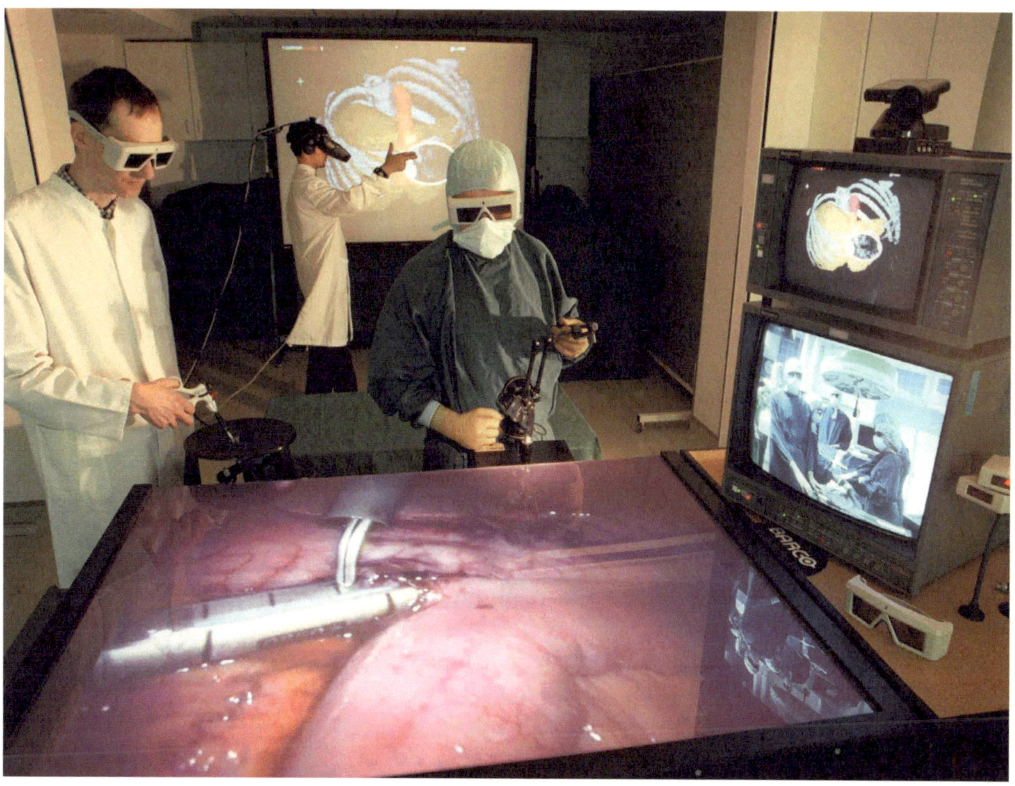

Fig. 8. Realistic simulations of surgical procedures

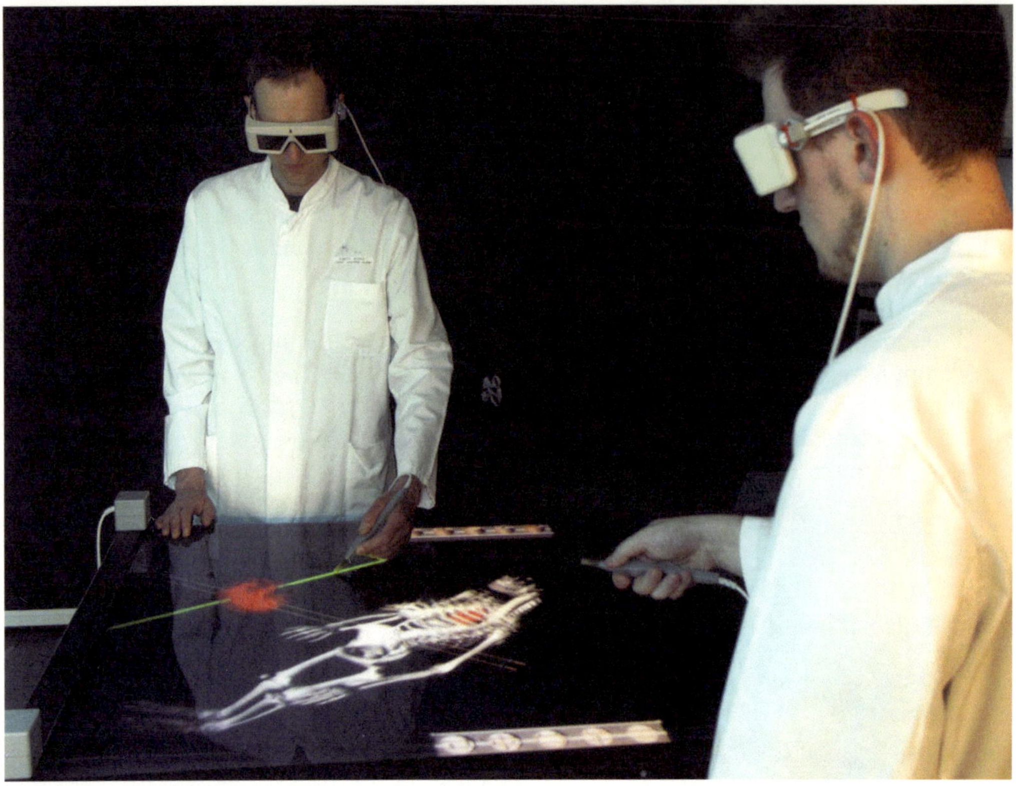

Fig. 9. Surgical Table: Simultaneous display of two opposite tracked views of the same data set (double-tracked mode)

4.2 Haptic feedback

Haptic feedback for touching and navigation of virtual objects with simultaneous stereoscopic visualisation in a distributed network environment has been implemented (Graschew, 2005b). This allows multiple users to feel the shape and surface structure of an organ with simultaneous stereoscopic visualisation and tracking of the user for surgical training.

Client-server architecture allows for distributed usage of the simulation. The server manages the 3-D scene graph by VRML loading and Java-3D scene graph building. Changing of the scene graph by a client is enabled by the synchronisation of the 3-D data. This architecture allows for navigation through the environment by each client. The task of making the objects touchable is achieved by the integration of the PHANTOM haptic device, a high precision 3-D force-feedback system for touching and manipulating the virtual objects (see Fig. 10). The schematic setup for a client with haptic integration is depicted in Fig. 11. The 3-D data are transferred and mapped to the haptic device. The simulation utilises the dynamic data from the PHANTOM haptic device.

A 3-D graphic card and a monitor with an active LCD-shutter in combination with polarising glasses allow the stereoscopic display of selected 3-D objects (e.g. spinal cord, brain, heart, etc.). The head movements of the user are tracked by an IR-tracking system enabling a visualisation of the object with the correct perspective according to the actual

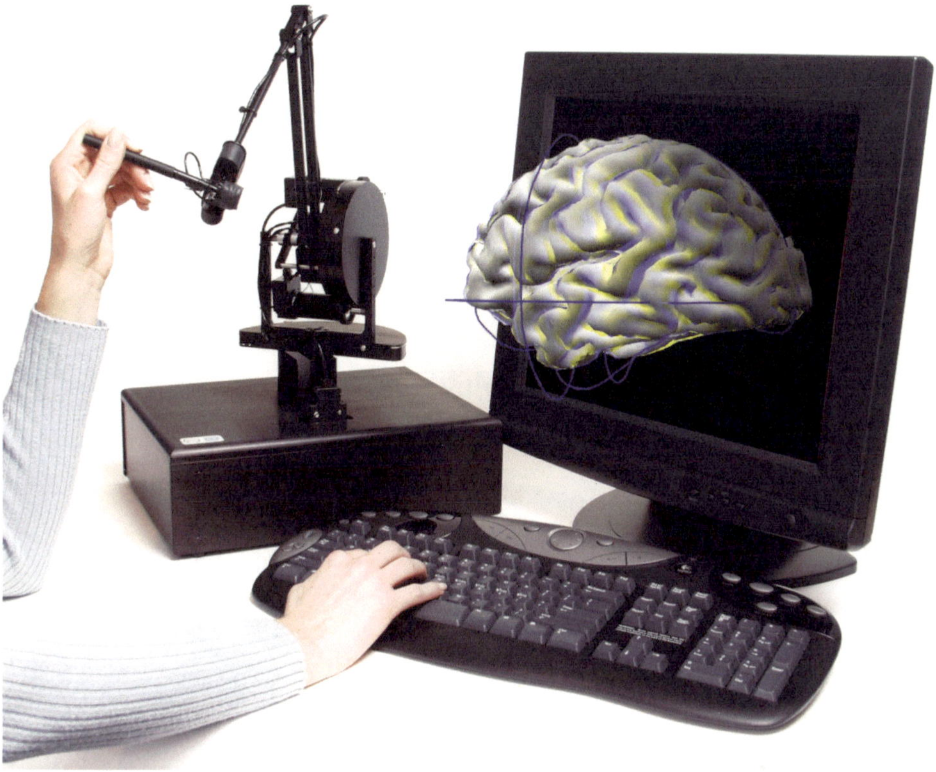

Fig. 10. Phantom haptic device

position of the user. With the PHANTOM haptic device it is possible to rotate and translate the object. Also with the PHANTOM it is possible to navigate a small pointer on the screen around the object and feel the surface structure at the tip of the pointer. Through natural access pathways it is also possible to navigate inside the object.

4.3 Stereoscopic and high-definition visualisation

Stereoscopic visualisation has been realised to achieve a better spatial coordination for the surgeon where he has to rely on video images instead of on his direct sight. As medical stereoscopic video sources a 3D camera integrated into the operating light is used to transmit images from the site of operation in open surgery. A 3D surgical microscope can visualise structures as small as 50 micrometers and gives the surgeon a magnified view e. g. in vascular surgery. For minimally invasive surgery a 3D laparoscope gives the surgeon a stereoscopic view inside the body of the patient.

High quality and high definition cameras have been adapted to different medical imaging devices and tested for medical purposes. For example a single definition 3-chip-CCD camera and an HDTV camera have been compared in a microscope for telepathology revealing greater details in the HD image of a pathological slide. Also a stereoscopic surgical microscope has been equipped with a pair of high definition 3-chip-CCD cameras with a special HDTV optical adapter yielding a higher contrast image. The use of HD-video systems in endoscopic and laparoscopic surgery leads to improved surgical dexterity

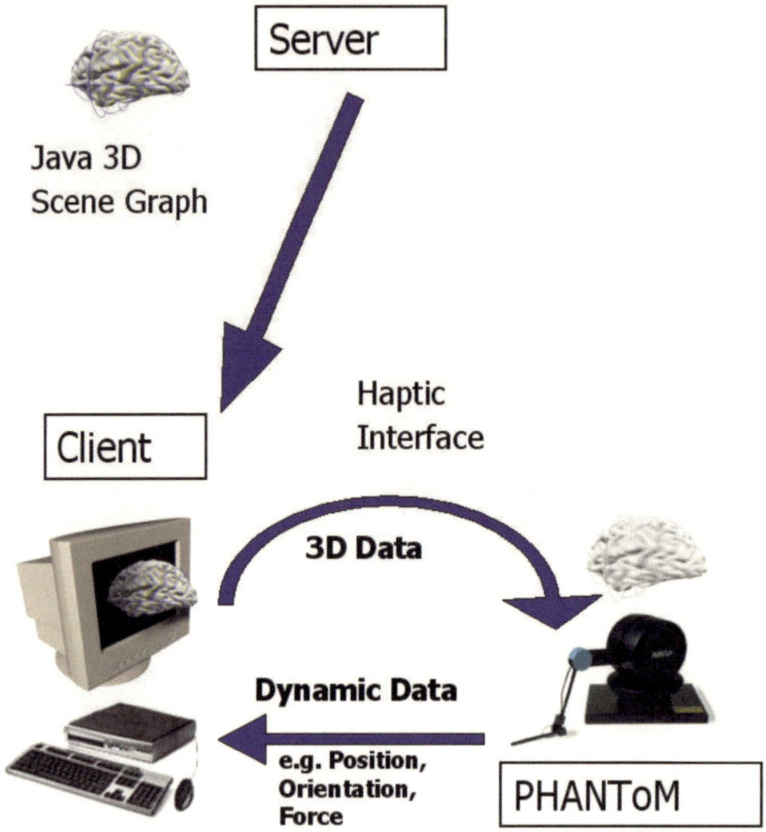

Fig. 11. Client with haptic integration

compared to 3-chip-CCD video systems as the surgeon has to visually judge tissue alterations, van Bergen 2000; Hagiike 2007).

Applying more and more effective compression techniques real-time transmission of stereoscopic medical video also live from the operating room using less bandwidth has become available. The real time transmission of uncompressed medical HD video would require a bandwidth of approximately 1000 Mbit/s. For the clinic-external transmission via existing networks a compression of the video data is required. The implementation of a codec for the coding of medical video data with HD resolution is in preparation.

The requirements for stereoscopic and HD video transmission are met by the WoTeSa/ WinVicos communication system (see section 2).

5. Conclusions and perspectives: virtual hospitals and the medical workplace of the future

Telemedicine networks and services are crucial to support ubiquitous access to healthcare. Appropriate enabling technologies must be deployed and interconnected via networks with an appropriate design. In this chapter we have presented WoTeSa/WinVicos as a flexible high-end module for real-time interactive telemedical services. Besides video communication in medically expedient quality, the provision of interactivity for the remote control of medical equipment is indispensable. Both video communication and interactivity require a (nearly) real-time mode of bi-directional interactions. Various examples have been given of particular networks and services that have been deployed, each to support medical telepresence in specific functional scenarios (DELTASS MEDASHIP and EMISPHER).

However, despite substantial improvements that have been realised, these developments bear the risk of creating and amplifying digital divides in the world. To avoid and counteract this risk and to fulfil the promise of Telemedicine, namely ubiquitous access to high-level healthcare for everyone, anytime, anywhere (so-called ubiquitous Healthcare or u-Health) a real integration of both the various platforms (providing the "Quality-of-Service", QoS) and the various services (providing the "Class-of-Service", CoS) is required (Graschew et al., 2002; Graschew et al., 2003b; Wootton et al., 2005; Rheuban & Sullivan 2005; Graschew et al., 2006a). A virtual combination of applications serves as the basic concept for the virtualisation of hospitals. Virtualisation of hospitals supports the creation of ubiquitous organisations for healthcare, which amplify the attributes of physical organisations by extending its power and reach. Instead of people having to come to the physical hospital for information and services the virtual hospital comes to them whenever they need it. The creation of Virtual Hospitals (VH) can bring us closer to the ultimate target of u-Health (Graschew et al., 2006b).

The methodologies of VH should be medical-needs-driven, rather than technology-driven. Moreover, they should also supply new management tools for virtual medical communities (e.g. to support trust-building in virtual communities). VH provide a modular architecture for integration of different telemedical solutions in one platform (see Fig. 12).

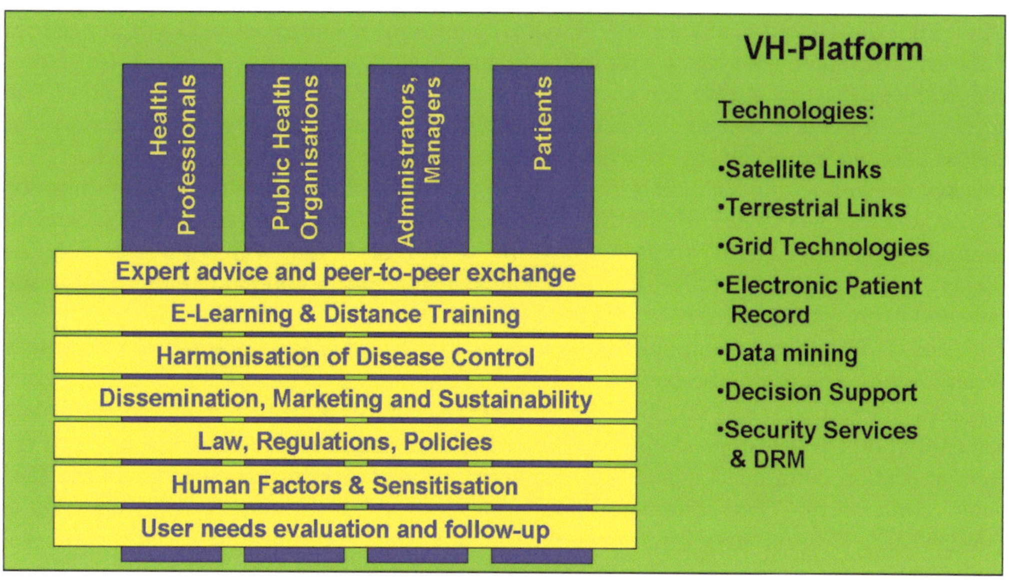

Fig. 12. Concept for the functional organisation of Virtual Hospitals (VH): The technologies of VH (providing the "Quality-of-Service", QoS) like satellite-terrestrial links, Grid technologies, etc. will be implemented as a transparent layer, so that the various user groups can access a variety of services (providing the "Class-of-Service", CoS) such as expert advice, e-learning, etc. on top of it, not bothering with the technological details and constraints.

The technology supporting this platform (in Fig. 12 represented as a green basic layer) should be implemented as a transparent layer, so that the end-users do not need to bother with technological details and constraints. These technologies will include both satellite and terrestrial communication links with seamless transitions between the various segments. Due to the distributed character of VH, data, computing resources as well as the need for these are distributed over many sites. Therefore, Grid infrastructures and services become useful for successful deployment of services like acquisition and processing of medical images (3D patient models), data storage, archiving and retrieval (especially for evidence-based medicine) [27]. Also generic technology tools like electronic patient records and data mining & decision support systems have to be included, as well as tools for security services and data privacy & ownership management. It is also obvious that the population of end-users (in Fig. 12 represented as blue columns) will quite heterogeneous and will include different categories such as health professionals, administrators and managers, public health organisations, as well as patients and citizens. Each of these groups must get tailored access to the various services to be provided. These services (in Fig. 12 represented as yellow rows) not only include the "classical" (tele-) medical services like consultation and exchange, education and training, etc., but must also address other key factors that are essential for successful realisation of u-Health: dissemination and marketing (to expand the number of stakeholders), sustainability (both in an economic and a social sense), law, regulations & policies (for liability and reimbursement issues), human factors & technology sensitisation (trust-building in virtual communities, technology acceptance, change management). Finally, it seems crucial for long-term success of VH in daily routine to apply rigorous users' needs evaluations in a continuous and iterative manner.

Due to the distributed character of VH, data, computing resources as well as the need for these are distributed over many sites in the Virtual Hospital. Therefore, Grid infrastructures and services become useful for successful deployment of services like acquisition and processing of medical images (3D patient models), data storage, archiving and retrieval, as well as data mining, especially for evidence-based medicine (Graschew et al., 2006c).

One key element within VH will be the design, implementation, validation and optimisation of the medical workplace of the future (Project 2020) that shall integrate the various clinically required modalities into one integrated workplace that will provide each of the various user groups with tailored access to all relevant information at the right place and time and in an optimised form.

The project 2020 represents trend-setting tele-medical technology by the use of a high-tech system configuration on the basis of linked application-specific modules. The individual modules are spatially and functionally autonomous units carrying out the primary data acquisition and processing. The image recording and processing modules along with the communication equipment enable the display of all visual information in real-time (3-D video conference). This equipment and functional modules can be operated via a standardised, surgical user environment. The modules are linked to form a universal configuration (user environment peripheral operation, monitoring facilities, 3-D image display; see Fig. 13).

The further design, implementation, validation and optimisation of a surgical-oncological workplace 2020 in which the various clinically required modalities are to be integrated is an important component for peri-operative research. This medical workplace 2020 shall provide the users with all required information at the right time and place and most important in optimally processed form. Important for a workplace 2020 is an integration of the following aspects: high-resolution (HD) and stereoscopic visualisation; interactive real-time video communication with remote control of medical devices for tele-mentoring, tele-training and distributed collaborative work; virtual reality simulations with tracked visualisation and haptic feedback; optimised user interfaces for intraoperative use, etc. By a modular design of the workplace 2020 the various functional groups in the daily clinical routine gain a tailored access to all required medical information, video communication, simulation, etc. The corresponding application of modern technologies of interaction as well as the extensive integration of the various modalities contributes to a more efficient and effective tele-mentoring and tele-training and finally the dissemination of new treatment methods and concepts.

Finally, the possibility to get support from external experts, the improvement of the precision of the medical treatment by means of a real medical telepresence, as well as online documentation and hence improved analysis of the available data of a patient, all contribute to an improvement in treatment and care of patients in all circumstances, thus supporting our progress from e-Health and Telemedicine towards real u-Health.

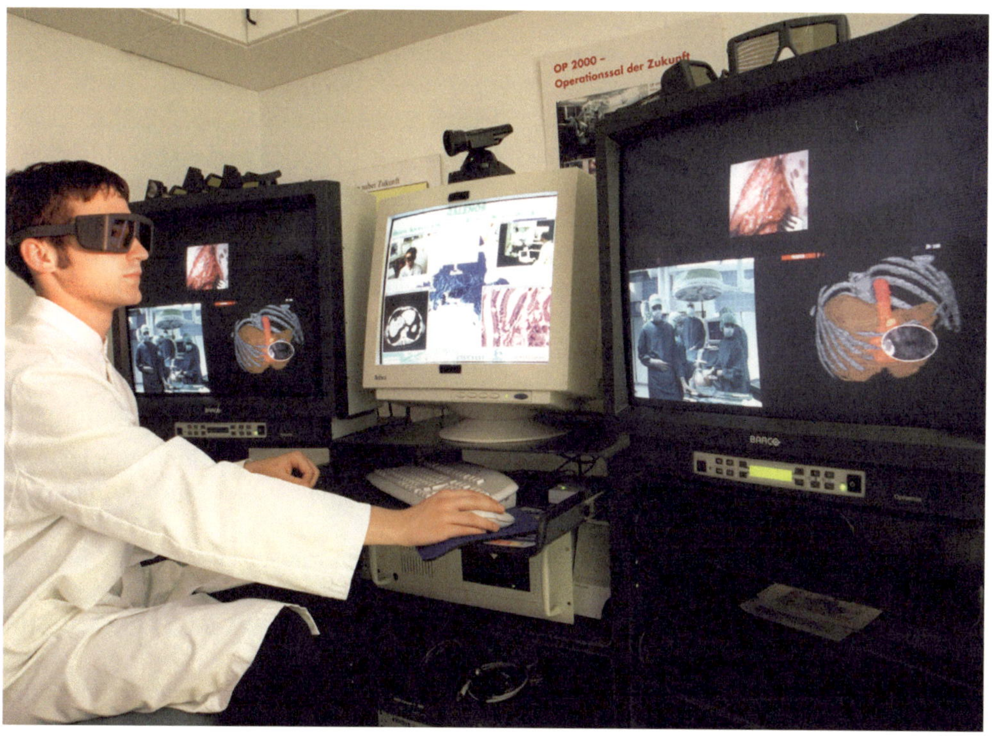

Fig. 13. Workplace 2020 for Surgical Oncology: Stereoscopic visualisation and real-time interactive video communication

6. References

Dario, C. et al. (2005). Opportunities and Challenges of eHealth and Telemedicine via Satellite. *Eur J. Med. Res., Vol. 10, Suppl I, Proceedings of ESRIN-Symposium, July 5, 2004, Frascati, Italy, (2005)*, pp. 1-52.

Doyle L., et al., (2008). A simulator to explore the role of haptic feedback in cataract surgery training. *Stud Health Technol Inform.* Vol. 132, pp. 106-111.

Eadie, L.H. et al., (2003). Telemedicine in surgery. *Br. J. Surg.*, Vol. 90, pp. 647-58.

Fröhlich B. et al., (1995). The Responsive Workbench: A Virtual Working Environment for Physicians. *Comput. Biol. Med.* Vol. 25, pp. 301-308.

Graschew, G. et al. (2000). Interactive telemedicine in the operating theatre of the future. *J Telemedicine and Telecare* Vol. 6, Suppl. 2, pp. 20-24.

Graschew, G. et al. (2002a). Broadband Networks for Interactive Telemedical Applications, *APOC 2002, Applications of Broadband Optical and Wireless Networks, Shanghai 16.-17.10.2002, Proceedings of SPIE,* Vol. 4912, pp. 1-6.

Graschew G., et al., (2002b). High immersive Visualisation and Simulation in the OP 2000 – Operating Room of the Future. *Proceedings of the 5th IASTED Conference, Computer Graphics and Imaging* p.266-268.

Graschew, G. et al. (2003a). Telemedicine as a Bridge to Avoid the Digital Divide World, *8. Fortbildungsveranstaltung und Arbeitstagung Telemed 2003, Berlin, 7.-8. November 2003, Tagungsband,* pp. 122-127.

Graschew, G. et al. (2003b). Telepresence over Satellite, *Proceedings of the 17th International Congress Computer Assisted Radiology and Surgery, London, 25.-28.6.2003,* International Congress Series, Vol. 1256, ed. H.U. Lemke et al., pp. 273-278.

Graschew, G. et al. (2004a). Interactive Telemedicine as a Tool to Avoid a Digital Divide of the World, In: *Medical Care and Compunetics 1,* L. Bos (Ed.), pp. 150-156, IOS Press, Amsterdam.

Graschew, G. et al., (2004b). MEDASHIP – Medizinische Assistenz an Bord von Schiffen, In: *Telemedizinführer Deutschland, ed. 2004,* A. Jäckel (Ed.), Deutsches Medizin Forum, Ober-Mörlen, Germany, pp. 45-50.

Graschew, G. et al., (2005a). Überbrückung der digitalen Teilung in der Euro-Mediterranen Gesundheitsversorgung – das EMISPHER-Projekt, In: *Telemedizinführer Deutschland, ed. 2005,* A. Jäckel (Ed.), Ober-Mörlen, Germany, pp. 231-236.

Graschew G. et al., (2005b). Java-3D Based Virtual Environment for Teaching and Training. *Proceedings of the 13th International Congress of the European Association for Endoscopic Surgery – EAES,* p. 125.

Graschew, G. et al., (2006a). VEMH – Virtual Euro-Mediterranean Hospital für Evidenz-basierte Medizin in der Euro-Mediterranen Region, In: *Telemedizinführer Deutschland, Ausgabe 2006,* A. Jäckel (Ed.), Medizin Forum AG, Bad Nauheim, Germany, pp. 233-236.

Graschew, G. et al., (2006b). New Trends in the Virtualization of Hospitals – Tools for Global e-Health, In: *Medical and Care Compunetics 3,* L. Bos et al. (Eds.) Proceedings of ICMCC 2006, The Hague, 7-9 June 2006, IOS Press, Amsterdam, pp.168-175.

Graschew, G. et al., (2006c). Virtual Hospital and Digital Medicine – Why is the GRID needed?, In: *Challenges and Opportunities of HealthGrids,* V. Hernandez et al. (Eds.) Proceedings of HealthGrid 2006, Valencia, 7-9 June 2006, IOS Press, Amsterdam, pp.295-304.

Graschew, G. et al., (2008). DELTASS - Disaster Emergency Logistic Telemedicine Advanced Satellites System - Telemedical Services for Disaster Emergencies. *International Journal of Risk Assessment and Management* Vol. 9, pp. 351-366.

Graschew, G. et al., (2009). *New developments in network design for telemedicine.* Hospital IT Europe, Vol. 2 No. 2, pp. 15-18.

Guillen, S. et al., (2002). User satisfaction with home telecare based on broadband communication. *J. Telemed. Telecare,* Vol. 8, pp. 81-90.

Hagiike M. et al., (2007). Performance differences in laparoscopic surgical skills between true high-definition and three-chip CCD video systems. *Surg Endosc.* Vol. 21, pp. 1849-1854.

Hellier D. et al., (2008). A modular simulation framework for colonoscopy using a new haptic device. *Stud Health Technol Inform.* Vol. 132, pp. 165-170.

Hu J., et al., (2006). Effectiveness of haptic feedback in open surgery simulation and training systems. *Stud Health Technol Inform.* Vol. 119, pp. 213-218.

Lacroix, L. et al., (2002). International concerted action on collaboration in telemedicine: recommendations of the G-8 Global Healthcare Applications Subproject-4. *Telemed. J. E-Health,* Vol. 8, pp. 149-157.

Lamata P. et al., (2006). Tissue consistency perception in laparoscopy to define the level of fidelity in virtual reality simulation. *Surg Endosc.* Vol. 20, pp. 1368-1375.

Latifi, R. et al., (2004). Telepresence and telemedicine in trauma and emergency care management. *Stud. Health Technol. Inform.,* Vol. 104, pp. 193-199.

Lemole G.M. Jr et al., (2007). Virtual reality in neurosurgical education: part-task ventriculostomy simulation with dynamic visual and haptic feedback. *Neurosurgery* Vol. 61, pp. 142-149.

Montgomery K., et al., (2005). User interface paradigms for patient-specific surgical planning: lessons learned over a decade of research. *Comput Med Imaging Graph.* Vol. 29, pp. 203-222.

O'Neill, S.K. et al., (2000). The design and implementation of an off-the-shelf, standards-based tele-ultrasound system. *J. Telemed. Telecare,* Vol. 6, suppl 2, pp. 52-53.

Pande, R.U. et al., (2003). The telecommunication revolution in the medical field: present applications and future perspective. *Curr. Surg.,* Vol. 60, pp. 636-640.

Rheuban, K.S. & Sullivan, E. (2005). The University of Virginia Telemedicine Program: traversing barriers beyond geography. *J. Long-Term Eff. Med. Implants,* Vol. 15, pp. 49-56.

Sable, C. (2002). Digital echocardiography and telemedicine applications in pediatric cardiology. *Pediatr-Cardiol.* Vol. 23, pp. 358-369.

Schlag, P.M. et al., (1999). Telemedicine - The New Must for Surgery. *Archives of Surgery* Vol. 134, pp. 1216-1221.

Smith, A.C. et al., (2004). Diagnostic accuracy of and patient satisfaction with telemedicine for the follow-up of paediatric burns patients. *J. Telemed. Telecare,* Vol. 10, pp. 193-198.

Testi D., et al., (2006). Efficacy of stereoscopic visualization and six degrees of freedom interaction in preoperative planning of total hip replacement. *Med Inform Internet Med.* Vol. 31, pp. 205-218.

van Bergen P. et al., (2000) The effect of high-definition imaging on surgical task efficiency in minimally invasive surgery: an experimental comparison between three-dimensional imaging and direct vision through a stereoscopic TEM rectoscope. *Surg Endosc.*, Vol. 14, pp. 71-74.

Wootton, R. et al., (2005). E-health and the Universitas 21 organization: 2. Telemedicine and underserved populations. *J. Telemed. Telecare*, Vol. 11, pp. 221-224.

15

Could There Be a Role for Home Telemedicine in the U.S. Medicare Program?

Lorenzo Moreno, Arnold Chen, Rachel Shapiro and Stacy Dale
Mathematica Policy Research
Princeton, NJ 08540,
USA

1. Introduction

Diabetes mellitus is a leading cause of mortality, morbidity, and health care costs among beneficiaries of the U.S. Medicare program. Serious and costly complications of diabetes include vision loss, kidney failure, nerve damage, coronary artery disease, cerebro-vascular disease, peripheral vascular disease, foot ulcers, lower extremity amputations, and infections. These complications often can be avoided through case management, monitoring, control of risk factors, and self-care (American Diabetes Association, n.d.[a], n.d.[b]). Unfortunately, geographic, linguistic, or cultural isolation keeps many Medicare beneficiaries from obtaining high-quality diabetes care. Isolation also may lessen beneficiaries' motivation to eat appropriately, exercise, and lose weight as advised by a physician. Beneficiaries most likely to suffer from diabetes and its complications, including those of African or Hispanic/Latino descent, also may be prone to isolation (Health Resources and Services Administation., n.d.).

Home telemedicine is the use of telecommunications technology to deliver diagnostic, monitoring, educational, and therapeutic services to health care users in their own homes. It may be a promising way to deliver such services to people living in medically underserved areas. Little is known about how well home telemedicine works for Medicare beneficiaries.

A congressionally mandated demonstration tested the clinical and cost outcomes of providing a particular type of home telemedicine service to a large number of Medicare beneficiaries who have diabetes and live in medically underserved areas of New York City and upstate New York. A consortium led by Columbia University College of Physicians and Surgeons and Columbia-Presbyterian Medical Center (the Consortium) performed the demonstration, which it called Informatics for Diabetes Education and Telemedicine, or IDEATel. Mathematica Policy Research was the independent evaluator. The Centers for Medicare & Medicaid Services (CMS) funded and oversaw the demonstration and evaluation. The demonstration was implemented in two four-year phases, from February 2000 to February 2008. Beneficiary enrollment began in December 2000.

Principal investigators for the Consortium have published results of their own analyses of the final effects of IDEATel on key clinical outcomes and costs (Shea et al., 2009); (Palmas et al., 2010). As in the independent evaluation (Moreno et al., 2009; Moreno et al., 2008), they found that the intervention positively affected participants' blood sugar, blood pressure, and lipid levels. These effects, however, must be considered in light of the intervention's acceptability to beneficiaries and potential cost savings to Medicare.

This chapter summarizes (1) participants' use of the telemedicine technology, (2) intervention effects on intermediate clinical outcomes, (3) intervention effects on the use and cost of Medicare services, and (4) costs of the demonstration during the two phases. It also discusses the policy implications of these findings in the context of recent U.S. health reform, particularly the potential role of home telemedicine in the Medicare program.

2. Demonstration overview

2.1 Goals

IDEATel's goals for participants were to (1) control blood sugar, high blood pressure, and abnormal lipid levels; and (2) reduce or eliminate obesity and physical inactivity. To help participants meet these goals, the Consortium designed an intervention to provide remote monitoring, case management, and web-based educational materials through a home telemedicine unit (HTU). IDEATel's goal for physicians was to increase provision of guideline-based diabetes care. To help physicians meet this goal, IDEATel diabetologists recommended guideline-based treatment adjustments when they believed changes were warranted. The Consortium also designed a web-based physician curriculum (Figure 1).

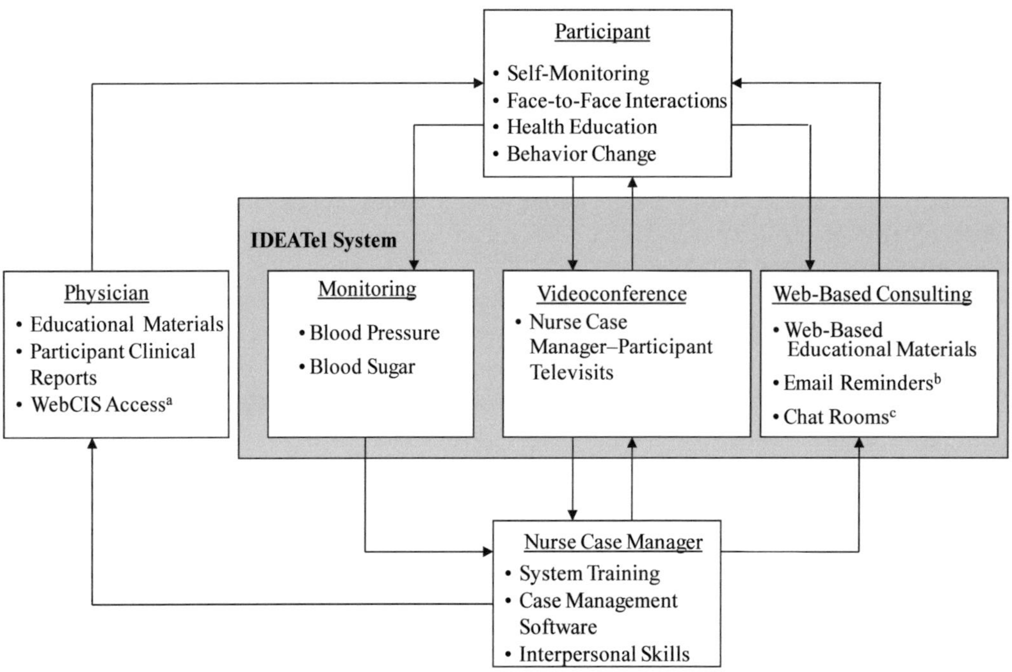

Source: Synthesis from Columbia University (1998) and other unpublished demonstration materials.
[a] WebCIS access only available in New York City.
[b] Email reminders were not systematically implemented in upstate New York.
[c] Chat rooms were not implemented in either site.
WebCIS = Clinical Information System, Columbia-Presbyterian Medical Center, New York.

Fig. 1. The IDEATel System Intervention

2.2 Recruitment

The Consortium first recruited primary care physicians in the demonstration target areas. Consenting physicians furnished lists of their Medicare patients to the Consortium, which screened patients for eligibility and attempted to recruit those who were eligible. Between December 2000 and October 2002, the demonstration recruited 1,665 eligible Medicare beneficiaries (775 in New York City and 890 in upstate New York) for Cohort 1 and randomly assigned them, in equal proportions, to a treatment or control group (Table 1). Between December 2004 and October 2005, the demonstration recruited 504 eligible Medicare beneficiaries (174 in New York City and 330 in upstate New York) for Cohort 2 and randomly assigned them to a treatment or a control group.

	Site		
Evaluation Group/Cohort	New York City	Upstate New York	Total
Cohort 1			
Treatment	397	447	844
Control	378	443	821
Total	775	890	1,665
Cohort 2			
Treatment	86	163	249
Control	88	167	255
Total	174	330	504

Source: IDEATel tracking-status file (Columbia University, 2007a).

Table 1. Distribution of Enrollees, by Site and Evaluation Group

Eligibility was limited to English- or Spanish-speaking Medicare beneficiaries age 55 or older who were being treated for diabetes by diet, oral medications, or insulin, and were living in a medically underserved or health professional shortage area in New York State. Beneficiaries with moderate or severe cognitive, visual, or physical impairment or with severe comorbid disease were excluded. Neither literacy nor prior computer experience were grounds for inclusion or exclusion. Consenting beneficiaries underwent a comprehensive in-person baseline assessment by Consortium staff that included a structured interview; measurements of body dimensions, weight, and blood pressure; blood and urine tests; and setup of a 24-hour ambulatory blood pressure monitor. The Consortium randomly assigned beneficiaries, in equal proportions, to a treatment or control group and sent laboratory results from the baseline assessments to the enrollees' physicians.

2.3 The Intervention

During the demonstration, control group members received diabetes care as usual from their primary care physicians. Treatment group participants also continued to see their primary care physicians, and they received a HTU. (Enrollees are eligible Medicare beneficiaries enrolled in the demonstration. Participants are enrollees in the treatment group, regardless of whether they received the intervention and used the services offered.)
For Phase I of the demonstration, the HTU (Generation 1) consisted of a personal computer with audio/video communication capabilities and devices for measuring blood sugar and blood pressure (Figure 2, right panel). For Phase II, the Consortium redesigned the HTU to

address several features that Cohort 1 participants had found unappealing, such as its large size and difficulty of use. The redesigned HTU (Figure 2, left panel) is known as Generation 2 or Generation 3, depending on the manufacturing date. The Generation 3 HTU had several advantages, such as a cast aluminum case, higher screen resolution, and smaller "footprint," that is, the table area it occupied (Columbia University, 2005).

Demonstration participants could use the HTU:

- To measure and monitor blood pressure and blood sugar and transmit their measurements to a nurse case manager; readings were stored in the HTU until participants performed an upload of the data (Generation 1 HTU) or the HTU transmitted them through periodic automatic uploads (Generation 2 and 3 HTUs)
- To communicate with a nurse case manager through audio/videoconferences known as "televisits"
- To access web-based chat rooms and educational materials available only to participants: chat rooms were implemented in both sites; Email reminders were not systematically implemented in the upstate site; and WebCIS access was operational only in New York City (U.S. Department of Health and Human Services, 2005).

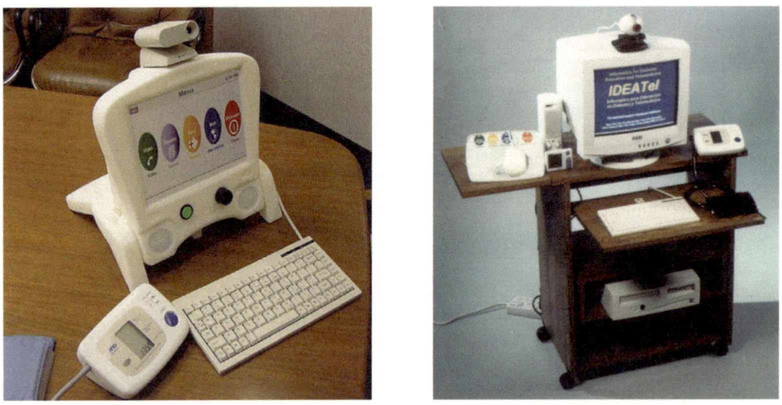

Generation 2 Generation 1

Source: Foster et al. (2006).

Fig. 2. The Generation 2 HTU and Its Predecessor

Televisits were a major component of the IDEATel intervention. By providing regular interaction between participants and nurse case managers at workstations in New York City or Syracuse, they were expected to help participants learn more about diabetes and self-care, improve their attitude toward their disease, and change their behavior. Televisits were to occur every two weeks, be scheduled in advance, and last about 30 minutes each.

2.4 Intended effects

Nurse education and coaching through televisits and self-tracking of progress through other HTU functions were expected to improve self-care behaviors such as monitoring blood sugar and blood pressure, and adhering to diet, exercise, foot care, and medication regimes. By giving physicians guideline-based recommendations, IDEATel also aimed to promote better prescribing patterns, which could improve physiologic outcomes. Better blood sugar control, weight loss, and improved fitness might help participants feel better in the short run. Improved control of blood sugar, lipids, blood pressure, weight loss, and improved fitness might help them avoid serious complications such as blindness, kidney failure, stroke, heart disease, and lower extremity infections and amputations in the long run. Better health, in turn, could reduce use of acute care services and Medicare costs.

3. Related research

Published studies of programs that use remote monitoring and web-based education to manage diabetes have generally used much smaller samples than IDEATel and have not focused on the Medicare population. Nonetheless, some diabetes management programs have demonstrated clinical effectiveness with relatively simple interventions. Aubert et al. (1998), The California Medi-Cal Type 2 Diabetes Study Group (2004), and Taylor et al. (2003) have used randomized experiments to test the clinical effects of providing nurse case management services to patients by telephone. All three of the tested interventions favorably affected hemoglobin A1c levels.

Other researchers have tested the effects of automated telephone systems on diabetes control. Piette et al. (2000) performed a randomized study of a computer system that called enrollees and asked questions in a recorded human voice. Enrollees responded by depressing buttons on a regular touch-tone telephone, prompting appropriate follow-up questions (Piette, 2000). Significant positive effects were found on self-reported self-care, self-efficacy, days of disability, communication with health care providers, and hemoglobin A1c. Delichatsios et al. (2001) found favorable effects on blood sugar control and satisfaction in a nonrandomized study of a similar intervention. Finally, several small studies of interventions featuring simple glucometers that allowed patients to record blood sugar measurements and upload them through a telephone modem showed favorable effects on diabetes-related behaviors and hemoglobin A1c (Ahring et al., 1992; Meneghini et al, 1998; Shultz et al., 1992).

Although not formally evaluated, many relatively inexpensive home telemedicine products are commercially available. Like the IDEATel HTU, such units use regular telephone lines and feature two-way videoconferencing, glucometers, blood pressure cuffs, and store-and-forward capability. Unlike the IDEATel HTU, however, these units are not PC-based, do not use the Internet, and do not allow for web browsing, electronic messaging, or software for tracking personal progress in diet, weight loss, or exercise (AmericanTeleCare, n.d.; HomMed, n.d.).

Few studies provide evidence about costs or both costs and clinical effectiveness. In 2004 the Congressional Budget Office (CBO) examined peer-reviewed studies for evidence of the cost-effectiveness of disease management in treating chronic illness (Congressional Budget Office, 2004). Thirty-one of the studies targeted diabetes and many featured telemedicine or another form of remote monitoring. Although many programs favorably affected process of care and intermediate outcomes, few studies measured effects on long-term health outcomes, health care use, and costs. Those attempting to address costs failed to account for the costs of the interventions themselves. Around the time of the CBO review, however, Villagra and Ahmed published the first-year results of a multistate diabetes management program sponsored by CIGNA HealthCare (Villagra & Ahmed, 2004). The intervention used telephone outreach by nurses, dietitians, or health educators; web-based education; remote monitoring devices; and mailed reminders and educational materials. Using two quasi-experimental methods, investigators found that, among members observed for at least 10 months, the intervention reduced overall health care costs by 8 to 25 percent per member per month (based on claims and encounter data), depending on the analytic method. Although these savings purportedly exceeded the cost of the intervention under both analytic methods, intervention costs were not reported. Moreover, since only 7 percent of the CIGNA subjects were age 65 or older, relevance to the Medicare program and comparability to IDEATel are limited.

4. Study methods

Mathematica researchers collected information through case studies of the IDEATel demonstration, including Consortium leadership and staff, participating physicians, and treatment group enrollees. The evaluation also drew on (1) annual, in-person surveys of treatment and control group enrollees; (2) log-use data of the interactions of participants with their HTUs; and (3) Medicare enrollment and claims data, all of which were collected by the Consortium. Table 2 summarizes the major features of the analysis.

Comparison	Key Measures Used	Primary Data Sources
Implementation analysis	Whether IDEATel was implemented as Congress intended	- Periodic site visits and telephone discussions with Consortium leadership and staff, participating physicians, and participants[a] - Demonstration documentation
Analysis of HTU	- Frequency of use of specific HTU functions and patterns of use over time across cohorts	HTU-use log data[b]
Impacts on behavioral, physiologic, and other health-related outcomes	- Enrollees' self-reported: communication with providers and behavior - Selected clinical and laboratory outcomes - Enrollees' health-related quality of life, and satisfaction with diabetes care	Annual, in-person survey data[b]
Impacts on use of Medicare-covered services and costs	- Medicare-covered service use - Medicare expenditures - Costs of implementing the demonstration	Medicare claims data[b] Demonstration documentation

Source: Columbia University (2007a, 2007b, 2007c, 2007d).

[a]Mathematica selected samples of physicians and participants who had consented to be interviewed from lists prepared by the Consortium following its IRB's guidelines.

[b]To ensure confidentiality, the Consortium collected these data and shared them with Mathematica *without* individual-level identifiers. The evaluation used Medicare Part A and Part B claims data; Part D had not yet been implemented during the period covered here.

Table 2. Analytic Approach Summary

The analyses were conducted separately for the New York City and upstate sites for two main reasons. First, some aspects of the intervention implementation at the sites were quite different. Specifically, the upstate intervention team solicited referring physicians' advance permission to adjust participants' diabetes treatment (for example, medication dosage), whereas the New York City team made recommendations to physicians and asked participants whether its suggestion was implemented. Second, enrollees from each site differed markedly on many major characteristics.

4.1 Qualitative description of the intervention implementation

To assess implementation of the demonstration, the analysis synthesized information from site visits, telephone calls, and demonstration documentation (U.S. Department of Health and Human Services, 2003, 2005). Site visits and telephone discussions with Consortium leadership and staff took place during fall/winter 2001, fall 2002, fall 2003, winter 2005, and winter 2007. The interviews with participating physicians and treatment group enrollees took place in winter 2007 (Foster et al., 2008).

4.2 Estimation of HTU use

To assess participants' interactions with the HTU, the analysis examined the time between home installation of the HTU and its first use, frequency of use, and patterns of use over time from log-use data. It also compared the experiences of Cohort 1 and Cohort 2 participants in the first two years after the start of HTU installation for each phase (December 2000 through February 2007 for Cohort 1 and December 2004 through February 2007 for Cohort 2), controlling for standard baseline characteristics. The analysis sample consisted of 753 Cohort 1 participants (out of 844) and 230 Cohort 2 participants (out of 249). For Cohort 1, the analysis excluded 50 participants whose records had a missing installation date, 6 who had dropped out before their HTUs were installed, 29 whose records did not specify the type of HTU they had received, and 6 whose records did not indicate when their HTU was upgraded from Generation 1 to Generation 2. For Cohort 2, the analysis excluded 17 participants whose installation date was missing and 2 whose records did not specify the type of HTU they had received.

4.3 Estimation of intervention effects

To assess impacts of the intervention on behavioral, physiologic, and other health-related outcomes, the analysis compared outcomes of treatment and control group enrollees using regression models that controlled for the baseline characteristics and baseline values for the outcomes in question. This analysis used the longitudinal survey data collected at baseline and at up to four follow-up annual interviews conducted for Cohort 1 through February 2007, the end of demonstration operations. Likewise, the analysis used the baseline and first annual interviews conducted through February 2007 for Cohort 2.

To assess impacts of the intervention on the use of Medicare-covered services and costs, the analysis compared outcomes of treatment and control group enrollees using regression models similar to those described above. This analysis used Medicare enrollment and claims data from 1999 through 2006.

In both the behavioral, physiologic, and health analyses; and the Medicare service use and cost analyses, enrollees were analyzed in the group to which they were originally randomized (in other words, these were intent-to-treat analyses). However, enrollees who dropped out of the study could not be included in the behavioral, physiologic, and health analyses for time points after the times they left the study, since they had no further survey and laboratory data. All randomized enrollees were included in the Medicare service use and cost analyses since Medicare claims data were available whether or not they had dropped out.

Finally, to assess the costs of the demonstration implementation, the analysis synthesized information from demonstration documents and market prices of products and services used in the demonstration, according to a methodology developed for the Phase I analysis (Starren et al., 2002;U.S. Department of Health and Human Services, 2005).

4.4 Sample characteristics

At baseline, Cohort 1 enrollees in the two sites differed in several ways. Compared with enrollees in the upstate site, New York City enrollees were more likely to be low-income, nonwhite, and Spanish-speaking (as opposed to English-speaking). New York City enrollees had fewer years of education than upstate enrollees and were less likely to have ever used a personal computer at baseline. In both sites, the treatment and control groups were similar on all characteristics, as expected with random assignment (U.S. Department of Health and Human Services, 2005).

In both sites, Cohort 1 and Cohort 2 enrollees differed in several ways. In New York City, Cohort 2 enrollees were younger, more likely to be Hispanic, less likely to have formal education, and less likely to have had prior experience with personal computers than Cohort 1 enrollees. In upstate New York, Cohort 2 enrollees were younger, but more likely to have had prior personal computer experience than Cohort 1 enrollees. In both sites, however, the Cohort 2 treatment and control groups were similar on all characteristics.

4.5 Enrollee attrition

By the fourth year of follow-up interviews, Cohort 1 sample sizes for health outcomes analyses declined substantially in both sites. The overall dropout rates in Cohort 1 were 30 percent in New York City and 58 percent upstate. As discussed in Section 5.3, the loss of these sample members substantially decreased the evaluation's ability to detect impacts. Loss of sample size also compromised the statistical power of the Cohort 2 analyses. After one year of follow-up interviews, the Cohort 2 attrition rate was 13 percent in New York City and 19 percent upstate. As with Cohort 1, however, numbers relative to the original sample were small, and there were no great differences between treatment and control dropouts in baseline characteristics.

Reasons for dropping out differed between treatment and control groups. There was a somewhat higher dropout rate among the treatment groups (33 percent in New York City, 64 percent in upstate New York) than the control groups (28 and 52 percent, respectively). In the New York City site, the rates of dropout in the treatment group because of death and "no reason recorded" were lower than in the control group, whereas the rates for "other reason" and, of course, HTU problems, were higher than in the control group. Although bias in the estimated impacts due to differences between treatment and control group enrollees who dropped out is unknowable, the potential for bias may be mitigated by the small numbers in any given category of reason for dropping out relative to the original sample size. Treatment and control group members also dropped out for different reasons in upstate New York. As in New York City, the rate of dropout in the treatment group because of death was lower than in the control group, while the rates of dropout for enrollee refusal and "too sick" were higher. But again, the numbers for individual reasons are small relative to the original sample. Finally, the intention-to-treat impact estimates based on Medicare claims data are not affected by differential dropout, since claims data are available for all enrollees whether or not they remained in the demonstration.

To assess further the possible effects of attrition on the estimates of program effects on health outcomes, the analysis compared the baseline characteristics of those who dropped out in Cohort 1 and those who remained. The analysis also assessed the sensitivity of a selected set of the calculated year 4 impacts to a range of favorable and unfavorable imputed outcome values for Cohort 1 enrollees who dropped out of the treatment or control groups. These comparisons and sensitivity analyses did not reveal major differences between treatment and control group members who dropped out, or indicate that results were sensitive to even extreme assumptions about the missing outcome values.

4.6 Limitations

Our evaluation has three main limitations. First, the demonstration was not designed to provide evidence on the marginal benefit of the intervention's components—use of the HTU and interactions with the nurse case managers. Thus, the evaluation cannot determine whether the clinical impacts of the demonstration resulted from the telemedicine intervention, the intensive nurse case management, or both (U.S. Department of Health and Human Services, 2005). Second, the high attrition rate in both sites limited any conclusions from the survey and in-person data. For instance, the high attrition rate in the upstate site between baseline and year 4 raises the possibility of bias of unknown magnitude and direction in the estimated impacts. The loss of sample in the New York City site also greatly reduced the evaluation's statistical power to detect impacts there. Finally, for Cohort 1, data on the fifth and sixth follow-up annual interviews were not available for enrollees whose annual interview data had not come up by the end of the study period (that is, February 27, 2007). Therefore, the analysis did not include these data. For Cohort 2, data on the second follow-up interview were available only for a small number of enrollees. As a result, the analysis did not use data from this round of in-person interviews.

5. Findings

5.1 IDEATel implementation

The IDEATel demonstration met requirements established by Congress for implementation. However, the intervention as delivered was neither as intensive nor as technologically sophisticated as originally designed, since the Consortium encountered unexpected challenges and deliberately departed from its plans in some areas. For example, it abandoned its intent to hold televisits every two weeks with all participants, as demonstration leadership argued that the nurse case managers should determine the appropriate frequency for each participant in their caseload. Likewise, the Consortium disavowed the premise that use of advanced HTU functions was central to the intervention, as leadership revised their hypotheses about the connection between these functions and participants' well-being and motivation to self-care. The most important unplanned departure resulted from the inability of a key subcontractor to deliver Generation 2 or 3 HTUs to most participants, which meant that only a few participants were able to experience the planned Phase II technological improvements in the newer units.

5.2 HTU use

Demonstration participants' use of the HTU was key for the success of the intervention. Because the intervention hinged entirely on the use of the HTU, participants who took a long time to learn to use the device, or used it infrequently, received correspondingly less intervention. To examine the intensity of the intervention and how it varied with length of time in the demonstration and across cohorts, the analysis examined use data recorded by participants during their interactions with the HTU.

5.2.1 HTU design, implementation, changes, and problems

5.2.1.1 Initial HTU design

During Phase I, The Consortium had difficulty engaging the participants in HTU use. Many participants had difficulty connecting to televisits. To connect with the Generation 1 HTU, participants had to answer a regular telephone call from a nurse, hang up, activate the HTU, and then answer a second call from the nurse using the HTU launch pad. This process confused many participants and could be interrupted by other incoming calls. Nurses and participants were frustrated that part of many televisits was devoted to connecting and other technical issues, rather than to the participants' clinical and behavioral progress. By the end of Phase I, staff said most participants who were still taking part in the intervention were able to connect to televisits. Between televisits, IDEATel participants were supposed to measure their blood sugar and blood pressure levels and share the information with their nurse case manager. With the Generation 1 HTUs, participants shared their measurements by uploading the data themselves. According to the nurse case managers interviewed late in Phase I, most participants were able to upload their blood pressure and blood glucose measurements, and many were able to monitor their clinical data. Sometimes, however, participants forgot to perform the upload or inadvertently uploaded the same data multiple times – the HTU gave no indication as to when transmission had succeeded.

Participants could also use the HTU to exchange email with nurse case managers and visit the web pages of the American Diabetes Association (ADA). According to the nurses, only about half the participants knew how to access email late in Phase I. Although the nurses thought about half the participants also knew how to access the ADA web pages, they believed few had done so. In addition, Consortium staff reported that few participants had used their HTUs to enter behavioral goals (such as for exercise), record their exercise activity, or send email to nurse case managers. Consortium staff said that chat rooms were never used, with one exception (U.S. Department of Health and Human Services, 2005).

5.2.1.2 Changes to the Initial HTU Design

The Consortium tried to increase participants' proficiency with the HTUs. It developed a video tutorial intended to gradually increase participants' facility, and expected that participants would use the HTUs more as their skills grew. However, by the third year of the demonstration, staff realized that HTU use was still not increasing. To understand participants' difficulties, an expert on human-machine interactions from Columbia University's Department of BioInformatics analyzed HTU use among a subset of participants who enrolled during the second year (Kaufman, Patel et al., 2003; Kaufman, Starren et al., 2003).

Based on the expert's findings, Consortium staff made several changes. They resolved software incompatibilities to increase the user-friendliness of the HTUs' screens; revised the video tutorial; and, most important, retrained all participants on the use of the HTU. Between July 2002 and January 2003, staff were able to train 203 of 359 participants in New York City (57 percent) and 350 of 379 in upstate New York (92 percent). The retraining effort required the hiring of a new staff member to train some participants in New York City in Spanish, and the rehiring of two nurses who originally installed the HTUs in upstate New York. In New York City, many participants reportedly were unavailable for this training or broke their appointments for it (U.S. Department of Health and Human Services, 2005).

5.2.1.3 HTU Redesign and Implementation Challenges

As with Phase I, the Consortium achieved most of its intended improvements with respect to the HTU. Unfortunately, most Cohort 1 participants never experienced the improvements. The redesigned HTU—the Generation 2—was much smaller and less cumbersome than its predecessor. The tabletop unit (pictured in Figure 2) consisted of a small flat screen, a large green answer button, a top-mounted camera, a pliable and "indestructible" keyboard, and a blood pressure cuff and glucose monitor. The unit featured built-in speakers and touch screen technology rather than a stand-alone launch pad.

In addition to being physically compact, the Generation 2 HTU was meant to be less technically demanding of participants. For example, participants connected to televisits simply by pressing a green answer button, and automatic data transmission ("data pulling") relieved participants of having to upload glucose and blood pressure readings. Finally, the Generation 2 HTUs were supposed to be programmed to turn on automatically at a time of the participant's choosing and ask the participant clinical questions in text format.

For both technical and financial reasons, newly enrolled Cohort 2 participants did not receive HTUs—or any form of intervention—as quickly as they had been told they would. Cohort 1 participants had no choice but to continue using their Generation 1 HTUs. Rather than wait out the supply shortage, the Consortium and its subcontractor began to design another model, the Generation 3 HTU. From the user's viewpoint, the Generation 3 HTU featured the same technical improvements as its immediate predecessor: simple connection to televisits, automatic clinical data uploads, and easy-to-navigate user interface.

Despite problems with HTU inventory, televisits continued to be the main component of the IDEATel intervention during Phase II. Unlike in Phase I, in which intervention teams initially sought to have televisits with participants every two weeks, there was no standard frequency for televisits during Phase II, according to Consortium staff. Instead, the nurse case managers determined an appropriate frequency for each participant in their caseload. In both demonstration sites, televisits every four to six weeks was said to be average.

5.2.1.4 Changed Expectations About HTU Use

Much of the difficulty with connecting to televisits was resolved in Phase II. The large green button on the Generation 2 HTU (or on the screen of the Generation 3 HTU) seemed an effective solution for most participants with these models, according to nurse case managers. However, some participants who had to keep their Generation 1 HTUs, and even a few with the newer models, never overcame their uncertainty about how to connect. Nurses reported that 10 to 15 percent of televisits were affected by poor transmission of audio or video data or by disconnections. Nurse case managers attributed this problem to aging telephone lines. When audio or video was inordinately poor, nurses opted to interact with participants by telephone rather than through the HTU.

Missed televisits, which had been a concern during Phase I, were not troublingly high during Phase II, according to nurse case managers. Except for a small number of participants the nurses described as "chronic missers," others participated in visits unless they were away or in the hospital. If participants were less likely to miss visits in Phase II than in Phase I, it may simply have been because, as noted, fewer visits were scheduled.

Participants with Generation 1 HTUs had to upload their stored blood sugar and blood pressure readings themselves. The Generation 2 and 3 HTUs, however, were programmed to transmit such readings automatically each day with no action by the participant. Nurse case managers said the newer procedure worked well, but not perfectly. If participants turned off or unplugged their HTUs between televisits, data were not transmitted.

By the time Phase II began, Consortium staff had drastically lowered their expectations about participants' use of advanced HTU functions, such as visiting the ADA web pages and exchanging email with nurse case managers. Access to ADA web pages that had been developed for IDEATel was discontinued in November 2003. Thereafter, participants could access only ADA pages available to the general public, but the Consortium did not track those visits. By that time, staff also tended to downplay the importance of these functions to participants' well-being and motivation for self-care. Nonetheless, the user interfaces of the Generation 2 and 3 HTUs were designed to be much easier to navigate than the interface of the Generation 1 HTU, which should have facilitated the use of advanced functions. According to interviews conducted in 2007, use of advanced functions was as rare in Phase II as it had been in Phase I, except for a few participants with prior internet experience.

5.2.2 HTU learning curves, and frequency and intensity of use

Cohort 1 members had steeper learning curves than their Cohort 2 counterparts. Since some HTU functions were more complex than others, comparing the learning curves in the two cohorts may suggest whether the redesign of the HTU resulted in a more user-friendly device. For several HTU functions, Cohort 1 participants took longer than their Cohort 2 counterparts to use their HTUs for the first time. For example, the median amounts of time for monitoring and uploading clinical readings were substantially higher for Cohort 1: 284 versus 179 days after installation for monitoring, and 19 versus 3 days for uploading (Moreno et al., 2005). In contrast, the median time to first measurement of blood sugar or blood pressure was the same for both cohorts (1 day), as was the time from HTU installation to the first televisit (23 and 21 days, respectively). Note that taking blood pressure and blood sugar measurements did not require logging into the HTU, and most participants had been using home blood pressure machines and home glucometers before the demonstration began. For complex functions, between 6 and 23 percent of Cohort 1 participants had learned how to use these functions 12 months after installation. For Cohort 2, these percentages ranged from 2 to 7 percent.

Cohort 1 participants were as likely as Cohort 2 participants to use the basic HTU functions during roughly the first 27 months after the start of HTU installation for each phase (December 2000 and December 2004). For example, in New York City, virtually all Cohort 1 participants (99 percent) participated in a televisit at least once during the follow-up period, compared with 97 percent among Cohort 2 participants—a difference that is not statistically significant. Likewise, in upstate New York, all Cohort 1 and 2 participants attended a televisit at least once during the follow-up period. In contrast, use of the complex HTU functions was rare for participants in both phases, although Cohort 1 participants in both sites were significantly more likely than their Cohort 2 counterparts to monitor clinical readings. Furthermore, Cohort 1 participants were also significantly more likely to read and send electronic messages in both sites and to enter behavioral goals in upstate New York. These differences are partly explained by the Consortium's decision to de-emphasize the use of complex HTU functions during Phase II, a result of the difficulties participants experienced during Phase I (U.S. Department of Health and Human Services, 2005).

Participants were asked to attend televisits every two weeks (about 24 times a year), and more often if necessary (Columbia University, 1998). The intensity of HTU use was higher for Cohort 2 than for Cohort 1 participants for five of the eight functions examined, although differences were statistically significant for only four (Table 3). For example, in New York City, Cohort 2 participants used the televisit function significantly more often than their Cohort 1 counterparts—about every 8 and 12 weeks, respectively. The frequency of self-monitoring recommended to each participant depended on the clinical circumstances and was determined by the nurse case managers, with support from the clinical guidelines and supervising diabetologists (U.S. Department of Health and Human Services, 2003). Likewise, in upstate New York, Cohort 2 participants attended televisits significantly more often than their Cohort 1 counterparts—about every five weeks versus every seven, respectively. Furthermore, in both sites, Cohort 2 participants measured their blood sugar and blood pressure significantly more often than Cohort 1 participants. Because of the data-pulling feature of the Generation 2 and 3 HTUs, Cohort 2 participants in both sites uploaded their blood pressure and blood sugar readings between seven and nine times more often, on average, than their Cohort 1 counterparts. For the complex functions, such as monitoring clinical readings, the between-cohort differences in the average frequency of use of HTU functions were small and not statistically significant.

HTU Function	Cohort 1	Cohort 2	Difference (*p*-Value[a])
Basic Functions			
Measure Blood Sugar			
New York City	161.1	208.6	47.5 (.048)
Upstate New York	237.0	386.2	149.2 (.000)
Measure Blood Pressure			
New York City	147.4	199.1	51.7 (.013)
Upstate New York	163.8	245.6	81.8 (.000)
Complex Functions			
Upload Clinical Readings			
New York City	9.3	128.5	119.2 (.000)
Upstate New York	14.7	169.4	154.7 (.000)
Monitor Clinical Readings			
New York City	5.5	6.8	1.3 (.697)

HTU Function	Cohort 1	Cohort 2	Difference (*p*-Value[a])
Upstate New York	8.7	6.7	- 2.0 (.737)
Participate in Televisits			
New York City	4.5	6.4	1.9 (.000)
Upstate New York	7.0	10.5	3.5 (.000)
Read Electronic Messages			
New York City	2.1	0.5	- 1.6 (.869)
Upstate New York	4.8	3.1	- 1.7 (.878)
Send Electronic Messages			
New York City	1.1	0.5	- 0.6 (.897)
Upstate New York	1.5	1.3	- 0.2 (.893)
Enter Behavioral Goals			
New York City	3.0	0.6	- 2.4 (.806)
Upstate New York	1.6	1.5	- 0.1 (.503)
Sample Size[b]	753	230	-

Source: IDEATel database on HTU use linked to the IDEATel tracking status file (Columbia University, 2007a, 2007b).

Notes: Estimates weighted based on length of enrollment between HTU installation and the dropout date or the cutoff date (February 15, 2003, for Cohort 1 and February 27, 2007, for Cohort 2). In Cohort 1, most participants used only Generation 1 HTUs; in Cohort 2, 226 participants used Generation 2 HTUs and 4 used Generation 1 HTUs. Excludes results for the following functions because no Cohort 2 participants used them: consult American Diabetes Association web pages, enter medications, and enter exercise activities.

[a]Controlling for participants' characteristics at baseline.

[b]The sample size varies by site and function.

HTU = home telemedicine unit.

Table 3. Mean Annual Number of Times HTU Function Was Used During the Intervention, by Cohort and Size

Cohort 1 participants used more functions than Cohort 2 participants (Table 4). In New York City, Cohort 1 participants used 4.3 HTU functions, on average, compared with 2.5 functions for Cohort 2. The averages for upstate New York are very similar (4.5 and 2.7, respectively). As noted, these differences are partly explained by the Consortium's decision to de-emphasize the use of complex HTU functions in Phase II due to the difficulties experienced in Phase I. Furthermore, by the end of the follow-up period, none of the Cohort 2 participants in both sites had used all the functions, though between 2 and 6 percent of Cohort 1 participants (New York City and upstate, respectively) had used all of them.

Cohort 2 participants in both sites had longer televisits, on average, than their Cohort 1 counterparts. In New York City, the average duration of a Cohort 2 televisit (29 minutes) was significantly higher, by about 5 minutes, than the Cohort 1 average. In the upstate site, the difference in the average duration of a televisit was smaller (about 2 minutes), but still significantly (statistically) longer for Cohort 2 participants relative to their Cohort 1 counterparts (33 and 31 minutes, respectively).

HTU Function	Cohort 1	Cohort 2	Difference (*p*-Value[a])
Any Function (Percentage)[b]			
New York City	99.6	99.3	- 0.3 (.602)
Upstate New York	100.0	99.9	- 0.1 (.580)
All HTU Functions (Percentage)[b]			
New York City	2.4	0.0	- 2.4 (.233)
Upstate New York	5.7	0.0	- 5.7 (.017)
Number of Functions Used [b]			
New York City	4.3	2.5	- 1.8 (.000)
Upstate New York	4.5	2.7	- 1.8 (.000)
Average Duration of Televisits (Minutes)[c]			
New York City	24.3	29.4	5.1 (.000)
Upstate New York	31.2	33.0	1.8 (.004)
Sample Size[d]	753	230	-

Source: IDEATel database on HTU use linked to the IDEATel tracking status file (Columbia University, 2007a, 2007b).

Notes: Estimates weighted based on length of enrollment between HTU installation and the dropout date or the cutoff date (February 15, 2003, for Cohort 1 participants and February 27, 2007, for Cohort 2 participants). In Cohort 1, most participants used only Generation 1 HTUs; in Cohort 2, 226 participants used Generation 2 HTUs and 4 used Generation 1 HTUs.

[a] Controlling for participants' characteristics at baseline.

[b] Excludes measurement of blood pressure and measurement of blood sugar, as neither function required system log-in. Also excludes consultations of American Diabetes Association web pages, because the Consortium did not collect data on these consultations after November 13, 2003.

[c] The number of participants participating in televisits varies by function.

[d] The sample size varies by site.

HTU = home telemedicine unit.

Table 4. Patterns of HTU Use During the Intervention, by Cohort and Site

The analysis of HTU use for Cohort 1 and Cohort 2 participants has four limitations. First, without a suitable control group to account for secular trends against which to compare changes in use in both cohorts, it is not possible to determine whether the redesign of the HTU is the sole factor behind the higher use by Cohort 2 participants of the array of HTU functions. Second, because communications between participants and providers are confidential, Mathematica was unable to determine whether any instances of HTU use were self-initiated or whether they occurred only after reminders from nurse case managers during televisits or in electronic messages. Furthermore, the use of the data-pulling feature in Generation 2 HTUs could have changed Cohort 2 participants' use of other functions by relieving them of the need to upload their glucose and blood pressure readings between televisits. Thus, it is unclear how much effort Consortium staff expended to generate the levels of use observed and how this varied by HTU type and cohort. Third, the sample size for Cohort 2 participants was small. Thus, it is likely that the estimates from this group are less robust than the estimates for the Cohort 1 sample. Finally, the Consortium stopped collecting data on use of the ADA web pages—an important intervention component—in November 2003. Therefore, it is not possible to assess the extent to which participants in both phases used these educational materials, particularly after Cohort 1 participants were retrained on HTU use during the third year of the demonstration.

5.3 Intermediate clinical outcomes

The intervention had substantial, statistically significant favorable impacts on blood sugar control and lipid levels in both demonstration sites. In New York City and upstate, blood sugar control was better in the treatment group than in the control group, and total cholesterol levels were about 5 to 6 percent lower, on average (Figure 3). In the upstate site only, the improvement in blood sugar control was greater for participants with poorly controlled blood sugar at baseline than it was for others. The intervention also affected in-person blood pressure measurements, but more so upstate. In New York City, mean systolic and diastolic readings were 2 percent lower in the treatment group than in the control group, although the difference was not statistically significant. Upstate, the mean differences were about 3 percent and were highly significant.

Although the Consortium prespecified blood sugar, blood pressure control, and lipid levels as the main study outcomes, it collected data on several other clinically important outcomes. According to our analysis, IDEATel did not affect ratios of microalbumin to creatinine (an indicator of kidney damage from diabetes), 24-hour ambulatory blood pressure measurements, body mass index, overweight or obesity, waist-to-hip ratio, or abdominal girth in either site. In addition, the intervention had no effects on mortality.

The attrition rate was high in both sites, especially among treatment group members (about 23 percent in New York City and 16 percent upstate between baseline and year 1). The substantial attrition rate among enrollees poses two serious problems. First, the reduction in sample size limits the power to detect impacts. For example, for a single comparison of treatment and control group means, the 30 percent loss of sample in the New York City site would result in minimum detectable differences (MDDs) roughly 25 percent greater than for the full sample, while the 58 percent loss of sample in the upstate site would increase the MDDs by about one-third. Second, and perhaps more important, depending on the mechanism for attrition, impacts calculated only on enrollees who remain in the study could be biased. Bias can occur if the dropout rate of enrollees with unmeasured characteristics that predict outcomes (for example, motivation or psychological distress) is greater in one intervention group than the other. Such differential dropout threatens the benefits of random assignment. Differential dropout cannot be directly ascertained. However, an examination of the recorded reasons for enrollee dropout and the characteristics of enrollees who dropped out, as well as sensitivity tests consisting of imputed possible values of outcome variables for those who dropped out surprisingly suggested no likelihood of bias.

5.4 Medicare service use and costs

IDEATel had no effects on treatment group members' use of Medicare-covered hospital, skilled nursing facility, or physician services. Upstate, however, use of home health care was statistically significantly higher for treatment group enrollees than for their control group counterparts. It also did not affect receipt of dilated eye examination, hemoglobin A1c testing, low-density lipoprotein testing, and urine microalbumin testing.

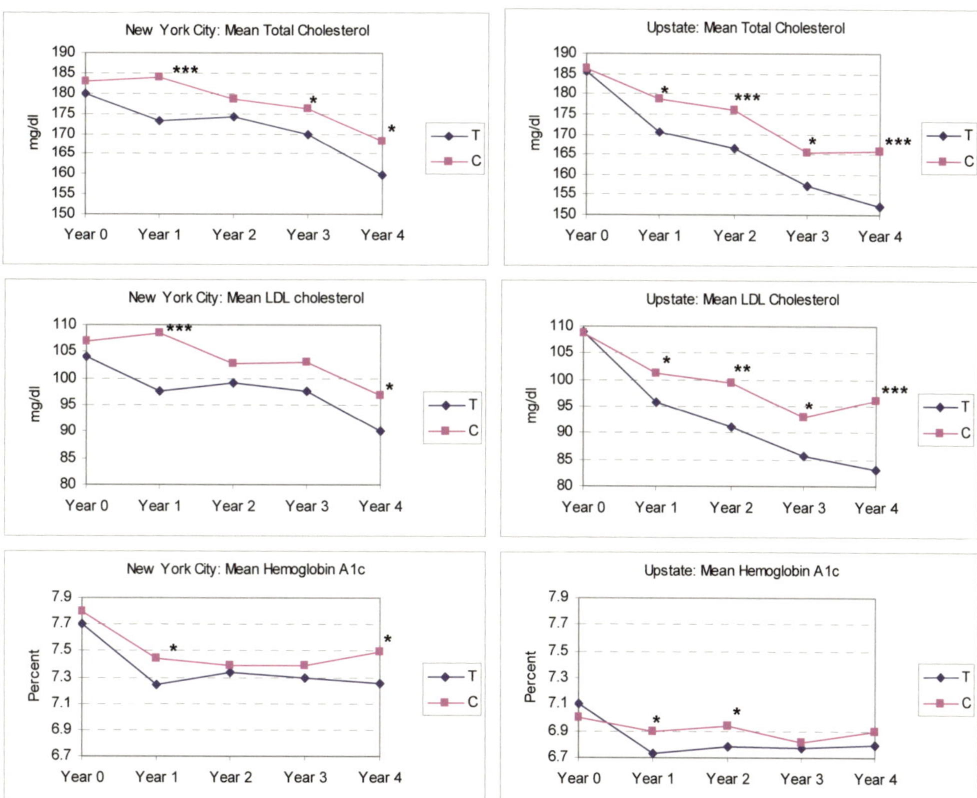

Source: IDEATel annual in-person interviews, conducted from December 2000 through October 2006 (Columbia University, 2007d).
*,**,*** Indicate treatment-control difference is statistically significant at the .05, .01, or .001 level, respectively.

Fig. 3. Impacts of IDEATel on Cohort 1 Enrollees' Selected Key Clinical and Laboratory Outcomes, Baseline to Year 4

The mean annual Medicare expenditures were higher for treatment group members than for control group members in both sites, but the differences were not statistically significant (Table 5). In New York City, the mean annual Medicare expenditures were $13,845 in the treatment group and $12,961 in the control group. Upstate, mean annual expenditures were $9,566 in the treatment group and $8,450 in the control group. By service type, statistically significant treatment-control differences were few. However, treatment group members had higher expenditures in all service categories except physician office visits, outpatient hospital, and laboratory services in New York City.

	New York City			Upstate New York		
Component/Service	Treatment Group	Control Group	Difference (*p*-Value)	Treatment Group	Control Group	Difference (*p*-Value)
Cohort 1 (Both Phases)						
Total Expenditures for Medicare-Covered Services	$13,845	$12,961	$884 (.476)	$9,566	$8,450	$1,116 (.094)
Total Intervention-Related Costs[a]	$8,662	0	n.a.	$8,662	0	n.a.
Total Costs	$22,507	$12,961	$9,546 (.001)	$18,228	$8,450	$9,778 (.000)
Cohort 2 (Only Phase II)						
Total Expenditures for Medicare-Covered Services	$11,906	$11,661	$245 (.931)	$6,450	$8,694	- $2,244 (.132)
Total Intervention-Related Costs	$8,437	0	n.a.	$8,437	0	n.a.
Total Costs	$20,343	$11,661	$8,682 (.000)	$14,877	$8,694	$ 6,183 (.000)
Cohort 1 Sample Size	379	358	-	446	442	-
Cohort 2 Sample Size	82	84	-	161	164	-

[a]Total demonstration service costs for Cohort 1 are based on the arithmetic average of demonstration costs for Phase I and Phase II, weighted by the average length of time that Phase I participants were enrolled during each phase.
n.a. = not applicable.

Table 5. Estimated Annual Per-Person Expenditures for Medicare-Covered Services, Demonstration Costs, and Total Costs

5.5 Demonstration costs

We estimated that the IDEATel intervention cost about $34.8 million or about 61 percent of the total demonstration budget. Depending on the study phase, between 11 and 15 percent of the total budget was for intervention design; between 46 and 50 percent was for implementation; and less than 1 percent was for closeout (for example, deinstalling HTUs when participants disenrolled or died). For Phase I, implementation costs ($12,905,572) divided by the number of treatment group enrollees (844) over the length of the intervention

(2 years) provides an estimate of the annual implementation cost per participant, or $7,645. For Phase II, implementation costs ($14,338,429) divided by the number of treatment group enrollees (514 treatment group members from Cohort 1 who were still participating in the demonstration at the beginning of Phase II [February 2004], and all 249 Cohort 2 treatment group members), gives a per-participant cost estimate of $7,029. To calculate the total annual costs per participant per cohort, the analysis assumed that Phase I lasted two years, as stated in the Consortium's original proposal, and that Phase II lasted an average of 2.67 years (three years for Cohort 1 and two years for Cohort 2 [Columbia University, 1998]). Design and closeout costs were depreciated over four years for Cohort 1 and over three years for Cohort 2 (U.S. Department of Health and Human Services, 2005). The final cost per participant is $8,662 for Cohort 1 (both phases), and $8,437 for Cohort 2 (only Phase II).

When the intervention's annual cost per participant is added to the annual Medicare expenditures of treatment group members, the treatment group's costs are about two and one-half times larger than the control group's costs. Thus, based on experiences of enrollees through December 2003, the demonstration substantially increases total costs. Even if the intervention had eliminated the treatment group's need for all other Medicare expenditures, that group's costs would have exceeded the control group's costs (upstate) or be within 5 percent of these costs (New York City).

5.6 Summary of findings

The IDEATel demonstration met Congressional implementation requirements. However, the intervention as delivered was neither as intensive nor as technologically sophisticated as originally designed, since the Consortium encountered unexpected challenges and deliberately departed from its plans in some areas. Had the Consortium retained its original target to hold televisits every two weeks with all participants—the most popular component of the intervention—participants might have been more motivated to use their HTUs and interact more frequently with their nurse case managers. In addition, this would have allowed nurse case managers to provide more guidance to participants on using other HTU functions, such as setting behavioral goals, which might have resulted in better clinical outcomes. Similarly, had the redesigned HTU been cheaper and less sophisticated, participants' acceptance of this technology might have increased and the costs of the demonstration might have been more reasonable.

IDEATel was clinically effective over the medium term in only one of two sites, which made it difficult to determine why it was more effective among participants upstate than in New York City or whether some demonstration features are essential for long-term impacts. The expectation that the demonstration could generate offsetting savings for Medicare services did not materialize, in spite of the six-year follow-up. The main driver of these costs was the size of the cooperative agreement allocated to the demonstration's operations, compounded with the use of very expensive HTUs. Table 6 summarizes the key findings from the evaluation of IDEATel.

While an ongoing program similar to IDEATel could potentially have lower costs, it would be virtually impossible for such a program to generate cost savings, particularly because the intervention-related costs of the demonstration were excessive by any standard. Given the absence of effects on costs or services, however, even a less expensive version of this demonstration would not produce sufficient Medicare savings to offset demonstration costs. Furthermore, while IDEATel had clinical impacts similar to those of other interventions for individuals with diabetes, it cost far more. For instance, *Project Dulce* (a diabetes case-management and self-management training program) had clinical impacts (derived from a comparison of program participants to a matched control group) similar in size to those produced by IDEATel. While the program was cost-effective according to commonly accepted standards, Project Dulce cost an estimated $662 to $1,537 per participant per year to implement—about an eighth the cost of IDEATel (Gilmer et al., 2007).

In sum, the results are clear: the IDEATel program cannot be cost neutral, given its large costs and the complete absence of any savings in traditional Medicare costs for hospitalizations and other covered services. Even if costs were halved and the intervention reduced hospitalizations by 50 percent (both highly unlikely scenarios), the program would still increase total costs to the government.

Outcome	New York City	Upstate
Implementation Analysis		
HTU Use	Cohort 1: Declined rapidly Cohort 2: Declined rapidly	Cohort 1: Constant through 2003, but declined thereafter Cohort 2: Declined rapidly
Impact Analysis		
Communication with Providers and Patient Self-Care	Cohort 1: Large positive impacts[a] Cohort 2: Large positive impacts in year 1	Cohort 1: Large positive impacts[a] Cohort 2: Large positive impacts in year 1
Clinical Outcomes	Cohort 1: Little or no impact[a] Cohort 2: No significant impacts in year 1	Cohort 1: Large and sustained impacts[a] Cohort 2: No significant impacts in year 1
Service Use and Expenditures	Cohort 1: No Medicare savings in any year except year 3 No effects on hospitalizations or service use, for either cohort	Cohort 1: No Medicare savings in any year No effects on hospitalizations or service use, for either cohort
Total Medicare Costs	The demonstration's high costs ($8,662 per participant per year for Cohort 1 and $8,437 per participant per year for Cohort 2) were not offset by any savings in Medicare Part A or Part B expenditures	

[a] Findings are for all four years for which follow-up survey data were available.

Table 6. Summary of Findings by Site

6. Discussion

6.1 Implications of the IDEATel evaluation for home-based telemedicine

Mathematica's overall findings about IDEATel are consistent with those from a CBO review of disease management programs for diabetes in which clinical improvements were not associated with long-run reduced costs (implied to be over a time frame of at least one year) (Congressional Budget Office, 2004). They are not consistent, however, with findings from a commercial diabetes management program that seemed to yield clinical improvements *and* cost savings in one year's time (Piette et al., 2001;Villagra & Ahmed, 2004). Because the

CBO-reviewed studies and the Villagra-Ahmed study rely on evaluation designs of different credibility and robustness, the above findings should be interpreted cautiously.

What mechanisms might have produced the modestly improved clinical outcomes? By providing participants free blood sugar and blood pressure meters, nurse case managers to encourage use of these meters, and a means of uploading the meter readings, the intervention set the stage for timely and aggressive treatment of diabetes symptoms. Specifically, the nurses conveyed concerns to supervising diabetologists. These physicians suggested different doses of guideline-recommended prescription drugs to participants' primary care physicians, who made the changes and participants responded favorably.

The problems with the HTU suggest that IDEATel's positive clinical effects may have been due more to the nurses' telephonic interactions with the patients than to the expensive HTU equipment. The intervention as implemented had limited acceptability among participants. For example, many participants found the HTU used during Phase I of the demonstration somewhat unappealing. In addition, participants found the HTU cumbersome or physically imposing (5 and 28 percent of Cohort 1 treatment group members refused installation between baseline and year 4 in New York City and upstate New York, respectively). They also found the more advanced functions difficult to perform (4 and 5 percent of Cohort 1 treatment group members left the study citing difficulty with the HTU between baseline and year 4 in New York City and upstate New York, respectively).

Although demonstration staff said participants who attended televisits enjoyed interacting with nurse case managers, participants attended televisits much less often than the Consortium requested (especially in New York City). Technical difficulties may have made the HTU more of a distraction than an asset for purposes of case management. As noted in section 4, the evaluation cannot definitively attribute the intervention's positive impacts to using the HTU, interacting with nurse case managers, or both because the demonstration was not designed to measure each component's marginal benefits. Nonetheless, these problems with the HTU suggest that this expensive component of the intervention may not have been the essential factor for producing the favorable effects on clinical indicators.

The finding that the intervention did not affect participants' use of Medicare-covered services, including diabetes-specific preventive services, was disappointing to program operators, but perhaps was not altogether surprising. First, televisits were not meant to substitute for regular physician visits, so no savings were expected in visits. Second, the provision of free annual hemoglobin A1c, lipid, and urine microalbuminuria testing to both the treatment and control groups during annual assessments would have blunted any between-group differences that might have arisen for these outcomes. It may also have attenuated effects on hospital use had these tests not been conducted for the control group absent the demonstration (to the extent that knowledge of problems with such indicators could lead to behavior or treatment changes that would ward off such exacerbations). Third, the demonstration's duration for Cohort 1 may have been too short to detectably reduce the need for hospitalizations or other health service use through the prevention of heart attacks, stroke, kidney failure, eye damage, and other complications. Fourth, enrollees may not have been at high risk for costly hospitalizations. Baseline hemoglobin A1c, lipid, and blood pressure levels suggested that enrollees were relatively well controlled in the three measures.

It is slightly disappointing that the intervention did not affect receipt of dilated eye exams; between 87 and 95 percent of control group enrollees received them, compared to between 88 and 98 percent of treatment group enrollees (in upstate New York and New York City, respectively). One would expect IDEATel nurse case managers to remind participants to have the exam, a widely accepted component of diabetes treatment guidelines. While nurses may have neglected to make reminders because they faced competing priorities during televisits or their case management software was not programmed to issue such reminders, this would not excuse such omission from their interactions. It could also be that participants ignored reminders, but this would suggest that the nurses were unsuccessful in developing enough trust and rapport with participants to encourage at least some of them to have this important exam. Baseline rates were also fairly high; perhaps physicians willing to participte in the study were already providing high quality care and beneficiaries willing to enroll were already adherent to recommended care. It may have thus been difficult for the intervention to effect substantial additional improvements above the already high baseline rates.

Given the absence of effects on service use, finding no effects on Medicare costs was not surprising. The higher Medicare expenditures for the treatment group may have been strictly a chance difference or may be because IDEATel identified the need for some health services among medically underserved beneficiaries. The expectation that the demonstration could generate offsetting savings for Medicare services did not materialize, in spite of the six-year follow-up. The main driver of these costs was the size of the cooperative agreement allocated to the demonstration's operations, compounded with the use of very expensive HTUs.

6.2 Potential role of home telemedicine in the Medicare program

Although the promise of home telemedicine has long been recognized by experts and policymakers, its use in the U.S. health care system is far from widespread, particularly in the Medicare program, the largest health insurer in the U.S. There are several studies that show that home telemedicine for Medicare can be efficacious, but they are limited by small sample sizes, inadequate length of follow-up, and inconclusive results (Hersh et al., 2006). Consequently, the failure of the IDEATel demonstration to provide a conclusive assessment of the potential of home telemedicine—improve access to care for Medicare beneficiaries with chronic conditions, provide cost-effective care to the Medicare population, and generate cost savings for the Medicare program—was disappointing for those expecting such changes in outcomes, such as the Agency for Healthcare Research and Quality, which sponsors a periodic systematic review of the effects of telemedicine for Medicare beneficiaries. Furthermore, in early 2008, at the end of the demonstration, the optimism among program developers, implementers, health care providers, and policymakers about whether and how home telemedicine could play a role in the Medicare program seemed to be fading away. This resulted primarily from the shift in emphasis from telemedicine to electronic health records that the federal government adopted starting in 2004.

A turnaround point for this impasse was the largest legislative push on health information technology (IT) ever in the U.S. In 2009, recognizing the unrealized potential of health IT to improve the quality and delivery of health care, Congress passed the Health Information Technology for Economic and Clinical Health (HITECH) Act as part of the American Recovery and Reinvestment Act. The goal of HITECH is to promote the adoption of health IT in public insurance programs, including the potential use of home telemedicine in Medicare to support key principles of the patient-centered medical home to improve health care quality and efficiency (Moreno et al., 2010). Recent health reform legislation (Patient

Protection and Affordable Health Care Act [P.L. 111-148]) offers promising prospects for home telemedicine, including an Innovation Center within CMS, the agency of the U.S. Department of Health and Human Services that administers Medicare. This center will test, evaluate, and expand in Medicare (as well as in Medicaid and the Children's Health Insurance Program) different payment structures and methodologies to reduce program expenditures while maintaining or improving quality of care, a role that telemedicine could fulfill. Other mandates of the health reform legislation that could directly or indirectly facilitate the adoption of home telemedicine in the program include a Federal Coordinated Health Care Office within CMS. The mission of this office is to more effectively integrate Medicare and Medicaid benefits and improve coordination between the federal government and states in order to improve access to and quality of care and services for dual-eligible beneficiaries (that is, those eligible for both Medicare and Medicaid), who typically have many care-coordination needs. There are many other health-reform legislative dispositions that could influence the adoption and use of home telemedicine, but we do not discuss them here because they are in early stages of development and implementation.

In sum, HITECH, the health-reform legislation, and other pre-HITECH legislation are intertwined and highly relevant to home telemedicine in the Medicare program. Despite our finding that IDEATel was unlikely to be cost-effective given that the demonstraton had modest clinical impacts at excessive cost, the concept of home telemedicine is still promising. One of the factors that has greatly enhanced the prospects of home telemedicine is the continous decline in health IT prices, such as those for smartphones, personal digital assistants, intelligent devices, and web-based applications. This unique alignment of policies and affordable technology raises hopes that there can be positive synergies in the immediate future to build a solid basis for home telemedicine in the Medicare program.

7. References

Ahring, K. K., Ahring, J. P., Joyce, C., & Farid, N. R. (1992). Telephone modem access improves diabetes control in those with insulin-requiring diabetes. *Diabetes Care,* 15(8), 971-975.

American Diabetes Association (a). Diabetes and seniors. Retrieved February 13, 2002, from www.diabetes.org/main/application/commercewf?origina=*.jsp&event=link(B4_4)

American Diabetes Association (b). Type II diabetes is preventable, major study shows. Retrieved February 13, 2002, from ada.yellowbrix.com/pages/ada/Story.nsp?story id=2754995&ID=ada

AmericanTeleCare, I. Products and services. Retrieved May 7, 2010, from www.americantelecare.com/prod_main.html

Aubert, R. E., Herman, W. H., Waters, J., Moore, W., Sutton, D., Peterson, B. L., Bailey, C. M., & Koplan, J. P. (1998). Nurse case management to improve glycemic control in diabetic patients in a health maintenance organization. A randomized, controlled trial. *Annals of Internal Medicine,* 129(8), 605-612.

California Medi-Cal Type 2 Diabetes Study Group. (2004). Closing the gap: Effect of diabetes case management on glycemic control among low-income ethnic minority populations: The California Medi-Cal Type 2 Diabetes Study. *Diabetes Care,* 27(1), 95-103.

Columbia University. (1998). Technical proposal for the IDEATel demonstration. New York: Columbia University.

Columbia University. (2005). Progress report: February 28, 2005–August 31, 2005. Revised April 25, 2006. Columbia University Cooperative Agreement no. 95-C-90998/2-01. Informatics, Telemedicine, and Education Demonstration Project. New York: Columbia University.

Columbia University. (2007a). Enrollees' tracking status database. New York: Columbia University.

Columbia University. (2007b). HTU-use log database. New York: Columbia University.

Columbia University. (2007c). Medicare enrollment and claims database. New York: Columbia University.

Columbia University. (2007d). Phase I and phase II annual, in-person interviews (including anthropometry measurements and laboratory results). New York: Columbia University.

Congressional Budget Office. (2004). An analysis of the literature on disease management programs. Washington, DC: U.S. Congress.

Delichatsios, H. K., Friedman, R. H., Glanz, K., Tennstedt, S., Smigelski, C., Pinto, B. M., Kelley, H., & Gillman, M. W. (2001). Randomized trial of a "talking computer" to improve adults' eating habits. *American Journal of Health Promotion,* 15(4), 215-224.

Foster, L., Moreno, L., Chen, A., & Shapiro, R. (2008). Third annual report on the Informatics for Diabetes Education and Telemedicine (IDEATel) demonstration: Phase II. Princeton, NJ: Mathematica Policy Research.

Foster, L., Shapiro, R., Chen, A., Black, W., & Moreno, L. (2006). First annual report on the Informatics for Diabetes Education and Telemedicine (IDEATel) demonstration: Phase II. Final report. Princeton, NJ: Mathematica Policy Research.

Gilmer, T. P., Roze, S., Valentine, W. J., Emy-Albrecht, K., Ray, J. A., Cobden, D., Nicklasson, L., Philis-Tsimikas, A., & Palmer, A. J. (2007). Cost-effectiveness of diabetes case management for low-income populations. *Health Services Research,* 42(5), 1943-1959.

Health Resources and Services Administration. Health professional shortage area guidelines for primary medical care/dental designation. Retrieved April 22, 2004, from www.hrsa.gov/shortage/hpsaguidepc.html

Hersh, W. R., Hickam, D. H., Severance, S. M., Dana, T. L., Krages, K. P., & Helfand, M. (2006). Telemedicine for the Medicare population: Update. *Evidence Report/Technology Assessment,* (131)(131), 1-41.

HomMed. How it works: The HomMed sentry and the HomMed central station. Retrieved May 5, 2004, from www.hommed.com/patients_families/how_it_works.asp

Kaufman, D. R., Patel, V. L., Hilliman, C., Morin, P. C., Pevzner, J., Weinstock, R. S., Goland, R., Shea, S., & Starren, J. (2003). Usability in the real world: Assessing medical information technologies in patients' homes. *Journal of Biomedical Informatics,* 36(1-2), 45-60.

Kaufman, D. R., Starren, J., Patel, V. L., Morin, P. C., Hilliman, C., Pevzner, J., Weinstock, R. S., Goland, R., & Shea, S. (2003). A cognitive framework for understanding barriers to the productive use of a diabetes home telemedicine system. AMIA Annual Symposium Proceedings. *AMIA Symposium,* 356-360.

Meneghini, L. F., Albisser, A. M., Goldberg, R. B., & Mintz, D. H. (1998). An electronic case manager for diabetes control. *Diabetes Care,* 21(4), 591-596.

Moreno, L., Chen, A., Foster, L., & Archibald, N. D. (June 10, 2005). Second interim report on the Informatics for Diabetes Education and Telemedicine (IDEATel) demonstration: Final report on phase I. Princeton, NJ: Mathematica Policy Research.

Moreno, L., Dale, S. B., Chen, A. Y., & Magee, C. A. (2009). Costs to Medicare of the Informatics for Diabetes Education and Telemedicine (IDEATel) home telemedicine demonstration: Findings from an independent evaluation. *Diabetes Care,* 32(7), 1202-1204.

Moreno, L., Peikes, D., & Krilla, A. (June 2010). The HITECH act and health information technology's potential to build medical homes. AHRQ Publication No. 10-0080-EF. Rockville, MD: Agency for Healthcare Research and Quality.

Moreno, L., Shapiro, R., Dale, S. B., Foster, L., & Chen, A. (September 5, 2008). Final report to Congress on the Informatics for Diabetes Education and Telemedicine (IDEATel) demonstration, phases I and II: Final report. Princeton, NJ: Mathematica Policy Research.

Palmas, W., Shea, S., Starren, J., Teresi, J. A., Ganz, M. L., Burton, T. M., Pashos, C. L., Blustein, J., Field, L., Morin, P. C., Izquierdo, R. E., Silver, S., Eimicke, J. P., Lantigua, R. A., Weinstock, R. S., & IDEATel Consortium. (2010). Medicare payments, healthcare service use, and telemedicine implementation costs in a randomized trial comparing telemedicine case management with usual care in medically underserved participants with diabetes mellitus (IDEATel). *Journal of the American Medical Informatics Association,* 17(2), 196-202.

Piette, J. D. (2000). Satisfaction with automated telephone disease management calls and its relationship to their use. *The Diabetes Educator,* 26(6), 1003-1010.

Piette, J. D., Weinberger, M., Kraemer, F. B., & McPhee, S. J. (2001). Impact of automated calls with nurse follow-up on diabetes treatment outcomes in a Department of Veterans Affairs health care system: A randomized controlled trial. *Diabetes Care,* 24(2), 202-208.

Piette, J. D., Weinberger, M., McPhee, S. J., Mah, C. A., Kraemer, F. B., & Crapo, L. M. (2000). Do automated calls with nurse follow-up improve self-care and glycemic control among vulnerable patients with diabetes? *The American Journal of Medicine,* 108(1), 20-27.

Shea, S., Weinstock, R. S., Teresi, J. A., Palmas, W., Starren, J., Cimino, J. J., Lai, A. M., Field, L., Morin, P. C., Goland, R., Izquierdo, R. E., Ebner, S., Silver, S., Petkova, E., Kong, J., Eimicke, J. P., & IDEATel Consortium. (2009). A randomized trial comparing telemedicine case management with usual care in older, ethnically diverse, medically underserved patients with diabetes mellitus: 5 year results of the IDEATel study. *Journal of the American Medical Informatics Association,* 16(4), 446-456.

Shultz, E. K., Bauman, A., Hayward, M., & Holzman, R. (1992). Improved care of patients with diabetes through telecommunications. *Annals of the New York Academy of Sciences,* 670, 141-145.

Starren, J., Hripcsak, G., Sengupta, S., Abbruscato, C. R., Knudson, P. E., Weinstock, R. S., & Shea, S. (2002). Columbia University's Informatics for Diabetes Education and Telemedicine (IDEATel) project: Technical implementation. *Journal of the American Medical Informatics Association,* 9(1), 25-36.

Taylor, C. B., Miller, N. H., Reilly, K. R., Greenwald, G., Cunning, D., Deeter, A., & Abascal, L. (2003). Evaluation of a nurse-care management system to improve outcomes in patients with complicated diabetes. *Diabetes Care,* 26(4), 1058-1063.

U.S. Department of Health and Human Services. (May 7, 2003). Report to Congress: First interim report on the Informatics for Diabetes Education and Telemedicine (IDEATel) demonstration. Washington, DC: DHHS.

U.S. Department of Health and Human Services. (December 18, 2005). Report to Congress: Second interim report on the Informatics for Diabetes Education and Telemedicine (IDEATel) demonstration: Final report on phase I. Washington, DC: DHHS.

Villagra, V. G., & Ahmed, T. (2004). Effectiveness of a disease management program for patients with diabetes. *Health Affairs* (Project Hope), 23(4), 255-266.

16

Development of a Portable Vital Sensing System for Home Telemedicine[1]

F. Ichihashi[1] and Y. Sankai[2]
[1]*Cyberdyne.Inc,*
[2]*University of Tsukuba, Graduate School of Systems and Information Engineering*
Japan

1. Introduction

Lifestyle diseases such as obesity, hypertension, hyperlipidemia, and diabetes lead to arteriosclerosis, which is one of the risk factors for developing cardiac diseases and cerebrovascular diseases. Because these lifestyle diseases can lead to chronic diseases, both prevention and early detection have become one of the most critical issues [1-4].
In order to prevent arteriosclerosis, aerobic exercise of moderate intensity is important. It has been reported that physical activity is not only a way of preventing life style-related diseases but decreases the mortality of the elderly [5-7] and prevents decline in bodily functions [8-10]. In Japan, the importance of physical activity in middle-aged and elderly people came to be recognized by Japanese researchers [11-13], especially as Japan is confronting with an aging society problem, a serious issue in Japan. According to the medium term variant projections by the National Institute of Population and Social Security Research's Population Projects for Japan, the percentage of the population over 65 years old will reach 26.0% by 2015. Therefore, it is of significance to maintain and promote the physical activity of middle-aged and elderly people.
To prevent or limit the consequences of lifestyle diseases and promote health condition among middle-aged and elderly people, a health management system providing effective exercise prescriptions is required. Since effective and safe prescriptions should be based on evidence from physical data, it is necessary to acquire such daily physical data and vital signs and to evaluate the suitability of this physical information for each user. Therefore, a home medical system to manage and evaluate daily physical activities, and to provide effective exercise prescriptions is desirable. Additionally, such a home medical system can be a provider of a number of healthcare services for those living in remote areas. In this case, the system needs to be a network-based system which enables the people to access the system through the Internet. The conceptual image of such a proposed system is shown in Figure 1 [14]. A medical data server is installed in a data center. The medical data server can handle a lot of physical data and exercise data from the people. Both potable vital sensing systems and exercise equipments are set in home and local community facilities such as fitness centers and healthcare centers. The measurement data are uploaded through the

---

[1] Based on the proceedings of the 29th Annual International Conference of the IEEE EMBS Cité Internationale, Lyon, France August 23-26, 2007

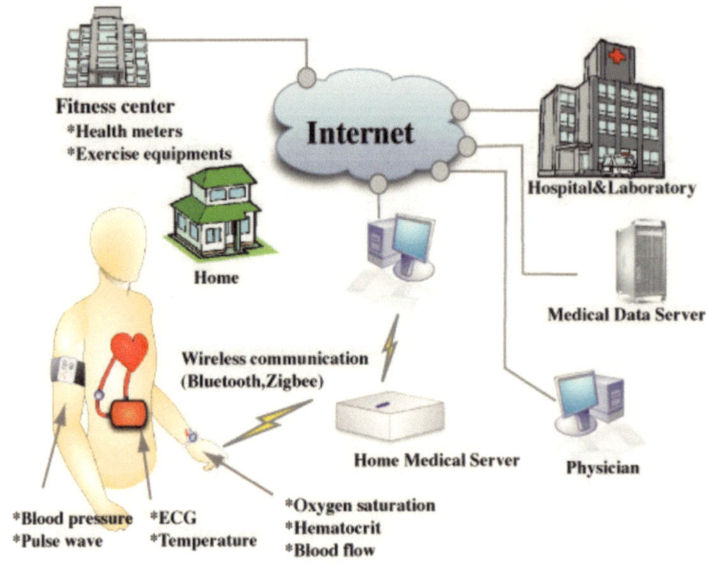

Fig. 1. The conceptual image of a home medical care system using vital sensing system

Internet, and stored on a medical data server. Moreover, an effective prescription program is established to analyze daily physical activity on the server.

To realize such a proposed system, it is necessary to develop a portable vital sensing system capable of measuring daily health conditions such as blood pressure, heart rate, electrocardiogram (ECG), body temperature, oxygen saturation, hematocrit and blood flow non-invasively and easily. Moreover, the medical information should be safely stored on local data server and remote data server. Thus, the purpose of this research is to develop a portable vital sensing system and a home medical server to establish home medical system.

2. Material and method

2.1 System configuration of a home medical system

A home medical system needs to meet highly integrated system requirements, including good portability, high reliability, seamlessly wireless communication and intelligent monitoring algorithm, because it can be used not only to basic health monitoring, but to a critical mission such as artificial heart and diabetes treatments [15,16]. The system architecture of a home medical system is shown in Fig. 2. The proposed home medical system consists of three main components including a home medical server, vital sensing units and a personal terminal. A home medical server can acquire both physiological data and physical data measured by respective portable vital sensing units with wireless communication, and can evaluate the patients' physiological conditions. Each vital sensor unit can be joined in a Wireless Personal Area Network (PAN) established by a home medical server. A Bluetooth PAN is called a piconet, and is composed of up to 8 active devices in a master-slave relationship. Moreover, a common component circuit for a vital sensing unit is independent of other diverse circuits to measure physiological data. It is possible to easily compose various types of vital sensing units like not only a custom sensor unit but also a commercial vital sensing unit with a wire communication line. A personal terminal (personal computer, Internet enabled PDA or cell-phone) is installed in user's home in order to check a current measurement data personally. In addition, a personal terminal enables users to access a remote medical data server through a home medical server. Therefore, users can check health condition from current to past, and diagnostic information form medical specialists.

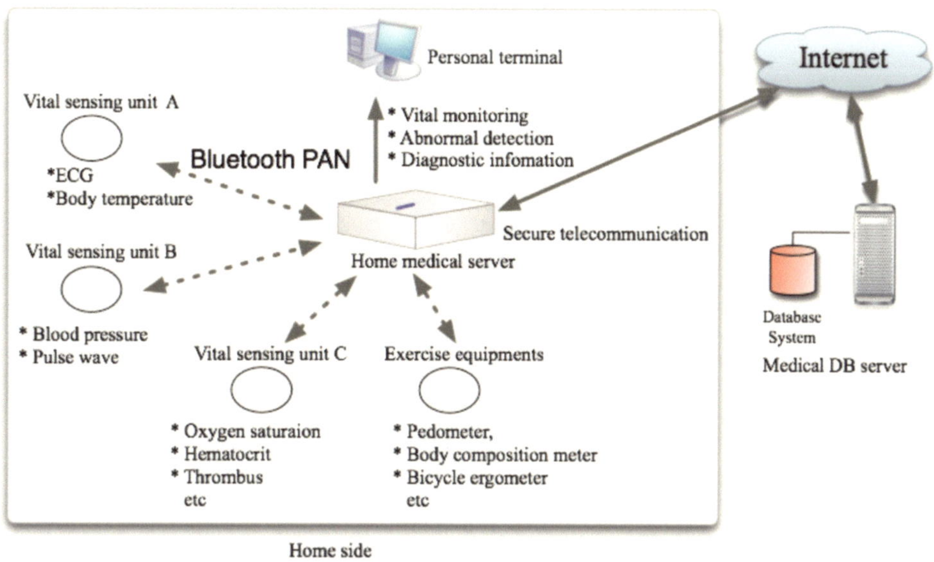

Fig. 2. System architecture of wireless vital sensing system at home

All measurement data are transferred to a remote medical database server by using a secure telecommunication technology, physicians are able to observe and evaluate the patients' condition from a remote place.

In consideration of using a vital sensing system at home, the noninvasive measurement items were decided. The set of physiological sensors described below.

- ECG sensor for monitoring heart activity
- Blood pressure sensor
- Pulse wave sensor for estimating arterial stiffness
- Body temperature sensor

Other physiological sensors and health meters may be added.

- Hematocrit sensor
- Oxygen saturation (SpO2) sensor
- Blood glucose sensor for diabetes patients
- Body composition meter
- Pedometer

2.2 Vital sensing unit

In order to acquire and communicate physiological data, a smart telecom unit was developed specifically for wireless network based data acquisition unit (Fig. 3). We integrated a wireless module (KC22, KC wirefree), a digital signal processor (dsPIC 30F3013, Microchip Technology Inc.) and a battery management circuit into an intelligent signal processing board that can be used as an extension of standard wireless sensor platform. The radio operating range of the Bluetooth module is class 2. Therefore, it is used up to 10 meters. The smart telecom unit has a digital I/O connector that allows two UART (Universal

Asynchronous Receiver Transmitter), I2C interface, and 5 analog input lines. The A/D converter on the smart telecom unit has a high resolution (12bits). A small Li-Ion battery was used as a power supply, whose width, height and thickness are 25 mm, 37 mm and 5 mm respectively. The capacity is 550 mAh.

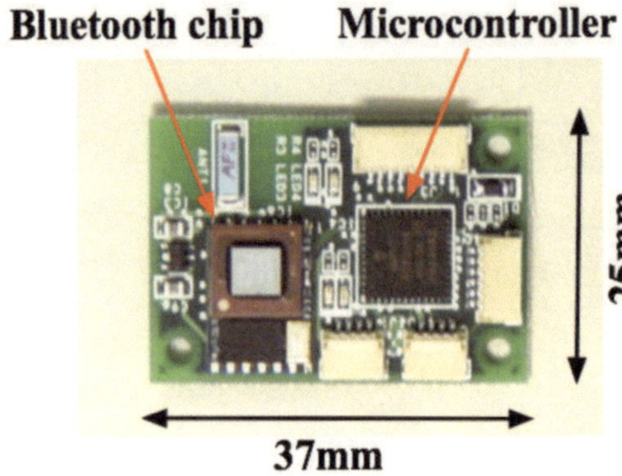

Fig. 3. A smart telecom unit with intelligent signal processing

1. *Blood pressure and pulse wave meter:*

A vital sensing system integrating both blood pressure meter and pulse wave sensor is shown in Fig. 4 and Fig. 5. The commercial wrist type blood pressure meter (HEM-637IT, OMRON Corporation) was used as a portable blood pressure meter. This blood pressure meter can communicate stored blood pressure data to a smart telecom unit with serial RS-232C port. Meanwhile, for measuring a pulse wave, a finger clip sensor with a photoplethysmograph was developed. A photoplethysmograph is a noninvasive method to measure a pressure pulse of finger or toe. The change in volume cased by the pressure pulse is detected by illuminating the skin with the light from a Light Emitting Diode (LED), and then measuring the amount of light reflected to a photodiode. A Infrared LED with a wavelength of 940nm was used. The Pulse wave was obtained from a patient's forefinger. As an anti-aliasing filter, a low-pass filter with cut-off frequency at 250 Hz was used in the end of a signal conditioning circuit. The signal digitized at a sampling rate of 1kHz with 12-bits resolution. Both blood pressure meter and pulse wave sensor connecting to a smart telecom unit, record data were transferred to a home medical server wirelessly.

2. *ECG and body temperature meter:*

The development of a vital sensing unit for measuring ECG and blood temperature is shown in Fig. 6 and Fig. 7. The vital sensing unit can measure both of two physiological parameters by attaching the body skin on left chest. The ECG sensor has two active electrodes and a capacitive ground within the bottom of the sensor case. The two active electrodes have their own preamplifier that transfers the displacement current into the voltage. An Ag-AgCl plated electrode was used as an ECG electrodes probe [17]. In order to measure the body temperature accurately, A small type platinum film thermal sensor (PTFC101A000, Labfacility Limited) was used, and was built in the bottom of the sensor case. This sensor is 2 mm * 2.3mm, which is a sufficient size to be built in the sensor case. Moreover, compared with a thermistor or thermocouples, a platinum thermal sensor has advantages in linearity and reproducibility. As an anti-aliasing filter, a low-pass filter with cut-off frequency at 250 Hz was used in the end of each signal conditioning circuit. The two signals were digitized at a sampling rate of 1kHz with 12-bit resolution.

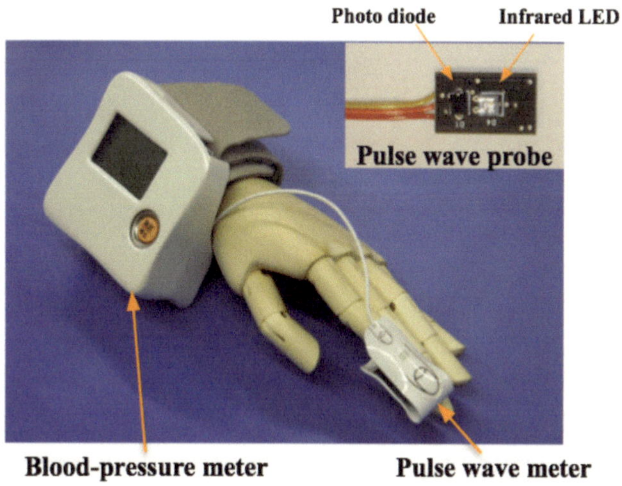

Fig. 4. The portable vital sensing unit for measuring blood pressure and pulse wave

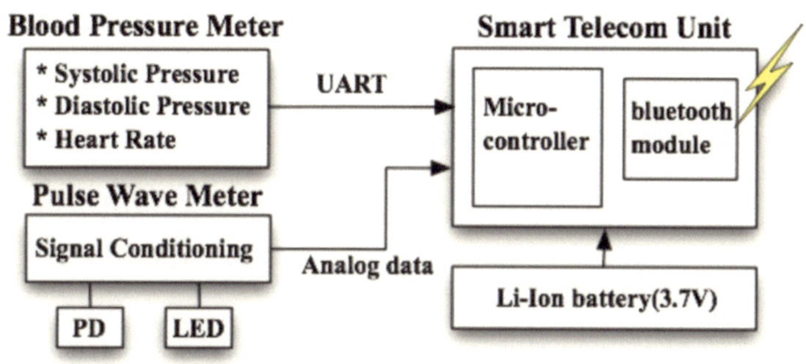

Fig. 5. Block diagram of the portable vital sensing unit (blood pressure and pulse wave meter)

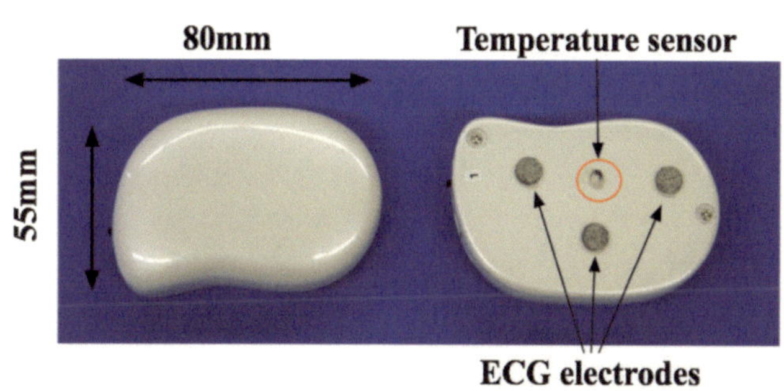

Fig. 6. A portable vital sensing unit for measuring ECG and body temperature. The left hand side is top view and the right hand side is bottom view.

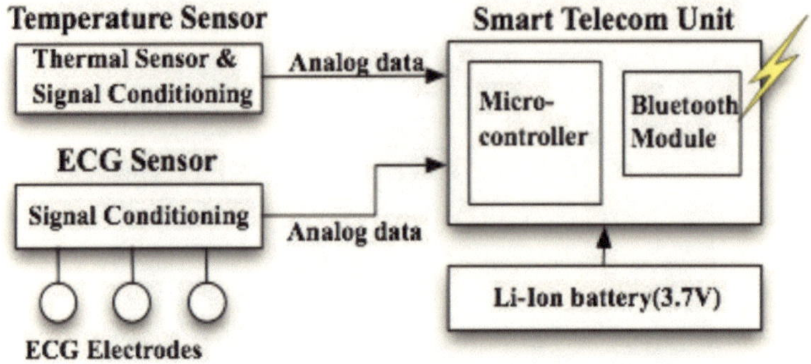

Fig. 7. Block diagram of the portable vital sensing unit (ECG and body temperature meter)

In order to calibrate the temperature sensor automatically, the two points calibration method was used. Generally, the relationship between the measured temperature and output voltage can be expressed as (1).

$$T_s = AV_s + B \tag{1}$$

where T_s is the temperature, V_s is the output voltage measured by a temperature circuit, A and B are constants dependent on the characteristics of the platinum thermal sensor and the measurement circuit. Although both a parameter "A" and "B" is unknown, two parameters are determined by using high-precision resistances.
The equations switching to each two reference resistance R_1 and R_2 are expressed by (2), (3).

$$T_1 = AV_1 + B \tag{2}$$

$$T_2 = AV_2 + B \tag{3}$$

where T_1 and T_2 are the temperature using R_1 and R_2 respectively, and V_1 and V_2 are the output voltages using to R_1 and R_2 respectively. Therefore, the unknown parameters A and B are determined by solving the simultaneous equation. These solving parameters describe below.

$$A = \frac{T_1 - T_2}{V_1 - V_2} \tag{4}$$

$$B = \frac{V_1T_2 - T_1V_2}{V_1 - V_2} \tag{5}$$

2.3 Home medical server

The home medical server consists of a small computer (MIU-Card 1001,Katoh Denki Co.Ltd Japan) of a size with 124mm*78mm*60mm and a weight of approximately 300g (Fig. 8) The Operating System is RT-Linux, which is globally accepted to be stable. The kernel and control program are installed in compact flush memory card (CF card) as a hard disk. CF card is strong against a shock compared with hard disk. And the home medical server has a wireless-LAN module to connect with Internet and a Bluetooth module to communicate portable vital sensing units. The server not only can transfer the measured data to a remote medical data server but can manage patient's condition by using its own diagnostic function. If an abnormal condition occurred, the home medical server can send the diagnostic information to remote medical server. Additionally, in order to protect user information through the Internet, cryptographic end-to-end secure sessions, that is Hypertext Transfer Protocol Security (HTTPS), that reduces risks by providing data confidentiality and integrity protection was established.

The medical data management server consists of a database system to handle user information and a web-based user interface to access diverse information like health conditions and prescriptions. The design of the system architecture of a medical data server is shown in Fig. 9. We adopt Tomcat and Apache as a web application deployment environment and PostgreSQL as a database system in consideration of the security, the easy development and deployment. Tomcat has a function that a comprehensive suite of tools and frameworks for quickly developing standards-based Web services and Java server applications. PostgreSQL offers high-speed access to structured data, fault tolerance

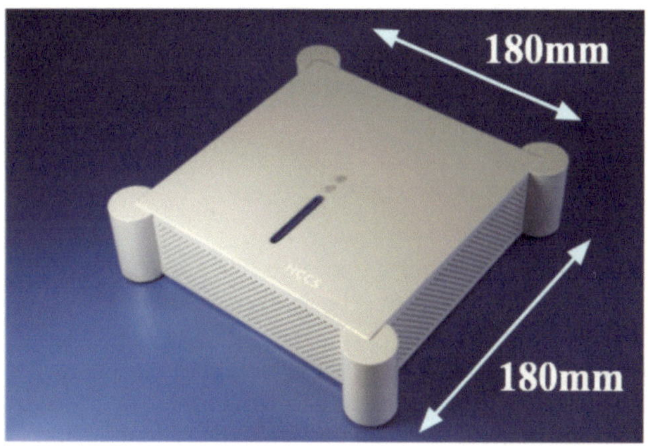

Fig. 8. Home medical server

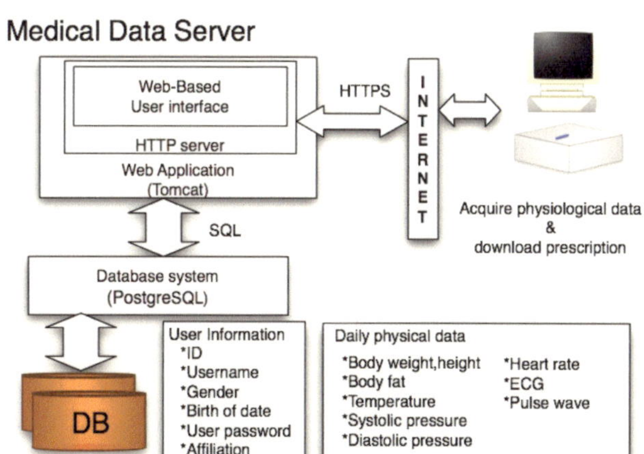

Fig. 9. System architecture of a medical data server for managing vital records

function, the clients never wait whenever the access is increasing and a unique multi-file journaling architecture ensures fault-tolerance and data integrity without compromising database performance.

The data viewer showing in Fig. 10 is able to monitor physiological data in real time. The waveform of ECG and pulse wave can be checked in the time of measurements.

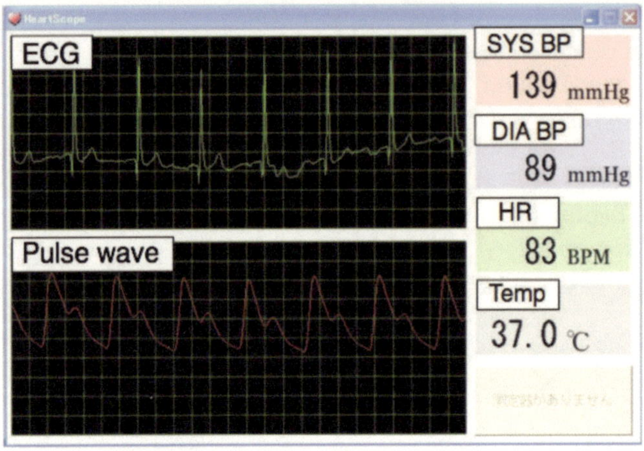

Fig. 10. Data viewer for portable vital sensing units

3. Result and discussion

3.1 Evaluation of measurement accuracy and stability

The vital sensing system was applied to a basic measurement test in order to evaluate its effectiveness.

Firstly, we evaluated the accuracy of the body temperature sensor by using a platinum thermal resister. The two coefficients were determined by using two points calibration method. The following coefficients were obtained at 40°C, A = 18.9 and B = -14.79. By using these parameters, an accuracy test was performed. In consideration of the range of human body temperature, temperature was controlled from 32°C to 45°C. The profile of controlled temperature was shown in Fig. 11. And the result of accuracy test was shown in Fig. 12. This figure shows the differences between a referenced temperature and a measured temperature. The maximal error was 0.3°C and the mean error was -0.08°C. Therefore, the result shows that the accuracy of a temperature sensor was suitable to measure a body temperature at the range from 32°C to 45°C. However, the response time of the temperature sensor was relatively long. It is because a thermal capacity increased, directly attaching the thermal sensor to the unit case.

Secondly, the stability of ECG and pulse wave was evaluated. The waveform of ECG measured by portable vital sensing system was shown in Fig. 13. According to this waveform, the hum noise level of ECG was quite low. Because Ag-AgCl electrodes were used, it is possible to maintain good electrical conductivity between the electrode and the skin without any conductive paste. As another reason, it is because of battery driven circuits. Compared with AC/DC power supply, DC battery supply dose not generate power-supply noise or hum noise. Therefore, it is suitable to measure a biological signal. However, the movement of the baseline was observed. The problem was mainly caused by

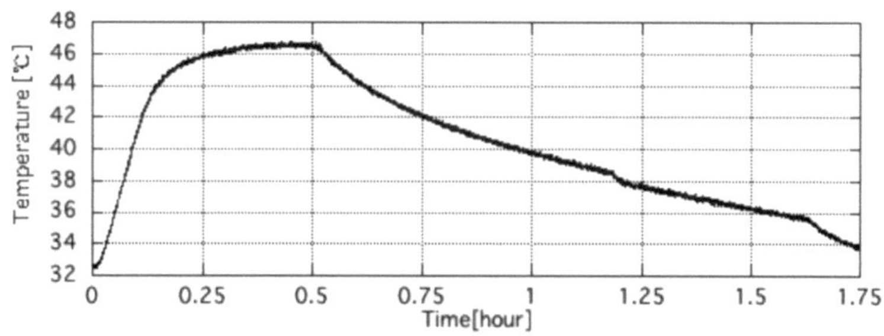

Fig. 11. The profile of a temperature accuracy test

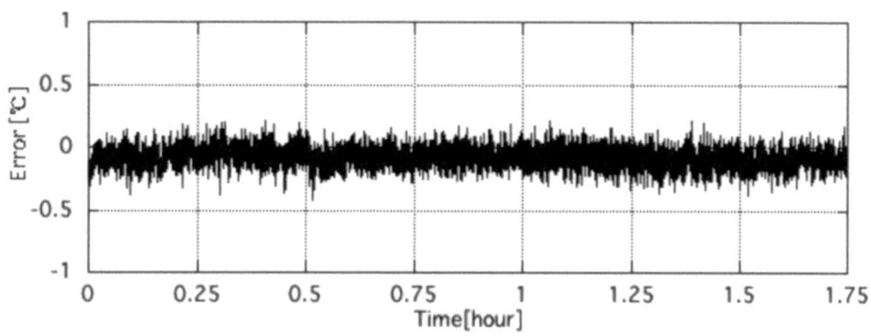

Fig. 12. The difference between a referenced temperature and a calibrated temperature using a platinum thermal sensor

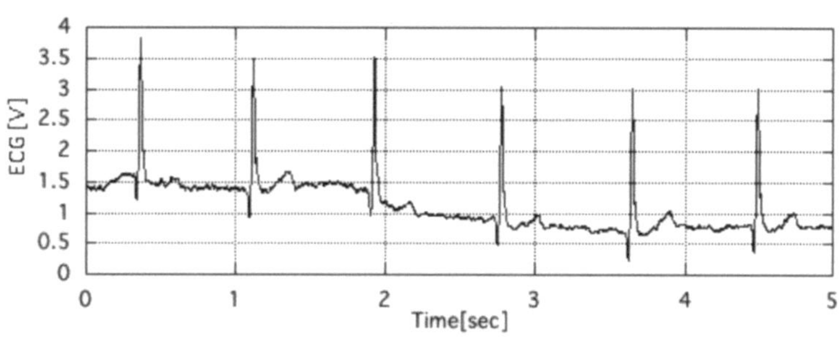

Fig. 13. The waveform of ECG measured by vital sensing system.

the change of electrical conductivity during breathing and body motion. In order to remove the baseline movement, a digital notch filter with notch frequencies at 0, 50 and its harmonics was implemented in the data acquisition program. An application of notch filter was shown in Fig.15 and Fig.16. Notch filter is generally a bond stop filter in a very narrow band. Since the designed notch filter was a comb type filter, having a frequency at o Hz, DC offset and baseline movement could be removed.

The waveform of pulse wave measured by a portable vital sensing system was shown in Fig. 14. It would be confirmed that it was stable to measure volume pulse wave by using a finger-type photoplethysmograph.

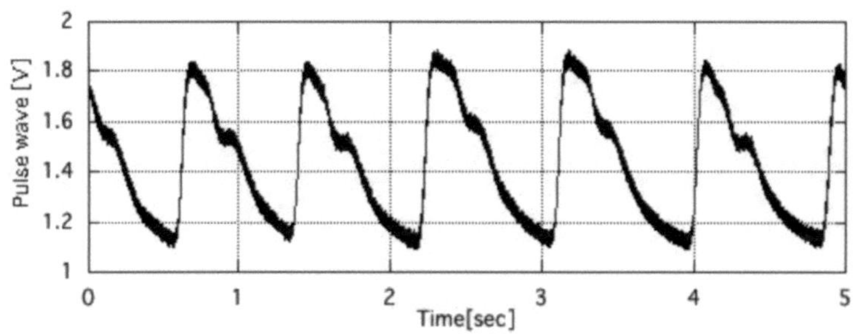

Fig. 14. The waveform of pulse wave measured by vital sensing system

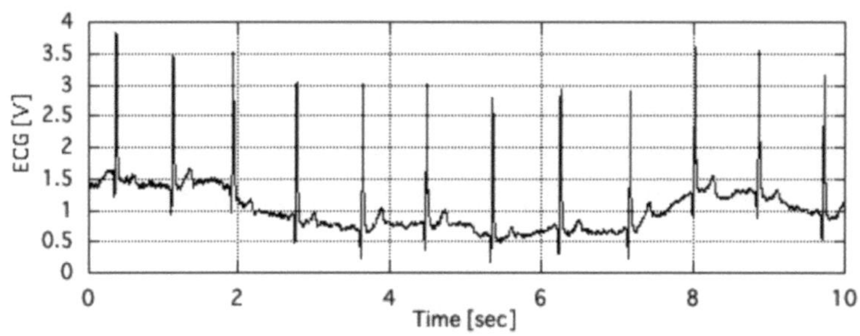

Fig. 15. The waveform of ECG without a notch filter

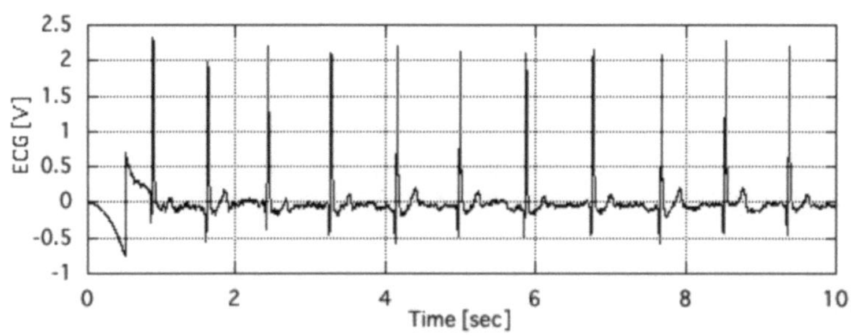

Fig. 16. The waveform of ECG with a digital notch filter: The designed notch filter has a notch frequency at 0 Hz, 50 Hz, and its harmonics.

3.2 Interoperability of home telemedicine

A home telemedicine system is a network-based and distributed information system to connect home patients to medical specialists. Therefore, it is of significance to consider interoperability of telemedicine systems. Regarding device connectivity to the home medical server, the proposed vital sensing system has the advantage of being easily connected to a Bluetooth PAN composed by the host medical server. However, considering network connectivity between a home medical server and a remote data server, more sophisticated system architecture is required in terms of data formats and communication protocols. Especially, HL7 (Health Level 7) which is a standard for exchanging information or DICOM (Digital Imaging and Communications in Medicine) which is a standard for medical imaging specification should be considered to improve interoperability of home telemedicine.

4. Conclusion

We developed a set of portable vital sensing system and a home medical server to establish a home telemedicine system. In order to develop a portable vital sensing system, physiological sensing circuit, digital signal processor and wireless communication device are integrated into a small electrical circuit, called "smart telecom unit" with a size of 25mm * 37mm. By using a smart telecom unit, noninvasive vital sensing units including blood pressure, electrocardiograph, pulse wave and body temperature were developed. Meanwhile, a home medical server consists of a small computer and virtual physiological model to estimate health conditions. These sensing units are able to communicate vital records to a home medical server, which can seamlessly connect to the Internet.

5. References

[1] M. Matsuda, "Effect of Exercise and Physical Activity on Prevention of Arteriosclerosis - Special Reference to Arterial Distensibility-," International Journal of Sport and Health Science, Vol. 4, pp.316-324, 2006.

[2] E. G. Lakatta, D. Levy, "Arterial and Cardiac Aging: Major Shareholders in Cardiovascular Disease Enterprises, Part I: Aging Arteries: A "Set Up"for Vascular Disease" Circulation, Vol. 107, pp.139-146, Jan, 2003.

[3] S. S. Najjar, A. Scuteri, and E. G. Lakatta, "Arterial Aging Is It an Immutable Cardiovascular Risk Factor?," Hypertention, Vol. 46, pp. 454-462, 2005.

[4] P. D. Tompson, D. Buchner, I. L Pina, G. J Balady, M. A. Williams, et al. "Exercise and physical Activity in the Prevention and Treatment of Atherosclerotic Cardiovascular Disease: A Statement From the Council on Clinical Cardiology (Subcommittee on Exercise, Rehabilitation, and Prevention) and the Council on Nutrition, Physical Activity, and Metabolism (Subcommittee on Physical Activity)," Circulation, Vol. 107, pp.3109-3116, 2003.

[5] G. A. Kaplan, T.E. Seeman, R. D Cohen, L.P. Kundsen, and J. Guralnik, "Mortality among the elderly in the Alameda County Study: behavioral and demographic risk factor," Am J Public Health, Vol. 777, pp.307-312, 1987.

[6] S. G. Leveille, J. M. Guralnik, L. Ferrucci, and J. A. Langlois, "Aging successfully until death in old age: opportunities for increasing active life expectancy," Am J Epidemiol, Vol. 149, No. 7, pp.654-664, 1999.

[7] G. E. Fraser, D. J. Shavlik, "Risk factors for all-cause and coronary heart disease mortality in the oldest-old. The Adventist Health Study," Arch Intern Med, Vol. 157, No. 19, pp.2249-2258, 1997.

[8] G. L. Burke, A.M. Arnold, D. E Bild, M. Cushman, L. P. Fried, et al. "Factors associated with healthy aging: the cardiovascular health study," J.Am.Geriatr.Soc, Vol. 49, pp.254-262, 2001.

[9] A. Z LaCroix, J. M Guralnik, L. F. Berkman, R. B Wallace, and S. Satterfield, "Maintaining mobility in late life. II. Smoking, alcohol consumption, physical activity, and body mass index," Am J Epidemiol, Vol. 137, pp.858-869, 1993.

[10] S. C. Wu, S. Y. Leu, and C.Y. Li, "Incidence of and predictors for chronic disability in activities of daily living among older people in Taiwan," Journal of the American Geriatric Society, Vol. 47, pp. 1082-1086, 1999.
[11] T. Yamauchi, T. Yamada, M.M. Islam, A. Okada, T. Takahashi, and N. Takeshima, "Effects of Well-rounded Exercise Program on Overall Fitness in Older Outpatients," Japanese Journal of Physical Fitness and Sports Medicine, Vol. 52 pp. 513-524, 2003.
[12] Y. Oida, Y. Kitabatake, T. Arao, H. Kohno, K. Egawa, T. Nagamatsu, Y. Nishijima, and H. Maie, "Effect of three years-intervention program on functional fitness and medical health status in community-dwelling elderly," Bulletin of the Physical Fitness Research Institute, Vol. 97 pp.1-13, 1999.
[13] A. Kubota, K. Ishikawa-Takata, and T. Ohta, "Effect of Daily Physical Activity on Mobility Maintenance in the Elderly," International Journal of Sport and Health Science, Vol. 3 pp. 83-90, 2005.
[14] F. Ichihashi, Y. Sankai, and S. Kuno, "Development of Secure Data Management Server for "e-Health Promotion System"," International Journal of Sport and Health Science, Vol.4, pp.617-627, 2006.
[15] E. kyriacou, S. Pavlopoulos, A. Berler, M. Neophytou, A. Bourka, A. Georgoulas, et al, "Multi-purpose HealthCare Telemedicine Systems with mobile communication link support",
[16] R. Kosaka, Y. Sankai, R. Takiya, T. Jikuya, T. Yamane, and T. Tsutsui, "Tsukuba Remote Monitoring System for Continuous-Flow Artificial Heart," Artif Organs.,Vol. 27, No. 10, pp.897-906, 2003.
[17] S. Nishimura, Y. Tomita, and T. Horiuchi, "Clinical Application of an Active Electrode Using an Operational Amplifier," IEEE Trans. Biomed. Eng., Vol. 39, pp.1096-1099, Oct, 1992.

17

Implementing the Chronic Disease Self Management Model in Vulnerable Patient Populations: Bridging the Chasm through Telemedicine

Cardozo Lavoisier J, Steinberg Joel, Cardozo Shaun, Vikas Veeranna, Deol Bibban and Lepczyk Marybeth
Wayne State University School of Medicine, Detroit, MI U.S.A.

1. Introduction

Vulnerable patient populations include those with chronic diseases, disability, the elderly, minorities and persons with limited health literacy. According to Healthy People 2000, despite recent progress in health care, there is a stagnation or decline in health care outcomes in these vulnerable patient groups. With the world population aging and the number of those over the age of 60 expected to grow to almost 2 billion by 2050 the prevalence of Chronic Disease (CD) will rise. So will the economic cost which currently is substantial and accounts for 46% of the global disease burden. Specifically in the United States, Chronic Diseases (CD's) will be responsible for 78% of all medical expenses. Unfortunately, the demographic imperatives of an aging society with the concomitant rise in disease burden will coincide with a decreasing provider base (Wooten et al., 2006). This will necessitate the adoption of different patient management models, to ensure cost effective patient monitoring within a continuum of care. Chronic Disease Self Management Programs (CDSMP) based on the Bandura's self-efficacy theory (Bandura 2004) focuses on teaching patients coping skills to include disease monitoring and understanding, skills to continue with normal living and strategies to improve emotional well being. Based on the Chronic Care Model, optimal care is achieved when a prepared, proactive practice team interacts with an informed, activated patient (Bordenheimer et al.2002). In the new paradigm patients with CDs become their own care givers, with health care providers acting as consultants in a supporting role. The Institutes of Medicine Report "Crossing the Quality Chasm" (1998) advocated continuous healing relationships, customized care with the patient in control, and an information system that flows freely to facilitate evidence based decision making. To achieve this, Healthcare Systems will have to shift from a Provider Centered to a Patient Centered System within the concept of Advanced Patient Centered Medical Homes, where patients are empowered as partners. The question therefore is can Telemedicine (TM) bridge the chasm by empowering patients, improving and supporting equal access, enhancing capacity, improving quality and cost effectiveness, reducing disease burden and supporting decision making, especially in vulnerable patient populations who have the greatest need and the highest disease burden. Within this context innovative use of technology (to include TM) has been adopted to facilitate seamless care, coordination of services and patient monitoring. The data to-date suggests that TM is a promising strategy with the potential to empower patients, change behaviors and attitudes, enhance knowledge and improve clinical outcomes. Moreover vulnerable populations such as older patients, those with limited health literacy, patients from rural areas and poor socio-economic status, appear to be willing to accept the use of technology to assist them in disease self management. This chapter will detail the history and the progress of TM and evaluate the current outcomes in Chronic Disease Management in vulnerable patients especially the elderly, those living in rural areas and minority populations especially those with low health literacy. We will also discuss the scope and potential of future novel TM advances which must emerge, as the challenge to tailor services to individual needs of the patients, the provision of continuous medical education to the patient and provider, within the complexities of the health care system become imperative.

2. History of telemedicine

The term "telemedicine" has a Greek origin from "tele" meaning at a distance and a Latin derivative for medicine "mederi" meaning "healing". A WHO definition of TM (1997) refers to "the delivery of healthcare services, where distance is a critical factor, by healthcare professionals using information and communications technologies for the exchange of valid information for diagnosis, treatment and prevention of diseases and injuries, research and evaluation, and for continuing education of healthcare providers, all in the interest of advancing health and their communities". Today TM refers to the use of communications and informational technologies for the purpose of providing clinical care, while the term "telehealth" includes the delivery of both clinical and non-clinical (medical education, research or administrative) services. While "e-health" is used as an umbrella term to cover telehealth, electronic medical records and other health informational technology. The relationship between the various terminologies associated with e-health is depicted in Figure 1.

The earliest form for communication at a distance was the use of smoke signals as a form of a communication system, a "preventive medicine" approach to warn people to stay away from a village afflicted with a serious disease. The history of present day TM dates to the early 1960's when the National Aeronautical and Space Agency (NASA) was able to measure astronaut physiological data in space, and successfully transmit it to earth. This galvanized NASA to support a project utilizing TM to deliver medical care (from 1972-75) to the Papago Indian Reservation in Arizona. NASA continued to fund TM projects in the late 1960's and early 1970,s and by 1975 there were 15 active TM projects. (Basher et al., 1975).

There are two different forms of technology used in TM, the first, also called "store and forward" which primarily transfers digital images and is used in tale-radiology (sending X-ray, MRI and CT scans), tale-pathology (pathology slides) and tale-dermatology (sending digital images of skin conditions for dermatologists to interpret). A second technology provides for a two-way interactive television when face to face consultation is needed. A number of subsequent variations have evolved to include video-conferencing, urban to rural links, capabilities to use an otoscope to examine the ear or use the electronic stethoscope to auscultate the heart from a distance and mobile TM systems termed mHealth.

The future vision as proposed by The Telemedicine Alliance formed under the European Commission is the development of a citizen-centered e-Health System (Figure 2).

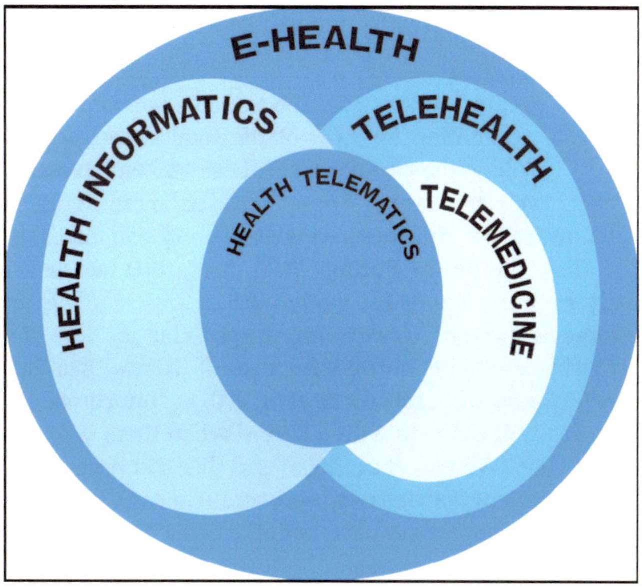

Fig. 1. The relationship between the various terminologies associated with e-Health.
Reproduced from: Telemedicine 2010: Visions For A Personal Medical
Medical Network-The Telemedicine Alliance-July 2004.

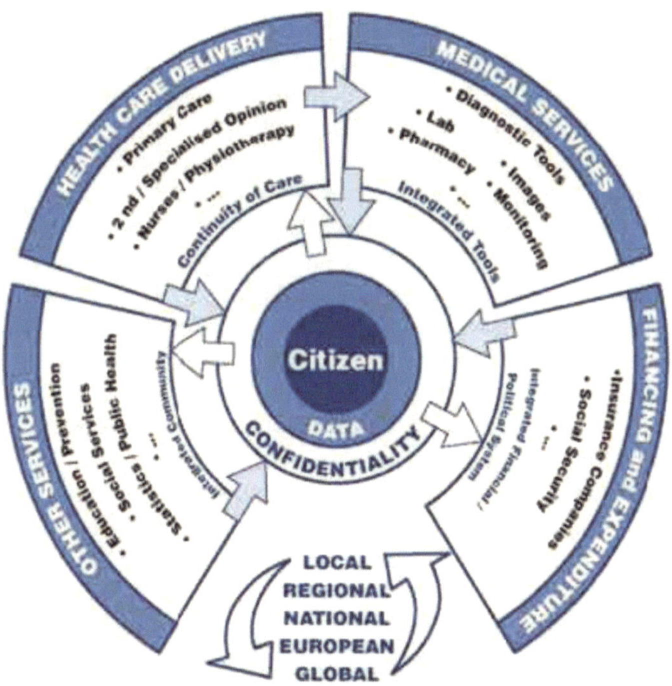

Fig. 2. The Vision For a Citizen-centered health care.
Reproduced from: Telemedicine 2010: Visions for A Personal Medical Network-The
Telemedicine Alliance-July 2004

3. Factors influencing the emerging growth of TM

3.1 The demographic imperative

The world population is ageing, tripling over the last 50 years and expected to rise to two billion by the year 2050, accounting for 21% of the total world population (Gavrilov & Heuveline 2003). In the US alone the population of those >65 will exceed 53 million by 2020 as the "baby-boomers swell the ranks. These baby boomers "will also accelerate the movement for greater awareness, self-care and wellness and will alter the traditional doctor patient relationship" (Institute for the Future, 2010). In Europe between 16 and 18% of the population is already over the age of 65, many with at least one CD and possibly more. Aging increases the prevalence of CDs currently responsible for 46% of the global disease burden and rapidly rising economic burden. As a result in most healthcare systems 5% of patients are responsible for 50% of costs (Berk et al, 2001). Unfortunately, as already stated the rising disease burden will coincide with a period when there is going to be a projected decline in the provider base (Wooten et al., 2006) and this will necessitate the development of novel approaches for patient management and access to care. In this context TM with its rapidly emerging technology appears to have both the capacity and the innovative potential to complement the growth and development of future healthcare delivery models.

3.2 Current healthcare system in need of change

The traditional system of healthcare delivery has focused on acute care where the patients admission is treated as a random event to be taken care of with the purpose of discharging the patient home when stable This may be appropriate for acute problems however with increasing longevity and rising prevalence of CD's the present model is distinctly unsuitable, it lacks a continuum and results in fragmentation of care leading to poor clinical outcomes and high cost. In addition a number of other factors are also driving the decision to consider alternative healthcare delivery modes; the culture and expectations of the baby boomers, the complexities of health care delivery, the need to monitor quality and the imperative to provide the tools to make seamless care a reality. As a result we are beginning to see a transition to the Chronic Care Disease Management Model practiced within a patient-centered health care delivery system, as the preferred option of care. This begins with a care transition program with a purpose to improve quality and safety during care hand offs. A recent position statement from the American Geriatrics Society defines transitional care as, " a set of actions designed to ensure the coordination and continuity of health care as patients transfer between different locations or different levels of care within the same location. Representative locations include (but are not limited to) hospitals, sub-acute and post-acute nursing facilities, the patient's home, primary and specialty care offices and long-term care facilities. Transitional care is based on a comprehensive plan of care and the availability of health care practitioners who are well trained in chronic care and have current information about the patient's goals, preferences and clinical status. It includes logistical arrangements, education of patient and family, and coordination among the health professionals involved in the transition. Transitional care, which encompasses both the sending and the receiving aspects of transfer, is essential for persons with complex care needs" (Coleman et al., 2003). TM can be the link to allow a seamless process from acute care through transitional care into a care continuum based on the Chronic Disease Care Model.

3.3 The increasing importance of the chronic care model

This is a system that empowers patients by allowing them to interact with providers, receive the necessary education to self-manage CDs and make decisions between the best options of care tailored to the patient's individual circumstance. The healthcare system has started to move from a physician-centered to a patient-centered system, wherein patients as knowledgeable partners interact with providers as mentors, to allow for disease self management with the aid of TM. The central tenet of the CDSMP is for the patient to be able to achieve the greatest possible physical ability and pleasure from life by "positively managing" illness (Lorig et al., 2006). According to the Chronic Care Model, optimal care is achieved in a proactive format wherein both patient and provider are well informed about the goals and care options (Bodenheimer et al., 2002). This is giving rise to a new paradigm in the management of CD with the patient acting as their own care-giver and the health care professional in the supporting role.

This partnership that emphasizes the concept of collaborative care and self-management requires an empowered patient with the necessary resources to solve their own problems with the aid of appropriate information (Holman et al., 2000). The success of the collaboration is based on the need of the patient having a high level of internal motivation and being less dependent on external (professional) motivation (Funnell et al., 1991).

The patient in turn as the manager has to decide what he/she wants to accomplish, examine alternate options as to how to achieve this, create a successful action plan and be able to make mid-course changes (problem solving) as necessary. Understanding and dealing with common disease symptoms and practicing different symptom management techniques while controlling the emotional overlay, is central to the process. Ultimately having the provider as mentor and the patient as manager is the basis for successful CDSMP.

The patient-physician partnership is becoming the new dyad, with the addition of patients as their own principal caregivers. To this effect Corbin and Strauss (1988) defined 3 sets of tasks patients with CDs have to learn: (1) medical management of the condition; (2) to create and maintaining new meaningful life roles and (3) to cope with the emotional fall out (anger, fear and frustration). A central tenant in self management is the development of self-efficacy it allows patients to solve patient identified problems. This requires a system with the capability of continuous patient education, disease monitoring and collaborative care where the provider can use TM as a resource. Current TM technology can bridge not only the chasm in the education continuum but also fill the gap between patient and provider. CDM programs are based on two pillars, a patient related and a professional directed intervention (Bodenheimer 1999; Kane et al., 2005).

The spectrum of self management extends from only providing written material to more extensive CDSMP designed to enhance self-efficacy.

Professional guidance requires an increased knowledge base and expertise necessary to support patient decision making skills. When an informed patient takes an active role in managing their health and providers feel prepared and supported with time and resources, the provider patient interaction can be more productive. It is becoming increasingly clear that patient education is a critical factor in disease management; it is an important determinant of treatment compliance and changes in behavior. There is evidence that programs teaching self management skills through TM are more effective than those that only provide patients with written disease information (Stromberg et al., 2006). For example, there is also evidence that TM Video education increases Congestive Heart Failure (CHF) self-care behaviors especially when symptoms are worsening (Albert et al., 2007). There are a number of interventions to promote self-care, skill development, behavior change, family support and redesign of systems of care. In all these aspects especially the latter, telehealth has a role in disease management as the focus shifts to providing care across the continuum and bridging the chasm between acute and chronic care.

3.4 The growing need to bridge the chasm and develop a care continuum through telehealth networks

The growth of telehealth technologies specifically home telemonitoring is a method to link acute, transitional and chronic care needs. In this regard Meystre (2005) concluded that long-term disease monitoring at home through TM represents a promising application of telemonitoring technology for the delivery of cost effective quality healthcare. A recent review of home telemonitoring for CDs showed a good level of accuracy and reliability of transmitted data (Pare et al., 2007). It also demonstrated the ability of TM to identify early changes and improvement in quality of life indices. In addition patients had positive attitudes to TM they expressed high levels of satisfaction, acceptance and compliance. Direct involvement by patients in their care was also associated with increased knowledge and awareness of disease leading to greater patient empowerment in management. Most studies have shown a reduction in cost of care with lower re-admission rates, decreased visits to emergency rooms and lower hospital length of stay. Specifically the Weight monitoring in HeART (Goldberg et al., 2003) trial demonstrated that daily reporting of weight and symptoms in patients with advanced CHF reduced mortality by 56.2%. Other studies have demonstrated that technology using video-conferencing and telephone-line transmission of weight, blood pressure and electrocardiograms were even more effective at reducing hospitalization and inpatient length of stay (Dang et al., 2009). Similar results were noted with improvement in self-efficacy and glycemic control using TM in older ethnically diverse patients with diabetes (Trief et al., 2009). TM is rapidly becoming the go to tool to bridge the chasm and improve quality of care especially for those with chronic illness while controlling cost.

4. Update on the current status of TM in vulnerable patient populations

4.1 TM in geriatrics

The rising cost of Medicare suggests that there is a need to move from a high-tech to a high-value practice system. Prevalence of CD increases with age, increased longevity (at the turn of the last century life expectancy was 47 years today it is 77), an astounding rise of 64% that has resulted in a population of 35 million over the age of 65 today. There are an estimated 64.4 million with cardiovascular disease (with 50 million having Hypertension, 13.2 million with Coronary Heart Disease, 7.8 million have had Myocardial Infarction, 5 million with Heart Failure and there are 4.8 million Strokes/year. Cardiovascular diseases including Strokes accounted for 40% of all deaths in the US in 2001 (AHA, 2004). The direct and indirect costs are substantial. Almost a fifth (19.6%) of Medicare beneficiaries discharged from hospital were re-hospitalized within 30 days and 34% within 90 days in 2004, at a cost of 17.4 billion dollars (Jenks et al., 2009) while 10% of reimbursement codes account for 90% of Medicare spending. The question therefore is can TM improve quality of care, reduce cost of care and is this technology applicable to older populations?

As regards improvement in essential hypertension, in a randomized controlled trial, direct links through TM to patient homes to monitor blood pressure, resulted in improved control

(Rogers et al., 2001), A number of studies have evaluated cost, Noel et al (2004) were able to show that non-invasive monitoring of patients with CHF, Diabetes and Chronic Lung Disease (supervised by a nurse manager) not only resulted in better disease outcomes but also reduced cost of care and increased patient satisfaction. Evidence also suggests that the elderly are able to manage computer based programs despite the fact that they as a group have lower access to computers at home. Other barriers to the use of computers by older persons such as low self-esteem, visual, auditory and mobility problems also need to be addressed when creating programs for the elderly (Hendrix 2000). These programs should have the capacity to be individualized to allow for choice of areas of interest that can be repeated and accessed at their learning pace using synchronized multimedia text, photos, animation and speech (Stromberg et al., 2002; Lewis 2003; Hendrix 2000). Even a single computer-based educational session on heart failure delivered to a group of older persons showed an increase in knowledge compared to a randomized similar group that only received the standard program (Stromberg 2002). As regards consultation for geriatric hospital patients, TM from an off-site location (while uncommon), could be of value for institutions with no geriatricians or for patients in rural hospitals. This modality has the potential to offer a service at a marginally increased cost with the added advantage of lowering the cost for the patient and doctor, by eliminating travel (Persaud et al., 2005). TM is now being used in dementia monitoring to support family caregivers and link home to their workplace (Mahoney 2009). Studies have been done in a variety of practice environments, inpatient, nursing home, consultation, triage, ambulatory care and community care (home care and wellness centers). While the literature supports the overall reliability, acceptance and cost effectiveness of TM in older populations recent reviews agree that "good quality studies are still scarce" (Whitten et al., 2002; Hailey et al., 2004; Pare et al., 2007; Dang et al., 2009). However with the current shortage of geriatricians which is expected to get worse and the rising prevalence of chronic diseases the role of TM in providing the continuum of care for older patients has to be advanced.

4.2 In rural areas

"The doctor will see you now. Please log On" describes how a two way video consult was able to diagnose that a patient on an oil rig was having pain secondary to a kidney stone, provide emergency treatment and have the patient air lifted for definitive management (Freudenheim 2010). With rapidly improving technology the distance between doctor and patient can be dramatically reduced to resemble a virtual in-office encounter. With up to a fifth of Americans living in areas where primary care physicians are scarce TM can make significant contributions. A number of organizations use TM to provide physician services to patients on oil rigs, psychiatric institutions and to prisoner inmates, at lower costs. As an example the State of California spends more than $40/day per inmate for health care, this includes the cost of guards and transportation for visits to outside doctors, the latter expenses would not be necessary with TM as a result of which there was a savings of $ 13 million (Bloch 2010). In a recent publication Kroenke et. al (2010) describes the effects of Telecare management of pain and depression in cancer patients. The intervention consisted of telephonic care management delivered by a nurse care manager at periodic intervals over 3 months coupled with a system of automated symptom monitoring.

This telecare management intervention resulted in significant improvements in both pain and depression when compared to usual care. The roles of TM in electrocardiography and echocardiography (Huffer et al., 2004), radiology and pathology, orthopedics (Couturier et al, 1998), psychiatry (Montani et al., 1997) and trauma care, in rural areas, are receiving greater attention (Latifi et al., 2009). There is also a role for TM in patient triage systems in a number of specialties. The benefit of these TM consultations is great especially if patient transfer poses a risk or the distance is great, a relevant factor given that a number of Americans (20%) live in places where primary care physicians are scarce or unavailable. A number of physician groups are addressing this need through TM and this mode of interactive TM is growing 10% annually in United States as Medicare, Medicaid and other agencies have begun to reimburse doctors and hospitals that provide care remotely to rural and underserved areas.

The combination of video-conferencing with TM has been reported to enhance the clinical interaction. In the ambulatory care TM requires the patient be introduced to the remote specialist, and the feasibility and efficacy of this process has been demonstrated in Neurology (Wiborg et el., 2003). While teleneurological examination via video conferencing in conjunction with tele-radiology (to examine brain scans) for stroke evaluation in pre-hospital triage and care is being increasingly utilized in rural areas (Audebert & Schwamm 2009). Another example of virtual outreach consultation is tele-psychiatry for rural nursing home residents which has been shown to be a cost-effective and is a medically acceptable alternative to face to face care (Rabinowitz et al., 2010).

Passive monitoring of indices for HTN, CHF, Diabetes and COPD have also shown positive clinical outcomes and savings in cost of care. In addition the technology (including video-conferencing) has been well accepted by patients. However, from the provider perspective the inability to elicit physical examination findings and/or only viewing images, leads to uncertainty and some dissatisfaction, a potential limitation to the use of TM.

4.3 In minority and low health literacy groups

Contrary to expectations patient populations deemed vulnerable to higher morbidity as a consequence of adverse psychosocial circumstances (the elderly, low socioeconomic status, minorities, underserved and disadvantaged) welcome collaborative care, they have the greatest potential benefit from information technology and are not as commonly believed disadvantaged by the "digital divide" (comScore study). While poor access to health care contributes to higher morbidity and mortality rates in minority populations, innovative solutions using technology have begun to show better outcomes and higher satisfaction rates. A case in point was demonstrated in the study in the Baby CareLink project (Safran 2003) in an Neonatal Intensive Care Unit (NICU). Here parents even remote from the NICU participated in decisions in the care of their premature infant, received customized education and information. The end result was better outcomes, lower cost, and greater patient and provider satisfaction rates. The cost effectiveness and feasibility of Telehealth was also shown in American Indians and Alaskan Native Subjects (Shore et al., 2007). This study compared direct costs of conducting structured clinical interventions via real-time interactive videoconferencing versus standard in-person methods, the latter proved to be more expensive.

Health literacy has been defined as "the degree to which the individuals have the basic capacity to obtain, process and understand basic health information and services needed to make appropriate health decisions" (Selden et al., 2000). A US health literacy survey done in 2003 estimated that 36% of the adult population had basic or below basic health literacy levels, which is defined as low literacy, this approximates to 87 million US adults (National Center for Education Statistics, 2006). Low health literacy plays a major role in determining the patient's outcome with maximal adverse impact on older people (Baker et al., 2007). To compound the problem numeracy skills (the ability to understand and use numbers in daily life, as in understanding and applying nutritional label information) are also low (Rothman et al., 2006). The high prevalence of low literacy in certain groups, those with limited education, certain racial and ethnic groups and the elderly may contribute to disparities in health care outcomes (Kirsch et al., 2002). Cardiovascular diseases constitutes the single largest entity of the chronic diseases afflicting 70 million Americans, with many of these patients above the age of sixty and prone to have low literacy levels. However a major barrier to improving patient education is that only 10% of the education material is written at the 8th grade level or below (Davis et al., 1990). One study found that more than 80% of the web site material on 37 non-prescription medicines was written at a grade 10th level (Wallace 2006).

The future challenge for TM is to develop material that is appropriate for this patient population. As stated in Healthy People 2010 adequate health literacy is necessary to provide individuals with the capacity to obtain, process and understand basic health information and services if they are to make individualized appropriate health decisions (Healthy People 2010). Currently the literature in this area specifically as it relates to the use of TM to overcome the barriers of health literacy remains sparse.

4.4 In chronic disease management

True disease management includes population identification processes, comprehensive needs assessment, pro-active health promotion, patient focused health management goals and education, self-care education, routine reporting and feedback with ongoing evaluation of outcomes (Disease Management). Studies have demonstrated the feasibility of group-based self-management processes among patients with congestive heart failure (Smeulders et al., 2009) and other chronic diseases (Lorig et al., 2003). Even limited heart failure self-care education by video can change patient behaviors (Albert et al., 2003), leading to fewer symptoms of volume overload. This study also showed that patients with better cognitive status benefited more from CDSMP as did those from lower education levels. Systems of care such as disease management and care-coordination can promote self-care because they facilitate transitions across care settings. A recent study (Maric et al., 2010) described the use of the Internet to remotely monitor patients with heart failure was described. Participants entered their weight and symptoms onto the Web for six months. Self-care, quality of life, 6-minute walk test and patient confidence showed sustained improvement.

In the Hypertension Intervention Nurse Telemedicine Study (HINTS) (Bosworth et al., 2007), the authors describe a novel multifactorial tailored behavioral and a medication management intervention control program, which was successful and feasible in the patient's home. More sophisticated technology such as video-conferencing and telephone line transmission of weight, BP and EKG's has been shown to be even more effective in reducing hospitalization rates, length of stay. (Woudend et al., 2008) and symptom reduction (Dawsky et al., 2008). Other workers (Dang et al, 2009) have evaluated the effects of the use of Home TM remote monitoring in the elderly with Heart Failure and concluded that the impact on healthcare utilization, mortality and cost appear to be positive in most cases. In their opinion the study by Clark et al (2007) had the strongest level of evidence in the meta-analysis, supporting the use of TM in the community setting for heart failure patients. Seto (2008) evaluated 11 articles using 10 different Heart Failure telemonitoring systems, for their economic impact. They concluded that TM requires an initial investment but it substantially reduces cost in the long term through decreased re-hospitalizations and patient travel costs. In a recent review of randomized controlled trials of structured telephone support or telemonitoring programs for patients with chronic heart failure versus usual care (Inglis et al., 2010), the authors concluded that telemonitoring was effective in reducing the risk of all-cause mortality, CHF related hospitalizations and that there was improved quality of life, reduced costs and it led to evidence-based prescribing.

A systematic review of home telemonitoring in diabetes, asthma, heart failure and hypertension covering 62 empirical studies from 1966-2008 (Pare et al., 2010), the author concluded that TM was a promising approach with a trend to better glycemic controls, significant improvements in asthma and control of hypertension however the studies were equivocal on heart failure. In a Diabetes study at a veteran hospital (Dang et al., 2007) care coordination facilitated by telemedicine resulted in improved glycemic controls and reduced resource utilization. A literature review of asynchronous and synchronous teleconsultation for diabetes care (Verhoeven 2010) from 1994 to 2009 concluded that despite the diversity and lack of quality in many studies, TM was feasible, cost-effective and reliable.

4.5 In home healthcare settings

In a systematic review of home telemonitoring for CD (Pare et al., 2010) an analysis of home telemonitoring for four disease categories (Diabetes, Hypertension, Chronic Pulmonary conditions and CHF) was done. In these studies most researchers (in the US and Europe) focused on exploring the benefits of TM. The consensus was that; (a) the data collected was accurate and consistently transmitted from the patients home, (b) the data appeared as reliable as that which would have been obtained from patient face to face examination, (c) that the findings related to the patient's attitudes and behaviors were consistent across all studies in that TM was well received, improved awareness, quality of life, fostered a sense of security and led to greater patient empowerment; however there was evidence of a decrease in patient compliance seen over time, (d) that TM is able to detect early changes in the patient's condition and (e) that there was a significant decrease in hospital admissions, emergency department visits and length of hospital stay.

The decrease in cost in terms of decrease in emergency visits, hospital admissions and length of stay were more consistent for pulmonary and cardiac diseases than for diabetes and hypertension. It also supported the fact that these findings were noted regardless of patient nationality, socioeconomic status or age, in those who complied with the program. Home-based case management directed by a nurse in conjunction with TM-case managed telemedicine (CMTM) is an effective intervention for enhancing the continuum of care (Speedie et al., 2008).

It has been shown to improve outcomes in those patients classified as high risk, in elderly veterans (Schofield, 2005), patients with chronic atrial fibrillation (Inglis et al., 2004), and diabetics (Chumbler et al., 2005). CMTM has also shown reduce cost of care, improve compliance, self-efficacy and patient education. We were able to show in a large study (851 recently discharged elderly patients followed up by TM for 2 months) that the majority showed improved quality of health perception, better disease understanding and high satisfaction rates. In addition we documented that treatment goals were met in 67%, patient compliance was 77%, and the average improvement in nine Quality of Care Measures (pain control, dyspnea, urinary incontinence, upper body dressing, bathing, toileting, transferring, ambulation/locomotion, medication management) was 66% (Cardozo & Steinberg, 2010)

5. Educational aspects of telemedicine

As mentioned previously, the WHO defines TM in the broad concept of "...delivery of healthcare services, where distance is a critical factor using information and communication technologies... for diagnosis, treatment, and prevention of diseases... and for continuing education...". In contemplating the application of TM for such an educational mission one could consider several logistical factors, including the choice of the specific technological platform or device used from the myriad of possibilities, the model of healthcare delivery in practice, the specific venues along the continuum of care (whether in the home, primary care clinic, non-institutional care setting, chronic long term care institutional care setting, hospital etc.) at which the educational event occurs, the educational content of the material, and the participants of the educational activity. Participants could include any members of the spectrum of individuals involved in the healthcare process, from patients (i.e. consumers) to healthcare professionals (i.e. providers), and may utilize the healthcare professional providers as a source of educational materials (i.e. teachers) directed at the targeted patient consumers (i.e. students).

While we may view the traditional educational landscape as populated by such patient consumer students taught by healthcare provider teachers, we must recognize the potential flexibility of these roles and the opportunities for reinforcing or recasting them through educational TM. In particular, the evolving models of CDSMP in the context of the Advanced Patient Centered Medical Home appear conducive to the anticipated goal of establishing TM as a potent educational tool to enhance outcomes, quality of care, and the healthcare experience for all participants. Virtual education, primarily in the various forms of online education gradually has established a presence in the conventional education process. Approximately 40% of public school districts in the United States offer at least one online class and some school districts instruct through virtual high schools, whose students exhibit high completion rates and performance on advance placement exams.

This integration of technology into the classroom spans the entire age range. A recent foundation sponsored symposium of public and private sector leading educators, innovators, researchers, and journalists, conclude that digital media provide a powerful learning tool especially at an elementary school level, and that the country, in an interdisciplinary manner should, " -build a coherent research and development effort, -use digital tools effectively and safely to help students read well, think critically, broaden geographical and cultural knowledge, and participate in collaborative learning communities, and to -advance digital equity to reach all children." (Shore 2008). Studies indicate that digital media can support social growth (more peer interaction around common interests; more collaborative projects); cognition (greater motivation to read, more opportunities for problem-solving); and health (through simulations and games, better understanding of the importance of healthy behaviors) (Bernholz 2006). Adult education also embraces virtual technology as reflected in the volume of online learning and matriculation opportunities.

As an early and committed proponent of the application of new technologies, the military recognizes the value of virtual reality simulations, creating the sophisticated virtual reality series titled Virtual Iraq, designed to provide soldiers with the skills necessary for deployment in regions of active conflict and also for therapeutic interventions such as treatment for Post Traumatic Stress Disorder (PTSD) (Rizzo et al., 2008).

The benefits of TM extend in to the realm of healthcare education. E-learning educational programs, in various electronic formats, directed toward patients, healthcare professionals, and healthcare professional trainees continue to gather acceptance and momentum. Many medical schools gradually present more material in an E-learning format, which may include simulated patient encounters, that encourages student self learning and facilitates self management of time and resources.

Healthcare professionals benefit from a growing repository of E-learning resources. In geriatrics education for example, some of these resources include the Portal of Online Geriatrics Education (Pogo-E), the Geriatric Web, The Online Geriatrics University (GeriU), Consortium of E-learning in Geriatrics (CELGI), and Geriatrics Resources on the Web (GROW). A few of the resources available in medical education include MedBiquitous, the International Virtual Medical School (IVIMEDS), Health Education Assets Library (HEAL), Competencies Across the Continuum of Health Education (CACHE), and the Multimedia Education Resource for Learning and On line Teaching (MERLOT). There are also exciting innovations in post-graduate health education and training where " surgical students geographically separated can collaboratively learn and interact with specialists, telemonitoring environments where trainees may be hand-held by geographically separated experts, and telesurgical planning environments where experts who are geographically separated may collaborate to plan surgery" (Conde et al., 2009).

As the concept, development, and implementation of TM emerges from the evolving economic and technology forces driving healthcare, patients will inevitably need to confront and contend with it. While TM will profoundly influence the practice of medicine, unavoidably impacting patients, innovative applications of TM may assist patients in successfully navigating our turbulent healthcare system. One TM application occurs in the form of computer based systems that attempt to allow patients to access and exchange health information, facilitate decision making, provide social and emotional support, and encourage behavior changes that promote health and well being (Calvin et al., 2009). This type of system integrates well into the CDSMP and Advanced Patient Centered Medical Home concepts. These types of systems allow patients to review their medical history, review information about diseases and their treatment, and communicate electronically with healthcare providers ultimately resulting in self management decisions. Health care delivery systems will need a change in format if it is to benefit from evolving telehealth applications. As an example the State of Arkansas has a telehealth program called "Antenatal and Neonatal Guidelines, Education and Learning System and Peds Place", an outreach program that has reduced cost and improved community health outcomes (Hall et al., 2008; Hall et al., 2009).

When used effectively these systems reduce hospital admission and mortality rates, and enhance patient health outcomes and quality of life for common chronic diseases such as congestive heart failure. Patients however may not accept TM applications. Barriers may prevent some patients from engaging these potentially empowering models of TM. User acceptance of technology depends on many factors including individual (demographic, health status, diagnostic/treatment intervention factors), human-technology interaction, organizational, social, task, and environmental factors (Karsh & Holden 2007).

While research has gathered abundant information about these factors outside of TM applications, much remains unknown about these in the patient user TM context. The limited patient acceptance data available, which mostly concerns only certain demographic factors, describes an inconsistent effect on age and no apparent effect on gender. Higher education and familiarity with computer technology appears to favor acceptance (Calvin et al., 2009). Sensory, motor, and cognitive functional limitations may interfere with acceptance (Lober et al., 2000). The few studies available concerning patient trust suggest it exerts a prominent influence (Song & Zahedi 2007). The inevitable presence of TM in the future of healthcare demands the need for a greater deal of further research to design successful patient empowering, user friendly, and medically outcome enhancing TM systems.

6. Future trends and Global issues in TM

During the last decade the pace of application in technology for diagnosis and management has been rapid, however the same needs to occur in the field of health information services to allow for effective collaborative care and participatory decision making process. The consumer (the patient) must be involved in the decisions about their health care by becoming an empowered partner (through shared information) for disease self management.

The European Union has developed a vision to convert traditional health strategies to e-health. With this in mind they have formed a TM-Alliance consortium in 2005 with the purpose to study the challenges and assess opportunities presented by e-health. The Alliance speaks to empowering patients, to improving and supporting equal access, building capacity, increasing quality and value, reducing travel burden and supporting decision making (Telemedicine 2010). In effect, to enhance the move towards citizen-centered healthcare. In the NIH Conference on the Future of Telehealth (NCRR's 2009-2013 Strategic Plan) a new model for collaborative efforts to harness information and communication technologies to expand the scope and reach of clinical and translational research, reduce health disparities and put science to work in the service of healthcare reform was proposed (Doarn et al., 2010).

It is also clear the while CD management is important Disease Prevention will become equally important. The WHO reports that "at least 80% of premature deaths from heart disease and stroke could be avoided through effective reduction of risk factors (WHO 1998). This needs to be viewed in the context that in 2005 over 861,826 deaths in the US were due to Cardiovascular Diseases, accounting for 32.5% of all deaths (Rosamond et al., 2008) while in Europe there were over 4.35 million deaths (49% of all deaths) each year (Peterson et al., 2005). Preventive approaches will require patients to take responsibility for self management and TM can both provide them with access to the education and the means to record and report data. In this regard the concept of a "virtual doctor's office" or a "virtual waiting rooms" to provide patients with 24 hour access to physicians for non-life-threatening consultations, is gaining momentum (Freudenheim 2010).

Home devices such as motion-detectors, medicine-cabinet and door opening monitors and event detectors (to record falls, blood pressure drops, heart rhythm changes) are available to create a "smart home", a virtual "assisted living" arrangement. These devices can identify risk factors, monitor health and onset of disease (Novak et el., 2004), or in cardiovascular disease to predict impending heart failure, arrhythmias or sudden death (Myerfeldt et al.,

2002), or in continuous electrocardiographic monitoring to diagnose unstable sleep patterns and sleep apnea (Kesek et al., 2009). Innovations such as the iBrain that uses a small probe to monitor electrical brain activity through a single electrode to measure neurological function has the potential to revolutionize the diagnosis and management of sleep disorders, seizures, drug effects, recovery from brain trauma and the course of neurodegenerative disorders including Alzheimer's disease. (Darce 2010). While a prototype device to monitor brainwaves and provide patients in-real time with warning of an impending seizure are in the testing phase (Hamblen 2010) and if found to be effective it would have a significant effect on the management of epilepsy. Other digital devices with the potential to diagnose early cancers, monitor cardiac markers, detect infectious diseases and other illnesses and transmit the data to physicians are in the offing. There are also telemonitoring devices embedded into belts, clothing or watches under investigation.

A variant of TM is the emerging mobile communications and network technologies for healthcare systems, termed mHealth. Currently 64% of mobile users are in emerging markets, it is estimated that by 2012, 50% of individuals in remote areas will have access to mobile phones. A mobile TM system can use attachments turning phones into microscopes to diagnose diseases such as tuberculosis and malaria. Major efforts in countries like India to enhance medical telecommunications via mHealth are underway though it will take time to reach a critical mass for a successful national TM network (Ganapathy et al., 2007).

The advent of Electronic Medical Records (EMR) does provide the opportunity to link with TM and provide a method to follow the dynamic changes between a patient's physiological responses and their interactions with the environment of care. Specifically, portable TM devices have been shown to have a positive role in monitoring patients with gait disturbances (Mudge et al., 2007), or in measuring the degree of patient social interaction through sociometric devices (Sung et al., 2005) an important TM advance given that increase social interaction and engagement is associated with slower cognitive decline (Barnes et al., 2004) and decreased fall risk (Baker et al., 2008).

It also provides the opportunity to establish mobility patterns (Gonzalez et al., 2008), aid in the management of Parkinson's disease by using accelerometer data (Patel et al., 2007) and to detect social isolation (Peel et al., 2005). Specific tools such as Asthmapolis are now available to help physicians and patients record, track and self manage their asthma in near-real-time through TM (Community Health Data Initiatives, 2010).

All these advances and the potential of TM has not gone un-noticed by the Federal Government in the United States. The Department of Health and Human Services (DHHS) has allocated funds towards the further development of rural TM. The State and Local Information Technology spending is expected to reach $ 10 billion by 2015. Of note," The New Wave Medicaid Management Information System" expects the Information Technology market to grow by 19% over the next 5 years, up from $ 8.3 billion in 2010 (The New Wave Medicaid Management System, 2010).

In April 2010 the DHHS announced the Open Government strategy to expand the availability to the public of health data to allow patients to make informed health care decisions when choosing their hospital (Conway & Van Lare 2010). While The Veteran's Health Administration which has the largest telehealth program in the world (with over 40,000 veterans enrolled) is well advanced in both the delivery of telehealth based treatment and researching the evidence based outcomes of TM (Darkins et al., 2008).

7. Conclusion

TM is coming of age. The rapid expansion seen in the last decade has followed the realization that increasing longevity with the concomitant rising prevalence of CDs necessitates the development of alternate models of health care access, delivery and management. I addition the need to change from a system that primarily focuses on acute care to one that facilitates the transition of care into a continuum is imperative for effective management of CDs. The process of developing a care continuum is further complicated by the impending decrease in the medical provider base and the unique culture that the baby boomers will bring as they enter the ranks of the elderly. A culture that expects health care to be individualized, one that encourages self care and self efficacy as practiced within a Chronic Disease Self Management System. Current advances in TM coupled with the increasing global access to the Internet, wider availability of mobile phones is setting the stage for TM to become the communication link to bridge the chasm between acute and chronic care and provider and patient even if geographically separated. We believe that TM will increasingly assume a major role in the practice of medicine in the 21st Century especially as it pertains to the care of vulnerable patient populations and the provision of continuous medical education to patients, to all level of medical trainees and providers in practice. The need to bring care to the patient in their home and other living environments in the "virtual" format will have increasing relevance. Governments, Health Care Systems and Corporations are looking at TM as a means to greater medical access to personalized health care, one that also improves quality, reduces cost and adds value to the service provided. The current positive outcomes seen with the incorporation of TM coupled with its general acceptance by patients bodes well for the future.

8. Acknowledgement

The manuscript reviewed and contributions from Dr. Luis Afonso, Division of Cardiology, Wayne State University School of Medicine are particularly appreciated.

9. References

Healthy People 2000: Citizens Chart the Course (1990). Institute of Medicine, National Academy Press, Washington, DC.

Wooten R.; Dimmick, S.L. & Kvedar J.C. editors. (2006). In: Home telehealth: Connecting care with community. The Royal Society of Medicine Press, Oxon, pp 1-7.

Bandura, A. (2004). Health Promotion by Social Cognitive Means. Health Education & Behavior; 31(2): 143-64.

Bodenheimer, T.; Wagner, E.H. & Grumbach, K. (2002). Improving Primary Care for Patients with Chronic Illness. Journal of the American Medical Association; 288: 1775-1779.

Institute of Medicine. (2001). Crossing the Quality Chasm: A New Health System for the 21st. Century. National Academy Press; Washington, D.C.

World Health Association (1997). Health Telematics Policy: Report of WHO Group Consultation on Health Telematics. Geneva, Switzerland: December, 11-16, 1997

The Telemedicine Alliance- Battrick, B. Editor. (July 2004).Telemedicine 2010: Vision For A Personal Medical Network- ESA Publications Division. ESTEC, PO Box 299,2200AG Noordwijk. The Netherlands. ISSN: 0250-1589. ISBN: 92-9092-799-2.

Basher R.L.; Armstrong, P.A. & Youssef, Z.I. (1975). Telemedicine: Exploration in the use of Telecommunications in Health Care. Springfield, Illinois: Charles C. Thomas

Gavrilov, L.A.; & Heuveline, P. (2003). Aging of population. 2003. Available at:http://longevity-science.org/population_htm.

Institute For The Future. (2000). Health and Health Care 2010. San Francisco, CA: Jossey-Bass Publications.

Berk, M.L. & Monheit, A.C. (2001). The Concentrations Of Healthcare Expenditures Revisited. Health Affairs; 20: 9-18.

Coleman, E.A; & Boult, C.E. on behalf of the American Geriatrics Society Health Care Systems Committee. (2003). Improving the Quality of Transitional Care for Persons with Complex Care Needs. Journal of the American Geriatrics Society; 51(4): 556-557

Lorig, K.; Sobel, D. & Gonzalez, V., et al (2006). Living a Healthy Life with Chronic Conditions. Third Edition. Bull Publishing Company, Boulder, CO.

Holman, H. & Lorig, K. (2000). Patients as Partners in Managing Chronic Disease. British Medical Journal; 320:526-527.

Funnell, M.M.; Anderson. R.M & Arnold, M.S., et al. (1991). Empowerment: an idea whose time has come in Diabetes Education. Diabetes Educator; 17:37-41.

Corbin, J. & Strauss, A. (1998). Unending Work and Care: Managing Chronic Illness at Home. San Francisco, Calif: Josey-Bass Publishers.

Bodenheimer, T. (1999). Disease management-Promises and pitfalls. New England Journal of Medicine; 340 (15): 1202-1205.

Kane, R.L.; Priester, R. & Totten, A.M. (2005). Meeting the challenge of chronic illness. Baltimore. The John Hopkins University Press.

Stromberg, A.; Dahistrom, U. & Fridlund, B.(2006). Computer-based education for patients with chronic heart failure: A randomized, controlled, multicentric trial of the effects on knowledge, compliance and quality of life. Patient Education and Counseling; 64 (1-3): 128-135.

Albert, N.M.; Buchsbaum, R. & Li, J. (2007). Randomized study of the effect of video education on heart failure healthcare utilization, symptoms, and self-care behaviors. Patient Education and Counseling, 69 (1-3): 129-139.

Meystre, S. (2005). The current state of telemonitoring: a comment on the literature. Telemedicine Journal and E-Health; 11(1): 63-69.

Albert, N.M.; Buchsbaum, R. & Hall, M.D., et al (2003). Does heart failure self-care education by video change patient behaviors? Journal of Cardiac Failure 2003; 9(5); S101.

Pare, G.; Jaana, M. & Sicotte, C. (2007). Systematic Review of Home Telemonitoring for Chronic Diseases: The Evidence Base. Journal of the American Medical Informatics Association; 14(3): 269-277.

Goldberg, L.R.; Piette, J.D. & Walsh, M.N., et al (2003). Randomized trial of a daily electronic home monitoring system in patients with advanced heart failure: The

Weight Monitoring in Heart failure (WHARF) trial. American Heart Journal; 146: 705-712.

Dang, S.; Dimmick, S. & Kelkar, G. (2009). Evaluating the evidence base for the use of Home Telehealth Remote Monitoring in Elderly with Heart Failure. Telemedicine and e-Health; 15(8): 783-96.

Trief, P.M.; Teresi, J.A., & Eimicke, J.P. et al (2009) Improvements in diabetes self-efficacy and glycaemic control using telemedicine in a sample of older, ethnically diverse individuals who have diabetes: the IDEATel project. Age and Ageing; 38(2); 219-225.

American Heart Association. (2004). Heart disease and Stroke statistics:2004 update; available at, www.americanheart.org/downloadable/heart/1078736729696hds stats 2004 update REV3-19-04-pdf.

Jenks, S.F.; Williams, M.V. & Coleman, E.A. (2009). Rehospitalizations among patients in the Medicare Fee for Service Program. New England Journal of Medicine; 360: 1418-28.

Rogers, M.A.; Small, D. & Buchan, D.A. et al. (2001). Home monitoring service improves mean arterial pressure in patients with essential hypertension. A randomized controlled trial. Annals of Internal Medicine; 134: 1024-32.

Noel, H.C.; Vogel, D.C. & Erdos, J.J. et al (2004). Home telehealth reduces health costs. Telemedicine Journal of E Health; 10: 170-83.

Hendrix, C.C. (2000). Computer use among elderly people. Computers in Nursing; 18: 62-68.

Stromberg, A.; Ahlen, H, & Fridlund, B. et al (2002). Interactive education on CD-ROM. A new tool in education of heart failure patients. Patient Education and Counseling; 46, 75-81.

Lewis, D. (2003). Computers in patient education. Computers, information, nursing; 21(2):88-96.

Persaud, D.D.; Jreige, S. & Skedgel, C. et al (2005). An incremental cost analysis of telehealth in Nova Scotia from a Societal perspective. Journal of Telemedicine and Telecare; 11: 77-84.

Mahoney, D. (2009). Linking homecare and the workplace through innovative wireless technology. Home Health Care Management Practice; 16: 417-428.

Whitten, P.; Mair, F. & Haycox, A. et al (2002). Systematic review of cost effectiveness studies of telemedicine interventions. British Medical Journal; 324: 1437-7.

Hailey, D.; Ohinmaa, A. & Roine, R. (2004). Study quality and evidence of benefit in recent assessments of telemedicine. Journal of Telemedicine and Telecare; 10: 318-24.

Freudenheim, M. (2010). The Doctor will see you now. Please log on. New York Times. May 30, 2010.

Bloch, C. (Editor) Telemedicine Care for Prisoners. Federal Telemedicine News. Sunday, February, 21st, 2010.

Kroenke, K.; Theobald, D. & Wu, J. et al (2010). Effects of Telecare management on pain and depression in patients with cancer; a randomized trial. Journal of the American Medical Association; 304(2): 163-171.

Huffer, L.L.; Bauch, T.D. & Furgerson, J.L. et al (2004). Feasibility of remote tele-echocardiography with satellite transmission and real-time interpretation to support medical activities in the austere medical environment. Journal of the American College of Echocardiography; 17: 670-4.

Couturier, P.; Tyrrell, J. & Tonetti, J. et al (1998). Feasibility of orthopedic teleconsulting in a geriatric rehabilitation service. Journal of Telemedicine and Telecare; 4 (suppl 11): 85-7.

Montani, C.; Billaud, N. & Tyrrell, J. et al (1997). Psychological impact of a remote psychometric consultation with hospitalized elderly people. Journal of Telemedicine and Telecare; 3(3): 140-5.

Latifi, R.; Hadeed, G.H. & Rhee, P. et al (2009). Initial experience and outcomes of telepresence in the management of trauma and emergency surgical patients. American Journal of Surgery; 198(6): 905-910.

Wiborg, A.M.D. & Widder, B.M.D.P. for the TSG. (2003). Teleneurology to provide Stroke Care in Rural areas. The Telemedicine in Stroke in Swabia (TESS) Project. Stroke; 34: 2951-6.

Audebert, H.S. & Schwamm, L. (2009). Telestroke: Scientific Results.Cerebrovascular Diseases; 27 (suppl 4): 15-20.

Rabinowitz, T.; Murphy, K.M. & Amour, J.L. et al (2010). Benefits of a TelepsychiatryConsultation Service for Rural Nursing Home Residents. Telemedicine and e-Health; 16 (1): 34-40.

comScore study; http;//www.comscore.com/news/cs_hispanic_050702.htm.

Safran, C. (2003). The collaborative edge: Patient empowerment for vulnerable populations. International Journal of Medical Informatics; 69(2-3): 185-190.

Shore, J.H.; Brooks, E. & Savin, D.M. et al (2007). An economic evaluation of Telehealth data collection with rural populations. Psychiatric Services; 58; 830-835.

Selden, C.R.; Zorn. M, Ratzan, S. et al compilers. (2000). Health Literacy. NLM Pub. No. CMB 2000-1. Bethesda, MD: National Library of Medicine.

National Center for Education Statistics, 2006. The Health Literacy of America's Adults: Results from the 2003 National Assessment of Adult Literacy. Washington, DC: U.S. Department of Education. NCES 2006-483.

Baker, D.W.; Wolf, M.S. & Feinglass, J. et al (2007). Health Literacy and mortality among elderly persons. Archives of Internal Medicine; 167(14): 1503-9.

Rothman, R.L.; Housman, R. & Weiss, H. et al (2006). Patient understanding of Food Labels: The role of Literacy and Numeracy. American Journal of Preventive Medicine; 31; 391-398.

Kirsch, I.S.; Jungeblut, A. & Jenkins, L. et al (2002). A. Adult Literacy in America: A first look at the findings of the National Adult Literacy Survey. 3rd Edition. Volume 201 Washington DC; National Center for Education, US Department of Education. NCES, 1993-275

Davis, T.C.; Crouch, M.A. & Willis, G. et al (1990). The gap between patient reading comprehension and the readability of patient education materials.
Journal of Family Practice; 31(5): 533-538.

Healthy People 2010. Health literacy. Available at http://www.healthypeople.gov/Document/pdf/uih/2010 uih.pdf

Wallace, L. (2006). Patient's health literacy skills: the missing demographic variable in primary care research. Annals of Family Medicine; 4: 85-86.

Disease Management Association of America. Definition of disease management. Available at: http://www.dmaa.org/phi_defenition.asp.

Smeulders, E.S.T.F.; van Haastregt, J.C.M. & Janssen-Boyne, J.J.J. et al (2009). Feasibility of a group-based self-management program among congestive heart failure: Heart & Lung: The Journal of Acute and Critical Care; 38(6): 499-512.

Lorig, K.R.; Ritter, P.L. & Gonzalez, V.M. (2003). Hispanic chronic disease self-management: a randomized community-based outcome trial. Nursing Research; 52(6): 361-369.

Maric, B.; Kaan, A. & Araki, Y. et al (2010). The Use of the Internet to remotely Monitor Patients with Heart Failure. Telemedicine and e-Health; 16(1): 23-33.

Bosworth, H.B.; Olsen, M.K. & McCant, F. et al (2007). Hypertension Intervention Nurse Telemedicine Study (HINTS): Testing a multifactorial tailored behavioral/educational and a medication management intervention for blood pressure control. American Heart Journal; 153(6); 918-924.

Woudend, A.K.; Sherrard, H. & Fraser, M. et al (2008). Telehome monitoring in patients with cardiac disease who are at a high risk of readmission. Heart Lung; 37: 36-45.

Dawsky, K.H.; Vasey, J. & Bowles, K. (2008). Impact of telehealth on clinical outcomes in patients with heart failure. Clinical Nursing Research; 17: 182-189.

Dang, S.; Dimmick, S. & Kelkar, G. (2009). Evaluating the evidence base for the use of home telehealth remote monitoring in elderly with heart failure. Telemedicine Journal of E Health; 15(8): 783-796.

Clark, R.A.; Yallop, J.J. &, Piterman, L. et al (2007). Adherence, adaptation and Acceptance of Elderly Heart Failure patients to receive health care via telephone monitoring. European Journal of Heart Failure; 9: 1104-1111.

Seto E. (2008). Cost comparison between telemonitoring and usual care of heart failure. A systematic review. Telemedicine Journal of E Health; 14(7): 679-86.

Inglis, S.C.; Clark, R.A. & McAlister, F.A. et al (2010). Structured telephone support or telemonitoring programmes for patients with chronic heart failure. Cochrane database of Systematic Reviews, Aug 4; 8: CD007228.

Pare, G.; Moqademm K.& Pineau, G. et al (2010). Clinical effects of home telemonitoring in the context of diabetes, asthma, heart failure and hypertension: a systematic review. Journal of Medical Internet Research; 12(2): 2010

Dang, S.; Ma, F, Nedd, N. & Aguillar, E. et al (2007). Care coordination and telemedicine improves glycemic control in ethnically diverse veterans with diabetes. Journal of Telemedicine and telecare; 13(5): 263-267.

Verhoeven, F.; Tanja-Dijkstra, K. & Nijland, N. et al (2010). Asynchronous and synchronous teleconsultation for diabetes care: a systematic literature review. Journal of Diabetes Science Technology; 4(30): 666-684.

Speedie, S.M. Ferguson, A.S. & Sanders, J. et al (2008). Telehealth: The promise of a new care delivery models. Telemedicine Journal of E Health; 14(9): 964-967.

Schofield, R.S.; Kline, S.E. & Schmalfuss, C.M. et al (2005). Early outcomes of a care coordination-enhanced telehome care program for elderly veterans with chronic heart failure. Telemedicine Journal of E Health; 11(1): 20-27.

Inglis, S.; McLennan, S. Dawson, A. et al. (2004). A new solution for a new problem? Effects of a nurse-led, multidisciplinary, home-based intervention on readmission and mortality in patients with chronic atrial fibrillation. Journal of Cardiovascular Nursing;19: 118-127.

Chumbler, N.R.; Vogel, W.B. & Garel, M. et al (2005). Health services utilization of care coordination/home telehealth program for veterans with diabetes. A matched-cohort study. Journal of Ambulatory Care Management; 28: 230-240.

Cardozo, L. & Steinberg, J. (2009). Telemedicine for recently discharged older patients. Telemedicine and e-Health; 19(1); 49-55.

Shore, R. (2008). Challenge Paper: The Power of Pow! Wham!: Children, Digital Media and Our Nation's Future. Three Challenges for the Coming Decade. New York: the Joan Ganz Cooney Center at Sesame Street.

Bernholz, L. (2006). Pedagogy, playstations, and the public interest. San Francisco: Blueprint Research & Design.

Rizzo, A.A.; Grapp, K. & Perlman, K. et al (2008). Virtual Iraq: initial results from a VR exposure therapy application for combat-related PTSD. Student Health Technological Information; 132: 420-425.

Conde, J.G.; De, S. & Hall, R.W. et al (2009). Telehealth Innovations in Health Education and Training. Telemedicine and e-Health; 16 (1): 103-106.

Hall, R.; Bronstein, J. & Fallon, J. et al (2008). Can telemedicine be used to improve neonatal and infant mortality in a Medicaid population in a rural state?(Abstract) (2008). Pediatric Academic Society.

Hall. R.; Hall-Barrow, J. & Garcia-Rice, E. Neonatal regionalization through telemedicine using a community based research and education core facility. Proceedings of the 11th RCMI International Symposium on Health Disparities, Dec 1-4, 2009, Honolulu, HI

Karsh, B. & Holden, R.J. (2007). New Technology implementation in healthcare in: Carayon P. Editor Handbook of Human Factors and Ergonomics in Healthcare and Patient Safety. Mahwah, NJ Lawrence Erlbaum Associates pp. 393-410

Calvin, K.L. & Karsh, B. (2009). A Systematic Review of Patient Acceptance of Consumer health Information Technology. Journal of the American Informatics Association; 16(4): 550-560.

Lober, W.B.; Zierler, B. & Herbaugh, A. et al (2006). Barriers to the Use of a Personal Health Record by an elderly population. Presented at the Annual Symposium of theAmerican Medical Informatics Association.

Song, J. & Zahedi, F.M. (2007). Trust in Health Infomediaries. Decision. Support Systems; 43(2):390-407.

Doarn, C.R.; Portilla, L.M. & Sayre, M.H. (2010). NIH Conference on the future of telehealth: essential tools and technologies for clinical research and care-a summary. Telemedicine Journal and e-Health; 16(1): 89-92.

The WHO Health Report 1998. Life in the 21st Century, WHO Press.

Rosamond, W.; Flegal, K. & Go, A. et al. (2008). Heart disease and stroke statistics-2008 update. A report from the American Heart association Statistics Committee and Stroke Statistics Subcommittee. Circulation; 117: e25-e146.

Peterson, S.; Peto, V. & Rayner M et al. (2005 Edition). European Cardiovascular Disease Statistics, European Heart Network and the British Heart Foundation, London.

Novak, V.; Young, A.L.L. & Lepicovsky, L. et al (2004). Multimodal pressure-flow method to assess dynamics of cerebral autoregulation in stroke and hypertension. Biomedical Engineering; 3: 39.

Meyerfeldt, U.; Wessel, N. & Schuttel, H. et al. (2002). Heart rate variability before onset of ventricular tachycardia. Differences between slow and fast arrythmias. International Journal of Cardiology; 84: 141-151.

Kesek, M.; Franklin, K.A. & Sahlin, H. et al (2009). Heart rate variability during sleep and sleep apnea in a population based study of 387 women.Clinical Physiology and Functional Imaging; 29: 309-315.

Darce, K. (August 25th. 2010). Union Tribune, Hamblen, M. (August 31st, 2010). Bloomberg Businessweek.

Ganapathy, M. & Ravindra, A. (2008). mHealth: A Potential tool for Health Care Delivery in India. Presented at Making the e-Health Connections: Global Partnerships, Local solutions conference of 2008, Bellagio, Italy.

Mudge, S.; Stott, A.S. & Walt, S.E. (2007). Criterion validity of the StepWatch Activity Monitor as a measure of walking activity in patients after a stroke. Archives of Physical Medicine and Rehabilitation; 88: 1710-1715.

Sung, M.; Marci, C. & Pentland, A. (2005). Wearable feedback system for rehabilitation. Journal of Neuroengineering and Rehabilitation, 2: 17.

Barnes, I.I.; Mendes de Leon, C.E. & Wilson, R.S. et al (2004). Social resources and cognitive decline in a population of older African Americans and Whites. Neurology; 63: 2322-2326.

Baker, P.S.; Bodner, E.V. & Allman, R.M. (2003). Measuring life-space mobility in community-dwelling older adults. Journal of the American Geriatrics Society; 51: 1610-1614.

Gonzalez, M.C.; Hidalgo, C.A. & Barabasi, A.L. (2008). Understanding individual human mobility patterns. Nature; 453: 779-782.

Patel, S.; Lorincz, K.& Hughes R et al. (2007). Analysis of feature space for monitoring person's with Parkinson's disease with application to a wireless wearable sensor system. Conference Proceedings IEEE Engineering Medical Biology Society 2007; 6291-6294.

Peel C, Sawyer Baker P, et al. (2005). Assessing mobility in older adults. The VAB study of Aging Life-Space Assessment. Physical Therapy; 85: 1008-1119.

Community Health Data Initiatives launches. (2010, June 2nd) Federal News Radio. http://www.federalnewsradio.com/?nid=376&sid=1971025

The New Wave Medicaid Management System (2010). MMIS spending from 2010-2015. Input State & Local Industry Insights.

Conway, P.H. & VanLare, J.M. (2010). Improving access to health care data. The open government strategy. Journal of the American Medical Association; 304(9): 1007-1008.

Darkins, A.; Ryan, P. & Kobb, R. et al (2008). Care coordination / Home Telehealth: The systematic implementation of Health Informatics, Home Health & Disease Management to support the care of Veterans with chronic conditions. Telemedicine Journal of E Health: 14: 1118-1126.

18

The Spanish Ministry of Defence (MOD) Telemedicine System

Alberto Hernandez Abadia de Barbara
Servicio de Telemedicina
Hospital Central de la Defensa "Gomez Ulla", Madrid
Spain

1. Introduction

Telemedicine is an important tool for the medical deployments of the International Missions. The Medical Treatment Facilities (MTFs) and the medical evacuation means (terrestrial and rotatory wing ambulances) are the main components of the military medical evacuation chain in the Operational Areas. The right diagnosis and the adequate treatment for casualties (battle and non battle injured) are key points which together with a rapid evacuation timing assure a high quality medical support on the field.

Tactical and strategical medical evacuations (MEDEVAC) are carried out to move the patients to the right places to be treated. The Role 3 units (campaign hospital) have many different medical specialists, but these units do not have the complete crew of the Role 4 (Hospitals in national territories).

The Telemedicine systems provides the capability to connect on real time the Role 4 units with their lower ones, but nowadays the whole MTFs have to be interconnected to support the medical deployment and to get medical information from the field. For these reasons the different MoDs are working to improve their Telemedicine systems and to be able to interconnect them.

The Military Medical Communications and Information Systems of NATO countries are being developed under the idea to interconnect with a common system, the MEDICS, which is the NATO common platform to obtain, to transmit and to store the medical information on the field.

The information and communication technologies are going to be applied in all echelons of the medical deployments. In this document is described the state of the Spanish Military Medical Systems and some of the projects which are being carried out to improve the system.

The Spanish MOD is actually carrying out several outland humanitarian missions all over the world. Troops are deployed in Afghanistan, the Lebanon…., almost all the missions are operating in politically unstable countries where skirmishes and terrorist attacks are frequent, and in hostile and hard-to-reach areas where environmental and hygienic conditions may be a potential source of disease. Providing the troops with the adequate medical support is hence of paramount importance. Unfortunately this is not an easy task, since medical people deployed in the operation area need assessment very often.

Consequently it is imperative to provide the medical people in the operation area with a decision support system to improve and speed up the quality of diagnostics and to fulfill the main goals of a medical mission, namely, the prevention of disease, treatment of sick and injured patients, and patient evacuation and hospitalization. Governments are making a great effort to equip their troops with telemedicine systems relying on the latest information and communication technologies. However, these systems must be able to operate together in a common framework; for this reason NATO (North Atlantic Treaty Organization) is dealing with integration and convergence of all the national standards into a new unique telemedicine system common to all member states.

Figure 1 shows the big picture of medical care principles and campaign logistics. The evacuation process goes through four steps: ROLE1 through ROLE4. Roles 1 through 3 are situated in the deployment area, whereas Role 4 is in the home or host country.

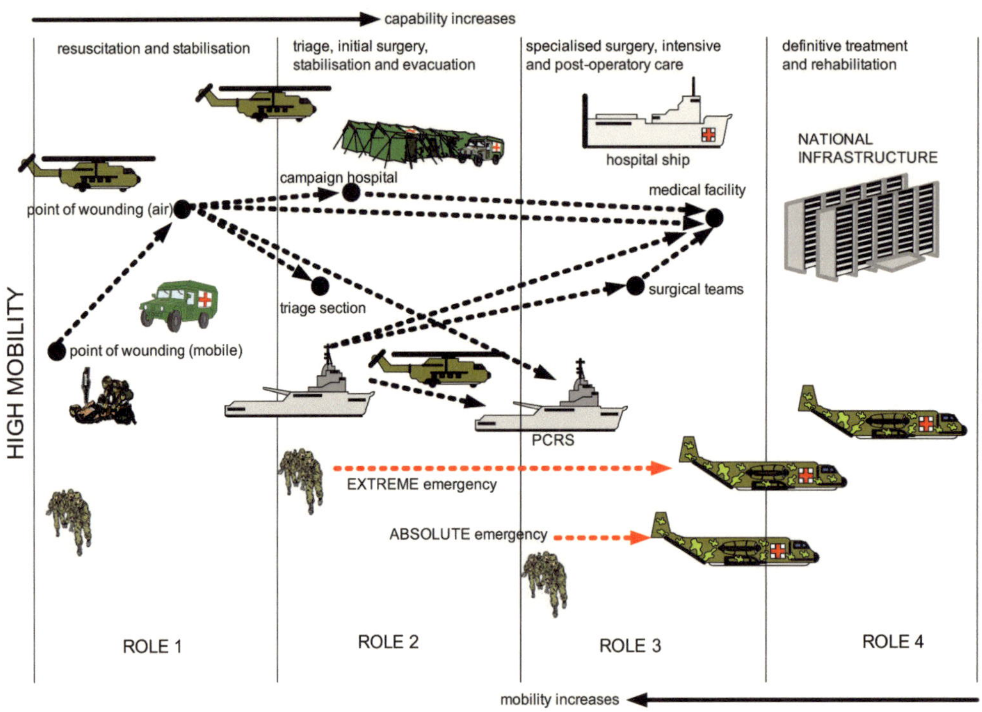

Fig. 1. Campaign Logistics and Evacuation Process.

Hence medical care is provided progressively ranging from first aid (ROLE 1) to definitive care and rehabilitation (ROLE 4), as the patient is evacuated rearward in the medical support chain. Tasks, structure and equipments of the medical teams involved at the different levels of the evacuation chain are very different. At ROLE 1 the first aid is provided by highly mobile medical teams whose main goal is immediate lifesaving, patient resuscitation and stabilization of the vital functions. Subsequently, patients are evacuated to a triage section where they are classified according to the severity of their clinical status. If they deserve intensive cares or specialized surgery already at an early stage, they are immediately evacuated to the upper levels of the evacuation chain. Otherwise, cares are provided by the campaign hospital.

The infrastructure at ROLE 2 Light Maneuver level allows damage control surgery, whereas specialized surgery may be only performed at ROLE 3 level.

The evacuation process is extremely complex since it may require the cooperation and coordination among land, sea and air forces, and the units deployed in the MTFs (Medical Treatment Facilities) at different roles. In addition, medical, transportation and rescue units involved in the process may not only belong to different DOBs (Deployed Operating Bases), but also to different States of the Allied Forces that are carrying out the mission. This further complicates the evacuation process; also, the evacuation must comply with the timelines established by AJP 4.10 NATO Medical Support Doctrine. According to this document, the patient must be provided with advanced trauma care within one hour from the first aid, with damage control surgery within two hours, and with primary surgery within four hours from the first aid.

To accomplish with such strict requirements the use of the modern information and communication technologies is compulsory. It is possible to apply to each role one or more technologies to support and improve communication and information flow between all the agents implied in the rescue and evacuation process. Figure 2 depicts the technological scenario that characterizes the different levels of the medical evacuation chain.

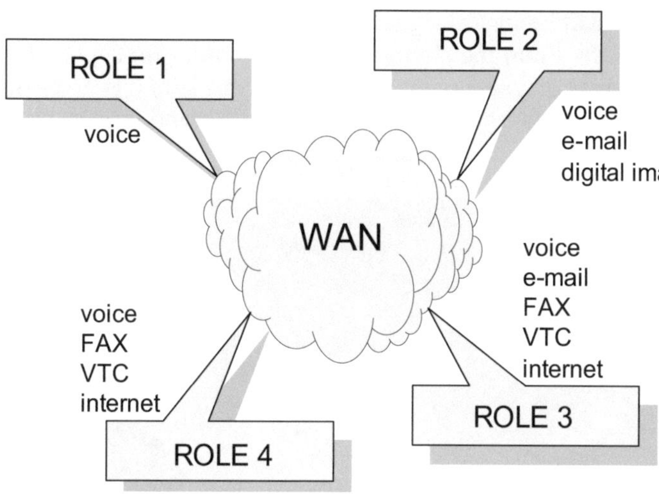

Fig. 2. Teleconsulting Capabilities.

Each role has different technological capabilities that increase with the complexity of the task that has to be carried out. The interaction among roles is guaranteed by a Wide Area Network (WAN). The spectrum of adopted technologies is broad and ranges from dedicated two-way voice channel (telephone or radio), fax and e-mail, to mail systems with support for large attachments (motion picture MPEG, digital pathology JPEG, or digital radiography DICOMM), real-time videoconferencing systems (VTCs) and distributed web-based platforms with multimedia and streaming video support.

The Spanish Government is currently developing, through projects SISANDEF (Spanish MEDICS) and SALVANY (RIS-PACS) its own telemedicine platform covering roles 3 and 4. Project deadline is 2012, but the system at role 3 level will be operating in 2011. Hence one of the goals of this paper is to define system requirements and specifications at the lower levels of the evacuation chain, namely roles 1 and 2. The system must be suitable to operate in critical scenarios and must comply with the highly mobility requirement of role 1 and 2 levels. Consequently it must be robust, low power-consuming, light and secure.

Electronic devices and communications networks have increased their presence in the latest years in almost all aspects of life, even in the medical field. On this way, the medical instruments are being useful tools for the personal health care to diagnose and to treat patients at hospitals or ambulatories centres. Telemedicine is the application of information and communication technologies to the medical diagnostics and therapies. The purpose is to allow the diagnostic of patients at the distance by means of Teleconsultations. The Spanish Ministry of Defence Telemedicine System (SMDTS) has an extended network to provide medical supports for the troops deployed outside the national territory.

Telemedicine systems have to implement tools between the network points that allow the personal communication and the transmission of patient's explorations results. In addition, it should be possible the record of all the material produced during the teleconsultations (videos, conversations, images, signals…). The Spanish Ministry of Defence Telemedicine System fulfils with a lot of features that make the system to be a worldwide leading reference in this field. However, it is wanted to increase the system effectiveness in relation with Telemonitoring capacities, that is, the transmission and storage of biomedical signals.

Telemonitoring is a key important aspect in a telemedicine system. It consists on the transmission and storage of biological signals, images or videos from the explorations. That information can be attached into the electronic health recorder (EHR) of each patient to be accessed lately, for medical diagnostics or studies. With this aim, it is necessary the creation of applications that collect data from the monitoring devices and transmit them to a central database.

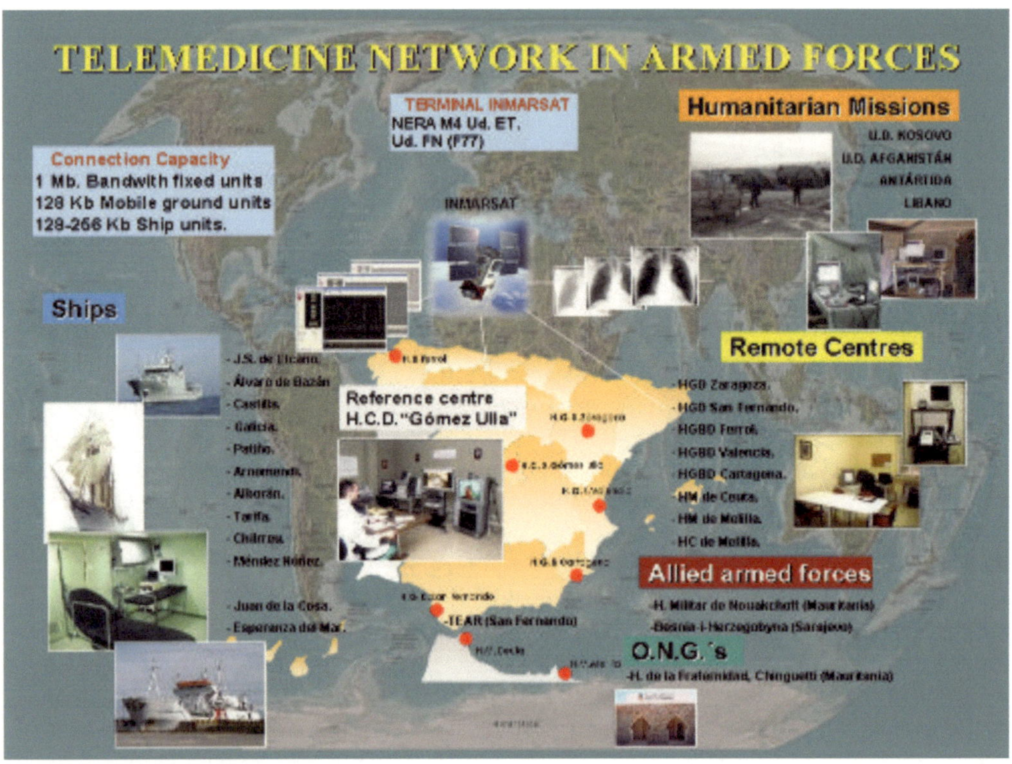

Fig. 3. A view of the SMDTS.

The scheme of the system consists on a reference centre (the CHD in Madrid, with back-up centre in the Military Hospital in Zaragoza), that provides the medical support to the rest of the points in the network, the remote centres. Those remote points are care units placed in ships, international missions or other military centres. Each one of these points has a telemedicine station used to communicate with the reference centre for advanced medical consultations.

The system uses an intranet for the communication, this is, a private and dedicated circuit that provides privacy, confidentiality and security to the connections. Depending on the emplacement, the bandwidth available for the consultations varies and it has influence in the quality of the communication and in the video and data transmission. For example, ships and not fixed emplacement connect by satellital modems with low bandwidth (up to 256 kbits/seg). The Spanish MoD has a satellital network that is used for medical purposes.

2. Equipments

The remote centres have a medical monitoring solution with a lot of tools to carry out a great variety of explorations on patients. They are fitted with the following equipment:

- Videoconference Camera.
- TV monitors.
- Personal Computer.
- X-ray picture scanner.
- Vital Signs monitor.
- Electrocardiography recorder.
- Router.
- High resolution external exploration camera.
- Ultrasound explorer machine.

As several of the TM stations are located in mobile units, the devices are assembled in a rugged box that makes easier the transportation and the storage of the equipments as well as acting like a protection container.

The reference centre must work as the link between the doctors in the hospital and the patients in the remote centres so that the devices installed in the HCD are oriented to reception, visualization, diagnostic and storage of the consultations. These are the devices and tools implemented:

- Videoconference camera.
- Plasma Monitors.
- DVD recorder.
- Ultra High resolution monitor for radiological images.
- Personal Computers.
- Email consultation inbox.
- LAN access - IP serial converter (reception of Telemonitoring signals).
- Surgical assistant tool.

With these devices it is possible:

- Audiovisual conference at real time.
- Visual Explorations: general explorations, endoscopies, teledermatology, teleotolaryngology…
- Diagnostic imaging (as fixed as dynamic): radiology, ultrasound explorations, Computerized tomography (TC), MRIs, PET-CT ...

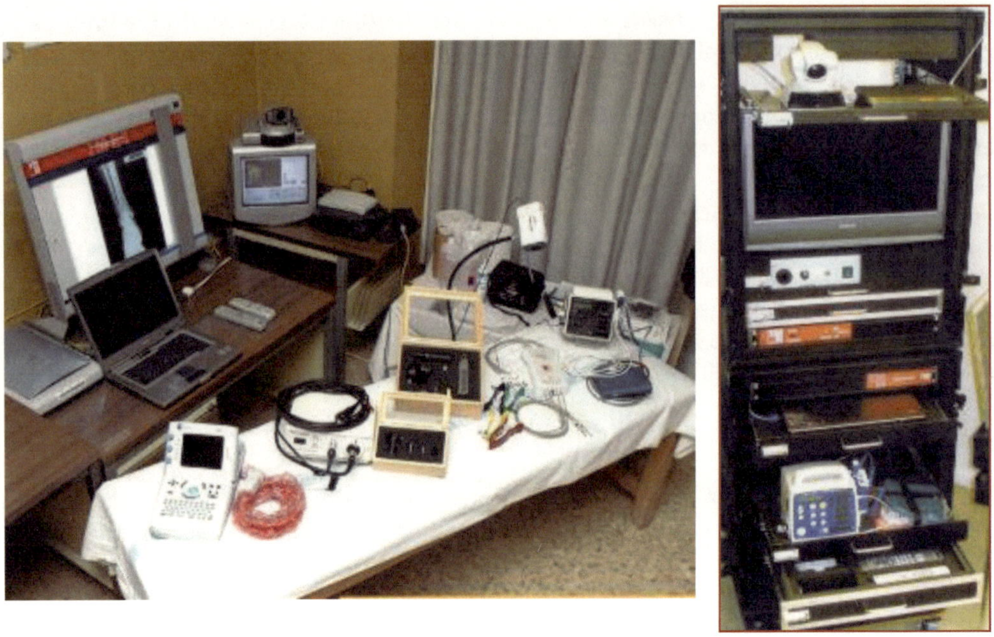

Fig. 4. Remote centres telemedicine equipments.

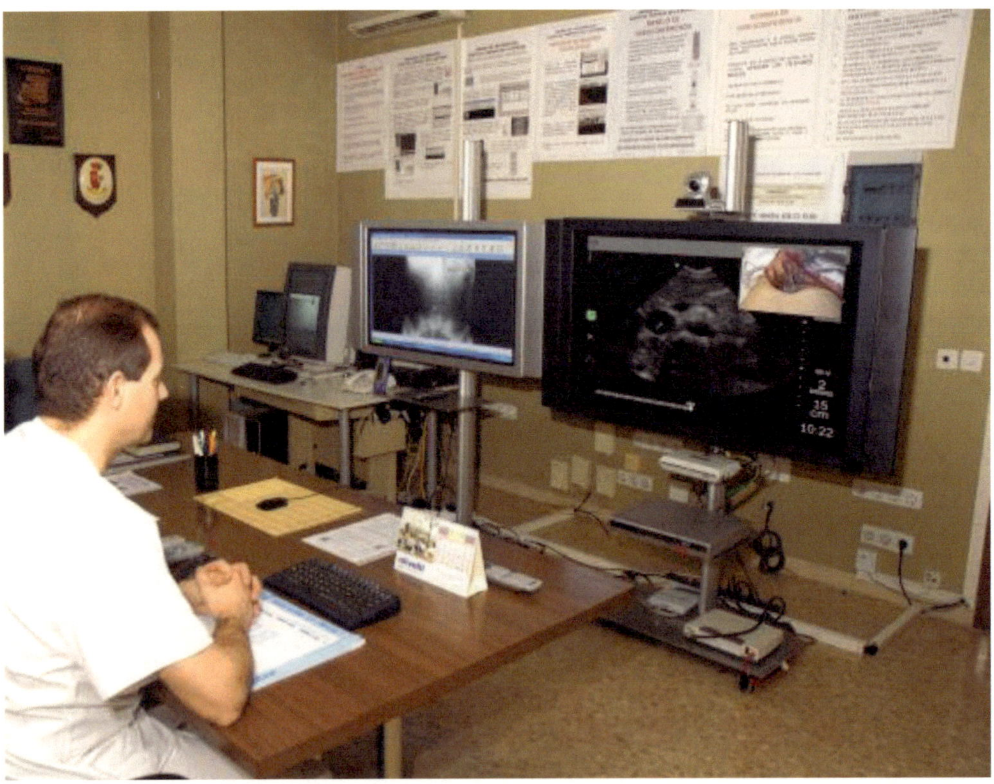

Fig. 5. The Spanish Military Telemedicine Reference Centre.

- Telemonitoring of Vital Signs: 12 leads Electrocardiogram, Heartbeat, Blood pressure, oxygen saturation…
- Consultations by email.
- Surgical indications for the remote centre with the virtual assistant board.
- Recording of consultations.

3. Operative mode

The system allows two types of consultations:

- ***"Asynchronous" or "Storage and forward"*:** The data are received and storage to be analyzed and diagnosed later. The doctors analyze the content and the response is sent back to the applicant. It is used to attend not urgent consultations. This service has a response time up to 24 hours.
- ***"Synchronous" or "Real time"*:** The remote centres establish a videoconference with the HCD. The specialists are requested to come to the Telemedicine Service and to attend the consultation. During the connection, the data are sent to the centre simultaneously.

The following table shows a resume of the type of teleconsultations:

System	Priority
Videoconference + data	Urgent/planned
Radio / phone	Urgent/planned
Email	Not at real time

4. Teleconsultation procedure

The reference centre is one of the points which are always connected to the intranet, waiting for incoming calls. When a remote centre wants to come into the net the router must link up the communication that allows the station works as a point of the system. When the consultations only require videoconference, the available bandwidth is used completely, but, in the case that the consultations required the digital transmission of medical data (X-ray, telemonitoring of vital signs) it is reserved a minimal bandwidth for its transmission.

Once the station has connection to the intranet, the different operations can be performed. Sometimes is not always necessary to establish a call for the consultations, and the e-mail results enough to send questions or to attach data as pictures or videos. For example, the X-ray images are sent to the reference centre before the consultation is carried out, with a PC application that collects the image and then send it to one inbox in the HCD. In the case of the Ultrasound or visual explorations, the way to send the video is connecting these equipments to the external input of the videoconference camera. This device digitalizes the analogue signals and it sends these ones as images of the videoconference. The videoconference is recorded in the HCD with the DVD recorder, to have a register of all the consultations.

When explorations require Vital Signs monitoring and ECG signals, it is necessary to activate the transmission a perfect synchronization between the remote station and the HCD. Otherwise, the application collapses and the reception of data do not work correctly. For this reason these explorations only can be carried out on live, when a call is activated to have communication between the two points. The application that collects data from the electromedical devices is a customization because the SV monitor installed does not have a

computer application, and the ECG computer tool given out by the manufacturer is only for local use, not to transmit the signals. The devices are connected by a com port to the computer, and in order to transmit the signals what is done is to make virtual the input com ports and to duplicate each of them. Then, the local application connects to one of the dual port, and the other port is used to collect the data and to encapsulate the information into IP packets. These IP packets are sent to the reference centre and the LAN access IP-serial converter extracts the data from the packets, and it puts them in its output com ports. The PC in the reference centre connects to this output com ports which simulate the acquisition equipments on the destiny, and the application reads the signal from these ports.
The Spanish MoD Medical Deployments are demanding new features to the Telemedicine System to achieve higher performance on the teleconsultations. The current system presents limited capacities and capabilities to transmit and storage efficiently biomedical signals. Nevertheless, the system should be able to transmit and to record the monitored information automatically in a database together with the patient's electronic health records. On this way, the results can be consulted lately or they can be used to perform data mining to extract statistical information. That is because it is necessary the creation of one application capable to acquire the signals from the monitoring devices, to visualize on graphical interfaces and to storage these in a central database (repository). This is called Telemonitoring, and it would add complete functionality to the SMDTS on creating an electronic register of all the consultations.
On a different aspect, the communications channels are a key factor in the Telemedicine Systems. The SMDTS counts with a wide variety of media channels through them the remote centres can connect with the HCD, i.e. satellital connections, military intranet, and internet connection with fixed IP address. To enhance the privacy and security of the system, the Telemedicine Network can be framed under a VPN that would protect the traffic of its applications.

5. Network traffic management

When it is necessary exchange information through a network, we have to take in consideration the security and the priority of the data. The router is the element that is in charge of the network access and the packet exchange. The Telemedicine network will be based in different remote points working as Local Area Network (LAN) but connecting through a WAN (Wide Area Network).
Creating a VPN (Virtual Private Network) to work across the remote points and the reference centre (the central database), the system would guarantee the privacy, the authenticity and the integrity of the data. The routers provide the possibility to create a tunnel link between two routers. AES encryption support has been introduced. The data encryption is carry out over the router input/output packets, so all the communications (videoconference and PC applications) will be encapsulated under the same SA (Software Application). The remote point's router has to connect to the VPN server that will be installed in the HCD to access into the Telemedicine VPN (TVPN). The same VPN server can attend several VPN clients, so that, several remote points can access within the Telemedicine Intranet at the same time.
The remote centre equipments with communication capacities (this is the videoconference camera and the PC) has one IP fixed address. These elements are connected to the router to exchange data with other points in the net. The routers provide traffic management tools to control the workflow. In example, data packets of VS (Vital Signs) and ECG

(Electrocardiography) applications have higher priority than others frames because those applications need a constant data flow to run correctly. To organize the applications traffic, it is necessary to define some rules by which the router will manage the packet streams (QoS). However, the IPsec encryption has problems to provide QoS correctly, because the TCP/UDP header packet information is encrypted before that the QoS acts over the frame. The command "QoS pre-classify" allows to the IOS to create a temporary copy of a packet in memory to be used for classification so that QoS actions can be performed on the final packet after encapsulation and/or encryption.

6. Standardizing the Telemonitoring System - ISO/IEEE 11073

The problem developing Telemonitoring applications are mainly the communications with the medical devices, and to extract, to sent and to store the medical data. The devices exchange data using proprietary protocols with communication paradigm and format defined by each manufacturer. This inconvenient makes complicated the creation of applications to manage the devices and the replacement and updating of devices in the systems.

The International Organization for Standardization (ISO) and the Institute of Electrical and Electronics Engineers (IEEE) proposed the ISO/IEEE 11073 Point of Care Medical Device Communication (PoCMDC) as a set of standards which purpose is to standardize the communications of medical devices supporting interoperability, transparency, plug-and-play, and easy of use and configuration.

ISO/IEEE 11073 standards enable communication between medical devices and external computer systems. The primary goals are to:

- Provide real-time plug-and-play interoperability for patient-connected medical devices.
- Facilitate the efficient exchange of vital signs and medical device data, acquired at the point-of-care, in all health care environments

In the standard, the interoperability at local level is solved with a central element to which all devices are connected, the *gateway*. This element acts as a main connection and it controls the interaction with the different medical devices, creating a patient network. Besides, this gateway has to connect the patient network with the Telemonitoring server to transmit the signals.

With the purpose of improving the medical support that the Spanish Ministry of Defence Medical Corp (SMDMC) provides to the personnel deployed on international missions, the Spanish Central Hospital of Defence "Gomez Ulla" started the Spanish Ministry of Defence Telemedicine Unit (SMDTU) activities on 1996. The system was designed in such a way that the CHD served as the core centre of the network (the reference centre) where all medical specialities are supported. When the medical personnel deployed (the remote points) requested advanced medical support, they could connect to the reference centre.

First communications in the early services were based on calls made by means of analogue videophones which allowed the establishment of calls along with video transmission using the switched circuit network. The development of data packet networks and the proliferation of communication tools for these networks permitted to include medical and communication devices which accomplished more variety, accuracy and reliable diagnostics. The wide variety of available features to diagnose, have consolidated the service as a new diagnostic tool by means of the specialists can give out better support to the missions. However, new needs are required to the system in order to achieve much more performance and easiness of Telemonitoring from the remote centres.

Telemonitoring seems to have a great functionality as a tool for remote medical diagnostics, avoiding the transportation of patients from remote centres. It implies to save a big amount of money because of medical transportation. Besides, telemonitoring could be applied for home-care in patients with scheduled consultations at care centres. But what is important to extend these kinds of medical tools, is the standardization of the medical devices and their communication protocols. For this purpose there is a working group into the IEEE organization developing the standard IEEE 11073, which concerns to the interoperability and data exchange between medical devices.

Another aspect to take in account is the communication link. The system is used in the military environment and the medical field; both require confidentiality and security during the information exchange. A private network provides these features. Virtual Private Networks (VPN) allow the establishment of private connections over the public networks (Internet, ATM) reducing the cost of the communications and holding similar capacities.

7. Projects on development:

7.1 The tactical telemedicine system:

This paper describes also the work-in-progress carried out by the Central Hospital of Defence "Gomez Ulla" toward the design of new devices for the military telemedicine system that is intended to give support to the medical people in the deployments. Previous studies have demonstrated that a decision support system is a major concern since 50% of the diagnostics performed in the operation area need reassurance. Consequently, such a system will help to improve considerably the quality of the diagnostics and to reduce the management and evacuations costs.

Following the NATO inputs the Spanish Ministry of Defence is developing a telemedicine system to be interoperable with this three main concepts:

1. Patient tracking:
   A system that has to be able to track the casualties into the evacuation chain, following their way along the Medical Treatment Facilities (MTFs) deployed into the areas of operation.
2. Patient regulating:
   With the information acquired from every patient tracing, the Medical Advisors have to decide where to redirect the casualties (to the right MTF considering the casualties classification and the level of operativeness of these units).
3. Disease surveillance:
   The system has to give epidemiological information about the difference diseases and kind of wounds which are detected into the operational area.

With this aim a system that accomplishes these features is under development. Some aspects of this project are going to be described on this document:

The hardware/software platform we describe will integrate the services and functionalities available from the existing e-health infrastructure and provide the medical people with a decision support system in remote and hard-to-reach areas. The specific aims are:

1. To design and implement a low-power Military Medical Information Carrier (MMMIC). A MMIC is a device that is intended to hold personal medical information that may be accessed by a medic through a specialized terminal, namely a MMMDA (Military Medical Digital Assistant).
2. To provide the MMDA with the software capability to interact with the MMIC and its local database of patient information. It is anticipated that our design will contribute to

improve the efficiency in the use of communication resources in telemedicine. In a bigger scope, this project should enhance our understanding of the limitations that hardware and software impose on the operation in critical scenarios.

System Overview

Our main goal is to design a complete network hierarchy of cooperating wireless, ad-hoc and hand-held devices for military telemedicine use at role 1, role 2 (light maneuver and enhanced) and role 3 levels of the evacuation chain. The network will integrate the services and functionalities available from the existing e-health infrastructure and provide the medical people with a decision support system in remote and hard-to-reach areas. Such network is formed by three classes of devices:

1. Military Personal Tag (MPT).
2. Military Medical Information Carriers (MMICs), and
3. Military Medical Digital Assistants (MMDAs).

These devices cooperate with a wireless ad-hoc network. A mobile, wireless, ad-hoc network is a collection of mobile nodes that are dynamically and arbitrarily located in a certain region. The dynamic character of the nodes implies that the interconnections among them, the network actual topology, may change with time frequently.

The main feature of these networks is that routing is performed by the nodes in the absence of a fixed infrastructure. The nodes act as routers which discover and maintain routes to other nodes in the network. The network itself emerges as the result of a collective effort of self-configuration of the nodes deployed.

There are several strategies to solve the routing problem in these networks. We will be specifically concerned with source-initiated, on-demand routing. This type of routing creates routes only when desired by the source node. When a node requires a route to a destination, it initiates a route discovery process within the network. This process is completed once a route is found or all possible route permutations have been examined. Once a route has been established, it is maintained by some form of route maintenance procedure until either the destination becomes inaccessible or the route is no longer desired.

Since mobile nodes are required to probe their surroundings trying to find routing nodes, and nodes are essentially hand-held terminals operated with batteries, power consumption is of paramount importance in the operation of these networks.

Ad-hoc networks have been proposed in many communications and remote-sensing settings. Among the emerging research topics, sensor database, sensor information storage and sensor network programming deserve particular attention.

<u>System Architecture</u>

A MMIC is a battery-operated device that is intended to replace "dog tags" and to hold medical information that may be accessed by a physician through a specialized terminal, namely a MMDA or a pocket PC through a RF (Radio Frequency) channel. The use of a wireless instead of a hardwired link (such as universal serial bus-USB or secure digital-SD) is motivated by the following reasons:

1. A wireless link is not affected by the operating conditions. In fact, external agents such as sweat, water, sand and mud may deteriorate a physical, plug-based, connection;
2. A physical connector increases the ruggerisation costs and complicates package and shield design;

3. The use of communication ports such as USB or SD implies the integration in the system of a controller unit with its own firmware and software. This, in turn, increases system complexity and requires more memory leading to increased costs and power consumption.

On the other hand, a wireless link is intrinsically unsafe; although this problem may be tackled by reducing MMIC emission radius to a few meters. This, in turn, helps to reduce power consumption as well.

The MMIC must have the following features:

1. A baseband processor to run the communication stack;
2. A RF module to implement wireless communications in the desired band;
3. A visual external interface with patient and communication status information.

The external interface is implemented by a set of five LEDs (Light Emitting Diodes) placed on both sides of the MMIC package. The diodes implement a color code whose meaning is represented in Table 1.

Diode	Meaning
Blue (flashing)	MMDA in the MMIC range
Blue (fixed)	Link established between MMIC and MMDA
Red	Patient status: critical
Yellow	Patient status: severe
Green	Patient status: soft
White	Patient status: recovered

Table 1. MMIC Visual Interface Color Code.

The patient status diodes may be adequately programmed by the physician by means of the MMDA, once a link with the patient has been established.

The MMIC must be capable to operate at very low voltages to minimize power consumption.

The MMIC operates on the patient side and stores all its clinical information in a local non-volatile memory. In addition, the device must have the capability to communicate with other MMICs or with MMDAs through a RF channel. This capability is implemented both in hardware and in software.

Device drivers implement the glue layer between the physical interface and the upper levels. They are a set of assembly language routines that control directly the hardware resources. These routines are then invoked by the system library and interrupt management routines to implement complex functions. This approach guarantees independence between hardware and software and hence full software compatibility between the protocol stack and processor future versions.

The MMDA operates on the medic side.

The major design concerns in the development of the system are:

1. **Technology**. Since the goal is to implement an analogue RF and digital baseband processor into a single chip, there exist severe restrictions on the fabrication process to use. This, in fact, limits the choice to expensive analogue and mixed-signal processes that must also provide the designer with the capability to embed RAM and ROM memories on chip.
2. **Area occupation**. The RF transceiver must be almost completely integrated in a single chip reducing as much as possible the number of external components to reduce the

overall fabrication costs. Nevertheless, integrated analogue components such as capacitors and inductors occupies large areas subtracting die area to the digital baseband, so chip floorplanning must be carefully carried out.

3. **Packaging**. Also packaging is a major concern in the design. In fact, medical information must be stored in a non-volatile memory, namely a flash memory. The use of a flash memory guarantees high storage densities, speed and versatility, since this kind of memory may be programmed and erased on-the-fly. Nevertheless, for technological reasons, flash memory may not be implemented on the same silicon substrate that hosts baseband processor and RF module.
4. **Power consumption**. The device must be battery-operated, so power consumption and battery lifetime are major design concerns. This implies that a trade-off must be found among chip-core operating voltage, transmission and reception bandwidths, device operating frequency, and device operating range.
5. **Modulation scheme**. The modulation scheme of the RF front-end is a crucial part of the design since it determines hardware complexity, power efficiency and transceiver bandwidth. Complex modulation schemes may also affect digital hardware and protocol stack.

Communication architecture and medium access control

MMICs and MMDAs are wireless devices, so information interchange between them relies on a wireless communication link. Prior to discussing all the issues related to MMIC PHY (Physical) and MAC (Medium Access Control) layers and to communication and network architecture it is better to review briefly the main industrial standards for WPAN (Wireless Personal Area Network) and WLAN (Wireless Local Area Network). The main difference between a WLAN and a WPAN is, basically, the range of a wireless node. For a WPAN the transmitting range is up to 10 meters with transmission powers ranging from 1 to 100mW. For a WLAN the transmitting range is up to 100 meters with a transmission power between 100 and 300mW.

In this scenario we need a network with the following characteristics:

1. Support for ad-hoc and hand-held wireless devices;
2. High mobility and rapid deployment, and hence little or no infrastructure;
3. Low power consumption;
4. Ease of scalability;
5. Sufficient data rate to support the application and information interchange;
6. Support for the existing e-health infrastructure.

Figure 6 depicts the proposed network architecture at role 2 level.

The proposed architecture is hence a network hierarchy in which several ad-hoc and hand-held wireless devices cooperate. The lowest hierarchy level is the WPAN formed by MMIC devices that operate with the IEEE 802.15.4 protocol stack. The upper level is the WLAN formed by MMDA devices that relies both on IEEE 802.15.4 to interact with MMICs and on IEEE 802.11a/g to implement the WLAN and interact with a gateway wireless access point.

7.2 Tele Assistant (diagnostic and surgical procedures) System.

The Telemedicine Service has a system that is able to point or to draw over the dynamic images of the Video teleconference and send them back to the Remote Centre connected on real time.

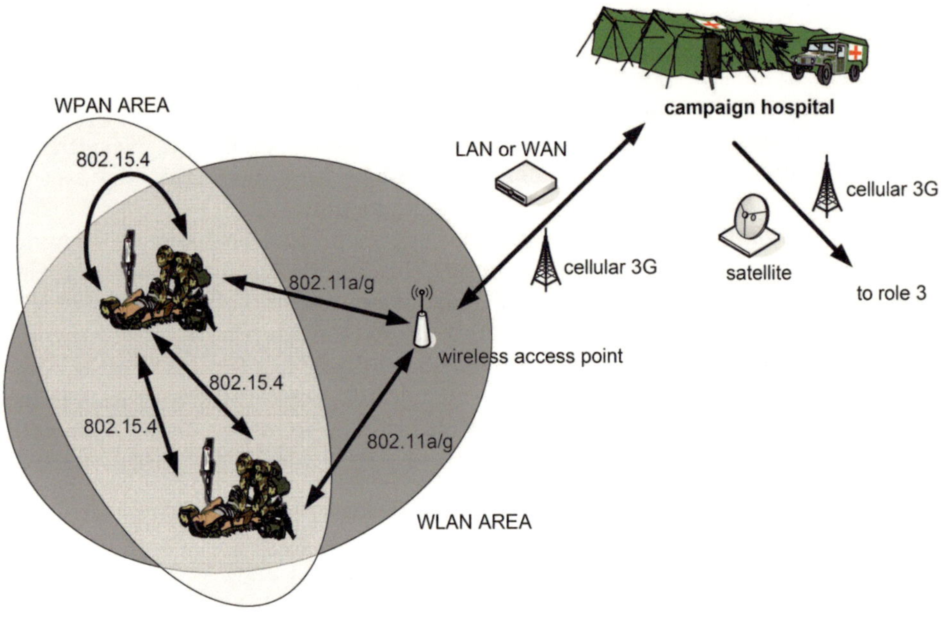

Fig. 6. Network Architecture at Role 2.

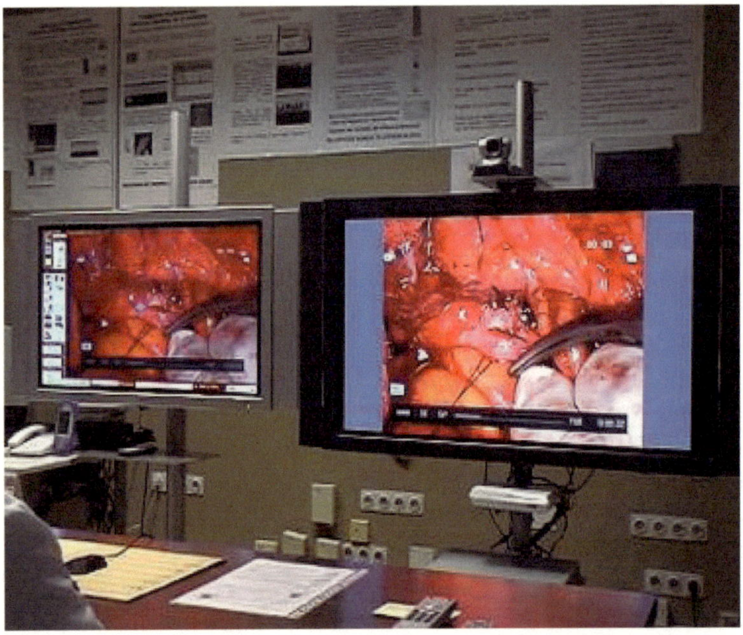

Picture 1. There is one view of the Tele Assistant system from the Reference Centre.

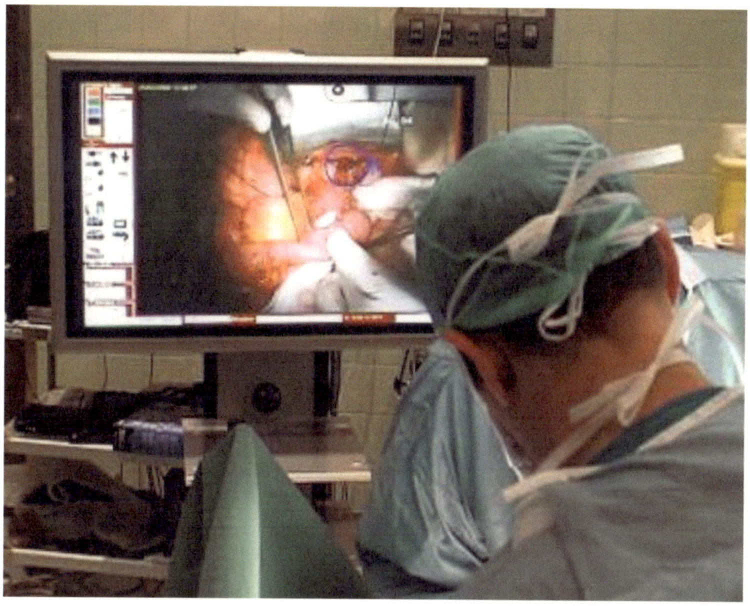

Picture 2. There is one view of the Tele Assistant system from the Remote Centre.

This is quite important for Telementoring purposes because it allows the specialist in the Reference Centre to show the medical personnel in the Remote Centre how to perform a diagnostic or therapeutic procedure on real time and to supervise it also.
This system is used for example to mark different points of interest in Tele Ultrasound examination on real time.
It was designed as a Tele Surgical Assistant System, but the experience showed to us that it was very useful for the majority of medical procedures.

7.3 Integration of an intelligent tele monitoring system.

Nowadays the monitoring vital signs devices have alarms (warnings) that can be set by the medical personnel to be activated when the values of these parameters arise to certain levels: The pulse rate may be set as 100 bites per minute as upper level and 60 as lower limit. When the cardiac frequency is higher than 100 of lesser than 60 an acoustic and visual alarms began to work warning about the situation.
This monitoring is quite important in Advanced Life Support because the Decision Making Process has to be on real time.
A next step is to include intelligent alarms for these devices with the aim to help the medical personnel about to realize as soon as possible, and with the highest accuracy what is going on in every moment during the management of critical casualties. One example of this kind of new monitoring could be that the devices would integrate the inputs from different vital signs: bradycardia + high blood pressure + irregular respiratory pattern = High intracranial pressure. This tool joint to a real time videoconference teleconsultation system is a powerful platform to mentor medical teams working on critical situations.

7.4 On call (cellular videoconference) medical specialist system.

The Reference Centre of the Telemedicine Service has a Gateway that transforms the Cellular Videoconference into ISDN (Integrated Services Digital Network) Videoconference.

This system gives the chance to access to the Reference Centre with a cellular phone with 3G (or upper) capability, videoconference and enough coverage.
We use this system from 2005 and its application is to telementor the people on duty at the Hospital taking care of the Telemedicine System if they had any trouble with the Teleconsultations.
It is quite useful because it allows us (Telemedicine Service personnel) to be on Telepresence 24/7 in our Reference Centre. We call it the "Big Brother" system.

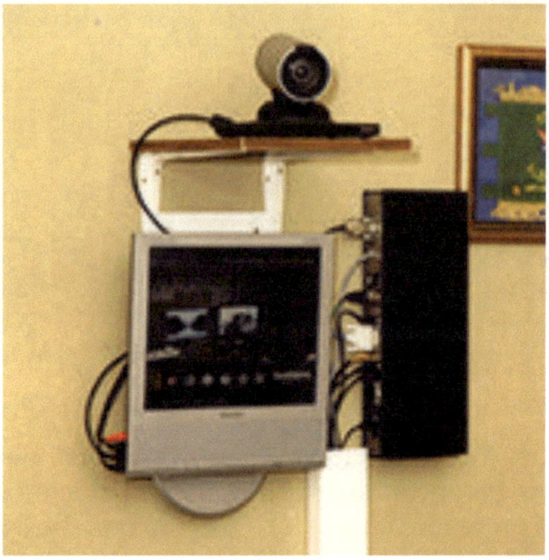

Picture 3. There is one view of the Big Brother Videoconference.

8. Tele mobile intensive care ambulance

The Medical Evacuation (MEDEVAC) is essential in every Prehospital Emergency Care System. The Medical Transportation of patients with the trained medical personnel and with the right materiel (electromedical devices) and proper vehicles assure the necessary conditions for a good care. Many times these MEDEVAC are carried out with critical or potentially critical care patients. In spite of the MEDEVAC personnel were ready for attending these kind of patients if they had the capability to connect in real time with the medical specialists who will receive the patients is quite useful. This is a way to receive Telementoring on real time (with Videoconference and vital signs transmission) and to show the status of the patients prior to the arrival to their hospitals of destination. This system improves the time and the quality of the Medical Information between different medical providers.
The "Hospital Central de la Defensa" has one ICU (Intensive Care Unit) ambulance with the capability to connect on moving with the Reference Centre of the Telemedicine Service. Two different communications are used: 3G cellular phone coverage and satellital communications. These terminals are installed into the ambulance (two antennas and to interfaces) and one laptop is integrated as a hub that connects the medical devices and the videoconference system with a software application that allows by a communications network (Internet or Intranet) to keep in contact the ICU ambulance and the Reference Centre.
This tool gives the chance to perform ultrasounds examinations from the ambulance being telementored and assessed by the medical specialist on duty who is going to receive the MEDEVAC.

The system has been tested with both communications system (satellital and 3G) with the aim to have always the chance to connect with the Hospital when it was necessary without geographical constrains.

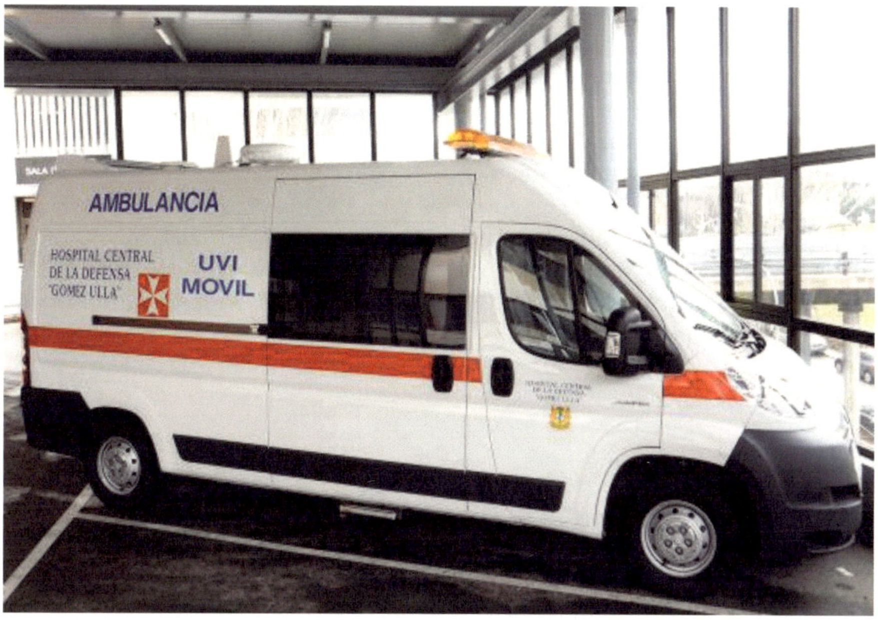

Picture 4. The ICU ambulance with the Telemedicine system integrated.

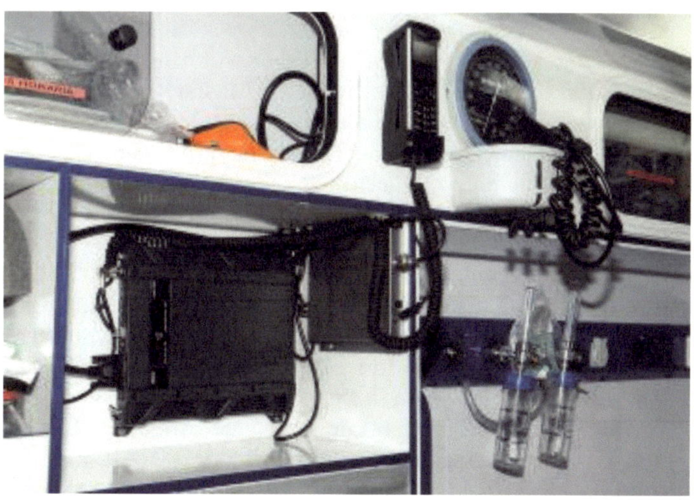

Picture 5. A view of the communication terminals inside the ICU ambulance.

9. Robotic tele ultrasound examinations:

Nowadays Teleultrasound is one of the most cost-effective techniques applied on Telemedicine. There are different ways of management in this field. This group began five years ago a trial with a Telementoring method in Teleultrasound using an agreed language

between the medical specialist provider (radiologist or cardiologist) and the Teleoperator (Nurse or Radiology Technician), on the idea that a well trained human being is a good interface for Teleultrasound.
There are some commands which are used by the specialist to telementor the medical personnel on the Remote Center on how to perform the ultrasounds examinations on real time: Move to, stop, freeze, spin, tilt to, bend to, compress and relax pressure.
The procedure is being applied with the Telemedicine System from the Remote Centres to the Reference Centre where the requested specialist are (radiologists, cardiologists, vascular surgeons or orthopedic surgeons mainly).
We are trying to make easier these explorations with the integration of robots. These robots can be attached to the ultrasound machine probe and then the specialist can move the probe remotely with a joystick from the Reference Centre (on real time), with direct visualization of the probe position over the patient´s body surface and with the ultrasound image simultaneously (dual video layout).
We are still on the testing phase of these devices, but we think that this will be a very helpful tool for these examinations.

10. References

NATO AJP 4.10.2, "*Allied Joint Doctrine for Medical Evacuation*", Ratification Draft, March 6th 2006.

NATO MC 326/2, "*Principles and Policies of Operational Medical Support*", April 7th 2004.

NATO MEDICS OCD, "*MEDICS: Medical Information and Coordination System*", Operational Concept Document, Edition 2.3, September 15th 2005.

NATO AMEDP-13, "NATO *Glossary of Medical Terms and Definitions*", Edition 1, February 2002.

MIMS STANAG, "*Standards for Development and Implementation of Medical Information Management and C3 Systems*", Study Draft 7, May 2004.

Sanchez Ruiz J, "Studing SACS platform as Telemonitoring solution for the Spanish Ministry of Defence Telemedicine System". Master Oficial en Tecnologías de la Información y Comunicaciones. Alcala University. Madrid 2010.

Kaplan I, Clikes I, "Telemedicine". ISBN 953-95168-0-3. Zagreb 2005.

Hernandez Abadia A, Hernandez Navarro M, "Telemedicina en la Sanidad Militar española". 233-243. "Telemedicina". ISBN 84-932521-2-3. Fundación Vodafone. Madrid 2004.

G. Aggelon, "*Mobile Ad-hoc Networks: From Wireless LANS to 4G Networks*", McGraw-Hill, 2004.

Barbier P, Alimento M, Berna G, Celeste F, Gentile F, Mantero A, Montericcio V, Muratori M. High-grade video compression of echocardiographic studies: a multicenter validation study of selected motion pictures expert groups (MPEG)-4 algorithms. J Am Soc Echocardiogr. 2007 May;20(5):527-36.

Ferrer-Roca O, Kurjak A, Mario Troyano-Luque J, Bajo Arenas J, Luis Merce A, Diaz-Cardama A. Tele-virtualsonography.J Perinat Med. 2006;34(2):123-9.

Burgul R, Gilbert FJ,. Undrill PE. Methods of measurement of image quality in teleultrasound. Br J Radiol. 2000 Dec;73(876):1306-12.

Chan FY, Soong B, Lessing K, Watson D, Cincotta R, Baker S, Smith M, Green E, Whitehall J. Clinical value of real-time tertiary fetal ultrasound consultation by telemedicine: preliminary evaluation.Telemed J. 2000 Summer;6(2):237-42.

Johnson MA, Davis P, McEwan AJ, Jhangri GS, Warshawski R, Gargum A, Ethier J, Anderson WW. Preliminary findings from a teleultrasound study in Alberta. Telemed J. 1998 Fall;4(3):267-76

19

A Telemedicine System for Hostile Environments

Ebrahim Nageba, Jocelyne Fayn and Paul Rubel
MTIC – EA4171, INSA-Lyon, Université Lyon 1, Lyon
France

1. Introduction

In telemedicine, a critical issue is to provide high quality healthcare services to persons located in rural areas and also in what is called hostile environments, e.g. isolated geographic areas such as high mountains resorts. These environments are potentially dangerous and difficult to reach. Moreover, in these particular environments, several factors must be considered during the telemedicine processes, especially in emergency situations. These factors could be for instance: the profiles and skills of the Rescue Team Members (RTM) or first aid persons, the technical characteristics of the telecommunication technologies embedded in the users' terminals, the availability of human and material resources and the accessibility to both the patient location and the required resources. All these factors should be taken into account to build a high performance telemedicine system. Most emergency telemedicine scenarios related to hostile environments are different, context-dependant and complex. For this reason, it is extremely difficult to define protocols or standards that meet the user needs in such environments. In addition, the decisions that should be made to orient a person who has a health problem are usually subjective and depend on the aptitude and skills of the actors who are involved in the medical tele-assistance process. From a telemedicine system point of view, the users need to perform multiple tasks in different scenarios. The management of these tasks will depend on the availability of the logistical, material and human resources that may be owned or managed by different healthcare institutions (Nageba et al., 2009). Thus, there is an essential need to design advanced telemedicine systems that are supported by knowledge models which capture knowledge about actors, tasks, resources, and organizations.

In general, the effectiveness of the healthcare services provided by the telemedicine systems is determined by many factors. The most important ones are the quality and availability of relevant information, where and when needed. However, telemedicine scenarios are various. Some of them are well know, viz patient remote monitoring (Healy et al., 2010), but other scenarios are contextual and more complex, e.g. patient tele-assistance or orientation in hostile environments like critical geographically and isolated areas where the assistant persons present next to the patient do not have enough knowledge to take the appropriate decisions (Nageba et al., 2007). This type of scenarios requires knowledge management to support the tasks and processes of medical tele-assistance.

In this chapter, we present our new Telemedicine system, called T-TROIE, standing for Telemedicine Tasks and Resources Ontology based system for Inimical Environments, which

takes into account the previous requirements to provide the healthcare professional with efficient decision making support tools. It implements a knowledge framework based on interrelated ontologies, a rule base and an inference engine (Nageba et al., 2008). T-TROIE handles contextual situations in both simple and complex scenarios using Telemedicine knowledge management. We define a "Telemedicine Task" as a set of activities ordered in sequenced steps within a telemedicine process, e.g. tele-assistance, tele-consultation, data searching, data access, message set up and transmission, etc. It is executed by a telemedicine system to provide the healthcare actors with data that are relevant to their requests.
The chapter is organized as follows. In the next section we explore some related works in the field of telemedicine, especially ontology or knowledge based telemedicine systems, in order to highlight their drawbacks and the needs these systems do not meet. In section 3 we present the telemedicine scenario we have adopted to demonstrate the feasibility of our proposed system, as well as the telemedicine process through a sequences diagram describing the user interactions with the system. In section 4 we give an overview of the T-TROIE architecture and of its components including a communication server, a task management server and a knowledge base. We detail some aspects of the T-TROIE realization and implementation in section 5.

2. Related works

Nowadays, ontologies have emerged as a significant instrument within the knowledge engineering community for defining flexible, scalable, personalizable and open models of concepts and interrelationships (Christopoulou and Kameas, 2004). The main advantage of an ontology resides in its ability to formally represent the knowledge in a given field and to interpret the data semantics. Currently, several ontology description languages are being used to formalize knowledge models.
The Ontology Web Language OWL (OWL, 2004), which has been adopted by the World Wide World Consortium (W3C), has the capacity of supporting semantic interoperability to exchange and share knowledge between different systems in various domains and of enabling automated reasoning. It is an expressive language based on RDF (Resource Description Framework), which has the capacity of supporting semantic interoperability to exchange and share knowledge between different systems in various domains and of enabling automated reasoning on contextual information with well defined declarative semantics. Thanks to XML and OWL, it becomes easy to align different ontologies structures. On the other hand, since XML has become very popular for data exchange and the fact that the ontology description languages RDF and OWL are based on XML, adopting OWL easies ontology model transformations in terms of data representation in different formats and makes the mapping between different ontology structures an easy process. In its turn, the Object Management Group (OMG) has specified an Ontology Definition Meta-model (OMG, 2009) which enables ontology modelling through the use of UML-based tools.
Despite of the diversity of scenarios, applications and services, we can classify telemedicine systems, from a system architecture point of view, into three main categories: the peer to peer P2P systems, such as the telemedicine system developed by the ARTEMIS project (ARTEMIS 2004), the Agent-based systems, such as the SAPHIRE project (SAPHIRE 2008), and the mobile systems, such as the EPI-MEDICS project (Fayn and Rubel, 2010).
From the electronic health record (EHR) access point of view, ARTEMIS (Dogac et al., 2006) has as objective to empower the sharing of the patients EHRs belonging to different

institutions by enabling the interoperability between the different existing standards, i.e. HL7, OpenEHR, and EHRcom (EN 13606). This approach is based on ontology mapping and on web services for data exchange. Another engineering approach has been developed within the scope of the ARTEMIS project to provide the exchange of meaningful clinical information among healthcare institutes through semantic mediation (Oemig and Blobel, 2009). The proposed framework provides the mapping of a source ontology into a target ontology with the help of a mapping tool producing a mapping definition which is then used to automatically transform the source ontology message instances into target message instances (Bicer et al., 2005). Smart Telehealth Home (STH) is an ontology-based model which takes advantage of the full potential of ontologies to describe the smart home domain, in order to provide an effective base for the development, the configuration and the execution of software applications (Latfi et al., 2007). The ontologies of STH (i.e. habitat ontology, person and medical history ontology, equipment ontology, behavior ontology and decision ontology) are employed to initialize Bayesian networks used for recognizing which activity is most likely to be performed by the patient at a given time and in a given place. In addition, an ontology-based model has been proposed for monitoring and assisting patient at home (Paganelli et al., 2008). The proposed model consists of several ontologies describing patient domain, home domain, alarm management and the social context ontology. The components of the proposed ontology-based model have been implemented by adopting standard technologies, i.e. internet protocols, XML and Web Services.

For areas that cannot be handled by existing telemedicine solutions, an approach has been proposed for creating scalable telemedicine networks based on Delay Tolerant Networking (DTN) using store-and-forward Voice-Over-IP (VoIP) (Scholl et al., 2009). DTN operates by leveraging mobility and local communications between participants in the network. Each member of the network communicates with other members when possible, for example when they are close enough for local wireless communications (using WiFi, Bluetooth, etc.), or when a long range link becomes available. Members store messages from each other and forward them later on when they establish connectivity with other members. This type of telemedicine network allows communication of non time-critical information between participants. However, in emergency scenarios where time is a critical factor, store-and-forward using VoIP is not an efficient solution. Additionally, a system for remote patient disease diagnosis and treatment has been proposed by Din (Din, 2010). It uses real time protocols, i.e. MPEG4/H.26X, for video and audio sessions and for connecting sophisticated medical equipments. Additionally, a High Definition TeleMedicine system (HDTM) architecture has been defined by Lu (Lu et al., 2010) that leverages the network as an intelligent transport and services platform that supports high-definition videoconferencing and audio telemetry.

The models and systems cited above present solutions based on the data captured by distributed sensors in pervasive environments, using common scenarios and standardized protocols. But, these research works neglect telemedicine scenarios problematics related to the availability and capability of heterogeneous resources in hostile environments where there are no sensors or pre-defined protocols to exchange data. Additionally, the works presented above ignore the need of knowledge management in order to provide the actors who lack the knowledge required to take the appropriate decisions, with efficient decision making support tools. In T-TROIE we have considered all the above issues to provide a more general and knowledge-based solution taking into account the specificities and diversities of contextual situations as well as the availability of the resources required to perform the telemedicine processes in hostile environments.

3. Patient orientation scenario in hostile environments

Figure 1 displays typical examples of telemedicine scenarios in different environments including home, hospitals, doctor's offices and other environments such as refuges in high mountains. The regulation center, hosting the T-TROIE system, constitutes a central point coordinating the communication among these environments. Let us take for illustration purpose a telemedicine scenario which concerns patient orientation in hostile environment such as high mountains resorts where telemedicine infrastructures and resources may be not available.

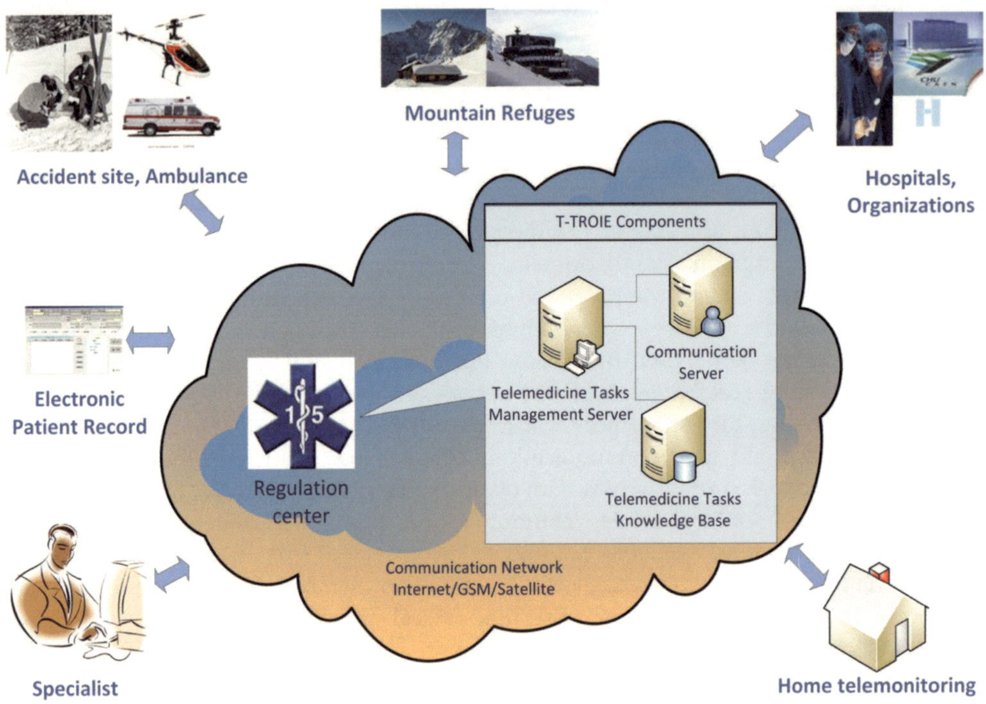

Fig. 1. Telemedicine applications scenarios in different environments

Let us suppose that a person has an accident or a heart attack while skiing or staying in a high mountains resort. The RTM or the person present next to the victim and/or the staff of the regulation center need to take a decision upon the patient orientation. This decision should consider several contextual factors such as the patient's clinical status, his social conditions, the hospital location, the availability and capability of different resources.

Using a telecommunication terminal, i.e. a Personal Digital Assistant (PDA) or a Smartphone, the RTM can connect to the T-TROIE system to perform the Patient Orientation telemedicine task. He or she should fill and submit a task form including patient personal information, e.g. first name, surname, security social number, the clinical status of the patient, e.g. heart attack, chest pain, high blood pressure, as well as the task parameters, such as, accident date, time and location.

To handle the contextual situation mentioned above, a telemedicine task, "Patient Orientation", has been defined to allow a healthcare professional or a RTM to take a decision for the transfer of the patient into an appropriate hospital that complies with the

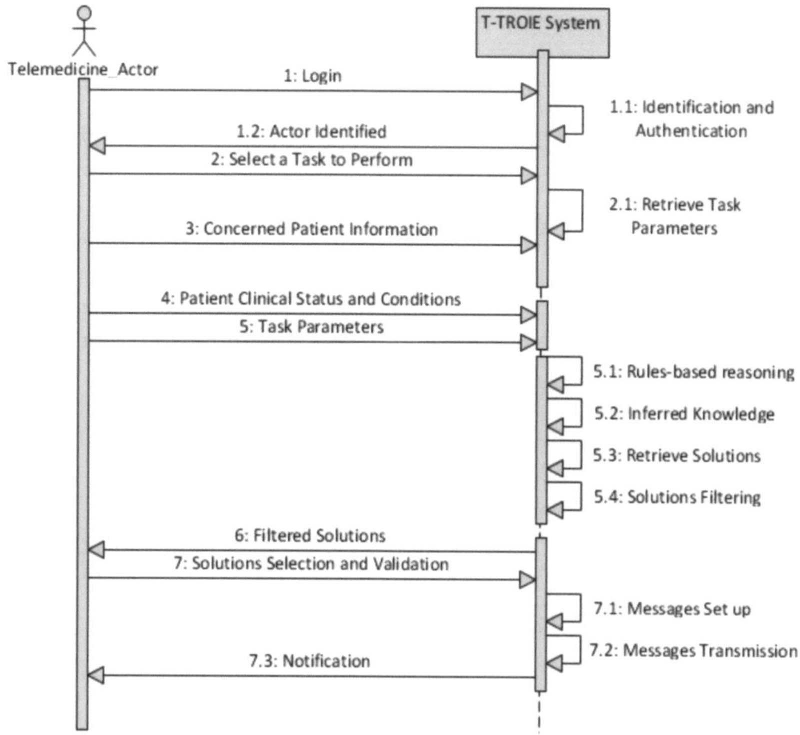

Fig. 2. Interaction diagram for a typical patient orientation scenario

patient contextual situation. We suppose that the patient has a heart attack. Depending on the clinical status of the patient, his context and the geographic location, T-TROIE will perform a rule-based reasoning and infer that the patient orientation task requires logistical resources such as an available bed in an intensive care unit and the material resources needed to perform some particular procedures like an angiography. T-TROIE will propose to the RTM a list of recipients including a general medical centre, an intensive care unit or a specialized hospital that have these resources available. Once the RTM has selected the solution that meets the context of the victim, T-TROIE will generate a set of messages that will be sent to the concerned recipient, i.e. an hospital. Then, T-TROIE will acknowledge the RTM that the selected hospital is ready to receive the patient. Figure 2 shows a sequence diagram representing the actor/system interactions and the exchanged messages.

The messages exchanged by the system are encapsulated in an XML format. The messages may be informative, for example to ask the intensive care unit to be ready to receive the patient, or provide a request for an advice, for immediate drug administration for instance, which requires a rapid response. The XML messages can include different types of data (i.e., patient's personal data, medical data such as blood pressure, symptoms descriptions, bio-signals like an ECG, and eventually a list of drugs or a digital picture of a wound).

4. T-TROIE architecture overview

Figure 3 displays the main components of the T-TROIE knowledge-based technical architecture to support the management and execution of context-dependent telemedicine tasks and processes taking into consideration the availability and capability of heterogeneous resources needed by the telemedicine processes. The architecture is composed of three main components: a Communication server, a Task Management server and a Knowledge Base.

4.1 The communication server

The communication server manages operations such as identification, authentification, and messaging. It operates as a mediator allowing users to manage their profile and access to data. The communication server also performs the exchange of the XML messages issued by the Task Management Server by taking into account the Message Transmission Policy (MTP) that we have defined. Based on the MTP, the communication server performs the following three major processes:

- Prioritize the messages coming from the Task Management Server according to the sender and receiver actors' profiles. For example, according to the MTP, the messages sent by an emergency physician must be assigned to a high priority.
- Stratify the messages in queues according to their priorities, i.e. a high priority message queue, a medium priority messages queue and a low priority messages queue.
- Apply message transmission rules, such as, *"send the first message in the high priority message queue; if there is no message in the high priority queue, send the first message in the medium priority message queue"*.

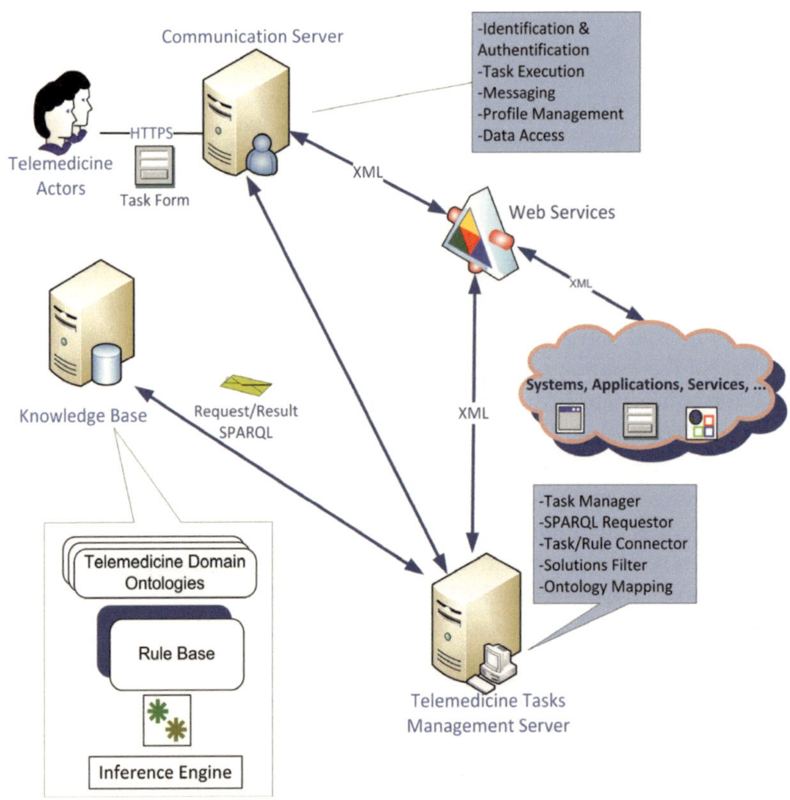

Fig. 3. General overview of the T-TROIE technical architecture

In addition, the communication server plays the role of a web server that responds to the HTTP requests issued by the users during the interactions with the system. It visualizes the different tasks forms generated by the task management server, forms that will be filled by the users who can also exchange messages with other actors in the telemedicine domain and manage their profiles. Moreover, the communication server allows other entities, i.e. systems, applications and services, to communicate with the T-TROIE system via web services protocols.

4.2 The task management server

The Tasks Management Server (TMS) is based on the W3C SPARQL Query Language for RDF (Prud'hommeaux and Seaborne, 2008). SPARQL permits to retrieve data from the ontology through queries such as SELECT, CONSTRUCT, ASK and DESCRIBE. It returns the query results in RDF. The main role of the TMS is to perform the following tasks:

- Link the identified actors with the tasks they can perform, for instance, a RTM can perform a patient orientation task, but he or she cannot perform a task which requires medical skills.
- Configure the form of the selected task by setting the required parameters. For example, if the actor selects the task patient orientation, TMS integrates in the task form several parameters such as the accident time, date and location.
- Select the rules which the inference engine will apply to infer the solutions needed by the users.
- Generate XML messages encapsulating different types of medical data, viz heart rate, systolic and diastolic blood pressure, body temperature, etc.
- Filter the solutions inferred by the inference engine according to different contextual factors related to location, actors' terminal technical characteristics, capability of human or material resources, etc.

4.3 The telemedicine knowledge base

The backbone of T-TROIE is the telemedicine knowledge base. As depicted in figure 3, this server consists of a set of interrelated ontologies describing the telemedicine domain, a rule base and an inference engine. We detail these components in the following sections.

4.3.1 Telemedicine domain ontologies

The ontologies we have created represent physical entities in the telemedicine domain such as Organization, Actor, Patient, Clinical Status, Resource and Location, as well as abstract entities such as Task, Service, Process, Message and Parameters. Figure 4 displays the different T-TROIE ontologies representing general concepts and their interrelationships in the telemedicine domain. Based on these ontologies, different contextual situations in various telemedicine scenarios can be easily handled. We provide hereafter a brief explanation of the main ontologies of T-TROIE.

- The Actor ontology represents classes of individuals such as healthcare professionals, i.e. General Practitioner, Specialist, Nurse, Emergency Physician, RTM, etc. A healthcare professional has the following data type properties: ID, name, general domain, specialty, location, etc.
- The Organization ontology describes healthcare institutions, i.e. hospital, medical center, insurance company, etc.

- The Resources are classified in two main classes: the material resource class, e.g. logistics, medical equipments, etc, and the communication resource class, e.g. server, laptop, smart phone, etc. The communication resource sub-ontology also describes resource properties such as brand description, memory size, screen size, resolution, embedded telecommunication technology, etc.
- The task ontology represents any activity to be performed by any actor in the telemedicine domain, whatever the actor is: a healthcare professional, a non medical staff, a patient or a patient's relative. The telemedicine tasks are classified in multiple categories, i.e. emergency, tele-consultation, tele-expertise, tele-radiology, etc.
- The Electronic Health Record ontology contains patient demographic information and patient medical data including medical history, allergy, risk factors, diagnostic summaries, ongoing pathology and treatment, etc.

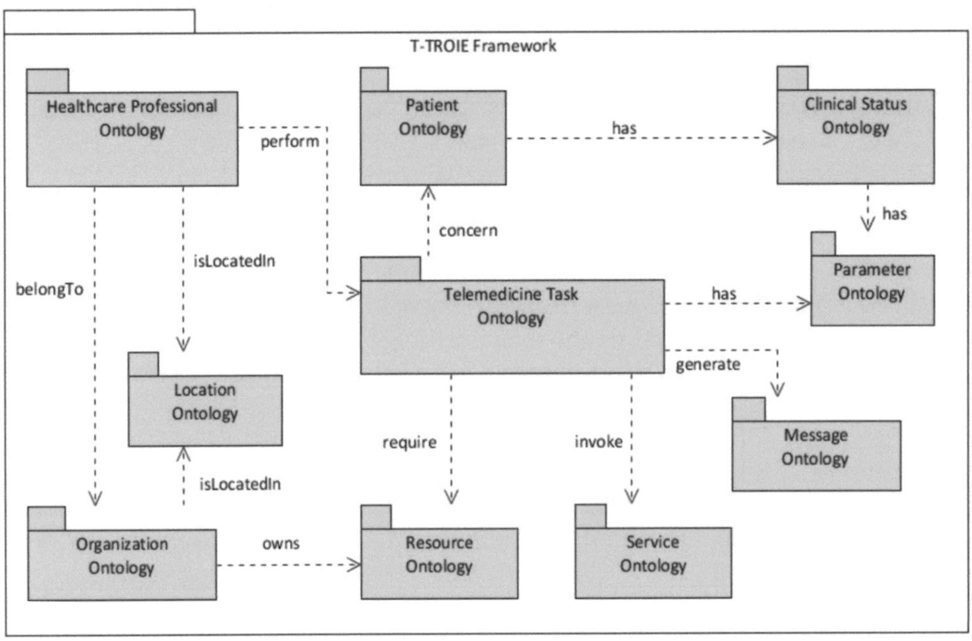

Fig. 4. T-TROIE ontologies and their interrelationships for the telemedicine domain

4.3.2 Rules for telemedicine tasks management

The rule base includes logical statements that specify how to handle the contextual situation by linking the context's elements such as the actors' profiles, the type of task, the patient clinical status and the resources required by the tasks. We distinguish two rule categories: (1) the management rules applied to infer the knowledge related to healthcare professionals, the telemedicine tasks, the different resources needed by the tasks and the organizations that manage or own these resources, (2) the communication rules enabling the designer to optimize message exchanges among different healthcare actors. The system designer defines a messages transmission policy including messages transmission priority levels according to the task type and to the actor's profile. For instance, messages generated by the patient orientation task have a higher priority level than the ones generated by a task like teleconsultation. In addition, messages generated by the tasks performed by an emergency physician or a RTM have a higher priority level than the messages generated by the tasks performed by a nurse. We provide rules examples in section 5.

4.3.3 Rules and context based reasoning

One of the key features of ontologies is that they can be processed by a reasoner which supports the decision-making process and provides the knowledge base with the capacity of reasoning by applying defined rules. Various existing logic reasoning mechanisms can be exploited to deduce decisions that shall support the tasks management in telemedicine applications. These decisions shall enable telemedicine processes optimizing the use of resources. Additionally, the decisions shall provide solutions to societal problems such as the patient orientation in emergency cases. An inference engine applies the defined rules using the knowledge represented by the ontologies to deduce facts related to the contextual situation. Furthermore, the reasoner allows to automatically infer the ontology classes hierarchy and easies ontologies consistency checking.

4.4 Web services based interoperation

Web services constitute an efficient way to access remote data. T-TROIE can communicate with other systems and applications via web services. Tasks may invoke several web services to retrieve data related to the patient, the resources and the environment. For example, in a task such as "Access to Patient EHR", the healthcare professional may need to access the patient's medical antecedents, current prescribed medicines, or risk factors. Patient medical data are distributed over multiple data sources, i.e. EHR hosts. Thus, the task "Access to Patient EHR" invokes the web services provided by the EHR hosts. Several issues concerning access rights, security, privacy, performance and ontologies mapping must be considered when using these web services.

5. T-TROIE realization and implementation

In this section, we briefly introduce the different tools which were used in the T-TROIE prototype implementation process. First, we present the protégé-based demonstrator which we have used to formalize the ontologies, define SWRL rules, carry out the rule-based reasoning and execute SPARQL requests. Next, we present an example of the graphic user interface of the web-based application.

5.1 Protégé-based demonstrator

We have used the Protégé version 3.4 Development Environment (PDE) (Protégé, 1997), for building the ontologies of T-TROIE, to define the data entry forms, and use this forms to acquire data as instances of the ontologies.

OWL has three increasingly-expressive sublanguages which are OWL-Lite, OWL-DL (Description Logics), and OWL-Full. To formalize the telemedicine domain ontologies we have used OWL-DL, which is much more expressive than OWL-Lite and includes additional DL that are flexible to automated reasoning. In OWL-DL, there are two main types of properties that can be defined. The first type is object property, e.g., *Organization owns Resources*. The second type is data type property, e.g., *Actor has Specialty*. The DL extension provides OWL with a rich set of primitives, i.e., intersection, union, complement, etc. It allows the ontology designer to define restrictions and conditions on the ontology classes. It is therefore possible to automatically determine the classification hierarchy and check for inconsistencies in an ontology that conforms to OWL-DL. To achieve this objective, we have used Pellet Reasoner (Pellet, 2007), which can be directly called from PDE, to check the ontologies consistency and to infer the classes hierarchy.

In fact, OWL has certain limitations which are related to the definition of composite properties. Efforts have been made by the W3 community to increase the expressiveness of OWL, particularly by developing a rule description language for the semantic web. W3C now recommends to use the Semantic Web Rule Language (SWRL, 2004), a combination of OWL-DL and OWL-Lite. We have used SWRL to create the rules used in our Telemedicine Task Ontology. The rules are written as antecedent-consequent pairs. In SWRL terminology, the antecedent refers to the rule body and the consequent refers to the head. The head and body consist of a conjunction of one or more atoms.

The rules definition process is an essential step in knowledge-based systems building. In T-TROIE, we have used the SWRL-TAP Protégé plug-in to manage the SWRL rules. Indeed, SWRL rules make T-TROIE ontologies semantically rich and facilitate the automation performed by the inference engine. We provide hereafter three examples of SWRL rules we have defined using SWRL-TAP to support tasks execution in the telemedicine domain.

Rule 1:

tele-onto:Task(?tele-onto:task) ∧ tele-onto:Patient(?tele-onto:patient) ∧ tele-onto:Heart_Attack (?tele-onto:heartAttack) ∧ tele-onto:Concernes(?tele-onto:task, ?tele-onto:patient) ∧ tele-onto:hasStatus(?tele-onto:patient, ?tele-onto:heartAttack) ∧ tele-onto:Coronarography_Equipment(?tele-onto:coronaroEquip) ∧ tele-onto:availability(?tele-onto: coronaroEquip, true)
→ tele-onto:requires(?tele-onto:task, ?tele-onto: coronaroEquip)

Rule 2:

tele-onto:Task(?tele-onto:task) ∧ tele-onto:Patient(?tele-onto:patient) ∧ tele-onto:Heart_Attack(?tele-onto: heartAttack) ∧ tele-onto:Concernes(?tele-onto:task, ?tele-onto:patient) ∧ tele-onto:hasStatus(?tele-onto:patient, ?tele-onto: heartAttack) ∧ tele-onto:IntensiveCareUnit(?tele-onto:icu) ∧ tele-onto:availability(?tele-onto:ice, true)
→ tele-onto:requires(?tele-onto:tas, ?tele-onto:icu)

Rule 3:

tele-onto:Rescue_Team_Member(?tele-onto:rtm) ∧ tele-onto:Task(?tele-onto:task) ∧ tele-onto:performs(?tele-onto:rtm, ?tele-onto:task) ∧ tele-onto:Message(?tele-onto:message)vtele-onto:generates(?tele-onto:task, ?tele-onto:message)
→ tele-onto:messagePriorityLevel(?tele-onto:message, "High ")

Rules 1 and 2 describe the following context: if the telemedicine task, patient orientation in our example, concerns a patient who has as clinical status "Heart Attack", the inference engine, according to these rules, shall infer that this task requires as material resources a coronarography equipment and an intensive care unit to be available in the hospital where the patient will be hospitalized. Rule 3 represents an example of the message transmission policy. When the RTM is performing a telemedicine task, then, the message generated by the task shall have a "high" priority level.

To perform the reasoning on the knowledge represented by the ontologies, we have used the Java Expert System Shell (JESS) protégé plug-in as an inference engine. There are three principal phases of reasoning with JESS. The first one converts OWL classes to JESS facts and converts SWRL rules to JESS rules. The second phase executes the reasoning. The last phase converts JESS inferred knowledge to knowledge described in OWL.

Figure 5 shows a snapshot of the Patient Orientation task interface, developed using Protégé, describing the task metadata, i.e. *Task Identifier, Task Description, Domain Speciality, etc.* This task is performed by a RTM and it concerns patient Mr.X being victim of a heart attack while skiing in the high mountains. Appling rules 1 and 2, the JESS inference engine infers that the patient orientation task requires as material resources a coronarography equipment and an available bed in an intensive care unit. As we have mentioned in the previously described scenario, Mr. X must be transported to an hospital which is close to the accident site and owns the needed material resources.

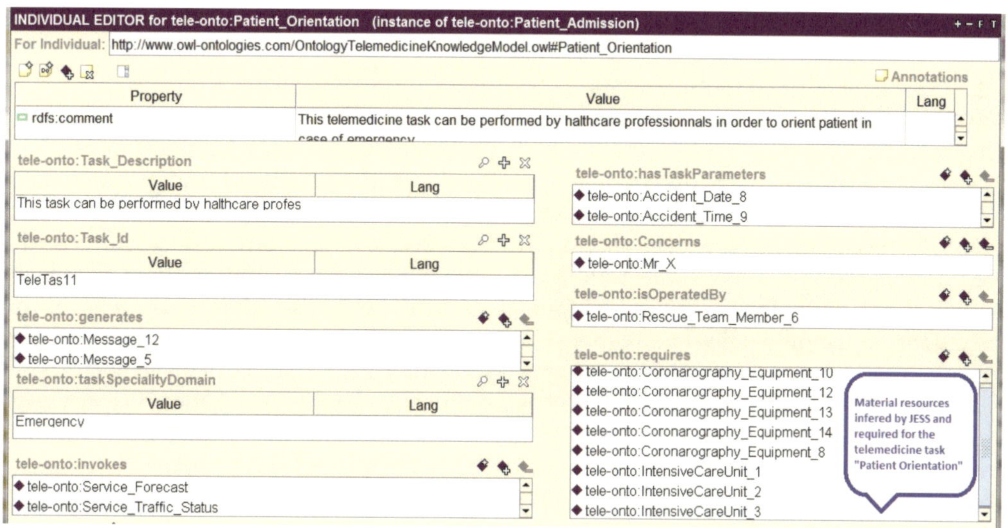

Fig. 5. Protégé-based interface representing patient orientation telemedicine task metadata including the required material resources inferred by the JESS inference engine.

A SPARQL query is executed to retrieve the appropriate hospitals, located in the same geographic area where the accident took place, and that have the required resources available (Figure 6). Once the RTM has selected one of these hospitals, messages, set with a high priority level, are generated and automatically sent to the selected hospital in order to notify it to be ready to receive the patient. Other services can be invoked to provide the rescue or the ambulance team with supplementary information that may be useful for the transportation like the road traffic status and the weather in case the patient is transported by helicopter.

5.2 T-TROIE web-base application

In order to make the application T-TROIE portable, usable and accessible from anyplace and on any material platform, we have developed a web-based prototype of T-TROIE implementing the main functionalities and services. In the next sections, we present an overview of the technologies we have used for the development of the web-based application. Then, we describe the main web-based user interface of the T-TROIE prototype.

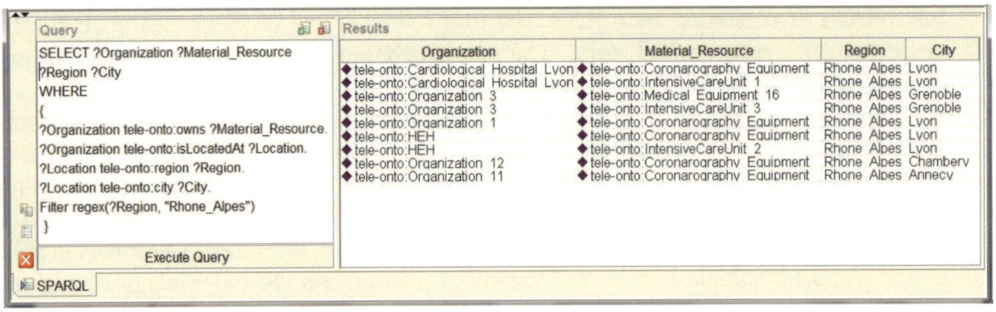

Fig. 6. Example of a SPARQL query used to sort out the list of hospitals which have the resources required by the patient orientation telemedicine task and the location of these organizations.

5.2.1 Overview of used technologies

For the T-TROIE prototype implementation, we have used the Java Object Oriented Programming language. Indeed, thanks to its portability and platform independence, Java enables applications to be executed independently of the hardware and the operating systems on which these applications are installed. In addition, we have used the RDF-based Jena API, developed by Hewlett-Packard (HP) (Jena 2009), which allows us to overcome the programming related to the syntactic analysis (parsing) and the writing of specific syntaxes (serialization). It facilitates the development of tasks and also allows us to focus on operations on the ontologies at a high level of abstraction, e.g. classes definition, ontologies instantiation, data-type and object-type properties setting and instances management.

The Servlet technology, Java Servlet API, has been used to handle the client HTTP requests. Multiple Servlets have been developed to create instances and to initialize them into the ontologies. Other web technologies like HTML, JavaScript, JSP (Java Server Page) and a Tomcat server have also been used for the development of the T-TROIE web application.

5.2.2 Web interface

Figure 7 displays the graphic user interface of the T-TROIE web-based prototype of the architecture presented in section 4, implementing the main telemedicine tasks used in hostile environments, i.e. Patient Orientation, Tele-expertise, Tele-consultation, and Access to medical data. The first step is the user identification (healthcare professionals, RTM, or patient relatives) in order to take advantage of the T-TROIE functionalities and to launch the tasks that are relevant with the user's profiles.

Once the user is identified, he or she can click, for example, on the task "patient orientation". A form related to this task appears asking the user to initialize data and information related to the running task (Figure 8). The users then enter the required data and submit the task form. Then, T-TROIE generates a list of hospitals which have the material resources required for the patient hospitalization, as we have seen in figure 5. In addition to the telemedicine tasks, healthcare professionals can manage their profiles and exchange messages with other telemedicine actors.

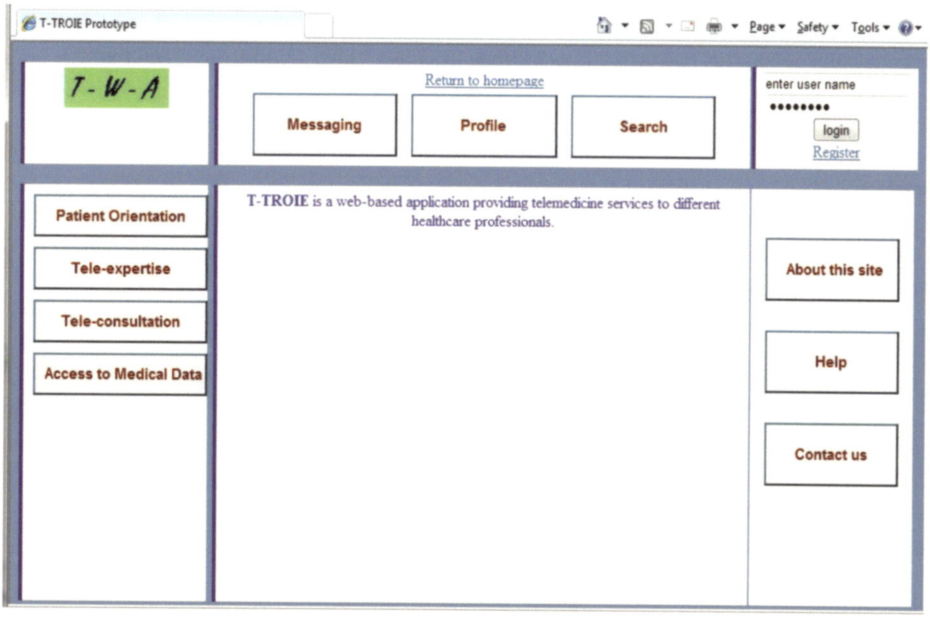

Fig. 7. Screenshot of the T-TROIE prototype web interface

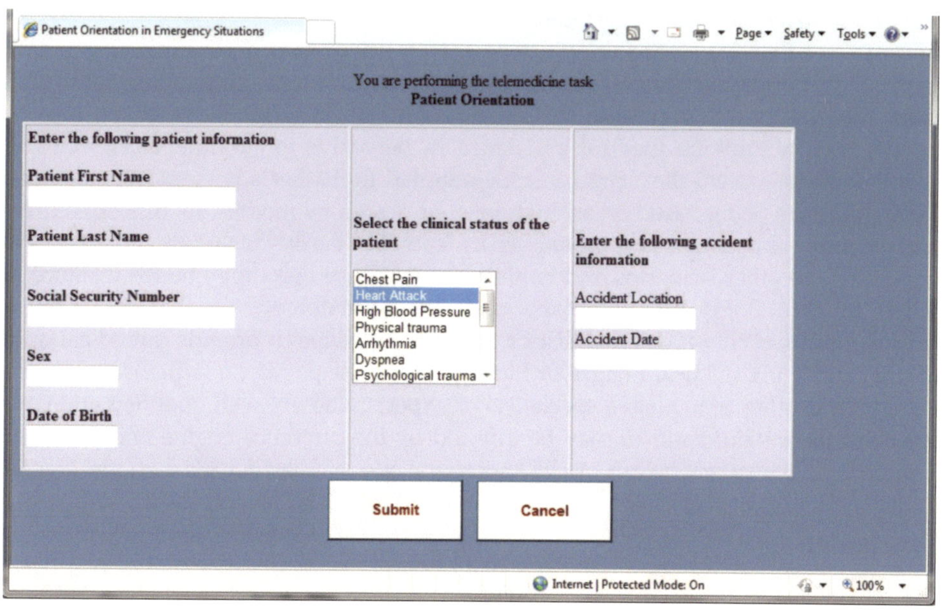

Fig. 8. Patient orientation task form example

6. Discussion

Numerous studies have reported about cases of cardiac death among sportsmen and active citizens, while others have demonstrated the relationship between mortality and the time delay to an appropriate treatment of the heart diseases (De Luca et al. 2004).

In general, the person who provides the first aid to a patient being subject to an accident or health troubles does not have the knowledge and the skills needed to take the appropriate decisions in terms of patient hospitalization. In addition, when a person is victim of a heart attack, by default, the ambulance service takes him to the nearest emergency center. This center may have the resuscitation equipment but it is not always able to perform an angiography, due to the lack of the needed resources. In this case, the ambulance team has to search another hospital which has the material and the human resources required by the angiography intervention and transfer the patient to this hospital. In some cases, patients die before arriving to the appropriate hospitals.

The high mountains or isolated areas emergency scenario example we presented as an illustration of such societal requirements demonstrates the need of providing an efficient and high quality tele-assistance to non skilled first aid persons located next to the patient who is subject to a health accident. Thus, it is extremely important to have a knowledge-based tool which links multiple telemedicine tasks with different types of resources required by these tasks, taking into account the availability and the capability of these resources. The T-TROIE knowledge-based telemedicine system we have developed answers the previous requirements. It has the capability to infer solutions adapted to different contexts in which multiple telemedicine tasks are performed.

The T-TROIE demonstrator has shown that the proposed knowledge-based architecture facilitates the design of complex medical tele-assistance processes and the management of telemedicine messages exchange and thus should contribute to the enhancement of the quality of pervasive telemedical services.

In contrast to other telemedicine solutions that were proposed to support pre-defined telemedical scenarios such as the continuity of care at home of patients with chronic diseases, the system we propose in this chapter aims to be generic enough for also being compliant with ubiquitous medical assistance in pervasive environment. T-TROIE is an open telemedicine system that may be easily adapted to further advances in healthcare. Its whole architecture being based on an high level of design by models, its functionalities can be persistently enhanced. Additional tasks can be easily included in the system, corresponding to other scenarios and environments. These tasks may be for instance Tele-expertise in cardiology, Tele-radiology and tele-dermatology, so that the healthcare professional can search which specialist or expert is available to provide a medical opinion or advice concerning medical images or bio-signals. Consequently, a sequence of solutions, including the profiles of available specialists or experts who are well qualified and capable to deal with the patient context, may be inferred by the inference engine and proposed to the requesting actor so that he can finally choose the one that best fits his own preferences.

7. Conclusion

In this chapter, we have presented T-TROIE, a knowledge-based system, supporting contextual situations handling in telemedicine environments, particularly in hostile environments like high mountains resorts. The proposed telemedicine system implements a knowledge base containing the basic interrelated ontologies in the telemedicine domain, such as healthcare professionals, healthcare institutions, resources, tasks, messages, and parameters.

The knowledge base we have implemented is generic, scalable and open to support different telemedicine applications and services. Representing the telemedicine activities by using an ontology of tasks facilitates the automation of the telemedicine processes. The knowledge base links each telemedicine task with the clinical status and the social conditions of the patient, as well as it links each task with the needed resources to provide a high quality medical tele-assistance.

We have implemented a T-TROIE prototype in the telemedicine domain to solve societal problems such as Patient Orientation in case of an hospitalization. The designed telemedicine domain ontologies have been formalized using the ontology description language OWL-DL. The key feature of T-TROIE resides in its capacity to perform reasoning taking into consideration the availability and capability of different resources required to perform various tasks and processes. T-TROIE has the ability of handling different contexts of use taking into account, on one side the clinical status and conditions of the patient and, on the other side, the availability and the capability of the required material, communication, and human resources.

Thus, the objective of T-TROIE is to enable an intelligent management of the tasks, processes and resources in different pervasive telemedicine services and applications by providing actors in the telemedicine domain with an efficient decision making support tool.

8. References

ARTEMIS: *A Semantic Web Service-based P2P Infrastructure for the Interoperability of Medical Information Systems,* (2004). Available at http://www.srdc.metu.edu.tr/webpage/projects/artemis

Bicer, V.; B. Laleci, G.; Dogac, A. & Kabak, Y. (2005). Artemis message exchange framework: semantic interoperability of exchanged messages in the healthcare domain. *SIGMOD Rec.,* Vol. 34, No. 3, (Sept 2005) 71-76

Christopoulou, E. & Kameas, A. (2004). Using Ontologies to Address Key Issues in Ubiquitous Computing Systems, In: *Lecture Notes in Computer Science, Ambient Intelligence,* Markopoulos; Eggen; Aarts & L. Crowley (EDs.) 13-24, Springer, ISBN 978-3-540-23721-1, Berlin Heidelberg

De Luca, G.; Suryapranata, H.; Ottervanger, J. P. & Antman, E. M. (2004). Time Delay to Treatment and Mortality in Primary Angioplasty for Acute Myocardial Infarction: Every Minute of Delay Counts. *Circulation,* Vol. 109, No. 10, (Mar 2004) 1223-1225

Din, I. U. (2010). Remote Patient Disease Diagnosing and Treatment Prototype for Third World/Remote Areas Using Real Time Protocols. *Proceedings of the 12th International Conference on Computer Modeling and Simulation,* pp. 659-664, ISBN 978-1-4244-6614-6, Cambridge, June 2010, IEEE Computer Society, New York

Dogac, A.; Laleci, G. B.; Kirbas, S.; Kabak, Y. et al. (2006). Artemis: deploying semantically enriched web services in the healthcare domain. *Inf. Syst,* Vol. 31, No. 4, (2005) 321-339

Fayn, J. & Rubel, P. (2010). Towards a Personal Health Society in Cardiology. *IEEE Trans. Inf. Technol. Biomed,* Vol. 14, No. 2, (Dec 2009) 401-409

Healy, P.; O'Reilly, R.; Boylan, G. & Morrison, J. (2010). Web-based Remote Monitoring of Live EEG. *Proceedings of the 12th International Conference On E-Health Networking, Application & Services,* pp. 169-174, Lyon France, July 2010, IEEE Computer Society, New York

Jena. (2009). Jena Semantic Web Framework. Available at *http://jena.sourceforge.net/*

Latfi, F., Lefebvre, B. & Descheneaux, C. (2007). Ontology-Based Management of the Telehealth Smart Home, Dedicated to Elderly in Loss of Cognitive Autonomy. *Proceedings of the 3rd International Workshop on OWL OWLED 2007: Experiences and Directions.* June 2007, Innsbruck Austria

Lu, W., Leung, H. & Estrada, E. (2010). Transforming Telemedicine for Rural and Urban Communities Telemedicine 2.0 – Any Doctor, Any Place, Any Time. *Proceedings of the 12th International Conference On E-Health Networking, Application & Services*, pp. 379-385, Lyon France, July 2010, IEEE Computer Society, New York

Nageba, E.; Fayn, J. & Rubel, P. (2007). A Generic Task-Driven Multi-Agent Telemedicine System. *Proceedings of the 29th Annual International Conference of the IEEE Engineering in Medicine and Biology Society EMBS*, pp. 3733-3736, Aug 2007, Lyon France, IEEE Computer Society, New York

Nageba, E.; Fayn, J. & Rubel, P. (2008). An Ontology-based Telemedicine Tasks Management System Architecture. *Proceedings of the 30th Annual International Conference of Engineering in Medicine and Biology Society*, pp. 1494-1497. Aug 2008, Vancouver BC Canada, IEEE Computer Society, New York

Nageba, E.; Fayn, J. & Rubel, P. (2009). A Model Driven Ontology-based Architecture for Supporting the Quality of Services in Pervasive Telemedicine Applications. *Proceedings the 3rd International Conference on Pervasive Computing Technologies for Healthcare,* pp. 1-8, Apr 2009, London UK, IEEE Computer Society, New York

Oemig, F. & Blobel, B. (2009). Semantic interoperability between health communication standards through formal ontologies. In: *Stud Health Technol Inform.,* Adlassnig, K.P.; Blobel, B.; Mantas, J. & Masic, I. (EDs), 200-204, IOS Press, ISBN 978-1-60750-044-5, Amsterdam, The Netherland

OMG. (2009). Ontology Definition Metamodel. Available at *http://www.omg.org/spec/ODM/1.0/*

Paganelli, F., Spinicci, E. & Giuli, D. (2008). ERMHAN: A Context-Aware Service Platform to Support Continuous Care Networks for Home-Based Assistance. *International Journal of Telemedicine and Applications,* Vol. 2008, No. 4 (Jan 2008), 1-13

OWL, Web Ontology Language Overview (2004). Available at *http://www.w3.org/TR/owl-features/..*

Pellet. (2007). Pellet: The Open Source OWL Reasoner. Available at *http://clarkparsia.com/pellet*

Protégé. (1997). The Protégé Ontology Editor and Knowledge Acquisition System. Available at *http://protege.stanford.edu/*

Prud'hommeaux, E. & Seaborne, A. (2008). SPARQL Query Language for RDF. Available at *http://www.w3.org/TR/rdf-sparql-query/*

SAPHIRE. (2008). SAPHIRE Project. Available at *http://www.srdc.metu.edu.tr/webpage/projects/saphire/*

Scholl, J., Lambrinos, L. & Lindgren, A. (2009). Rural Telemedicine Networks Using Store-and-Forward Voice-over-IP. In: *Stud Health Technol Inform.*, Adlassnig, K.P.; Blobel, B.; Mantas, J. & Masic, I. (EDs), 448-452, IOS Press, ISBN 978-1-60750-044-5, Amsterdam, The Netherland

SWRL: A Semantic Web Rule Language Combining OWL and RuleML (2004). Available at *http://www.w3.org/Submission/SWRL/*